WL 300

D1429146

Uncommon Causes of Movement Disorders

Uncommon Causes of Movement Disorders

Edited by

Néstor Gálvez-Jiménez
Chairman, Department of Neurology and Chief, Movement Disorders Program, Cleveland Clinic Florida, Weston, Florida, USA
Associate Clinical Professor of Neurology, Herbert Wertheim College of Medicine, Florida International University, Miami, Florida, USA

Paul J. Tuite
Associate Professor of Neurology and Director of Movement Disorders, University of Minnesota, Minneapolis, Minnesota, USA

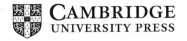
CAMBRIDGE
UNIVERSITY PRESS

CAMBRIDGE UNIVERSITY PRESS
Cambridge, New York, Melbourne, Madrid, Cape Town,
Singapore, São Paulo, Delhi, Tokyo, Mexico City

Cambridge University Press
The Edinburgh Building, Cambridge CB2 8RU, UK

Published in the United States of America by Cambridge University Press, New York

www.cambridge.org
Information on this title: www.cambridge.org/9780521111546

First published 2011

Printed in the United Kingdom at the University Press, Cambridge

A catalogue record for this publication is available from the British Library

Library of Congress Cataloguing in Publication data
Uncommon causes of movement disorders / [edited by] Néstor Gálvez-Jiménez, Paul J.Tuite.
  p. ; cm.
Includes bibliographical references and index.
ISBN 978-0-521-11154-6 (hardback)
1. Movement disorders–Etiology. 2. Diagnosis, Differential. I. Gálvez-Jiménez, Néstor. II. Tuite, Paul J.
[DNLM: 1. Movement Disorders–etiology. 2. Diagnosis, Differential. 3. Dyskinesias–etiology. WL 390]
RC376.5.U53 2011
616.8′3–dc22
2011006358

ISBN 978-0-521-11154-6 Hardback

Contents

Contents

Contributors

Alberto Albanese, MD
Professor of Neurology, Istituto Neurologico Carlo Besta and Università Cattolica del Sacro Cuore, Milan, Italy

Karine Auré, MD, PhD
Federation of Neurology and CRICM UMR-S UPMC, Inserm 975, Salpetriere Hospital, Paris, France

Selim R. Benbadis, MD
Professor of Neurology, University of South Florida, Tampa, Florida, USA

Jose Biller, MD, FACP, FAAN, FAHA
Department of Neurology, Loyola University Chicago, Stritch School of Medicine, Maywood, Illinois, USA

Matthew Bower MS, CGC
Certified Genetic Counselor, Institute of Human Genetics, University of Minnesota Medical Center, Fairview, Fairview Southdale Hospital, Minnesota, USA

Francisco Cardoso, MD, PhD
Professor of Neurology, Internal Medicine Department, The Federal University of Minas Gerais, Belo Horizonte, Minas Gerais, Brazil

Kelvin L. Chou, MD
Deep Brain Stimulation Clinic, Department of Neurology, University of Michigan, Ann Arbor, Michigan, USA

Rima M. Dafer, MD, MPH, FAAN
Department of Neurology, Loyola University Chicago, Stritch School of Medicine, Maywood, Illinois, USA

Praveen Dayalu, MD
Department of Neurology, University of Michigan, Ann Arbor, Michigan, USA

Michelle M. Dompenciel, MD
Department of Neurology, Cleveland Clinic, Weston, Florida, USA

Eissa Ibrahim Al Eissa, MD
University of South Florida, Tampa, Florida, USA

Alberto J. Espay, MD, MSc
Director of Clinical Research, James J. and Joan A. Gardner Center for Parkinson's Disease and Movement Disorders, UC Neuroscience Institute, Department of Neurology, University of Cincinnati, Cincinnati, Ohio, USA

Hubert H. Fernandez, MD
Head of Movement Disorders, Center for Neurological Restoration, Cleveland Clinic, Cleveland, Ohio, USA

Brent L. Fogel, MD, PhD
UCLA Program in Neurogenetics, Department of Neurology, David Geffen School of Medicine at UCLA, Los Angeles, California, USA

Steven Frucht, MD
Center for Parkinson's Disease and Other Movement Disorders, The Neurological Institute, Columbia University School of Medicine, New York, New York, USA

Victor S. C. Fung, MBBS, PhD, FRACP
Clinical Associate Professor and Director, The University of Sydney and Department of Neurology, Westmead Hospital, Westmead, New South Wales, Australia

Néstor Gálvez-Jiménez MD, MSc, MHSA, FACP, FAHA, FACA
Chairman and Associate Clinical Professor, Department of Neurology; Director, Movement Disorders and Fellowship Program, Cleveland Clinic Florida, Weston (Fort Lauderdale), Florida; Faculty Development and Associate Clinical Professor, Neuroscience Curriculum, Herbert Wertheim College of Medicine at Florida International University, Miami, Florida, USA

David Grabli, MD, PhD
Federation of Neurology and CRICM UMR-S UPMC, Inserm 975, Salpetriere Hospital, Paris, France

Era Hanspal, MD
Fellow in Movement Disorders, Columbia University, New York, New York, USA

Claire Henchcliffe, MD, DPhil
Department of Neurology and Neuroscience, Weill Medical College of Cornell University, New York, New York, USA

Nelson Hwynn, DO
Division of Neurology, Scripps Clinic, La Jolla, California, USA

Kurt A. Jellinger, MD
Professor of Neuropathology, Institute of Clinical Neurobiology, Vienna, Austria

Julia Johnson, MD
Division of Neurology, Duke University Medical Center, Durham, North Carolina, USA

Danita Jones, DO, MPH
Department of Neurology, Cleveland Clinic Florida, Weston (Fort Lauderdale), Florida, USA

Daniel Kantor, MD, BSE
Medical Director, Neurologique Foundation Inc., Ponte Vedra, Florida, USA

Ninith Kartha, MD
Department of Neurology, Loyola University Chicago, Stritch School of Medicine, Maywood, Illinois, USA

Jan Kassubek, MD
Department of Neurology, University of Ulm, Ulm, Germany

Taranum Khan, MD
Movement Disorders Program, Department of Neurology, Cleveland Clinic Florida, Weston (Fort Lauderdale), Florida, USA

Samuel Kim, BSc(Med), MBBS, FRACP
Department of Neurology, Westmead Hospital, Westmead, Sydney, New South Wales, Australia

Christine Klein, MD
Schilling Section of Clinical and Molecular Neurogenetics, Department of Neurology, University of Luebeck, Luebeck, Germany

Neeraj Kumar, MD
Department of Neurology, Mayo Clinic, Rochester, Minnesota, USA

Roger Kurlan, MD
Medical Director, Movement Disorders Program, Atlantic Neuroscience Institute, Summit, New Jersey, USA

Corneliu Luca, MD, PhD
Center for Parkinson's Disease and Movement Disorders, Department of Neurology, University of Miami Miller School of Medicine, Miami, Florida, USA

Ramon Lugo, MD
Fellow, Movement Disorders Program, Department of Neurology, Cleveland Clinic Florida, Weston (Fort Lauderdale), Forida, USA

Roneil Malkani, MD
Northwestern University, Parkinson's Disease and Movement Disorders Center, Chicago, Illinois, USA

Giacomo Della Marca, MD, PhD
Istituto di Neurologia, Università Cattolica del Sacro Cuore, Rome, Italy

Marcelo Merello, MD, PhD
Director, Neurosciences Department, Movement Disorders Section, Raul Carrea Institute for Neurological Research, FLENI, Buenos Aires, Argentina

Henry Moore, MD
Center for Parkinson's Disease and Movement
Disorders, Department of Neurology, University
of Miami Miller School of Medicine, Miami,
Florida, USA

Sarkis Morales-Vidal, MD
Department of Neurology, Loyola University Chicago,
Stritch School of Medicine, Maywood, Illinois, USA

Santiago Perez-Lloret, MD, PhD, CPI
Biomedical Research Coordinator, Movement
Disorders Section, Raul Carrea Institute for
Neurological Research, FLENI, Buenos Aires,
Argentina; Department of Clinical Pharmacology and
Neurosciences, Hospital and University Paul Sabatier
of Toulouse, and INSERM CIC9023 and UMR 825,
Toulouse France

Susan Perlman, MD
UCLA Program in Neurogenetics, Department
of Neurology, David Geffen School of Medicine at
UCLA, Los Angeles, California, USA

Elmar H. Pinkhardt, MD
Department of Neurology, University of Ulm, Ulm,
Germany

David E. Riley, MD
Movement Disorders Center, Neurological Institute,
University Hospitals and Case Western Reserve
University School of Medicine, Cleveland, Ohio, USA

Emmanuel Roze, MD, PhD
Federation of Neurology and CRICM UMR-S UPMC,
Inserm 975, Salpetriere Hospital, Paris, France

Daniel S. Sa, MD
Director, Movement Disorders Center, Marshfield
Clinic, Marshfield, Wisconsin, USA

Virgilio D. Salanga, MD
Department of Neurology, Cleveland Clinic, Weston,
Forida, USA

Michael J. Schneck, MD, FAAN, MBA
Department of Neurology, Loyola University Chicago,
Stritch School of Medicine, Maywood, Illinois, USA

Susanne A. Schneider, MD
Schilling Section of Clinical and Molecular
Neurogenetics, Department of Neurology, University
of Luebeck, Luebeck, Germany

David Shprecher, DO
University of Utah, Department of Neurology, Salt
Lake City, Utah, USA

Carlos Singer, MD
Center for Parkinson's Disease and Movement
Disorders, Department of Neurology, University of
Miami Miller School of Medicine, Miami, Florida,
USA

Mark Stacy, MD
Division of Neurology, Duke University Medical
Center, Durham, North Carolina, USA

Sylvia Stemberger, DI(FH)
Department of Neurology, Medical University of
Innsbruck, Innsbruck, Austria

Pichet Termsarasab, MD
Movement Disorders Center, Neurological Institute,
University Hospitals and Case Western Reserve
University School of Medicine, Cleveland, Ohio, USA

Paul J. Tuite, MD
Associate Professor of Neurology and Director of
Movement Disorders, University of Minnesota,
Minneapolis, Minnesota, USA

Marie Vidailhet, MD
Federation of Neurology and CRICM UMR-S UPMC,
Inserm 975, Salpetriere Hospital, Paris, France

Mary Vo, MD
Department of Neurology and Neuroscience, Weill
Medical College of Cornell University, New York,
New York, USA

Ruth H. Walker, MB, ChB, PhD
Department of Neurology, James J. Peters Veterans
Affairs Medical Center, Bronx, and Department of
Neurology, Mount Sinai School of Medicine,
New York, New York, USA

Gregor K. Wenning, MD, PhD, MSC
Head, Department of Clinical Neurobiology and
Consultant Physician, Parkinson and Movement
Disorder Centre, Department of Neurology, Medical
University of Innsbruck, Innsbruck, Austria

Cindy Zadikoff, MD, FRCPC, MSc
Assistant Professor of Neurology, Northwestern
University, Parkinson's Disease and Movement
Disorders Center, Chicago, Illinois, USA

Preface

This book came about when it became clear that a work on unusual movements or unusual causes of disorders of motor control was lacking, especially for neurologists, neurosurgeons and psychiatric specialists and physicians in training. Most available books are almost exclusively for movement disorders specialists; or the information related to these conditions is found scattered throughout the literature. In addition, many aspects related to movement disorders such as neuro-ophthalmologic problems, demyelinating diseases, neuromuscular disorders, gait and balance difficulties and the boundaries of epilepsy and neuropsychiatric diseases are beginning to be recognized as important in the field but are poorly discussed in most textbooks. We cover these areas extensively in this book. Along with our publishers we hope this work can begin to fill the gap. The book follows a sequence beginning with akinetic rigid syndromes and followed by hyperkinetic and miscellaneous disorders. With advances in the field, the scope of movement disorders now includes disorders of gait and balance, cerebellar conditions, dementing disorders with "extrapyramidal" signs, disorders of sleep, and movement conditions that overlap neuromuscular diseases or epilepsy conditions. Examples of such include cramps, fatigue, weakness, twitchy muscles/fingers/extremities, nocturnal jerks and movements, hypermotor behaviors and disorders of sleep.

The book features chapters on multiple system atrophy, progressive supranuclear palsy and corticobasal degeneration written by the teams headed by Professors Gregor Wenning, Carlos Singer and David Riley, respectively, who have been pioneers in the understanding of these disorders. The emerging area of apraxias in movement disorders was superbly written by Roneil Malkani and Cindy Zadikoff. Wilson disease is reviewed by Dr. Neeraj Kumar from the Mayo Clinic, in which he demonstrates his expertise in the diagnosis and treatment of such conditions. Continuing progress in neurodegeneration with brain accumulation is reviewed by Dr. Paul Tuite and Mr. Bower from the University of Minnesota. In this review, the authors make simple to the reader what is normally a complex disorder and demonstrate their accumulated expertise in this group of disorders. Dementia with parkinsonism and impulsive and compulsive behaviors are reviewed by Drs. Praveen Dayalu and Kelvin Chou, and by Drs. Nelson Hwynn and Hubert Fernandez, respectively.

We were extremely lucky to have Professor Kurt Jellinger revisit pallidal and thalamic atrophies, a topic that was last reviewed by him many years ago in the *Handbook of Neurology* edited by Bruyn. This timely review puts into current perspective the advances in this rarely discussed area. Professor Alberto Albanese and Professor Giacomo Dell Marca introduce us to restless legs syndrome and sleep-related disorders, areas in which both authors are very well known. Professor Christine Klein has made seminal contributions to the understanding of genetics in movement disorders. She and her team provide an up to date introduction to dystonic syndromes, focusing on the emerging genetics of dystonia.

Other dyskinesias such as hemifacial spasm, tardive dyskinesias and other drug-induced movement disorders are reviewed in detail by Danita Jones and Néstor Gálvez-Jiménez of the Cleveland Clinic in Florida and Santiago Perez-Lloret and Marcello Merello from Buenos Aires, Argentina, respectively. Drs. Jones and Gálvez-Jiménez introduce us to a practical anatomy of the facial nerve, its pathophysiology and unusual causes of hemifacial dyskinesias. Professors Perez-Lloret and Merello provide the reader with a practical overview of drug-induced movement disorders and tardive syndromes.

Nonhereditary choreas and neuroacanthocytosis are introduced by two very well-recognized experts in the field. Dr. Francisco Cardoso from Brazil reviews his experience in nonhereditary choreas, and Dr. Ruth Walker from New York presents her experience in neuroacanthocytosis.

Tremor and myoclonus are superbly reviewed by Drs. Mark Stacey and Julia Johnson and by Drs. Steven Frucht and Era Hanspal, respectively. Dr. Stacey's and Dr. Frucht's groups have made seminal contributions in movement disorders, especially in tremor and myoclonus. We were very fortunate to have them participate in this project.

Dr. Roger Kurlan's expertise in tics and Tourette syndrome is demonstrated in his review of the topic. The complex area of cerebellar disorders is superbly covered by Dr. Susan Perlman and her team from UCLA. Unusual gait disorders and psychogenic movement disorders are discussed by Dr. Victor Fung and Mr. Samuel Kim from Adelaide Australia and by Dr. Alberto Espay from Cincinnati, Ohio.

Stiff person syndrome is reviewed by Dr. Daniel Sa from the Marshfield Clinic. Hereditary spastic paraplegias are summarized by Drs. Ramon Lugo, Taranum Khan and Néstor Gálvez-Jiménez from the Cleveland Clinic in Florida and by Mr. Matthew Bower from the University of Minnesota.

Miscellaneous disorders that overlap other areas of neurology including cramps, contractures and myalgias are covered by Drs. Virgilio Salanga and Michelle Dompenciel, neuromuscular clinicians with extensive expertise in the field and in general neurology. This chapter represents the twilight zone between neuromuscular diseases and movement disorders. Similarly, the boundaries between epilepsy and movement disorders are continuously being revised in the light of novel information about cortical and deep brain structures such as the basal ganglia and thalamus. This area is succinctly reviewed by Drs. Selim Benbadis and Eissa Ibrahim Al Eissa. Dr. Benbadis's team from Tampa has made numerous contribution to the field of epilepsy, abnormal movements and psychogenicity.

In addition, neuro-ophthalmologic alterations in patients with movement disorders are reviewed by authorities in the field such as Professors Jan Kassubek and Elmar Pinkhardt; while cerebrovascular diseases and movement disorders, and demyelinating diseases resulting in abnormal movements are covered by Professor Jose Biller and his team from Loyola University, and by Dr. Daniel Kantor from Gainsville, Florida, respectively. These three topics complete the miscellaneous movement disorders that are rarely discussed and summarized in a work of this nature.

As editors we found the preparation of this work a very humbling experience and daily lessons were learned during the preparation and coordination of the work. We are extremely grateful to all contributors for their willingness to take the time from busy personal and professional lives to write these papers summarizing their area of expertise and for their patience during the preparation of this work.

Finally. N. G.-J. would like to thank Ms. Pauline Braathen and the Pauline Braathen fund for their unyielding support of his activities. None of this work would have been possible without their support.

Néstor Gálvez-Jiménez
Paul Tuite

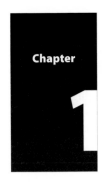

Multiple system atrophy

Sylvia Stemberger and Gregor K. Wenning

History

Multiple system atrophy (MSA) is a progressive neurodegenerative movement disorder characterized by a variable combination of autonomic failure, poorly levodopa-responsive parkinsonism, cerebellar ataxia and pyramidal symptoms. Neuronal cell loss in the basal ganglia, cerebellum, pontine and inferior olivary nuclei, pyramidal tract, intermediolateral cell column and Onuf's nucleus as well as gliosis and α-synuclein containing glial cytoplasmic inclusions (GCIs) are typically observed [1]. MSA is an orphan disease (prevalence rate 4.4/100 000; incidence rate 3/100 000 per year [2,3]) equally affecting men and women; it usually starts in the sixth decade and progresses relentlessly, with death occurring after an average of 9 years [4].

Up to 1969, three cardinal presentations of MSA including striatonigral degeneration (SND), sporadic olivopontocerebellar atrophy (OPCA), and the Shy–Drager syndrome (SDS) were regarded distinct entities until Graham and Oppenheimer recognized their substantial clinicopathological overlap and proposed MSA as umbrella term [5]. Ubiquitin-positive GCIs were first reported in 1989 [6] and subsequently confirmed as cellular marker of MSA regardless of the phenotypic presentation. α-Synuclein immunostaining of GCIs was first described in the late 1990s. Following this discovery, MSA has been regarded as α-synucleinopathy along with Parkinson disease (PD), dementia with Lewy bodies and pure autonomic failure (PAF). Quinn proposed the first set of diagnostic criteria and distinguished the motor subtypes MSA-P and MSA-C, although there was unintended overlap. Further, he allowed an abnormal external sphincter electromyogram (EMG) as diagnostic criterion, thereby creating practical difficulties [7]. For these reasons a consensus conference was convened in 1998 that proposed exclusively clinical guidelines for the diagnosis of MSA. Subdivision into MSA-P and MSA-C was recommended based on the predominant motor feature at presentation [8]. Based on improvements of early diagnosis by defining warning signs (red flags) and sensitive neuroimaging indices, the consensus guidelines were revised 10 years later [9]. A unified MSA rating scale (UMSARS) quantifying disease severity has been established and validated in the meantime by the European MSA Study Group (EMSA-SG) [10]. UMSARS has been applied in the EMSA natural study, confirming the rapid progression of autonomic failure, cerebellar ataxia and parkinsonism (G. K. Wenning *et al.*, unpublished data). Animal models have become available as preclinical testbeds for translational neuroprotection and neuroregeneration studies [11]. The first clinical trials have been conducted by two independent consortia using minocycline (EMSA-SG) [12] and riluzole (Neuroprotection and Natural History in Parkinson-Plus Syndromes [NNIPPS]) [13]. Other international networks have been established in the last few years including NAMSA (North American MSA Study Group) [14], JAMSAC (Japanese MSA Consortium) and CNMSA (Chinese MSA Study Group). Globalization of MSA research has led not only to the aforementioned trial activities but also to the first genetic breakthrough by indentifying variants in the α-synuclein gene and their association with increased disease risk in a large population of MSA patients [15]. In addition several pedigrees with monogenic MSA but yet unidentified loci have been reported [16].

Clinical findings

Clinically, cardinal features include autonomic failure, parkinsonism, cerebellar ataxia, and pyramidal signs in any combination (Table 1.1). Two major motor presentations can be distinguished. In the western hemisphere

Uncommon Causes of Movement Disorders, ed. Néstor Gálvez-Jiménez and Paul J. Tuite. Published by Cambridge University Press. © Cambridge University Press 2011.

Table 1.1. Clinical presentation of MSA according to the EMSA Registry.

437 patients (53% male; mean age at disease onset 58 years; mean disease duration 5.8 years; 68% MSA-P; 32% MSA-C)

Autonomic failure
- Urinary symptoms (83%)
  - Urge incontinence (73%)
  - Incomplete bladder emptying (48%)
  - Erectile failure (84%)
- Orthostatic hypotension (75%; syncope 19%)
- Chronic constipation (33%)

Parkinsonism
- Bradykinesia and rigidity (93%)
- Postural instability (89%)
- Rest tremor (33%)
- Freezing of gait (38%)

Cerebellar ataxia
- Gait ataxia (86%)
- Limb ataxia (78%)
- Ataxic dysarthria (69%)

Pyramidal signs
- Babinski sign (28%)
- Generalized hyperreflexia (43%)

Neuropsychiatric features
- Depression (41%)
- Hallucinations (5.5%)[a]
- Dementia (4.5%)[a]
- Insomnia (19%)
- Daytime sleepiness (17%)
- Restless legs (10%)

Modified according to Koellensperger and Wenning [17].
[a] Patients were entered on the basis of expert opinion regardless of diagnostic criteria.

parkinsonian features predominate in 60% of patients (MSA-P subtype, Figure 1.1), cerebellar ataxia is the major motor feature in 40% of patients (MSA-C subtype) [17]. The reverse distribution is observed in the eastern hemisphere [18,19]. MSA-associated parkinsonism is dominated by progressive akinesia and rigidity, whereas tremor is less common than in PD. Postural stability is compromised early on; however, recurrent falls at disease onset are unusual in contrast to progressive supranuclear palsy. The cerebellar disorder of MSA is composed of gait ataxia, limb kinetic ataxia, and scanning dysarthria, as well as cerebellar oculomotor disturbances. Dysautonomia develops in

virtually all patients with MSA [20]. Early impotence (erectile dysfunction) is virtually universal in men, and urinary incontinence or incomplete bladder emptying, often early in the course or as presenting symptoms, are frequent. Orthostatic hypotension is present in two-thirds of patients [17]. Progressive hypohidrosis is also prominent.

The clinical diagnosis of MSA rests largely on history and physical examination. The revised consensus criteria [9] specify three diagnostic categories of increasing certainty: possible, probable, and definite. Whereas a definite diagnosis requires neuropathological evidence of a neuronal multisystem degeneration (SND, OPCA, central autonomic degeneration) and abundant GCIs [21], the diagnosis of possible and probable MSA is based on the presence of clinical and imaging features (Tables 1.2–1.4). In addition, supportive features (warning signs or red flags) as well as nonsupportive features may be considered (Tables 1.5 and 1.6).

Natural history and progression

The disease affects men and women alike. It usually starts in the sixth decade and progresses relentlessly until death on average 9 years after disease onset [4,13,23]. There is a considerable variation of disease duration, with survival times of up to 15 years or more. Predictors of poor outcome include female sex, older age at onset, autonomic failure and rapid progression [24]. The motor variants of MSA are associated with similar survival [25], although disease progression is more rapid in MSA-P than in MSA-C patients [18]. Most MSA patients succumb to sudden death reflecting central cardiovascular or respiratory disturbances due to loss of serotonergic neurons in the ventrolateral medulla [26]. Other causes of death may include aspiration pneumonia or pulmonary embolism.

The recent natural history study by the EMSA-SG applied the unified MSA rating scale (UMSARS) [10] and confirmed rapid progression with an average increase of UMSARS I scores (reflecting activities of daily living) by 16.8% in the first 6 months compared with baseline. Further, UMSARS II (motor examination) scores increased by 26.1% and UMSARS IV (global disability) scores by 12.5% [27].

Investigations

The diagnosis of MSA rests on both history and neurological examination. Additional investigations may be performed according to the consensus criteria

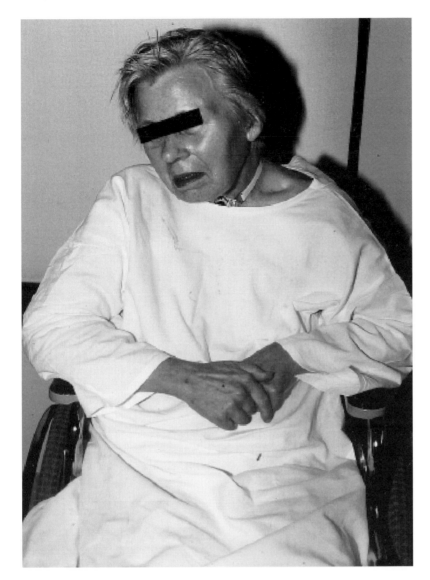

Figure 1.1. MSA-P patient with non-L-dopa-responsive akinetic-rigid parkinsonism and early development of the "wheelchair sign." In addition, the patient showed a disproportionate antecollis and a pronounced inspiratory stridor that caused respiratory failure leading to tracheostomy. (Reproduced from Wenning *et al.* [142] with kind permission of Springer Science+Business Media.)

(Table 1.7). These include cardiovascular autonomic function tests, external sphincter EMG and neuroimaging. However, previous studies have largely been conducted in patients with advanced MSA and therefore the diagnostic validity of additional testing in early MSA remains to be determined.

Pathology

A definite diagnosis of MSA requires neuropathological evidence of glial cytoplasmic inclusions (GCIs) in association with selective neurodegeneration (Figure 1.2) [21]. Specifically, there is neuronal loss and gliosis of the striatum, substantia nigra pars compacta (SNc), locus ceruleus, cerebellum, pontine nuclei, inferior olives, intermediolateral columns and Onuf's nucleus [28]. This neurodegenerative pattern is characterized by astrogliosis, microglial activation, microgliosis and myelin loss [29–32].

Multiple system atrophy is a unique oligodendrogliopathy [33] with widespread and abundant GCIs (Papp–Lantos bodies) that were first identified in 1989 by Gallyas silver impregnation [6,34]. GCIs contain filamentous α-synuclein [1,6,35–38] linking MSA with the spectrum of neuronal α-synucleinopathies such as PD, dementia with Lewy bodies and pure autonomic failure. GCIs are argyrophilic flame-shaped aggregates[39] that in addition to α-synuclein comprise other constituents, identified to date by either

Table 1.2. Consensus criteria for the diagnosis of probable MSA.

A sporadic, progressive, adult-onset (>30 years) disease characterized by:

- Autonomic failure involving urinary incontinence (inability to control the release of urine from the bladder, with erectile dysfunction in males) or an orthostatic decrease of blood pressure within 3 minutes of standing by at least 30 mmHg systolic or 15 mmHg diastolic and
- Poorly levodopa-responsive parkinsonism (bradykinesia with rigidity, tremor, or postural instability) or
- A cerebellar syndrome (gait ataxia with cerebellar dysarthria, limb ataxia, or cerebellar oculomotor dysfunction)

Modified according to Gilman *et al.* [9] and reproduced from Wenning and Stefanova [22] (with kind permission of Springer Science+Business Media).

Table 1.3. Consensus criteria for the diagnosis of possible MSA.

A sporadic, progressive, adult-onset (>30 years) disease characterized by:

- Parkinsonism (bradykinesia with rigidity, tremor, or postural instability) or
- A cerebellar syndrome (gait ataxia with cerebellar dysarthria, limb ataxia, or cerebellar oculomotor dysfunction) and
- At least one feature suggesting autonomic dysfunction (otherwise unexplained urinary urgency, frequency or incomplete bladder emptying, erectile dysfunction in males, or significant orthostatic blood pressure decline that does not meet the level required in probable MSA) and
- At least one of the additional features shown in Table 1.4

Modified according to Gilman *et al.* [9] and reproduced from Wenning and Stefanova [22] (with kind permission of Springer Science+Business Media).

Table 1.4. Additional features of possible MSA.

Possible MSA-P or MSA-C

- Babinski sign with hyperreflexia
- Stridor

Possible MSA-P

- Rapidly progressive parkinsonism
- Poor response to levodopa
- Postural instability within 3 years of motor onset
- Gait ataxia, cerebellar dysarthria, limb ataxia, or cerebellar oculomotor dysfunction
- Dysphagia within 5 years of motor onset
- Atrophy on MRI of putamen, middle cerebellar peduncle, pons, or cerebellum
- Hypometabolism on FDG-PET in putamen, brainstem, or cerebellum

Possible MSA-C

- Parkinsonism (bradykinesia and rigidity)
- Atrophy on MRI of putamen, middle cerebellar peduncle, or pons
- Hypometabolism on FDG-PET in putamen
- Presynaptic nigrostriatal dopaminergic denervation on SPECT or PET

Modified according to Gilman [9] and reproduced from Wenning and Stefanova [22] (with kind permission of Springer Science+Business Media).

immunohistochemistry or mass spectrometry. These include for example ubiquitin, tubulin and p25α (Table 1.8) [29,33,40,41].

Localization of GCIs is widespread and their appearance has been correlated with severe neuronal loss as well as disease duration and severity [42,43]. The cellular inclusion pathology is not restricted to GCIs. Neuronal cytoplasmic inclusions (NCIs) and neuronal nuclear inclusions (NNIs) have also been observed, mainly restricted to the putamen, substantia nigra, inferior olivary nucleus, motor cortex, dentate gyrus and pontine nuclei [44–52].

Table 1.5. Supportive features (red flags) for a diagnosis of MSA.

- Orofacial dystonia
- Disproportionate antecollis
- Camptocormia (severe anterior flexion of the spine) and/or Pisa syndrome (severe lateral flexion of the spine)
- Contractures of hands or feet
- Inspiratory sighs
- Severe dysphonia
- Severe dysarthria
- New or increased snoring
- Cold hands and feet
- Pathological laughter or crying
- Jerky, myoclonic postural/action tremor

Modified according to Gilman [9] and reproduced from Wenning and Stefanova [22] (with kind permission of Springer Science+Business Media).

Table 1.6. Nonsupportive features for a diagnosis of MSA.

- Classic pill-rolling tremor
- Clinically significant neuropathy
- Hallucinations not induced by drugs
- Onset age after 75 years
- Family history of ataxia or parkinsonism
- Dementia on (DSM-IV)
- White matter lesions suggesting multiple sclerosis
- Pathological laughter or crying
- Jerky, myoclonic postural/action tremor

Modified according to Gilman [9] and reproduced from Wenning and Stefanova [22] (with kind permission of Springer Science+Business Media).

The factors triggering and maintaining progressive α-synuclein accumulation in oligodendrocytes are still unknown, but the finding of oligodendroglial p25α accumulation predating GCI formation as well as alterations of myelin basic protein support a primary oligodendrogliopathy [33,53–58].

Etiopathogenesis
Environmental factors

The underlying etiopathogenesis of MSA is still unclear, but complex interactions of genetic and environmental factors, similar to other sporadic neurodegenerative diseases, appear to be likely [59]. In a few controlled studies, an increased risk of developing MSA by occupational and daily habits, such as exposure to solvents, additives, plastic monomers, metals and various other toxins [8,60,61], as well as history of farming [59,61] has been observed. A recent study, however, questioned some of the associations [62].

In general, convincing findings from environmental studies, are hard to obtain to owing limiting factors such as recall (over-reporting of exposure) and selection bias (patients with severe diseases are less able to participate) [63]. Hence the role of environmental factors is far from clear.

Genetic factors

MSA seems to occur sporadically and, compared with PD, few families have been reported with a family history of MSA [64,65]. Lately, an autosomal recessive inheritance pattern of MSA was reported in Japan [16,66]. Furthermore, some studies suggest that MSA-like features are in close relation with various forms of spinocerebellar ataxia [67–71].

Several investigators addressed potential abnormalities of the α-synuclein gene in MSA due to its postulated etiologic role [6,33,36]. Early studies (including sequencing of SNCA coding sequence, gene dosage measurements, microsatellite testing and haplotype studies) had failed to identify significant associations with the α-synuclein gene owing to insufficient sample size [72–75]. A recent genome-wide association study by the EMSA-SG and associated consortia identified a number of single nucleotide polymorphisms (SNPs) within the α-synuclein gene that were associated with increased MSA disease risk [15]. These findings were recently confirmed in an independent patient cohort [76]; however, the genetic background of the control population appears to be of importance when interpreting disease risk [77]. Further, polymorphisms of genes involved in inflammatory processes, such as interleukin-1α, interleukin-1β, interleukin-8, intercellular adhesion molecule-1 and tumor necrosis factor showed elevated odds ratios in MSA cohorts compared with controls [78–82]. Polymorphism of genes involved in oxidative stress as well as the alpha-1-antichymotrypsin AA genotype (ACT-AA) were also related to MSA risk [83]. In contrast, other genes coding for apolipoprotein E, dopamine β-hydroxlyase, ubiquitin C terminal hydrolase-1, fragile x mental retardation 1 and leucine-rich kinase 2 showed no significant association [74].

Table 1.7. Additional investigations in MSA.

Investigation	Typical results
Cardiovascular autonomic function tests	Orthostatic hypotension ($\geq$20/10 mmHg systolic/diastolic blood pressure drop) Impaired reflex tachycardia Impaired heart rate variability Impaired Valsalva maneuver Impaired rise of plasma noradrenaline upon standing
Arginine/clonidine challenge test	Impaired release of growth hormone (controversial)
Thermoregulatory sweat test (TST), quantitative sudomotor axon reflex test (QSART)	Sudomotor dysfunction (an-/hypohidrosis) due to pre- and postganglionic sympathetic failure
Sympathetic skin response	Abnormal or absent
CSF	Increased neurofilament (light and heavy chain) level
External anal sphincter EMG	Denervation (nonspecific)
Transcranial sonography	Lentiform hyperechogenicity and nigral normoechogenicity
CCT	Unhelpful
MRI (1.5 tesla)	Basal ganglia abnormalities (putaminal atrophy/ hyperintense putaminal rim/ putaminal hypointensity, infratentorial signal change – hot cross bun sign), cerebellar and/or brain stem atrophy
MRI (DWI)	Increased diffusivity of putamen (posterior > anterior), rostral pons and middle cerebellar peduncle
MR volumetry	Regional volume loss (putamen in MSA-P, MCP, brainstem and cerebellum in MSA-C)
FP-CIT SPECT	Reduced striatal dopamine transporter binding
IBZM SPECT	Reduced striatal dopamine D2 receptor binding
F-Dopa-PET	Reduced striatal F-dopa uptake
C-Raclopride-PET	Reduced striatal dopamine D2 receptor binding
F-PK11195-PET	Microglial activation in basal ganglia and brainstem areas
FDG-PET	Reduced striatal, frontal, and infratentorial metabolism
MIBG scintigraphy	Preserved myocardial MIBG uptake

Animal models

The role of oligodendroglial α-synucleinopathy as a trigger of MSA-like neurodegeneration has been investigated in transgenic mice with targeted overexpression of human α-synuclein under the control of specific oligodendroglial promoters. Insolubility and hyperphosphorylation of α-synuclein reproduced the main feature of human GCI pathology in transgenic mice and further induced neuronal loss involving (i) axonal α-synuclein aggregation and axonal degeneration [84], (ii) mitochondrial dysfunction [42], (iii) microgliosis [85], or (iv) environmental oxidative stress [86,87]. The transgenic models with α-synuclein overexpression are useful experimental tools to study

basic mechanisms related to GCI-pathology in vivo; however, they also have well-recognized limitations such as not being able to replicate complete MSA-like degeneration and no documented MSA-like change in CNS neurotransmitter expression.

Management
Therapies

Currently, there is no effective neuroprotective therapy in MSA. Symptomatic treatment is largely restricted to parkinsonism and dysautonomia. Other features such as cerebellar ataxia appear to be unresponsive to drug treatment.

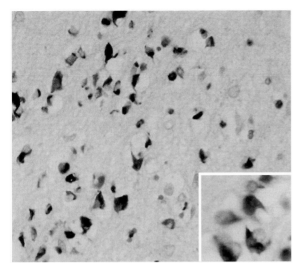

Figure 1.2. Argyrophilic glial cytoplasmic inclusions (GCIs) in the striatum of a patient with multiple system atrophy.

Table 1.8. List of protein constituents identified in GCIs from human MSA.

- α-Synuclein
- α-Tubulin
- Beta-tubulin
- 14-3-3 protein
- Bcl-2
- Carbonic anhydrase isoenzyme II[a]
- cdk-5 (cyclin-dependent kinase 5)
- Midkine
- DARPP32
- Dorfin
- Heat shock proteins Hsc70 and Hsp70
- Isoform of four-repeat tau protein (hypophosphorylated)
- DJ-1
- Mitogen-activated protein kinase (MAPK)
- NEDD-8
- Other microtubule-associated proteins (MAPs): MAP-1A and -1B; MAP-2 isoform 1, and MAP-2 isoform 4
- Phosphoinositide 3-kinase (PI3K)
- p25α/TPPP
- p25α/TPPP
- Transferrins
- Ubiquitin SUMO-1 (small ubiquitin modifier 1)

Modified from Wenning *et al.* [33]

[a] Known oligodendroglial marker

Neuroprotective therapy

A placebo-controlled double-blind pilot trial of recombinant human growth hormone (r-HGH) conducted by the EMSA-SG has shown a trend towards reduction of motor progression (measured both with the Unified Parkinson Disease Rating Scale [UPDRS] and UMSARS) but this failed to reach significance [88].

More recently, minocycline – an antibiotic with neuroprotective effects in a transgenic MSA mouse model [85] as well as models of related neurodegenerative disorders [89,90] – proved ineffective in a phase II neuroprotection trial by the EMSA-SG and the German Parkinson Network (KNP) [12].

The primary and secondary endpoints of the randomized-controlled double blind NNIPPS trial investigating the effects of riluzole, an antiglutamatergic agent, on mortality and progression in atypical parkinsonian disorders including MSA have been negative [13]. A small randomized controlled trial had already excluded symptomatic benefit of riluzole in a small series of MSA-P patients [91].

Rasagiline, a secondary cyclic benzylamine and indane derivative that provides irreversible, potent monoamine oxidase B (MAO-B) inhibition [92], has shown neuroprotective and neurorestorative activities in multiple in-vitro and in-vivo experiments [93–101]. Its disease-modifying effects in patients with Parkinson disease (the ADAGIO [Attenuation of Disease Progression with Azilect Given Once Daily] trial) [88,97,102–104] as well as data from a preclinical study on rasagiline treatment in a transgenic MSA mouse, resulting in behavioral improvement and neuroprotection in SNc, striatum, cerebellar cortex, pontine nuclei and inferior olives [105], make it a potent candidate for MSA therapy. A clinical trial (phase II) to assess efficacy, safety, and tolerability of rasagiline mesylate 1 mg in patients with multiple system atrophy of the parkinsonian subtype (MSA-P) has been initiated.

The success of further neuroprotection trials in MSA depends crucially on defining appropriate pathogenetic targets that are likely to mediate the progression of the disease [33].

Symptomatic therapy

Parkinsonism

Only a small number of randomized controlled trials have been conducted in MSA; the practical management is largely based on empirical evidence or single randomized studies.

Dopaminergic agents

L-Dopa is widely regarded as the antiparkinsonian therapy of choice in MSA, although a randomized controlled trial of L-dopa has never been performed. Despite MSA patients commonly being believed to be nonresponsive or poorly responsive to dopaminergic therapy, efficacy has been documented in up to 40%, often lasting for up to a few years [1]. However, the benefit is transient in most of these subjects, leaving 90% of the MSA-P patients L-dopa-unresponsive in the long term [27]. L-Dopa responsiveness should be tested by administering escalating doses over a 3-month period up to a least 1000 mg/day (if necessary and if tolerated). L-Dopa-induced dyskinesias affecting orofacial and neck muscles occur in 50% of MSA-P patients, sometimes in the absence of motor benefit [106].

No controlled trials with dopamine agonists are available; these compounds seem no more effective than L-dopa and are often poorly tolerated. Lisuride was effective in only one of seven MSA patients [107]. Heinz et al. reported benefit of continuous subcutaneous lisuride infusion in four patients with OPCA and severe signs of parkinsonism [108]. Goetz and colleagues, using doses of 10–80 mg daily of bromocriptine, reported a benefit in five patients who had previously responded to L-dopa and one patient who had failed to respond to L-dopa [109]. There are no reports on other ergolene or non-ergolene dopamine agonists such as pergolide, cabergoline, ropinirole or pramipexole.

Pathological hypersexuality predominantly linked to adjuvant dopamine agonist therapy has been reported in two patients with MSA [110].

MSA patients frequently report the appearance or worsening of postural hypotension after initiation of dopaminergic therapy, which may limit further increase in dosage.

Anticholinergic agents

Anticholinergics usually do not improve motor symptoms, but they may be helpful when sialorrhea is severe and disturbing.

NMDA (N-methyl-D-aspartic acid) receptor antagonists

Despite anecdotal benefit in single cases [10], a short-term open trial with amantadine at high doses (400–600 mg/day) in five patients with MSA unresponsive to

L-dopa was negative [111]. These disappointing results were confirmed more recently in a randomized placebo-controlled trial [112].

Selective serotonin reuptake inhibitors (SSRIs)

Paroxetine 30 mg t.i.d. has been shown to improve motor symptoms in a double-blind placebo-controlled randomized trial with 19 MSA patients [113].

Surgical therapy

Whereas ablative neurosurgical procedures such as medial pallidotomy fail to improve parkinsonism in MSA [114], bilateral subthalamic stimulation has been reported beneficial in four patients with MSA-P [115] although a poor response was seen in other cases [116,117]. At present there is no role for deep brain stimulation (DBS) procedures in the routine management of MSA patients.

Nonpharmacological treatments

Because of the poor efficacy of antiparkinsonian therapies in MSA, nonpharmacological interventions such as physiotherapy, speech and occupational therapy are all the more important. Indeed, a recent study showed substantial benefit of occupational therapy in a series of 17 MSA patients [118]. Treated patients showed a reduction of 20% in UPDRS-ADL scores as well as the PDQ-39 index score, whereas the control group deteriorated significantly over the 2-month study period.

Dystonia

Local injections of botulinum toxin are effective in orofacial as well as limb dystonia associated with MSA [119]. Severe dysphagia with the necessity of nasogastric feeding has been reported after treatment of disproportionate antecollis with botulinum toxin hence this type of treatment is not currently recommended [120].

In addition, local botulinum toxin injections into parotid and submandibular glands have been effective in PD-associated sialorrhea in two double-blind placebo-controlled trials [121,122]. In contrast to anticholinergics, central side-effects can be avoided.

Autonomic symptoms

Treatment of autonomic dysfunction is crucial to avoid complications such as ascending urinary tract infections or orthostatic hypotension, which could lead to falls. In addition, autonomic dysfunction is associated with reduced quality of life [123,124]. Unfortunately, most of the available therapies have not been evaluated in randomized controlled trials.

Orthostatic hypotension

Nonpharmacological options to treat orthostatic hypotension (OH) include sufficient fluid intake; high-salt diet; more frequent, but smaller, meals per day to reduce postprandial hypotension by spreading the total carbohydrate intake; and compression stockings or custommade elastic body garments. Ingestion of ~0.5 liter of water in less then 5 minutes substantially raises blood pressure in patients with autonomic failure including MSA [125,126]. During the night, head-up tilt not only reduces hypertensive cerebral perfusion pressure but also increases intravasal volume up to 1 liter within a week, which is particularly helpful in improving hypotension early in the morning. Constipation can affect the overall well-being and is relieved by an increase in intraluminal fluid, which may be achieved by macrogol–water solution [40].

Midodrine showed significant benefit in randomized placebo-controlled trials [127,128] in patients with OH but may exacerbate urinary retention. Another promising drug seems to be the norepinephrine precursor L-threo-dihydroxyphenylserine (L-threo-DOPS), which has been used for this indication in Japan for years and whose efficacy has now been shown by two double-blind placebo-controlled trials including patients with MSA [129,130].

The somatostatin analogue octreotide has been shown to be beneficial in postprandial hypotension in patients with pure autonomic failure [131], presumably because it inhibits release of vasodilatory gastrointestinal peptides [132]; importantly, it does not enhance nocturnal hypertension [131].

Urinary dysfunction

Whereas procholinergic substances are usually not successful in adequately reducing post-void residual volume in MSA, anticholinergics such as oxybutynin can improve symptoms of detrusor hyperreflexia or sphincter-detrusor dyssynergy in the early course of the disease [133]. However, central side-effects may be limiting. In a large multicentre randomized controlled study in patients with detrusor hyperreflexia, trospium chloride, a peripherally acting quaternary anticholinergic, has been shown to be equally effective with better tolerability [134]. However, trospium

has not been investigated in MSA and, further, it appears that central and peripheral anticholinergics are equally effective and tolerated in nondemented PD patients. At present, there is no evidence for ranking the efficacy and safety of anticholinergics in the management of detrusor hyperreflexia associated with MSA. Alpha-adrenergic receptor antagonists such as prazosin and moxisylyte have been shown to improve voiding with reduction of residual volumes in MSA patients [20].

The vasopressin analogue desmopressin, which acts on renal tubular vasopressin-2 receptors, reduces nocturnal polyuria and improves morning postural hypotension [135].

The peptide erythropoietin may be beneficial in some patients by raising red cell mass, secondarily improving cerebral oxygenation [136,137].

Surgical therapies for neurogenic bladder problems should be avoided in MSA because postoperative worsening of bladder control is most likely [133], but, for example, severe prostate hypertrophy with urinary retention and secondary hydronephrosis cannot be left untreated.

With postmicturition volumes >150 ml clean intermittent catheterization three to four times per day may be necessary to prevent secondary consequences. Permanent transcutaneous suprapubic catheter may become necessary if mechanical obstruction in the urethra or motor symptoms of MSA prevent uncomplicated catheterization.

Erectile dysfunction

After an initial report on the efficacy in the treatment of erectile dysfunction in PD [138]. Sildenafil citrate has been shown effective in a double-blind placebo-controlled randomized trial in patients with PD and MSA [104]. Since it may unmask or exacerbate OH, measurement of lying and standing blood pressure before prescription of sildenafil to men with parkinsonism is recommended. Erectile failure in MSA may also be improved by oral yohimbine or by intracavernosal injection of papaverine or a penis implant [133].

Inspiratory stridor

Inspiratory stridor develops in about 30% of patients. Continuous positive airway pressure (CPAP) may be helpful in some of these patients as long-term therapy [139–141]. A tracheostomy is rarely needed or performed.

Table 1.9. Pragmatic management of MSA.

Parkinsonism

1st choice: L-dopa (up to 1000 mg/day, if tolerated and necessary)

2nd choice: dopamine agonists (PD titration schemes)

3rd choice: amantadine (100 mg t.i.d.)

Dystonia (orofacial and limb, antecollis excluded)

1st choice: botulinum toxin

Cerebellar ataxia

None available

Autonomic symptoms

Orthostatic hypotension

1st choice: nonpharmacological strategies: elastic support stockings or tights, high-salt diet, frequent small meals, head-up tilt of the bed at night

If needed: add fludrocortisone (0.1–0.3 mg) at night

If needed: add midodrine (2.5–10 mg t.i.d.) (combined with fludrocortisone)

If needed: replace midodrine by ephedrine (15–45 mg t.i.d.) or L-threo-DOPS (100 mg t.i.d.)

Urinary failure – urge incontinence

Trospium chloride (20 mg bid or 15 mg t.i.d.)

Oxybutynin (2.5–5 mg bid to t.i.d.). NB: central side-effects

Urinary failure – incomplete bladder emptying

Postmicturition residue of >100 ml is an indication for intermittent self-catheterization

In the advanced stages of MSA a urethral or suprapubic catheter may become necessary

Erectile failure

1st choice: sildenafil (50–100 mg)

2nd choice: oral yohimbine (2.5–5 mg)

3rd choice: intracavernosal injection of papaverine

Palliative therapy

- Physiotherapy
- Occupational therapy
- Speech therapy
- PEG
- Botulinum toxin for sialorrhea
- CPAP (for prominent stridor)
- Tracheostomy (rarely needed)

Palliative care

Because the results of drug treatment for MSA are generally poor, other therapies are all the more important. Physiotherapy helps to maintain mobility and prevent contractures, and speech therapy can improve speech and swallowing and provide communication aids [118]. Dysphagia may require feeding by means of a nasogastric tube or even percutaneous endoscopic gastrostomy. Occupational therapy helps to limit the handicap resulting from the patient's disabilities and should include a home visit. Provision of a wheelchair is usually dictated by the liability to falls because of postural instability and gait ataxia but not from akinesia and rigidity per se. Psychological support for patients and partners needs to be stressed (see Table 1.9).

Conclusions

During the last decade substantial progress has been made in MSA research mainly through the combined efforts of international academic networks in Europe (EMSA-SG), North America (NAMSA-SG), and Japan, which provide the necessary infrastructure to study this rare and rapidly progressive disease. Future experimental and clinical research will be needed to unravel the etiopathogenesis of MSA, to identify targets for intervention, to develop robust motor and non-motor endpoints for phase III trials and to screen candidate neuroprotective and neurorestorative interventions in appropriate MSA models. These efforts will hopefully result in novel therapies able to tame the beast [7].

References

1. Wenning GK, Colosimo C, Geser F, Poewe W. Multiple system atrophy. *Lancet Neurol* 2004; **3**: 93–103.

2. Bower JH, Maraganore DM, McDonnell SK, Rocca WA. Incidence of progressive supranuclear palsy and multiple system atrophy in Olmsted County, Minnesota, 1976 to 1990. *Neurology* 1997; **49**: 1284–8.

3. Schrag A, Ben Shlomo Y, Quinn NP. Prevalence of progressive supranuclear palsy and multiple system atrophy: a cross-sectional study. *Lancet* 1999; **354**: 1771–5.

4. Wenning GK, Ben Shlomo Y, Magalhaes M, Daniel SE, Quinn NP. Clinical features and natural history of multiple system atrophy. An analysis of 100 cases. *Brain* 1994; **117**(Pt 4): 835–45.

5. Graham JG, Oppenheimer DR. Orthostatic hypotension and nicotine sensitivity in a case of multiple system atrophy. *J Neurol Neurosurg Psychiatry* 1969; **32**: 28–34.

6. Papp MI, Kahn JE, Lantos PL. Glial cytoplasmic inclusions in the CNS of patients with multiple system atrophy (striatonigral degeneration, olivopontocerebellar atrophy and Shy–Drager syndrome). *J Neurol Sci* 1989; **94**: 79–100.

7. Quinn N. Multiple system atrophy – the nature of the beast. *J Neurol Neurosurg Psychiatry* 1989; Suppl: 78–89.

8. Gilman S, Low P, Quinn N *et al.* Consensus statement on the diagnosis of multiple system atrophy. American Autonomic Society and American Academy of Neurology. *Clin Auton Res* 1998; **8**: 359–62.

9. Gilman S, Wenning GK, Low PA *et al.* Second consensus statement on the diagnosis of multiple system atrophy. *Neurology* 2008; **71**: 670–6.

10. Wenning GK, Tison F, Seppi K *et al.* Development and validation of the Unified Multiple System Atrophy Rating Scale (UMSARS). *Mov Disord* 2004; **19**: 1391–402.

11. Stefanova N, Tison F, Reindl M, Poewe W, Wenning GK. Animal models of multiple system atrophy. *Trends Neurosci* 2005; **28**: 501–6.

12. Dodel R, Spottke A, Gerhard A *et al.* Minocycline 1-year therapy in multiple-system-atrophy: effect on clinical symptoms and [11C] (R)-PK11195 PET (MEMSA-trial). *Mov Disord* 2010; **25**: 97–107.

13. Bensimon G, Ludolph A, Agid Y, Vidailhet M, Payan C, Leigh PN. Riluzole treatment, survival and diagnostic criteria in Parkinson plus disorders: the NNIPPS study. *Brain* 2009; **132**: 156–71.

14. Gilman S, May SJ, Shults CW *et al.* The North American Multiple System Atrophy Study Group. *J Neural Transm* 2005; **112**: 1687–94.

15. Scholz SW, Houlden H, Schulte C *et al.* SNCA variants are associated with increased risk for multiple system atrophy. *Ann Neurol* 2009; **65**: 610–4.

16. Hara K, Momose Y, Tokiguchi S *et al.* Multiplex families with multiple system atrophy. *Arch Neurol* 2007; **64**: 545–51.

17. Kollensperger M, Wenning GK. Assessing disease progression with MRI in atypical parkinsonian disorders. *Mov Disord* 2009; **24**(Suppl 2): S699–S702.

18. Watanabe H, Saito Y, Terao S *et al.* Progression and prognosis in multiple system atrophy: an analysis of 230 Japanese patients. *Brain* 2002; **125**: 1070–83.

19. Tsuji S, Onodera O, Goto J, Nishizawa M. Sporadic ataxias in Japan – a population-based epidemiological study. *Cerebellum* 2008; **7**: 189–97.

20. Sakakibara R, Hattori T, Uchiyama T *et al.* Are alpha-blockers involved in lower urinary tract dysfunction in multiple system atrophy? A comparison of prazosin and moxisylyte. *J Auton Nerv Syst* 2000; **79**: 191–5.

21. Trojanowski JQ, Revesz T. Proposed neuropathological criteria for the post mortem diagnosis of multiple system atrophy. *Neuropathol Appl Neurobiol* 2007; **33**: 615–20.

22. Wenning GK, Stefanova N. Recent developments in multiple system atrophy. *J Neurol* 2009; **256**: 1791–808.

23. Schrag A, Wenning GK, Quinn N, Ben Shlomo Y. Survival in multiple system atrophy. *Mov Disord* 2008; **23**: 294–6.

24. O'Sullivan SS, Massey LA, Williams DR *et al.* Clinical outcomes of progressive supranuclear palsy and multiple system atrophy. *Brain* 2008; **131**: 1362–72.

25. Ben Shlomo Y, Wenning GK, Tison F, Quinn NP. Survival of patients with pathologically proven multiple system atrophy: a meta-analysis. *Neurology* 1997; **48**: 384–93.

26. Tada M, Kakita A, Toyoshima Y *et al.* Depletion of medullary serotonergic neurons in patients with multiple system atrophy who succumbed to sudden death. *Brain* 2009; **132**: 1810–9.

27. Geser F, Wenning GK, Seppi K *et al.* Progression of multiple system atrophy (MSA): a prospective natural history study by the European MSA Study Group (EMSA SG). *Mov Disord* 2006; **21**: 179–86.

28. Jellinger KA. Neuropathological spectrum of synucleinopathies. *Mov Disord* 2003; **18**(Suppl 6): S2–12.

29. Rockenstein E, Crews L, Masliah E. Transgenic animal models of neurodegenerative diseases and their application to treatment development. *Adv Drug Deliv Rev* 2007; **59**: 1093–102.

30. Ishizawa K, Komori T, Sasaki S, Arai N, Mizutani T, Hirose T. Microglial activation parallels system degeneration in multiple system atrophy. *J Neuropathol Exp Neurol* 2004; **63**: 43–52.

31. Shimohata T, Ozawa T, Nakayama H, Tomita M, Shinoda H, Nishizawa M. Frequency of nocturnal sudden death in patients with multiple system atrophy. *J Neurol* 2008; **255**: 1483–5.

32. Schwarz J, Weis S, Kraft E *et al.* Signal changes on MRI and increases in reactive microgliosis, astrogliosis, and iron in the putamen of two patients with multiple system atrophy. *J Neurol Neurosurg Psychiatry* 1996; **60**: 98–101.

33. Wenning GK, Stefanova N, Jellinger KA, Poewe W, Schlossmacher MG. Multiple system atrophy: a primary oligodendrogliopathy. *Ann Neurol* 2008; **64**: 239–46.

34. Gallyas F, Wolff JR. Metal-catalyzed oxidation renders silver intensification selective. Applications for the histochemistry of diaminobenzidine and neurofibrillary changes. *J Histochem Cytochem* 1986; **34**: 1667–72.

35. Lantos PL. The definition of multiple system atrophy: a review of recent developments. *J Neuropathol Exp Neurol* 1998; **57**: 1099–111.

36. Spillantini MG, Crowther RA, Jakes R, Cairns NJ, Lantos PL, Goedert M. Filamentous alpha-synuclein inclusions link multiple system atrophy with Parkinson's disease and dementia with Lewy bodies. *Neurosci Lett* 1998; **251**: 205–8.

37. Tu PH, Galvin JE, Baba M et al. Glial cytoplasmic inclusions in white matter oligodendrocytes of multiple system atrophy brains contain insoluble alpha-synuclein. *Ann Neurol* 1998; **44**: 415–22.

38. Wakabayashi K, Yoshimoto M, Tsuji S, Takahashi H. Alpha-synuclein immunoreactivity in glial cytoplasmic inclusions in multiple system atrophy. *Neurosci Lett* 1998; **249**: 180–2.

39. Wenning GK, Jellinger KA. The role of alpha-synuclein and tau in neurodegenerative movement disorders. *Curr Opin Neurol* 2005; **18**: 357–62.

40. Eichhorn TE, Oertel WH. Macrogol 3350/electrolyte improves constipation in Parkinson's disease and multiple system atrophy. *Mov Disord* 2001; **16**: 1176–7.

41. El Fakhri G, Habert MO, Maksud P et al. Quantitative simultaneous 99mTc-ECD/123I-FP-CIT SPECT in Parkinson's disease and multiple system atrophy. *Eur J Nucl Med Mol Imaging* 2006; **33**: 87–92.

42. Shults CW, Rockenstein E, Crews L et al. Neurological and neurodegenerative alterations in a transgenic mouse model expressing human alpha-synuclein under oligodendrocyte promoter: implications for multiple system atrophy. *J Neurosci* 2005; **25**: 10689–99.

43. Ozawa T, Paviour D, Quinn NP et al. The spectrum of pathological involvement of the striatonigral and olivopontocerebellar systems in multiple system atrophy: clinicopathological correlations. *Brain* 2004; **127**: 2657–71.

44. Arima K, Murayama S, Mukoyama M, Inose T. Immunocytochemical and ultrastructural studies of neuronal and oligodendroglial cytoplasmic inclusions in multiple system atrophy. 1. Neuronal cytoplasmic inclusions. *Acta Neuropathol* 1992; **83**: 453–60.

45. Armstrong RA, Lantos PL, Cairns NJ. Spatial patterns of alpha-synuclein positive glial cytoplasmic inclusions in multiple system atrophy. *Mov Disord* 2004; **19**: 109–12.

46. Armstrong RA, Cairns NJ, Lantos PL. Multiple system atrophy (MSA): topographic distribution of the alpha-synuclein-associated pathological changes. *Parkinsonism Relat Disord* 2006; **12**: 356–62.

47. Kato S, Nakamura H. Cytoplasmic argyrophilic inclusions in neurons of pontine nuclei in patients with olivopontocerebellar atrophy: immunohistochemical and ultrastructural studies. *Acta Neuropathol* 1990; **79**: 584–94.

48. Nishie M, Mori F, Yoshimoto M, Takahashi H, Wakabayashi K. A quantitative investigation of neuronal cytoplasmic and intranuclear inclusions in the pontine and inferior olivary nuclei in multiple system atrophy. *Neuropathol Appl Neurobiol* 2004; **30**: 546–54.

49. Papp MI, Lantos PL. Accumulation of tubular structures in oligodendroglial and neuronal cells as the basic alteration in multiple system atrophy. *J Neurol Sci* 1992; **107**: 172–82.

50. Sakurai A, Okamoto K, Yaguchi M et al. Pathology of the inferior olivary nucleus in patients with multiple system atrophy. *Acta Neuropathol* 2002; **103**: 550–4.

51. Takeda A, Arai N, Komori T, Iseki E, Kato S, Oda M. Tau immunoreactivity in glial cytoplasmic inclusions in multiple system atrophy. *Neurosci Lett* 1997; **234**: 63–6.

52. Yokoyama T, Kusunoki JI, Hasegawa K, Sakai H, Yagishita S. Distribution and dynamic process of neuronal cytoplasmic inclusion (NCI) in MSA: correlation of the density of NCI and the degree of involvement of the pontine nuclei. *Neuropathology* 2001; **21**: 145–54.

53. Orosz F, Kovacs GG, Lehotzky A, Olah J, Vincze O, Ovadi J. TPPP/p25: from unfolded protein to misfolding disease: prediction and experiments. *Biol Cell* 2004; **96**: 701–11.

54. Jellinger KA, Seppi K, Wenning GK. Clinical and neuropathological correlates of Lewy body disease. *Acta Neuropathol* 2003; **106**: 188–9.

55. Jellinger KA. P25alpha immunoreactivity in multiple system atrophy and Parkinson disease. *Acta Neuropathol* 2006; **112**: 112.

56. Kovacs GG, Gelpi E, Lehotzky A et al. The brain-specific protein TPPP/p25 in pathological protein deposits of neurodegenerative diseases. *Acta Neuropathol* 2007; **113**: 153–61.

57. Lindersson E, Lundvig D, Petersen C et al. p25alpha Stimulates alpha-synuclein aggregation and is co-localized with aggregated alpha-synuclein in alpha-synucleinopathies. *J Biol Chem* 2005; **280**: 5703–15.

58. Song YJ, Lundvig DM, Huang Y et al. p25alpha relocalizes in oligodendroglia from myelin to cytoplasmic inclusions in multiple system atrophy. *Am J Pathol* 2007; **171**: 1291–303.

59. Brown RC, Lockwood AH, Sonawane BR. Neurodegenerative diseases: an overview of environmental risk factors. *Environ Health Perspect* 2005; **113**: 1250–6.

60. Nee LE, Gomez MR, Dambrosia J, Bale S, Eldridge R, Polinsky RJ. Environmental-occupational risk factors and familial associations in multiple system atrophy: a preliminary investigation. *Clin Auton Res* 1991; **1**: 9–13.

61. Vanacore N. Epidemiological evidence on multiple system atrophy. *J Neural Transm* 2005; **112**: 1605–12.

62. Vidal JS, Vidailhet M, Elbaz A, Derkinderen P, Tzourio C, Alperovitch A. Risk factors of multiple system atrophy: a case-control study in French patients. *Mov Disord* 2008; **23**: 797–803.

63. Stefanova N, Bucke P, Duerr S, Wenning GK. Multiple system atrophy: an update. *Lancet Neurol* 2009; **8**: 1172–8.

64. Soma H, Yabe I, Takei A, Fujiki N, Yanagihara T, Sasaki H. Heredity in multiple system atrophy. *J Neurol Sci* 2006; **240**: 107–10.

65. Wullner U, Schmitt I, Kammal M, Kretzschmar HA, Neumann M. Definite multiple system atrophy in a German family. *J Neurol Neurosurg Psychiatry* 2009; **80**: 449–50.

66. Wullner U, Abele M, Schmitz-Huebsch T *et al*. Probable multiple system atrophy in a German family. *J Neurol Neurosurg Psychiatry* 2004; **75**: 924–5.

67. Gilman S, Sima AA, Junck L *et al*. Spinocerebellar ataxia type 1 with multiple system degeneration and glial cytoplasmic inclusions. *Ann Neurol* 1996; **39**: 241–55.

68. Kamm C, Healy DG, Quinn NP *et al*. The fragile X tremor ataxia syndrome in the differential diagnosis of multiple system atrophy: data from the EMSA Study Group. *Brain* 2005; **128**: 1855–60.

69. Khan NL, Giunti P, Sweeney MG *et al*. Parkinsonism and nigrostriatal dysfunction are associated with spinocerebellar ataxia type 6 (SCA6). *Mov Disord* 2005; **20**: 1115–9.

70. Lee WY, Jin DK, Oh MR *et al*. Frequency analysis and clinical characterization of spinocerebellar ataxia types 1, 2, 3, 6, and 7 in Korean patients. *Arch Neurol* 2003; **60**: 858–63.

71. Nirenberg MJ, Libien J, Vonsattel JP, Fahn S. Multiple system atrophy in a patient with the spinocerebellar ataxia 3 gene mutation. *Mov Disord* 2007; **22**: 251–4.

72. Lincoln SJ, Ross OA, Milkovic NM *et al*. Quantitative PCR-based screening of alpha-synuclein multiplication in multiple system atrophy. *Parkinsonism Relat Disord* 2007; **13**: 340–2.

73. Morris HR, Vaughan JR, Datta SR *et al*. Multiple system atrophy/progressive supranuclear palsy: alpha-synuclein, synphilin, tau, and APOE. *Neurology* 2000; **55**: 1918–20.

74. Ozawa T. Pathology and genetics of multiple system atrophy: an approach to determining genetic susceptibility spectrum. *Acta Neuropathol* 2006; **112**: 531–8.

75. Ozawa T, Takano H, Onodera O *et al*. No mutation in the entire coding region of the alpha-synuclein gene in pathologically confirmed cases of multiple system atrophy. *Neurosci Lett* 1999; **270**: 110–2.

76. Al Chalabi A, Durr A, Wood NW *et al*. Genetic variants of the alpha-synuclein gene SNCA are associated with multiple system atrophy. *PLoS One* 2009; **4**: e7114.

77. Kim HS, Lee MS. Frequencies of single nucleotide polymorphism in alcohol dehydrogenase7 gene in patients with multiple system atrophy and controls. *Mov Disord* 2003; **18**: 1065–7.

78. Combarros O, Infante J, Llorca J, Berciano J. Interleukin-1A (-889) genetic polymorphism increases the risk of multiple system atrophy. *Mov Disord* 2003; **18**: 1385–6.

79. Furiya Y, Hirano M, Kurumatani N *et al*. Alpha-1-antichymotrypsin gene polymorphism and susceptibility to multiple system atrophy (MSA). *Brain Res Mol Brain Res* 2005; **138**: 178–81.

80. Infante J, Llorca J, Berciano J, Combarros O. Interleukin-8, intercellular adhesion molecule-1 and tumour necrosis factor-alpha gene polymorphisms and the risk for multiple system atrophy. *J Neurol Sci* 2005; **228**: 11–13.

81. Nishimura M, Kawakami H, Komure O *et al*. Contribution of the interleukin-1beta gene polymorphism in multiple system atrophy. *Mov Disord* 2002; **17**: 808–11.

82. Nishimura M, Kuno S, Kaji R, Kawakami H. Influence of a tumor necrosis factor gene polymorphism in Japanese patients with multiple system atrophy. *Neurosci Lett* 2005; **374**: 218–21.

83. Soma H, Yabe I, Takei A, Fujiki N, Yanagihara T, Sasaki H. Associations between multiple system atrophy and polymorphisms of SLC1A4, SQSTM1, and EIF4EBP1 genes. *Mov Disord* 2008; **23**: 1161–7.

84. Yazawa I, Giasson BI, Sasaki R *et al*. Mouse model of multiple system atrophy alpha-synuclein expression in oligodendrocytes causes glial and neuronal degeneration. Neuron 2005; **45**: 847–59.

85. Stefanova N, Reindl M, Neumann M, Kahle PJ, Poewe W, Wenning GK. Microglial activation mediates neurodegeneration related to oligodendroglial alpha-synucleinopathy: implications for multiple system atrophy. *Mov Disord* 2007; **22**: 2196–203.

86. Stefanova N, Reindl M, Neumann M *et al*. Oxidative stress in transgenic mice with oligodendroglial alpha-synuclein overexpression replicates the characteristic neuropathology of multiple system atrophy. *Am J Pathol* 2005; **166**: 869–76.

87. Ubhi K, Lee PH, Adame A *et al*. Mitochondrial inhibitor 3-nitroproprionic acid enhances oxidative modification of alpha-synuclein in a transgenic mouse model of multiple system atrophy. *J Neurosci Res* 2009; **87**: 2728–39.

88. Holmberg B, Johansson JO, Poewe W *et al*. Safety and tolerability of growth hormone therapy in multiple system atrophy: a double-blind, placebo-controlled study. *Mov Disord* 2007; **22**: 1138–44.

89. Zhu S, Stavrovskaya IG, Drozda M *et al*. Minocycline inhibits cytochrome *c* release and delays progression of amyotrophic lateral sclerosis in mice. *Nature* 2002; **417**: 74–8.

90. Casarejos MJ, Menendez J, Solano RM, Rodriguez-Navarro JA, Garcia dY, Mena MA. Susceptibility to rotenone is increased in neurons from parkin null mice and is reduced by minocycline. *J Neurochem* 2006; **97**: 934–46.

91. Seppi K, Peralta C, Diem-Zangerl A *et al*. Placebo-controlled trial of riluzole in multiple system atrophy. *Eur J Neurol* 2006; **13**: 1146–8.

92. Youdim MB, Gross A, Finberg JP. Rasagiline [*N*-propargyl-1*R*(+)-aminoindan], a selective and potent inhibitor of mitochondrial monoamine oxidase B. *Br J Pharmacol* 2001; **132**: 500–6.

93. Blandini F, Armentero MT, Fancellu R, Blaugrund E, Nappi G. Neuroprotective effect of rasagiline in a rodent model of Parkinson's disease. *Exp Neurol* 2004; **187**: 455–9.

94. Eliash S, Speiser Z, Cohen S. Rasagiline and its (*S*) enantiomer increase survival and prevent stroke in salt-loaded stroke-prone spontaneously hypertensive rats. *J Neural Transm* 2001; **108**: 909–23.

95. Eliash S, Shteter N, Eilam R. Neuroprotective effect of rasagiline, a monoamine oxidase-B inhibitor, on spontaneous cell degeneration in a rat model. *J Neural Transm* 2005; **112**: 991–1003.

96. Finberg JP, Takeshima T, Johnston JM, Commissiong JW. Increased survival of dopaminergic neurons by rasagiline, a monoamine oxidase B inhibitor. *Neuroreport* 1998; **9**: 703–7.

97. Huang W, Chen Y, Shohami E, Weinstock M. Neuroprotective effect of rasagiline, a selective monoamine oxidase-B inhibitor, against closed head injury in the mouse. *Eur J Pharmacol* 1999; **366**: 127–35.

98. Mandel SA, Sagi Y, Amit T. Rasagiline promotes regeneration of substantia nigra dopaminergic neurons in post-MPTP-induced Parkinsonism via activation of tyrosine kinase receptor signaling pathway. *Neurochem Res* 2007; **32**: 1694–9.

99. Waibel S, Reuter A, Malessa S, Blaugrund E, Ludolph AC. Rasagiline alone and in combination with riluzole prolongs survival in an ALS mouse model. *J Neurol* 2004; **251**: 1080–4.

100. Youdim MB, Amit T, Falach-Yogev M, Bar AO, Maruyama W, Naoi M. The essentiality of Bcl-2, PKC and proteasome-ubiquitin complex activations in the neuroprotective-antiapoptotic action of the anti-Parkinson drug, rasagiline. *Biochem Pharmacol* 2003; **66**: 1635–41.

101. Youdim MB, Weinstock M. Molecular basis of neuroprotective activities of rasagiline and the anti-Alzheimer drug TV3326 [(*N*-propargyl-(3*R*) aminoindan-5-yl)-ethyl methyl carbamate]. *Cell Mol Neurobiol* 2001; **21**: 555–73.

102. Hauser TK, Luft A, Skalej M *et al*. Visualization and quantification of disease progression in multiple system atrophy. *Mov Disord* 2006; **21**: 1674–81.

103. Hughes AJ, Daniel SE, Lees AJ. Improved accuracy of clinical diagnosis of Lewy body Parkinson's disease. *Neurology* 2001; **57**: 1497–9.

104. Hussain IF, Brady CM, Swinn MJ, Mathias CJ, Fowler CJ. Treatment of erectile dysfunction with sildenafil citrate (Viagra) in parkinsonism due to Parkinson's disease or multiple system atrophy with observations on orthostatic hypotension. *J Neurol Neurosurg Psychiatry* 2001; **71**: 371–4.

105. Stefanova N, Poewe W, Wenning GK. Rasagiline is neuroprotective in a transgenic model of multiple system atrophy. *Exp Neurol* 2008; **210**: 421–7.

106. Boesch SM, Wenning GK, Ransmayr G, Poewe W. Dystonia in multiple system atrophy. *J Neurol Neurosurg Psychiatry* 2002; **72**: 300–3.

107. Lees AJ, Bannister R. The use of lisuride in the treatment of multiple system atrophy with autonomic failure (Shy–Drager syndrome). *J Neurol Neurosurg Psychiatry* 1981; **44**: 347–51.

108. Heinz A, Wohrle J, Schols L, Klotz P, Kuhn W, Przuntek H. Continuous subcutaneous lisuride infusion in OPCA. *J Neural Transm Gen Sect* 1992; **90**: 145–50.

109. Goetz CG, Tanner CM, Glantz RH, Klawans HL. Chronic agonist therapy for Parkinson's disease: a 5-year study of bromocriptine and pergolide. *Neurology* 1985; **35**: 749–51.

110. Klos KJ, Bower JH, Josephs KA, Matsumoto JY, Ahlskog JE. Pathological hypersexuality predominantly linked to adjuvant dopamine agonist therapy in Parkinson's disease and multiple system atrophy. *Parkinsonism Relat Disord* 2005; **11**: 381–6.

111. Colosimo C, Merello M, Pontieri FE. Amantadine in parkinsonian patients unresponsive to levodopa: a pilot study. *J Neurol* 1996; **243**: 422–5.

112. Wenning GK. Placebo-controlled trial of amantadine in multiple-system atrophy. *Clin Neuropharmacol* 2005; **28**: 225–7.

113. Friess E, Kuempfel T, Modell S *et al*. Paroxetine treatment improves motor symptoms in patients with multiple system atrophy. *Parkinsonism Relat Disord* 2006; **12**: 432–7.

114. Lang AE, Lozano A, Duff J *et al*. Medial pallidotomy in late-stage Parkinson's disease and striatonigral degeneration. *Adv Neurol* 1997; **74**: 199–211.

115. Visser-Vandewalle V, Temel Y, Colle H, van der LC. Bilateral high-frequency stimulation of the subthalamic nucleus in patients with multiple system atrophy – parkinsonism. Report of four cases. *J Neurosurg* 2003; **98**: 882–7.

116. Lezcano E, Gomez-Esteban JC, Zarranz JJ *et al*. Parkinson's disease-like presentation of multiple system atrophy with poor response to STN stimulation: a clinicopathological case report. *Mov Disord* 2004; **19**: 973–7.

117. Santens P, Vonck K, De Letter M *et al*. Deep brain stimulation of the internal pallidum in multiple system atrophy. *Parkinsonism Relat Disord* 2006; **12**: 181–3.

118. Jain S, Dawson J, Quinn NP, Playford ED. Occupational therapy in multiple system atrophy: a pilot randomized controlled trial. *Mov Disord* 2004; **19**: 1360–4.

119. Muller J, Wenning GK, Wissel J, Seppi K, Poewe W. Botulinum toxin treatment in atypical parkinsonian disorders associated with disabling focal dystonia. *J Neurol* 2002; **249**: 300–4.

120. Thobois S, Broussolle E, Toureille L, Vial C. Severe dysphagia after botulinum toxin injection for cervical dystonia in multiple system atrophy. *Mov Disord* 2001; **16**: 764–5.

121. Lagalla G, Millevolte M, Capecci M, Provinciali L, Ceravolo MG. Botulinum toxin type A for drooling in Parkinson's disease: a double-blind, randomized, placebo-controlled study. *Mov Disord* 2006; **21**: 704–7.

122. Mancini F, Zangaglia R, Cristina S *et al.* Double-blind, placebo-controlled study to evaluate the efficacy and safety of botulinum toxin type A in the treatment of drooling in parkinsonism. *Mov Disord* 2003; **18**: 685–8.

123. Schrag A, Geser F, Stampfer-Kountchev M *et al.* Health-related quality of life in multiple system atrophy. *Mov Disord* 2006; **21**: 809–15.

124. Kollensperger M, Stampfer-Kountchev M, Seppi K *et al.* Progression of dysautonomia in multiple system atrophy: a prospective study of self-perceived impairment. *Eur J Neurol* 2007; **14**: 66–72.

125. Shannon JR, Diedrich A, Biaggioni I *et al.* Water drinking as a treatment for orthostatic syndromes. *Am J Med* 2002; **112**: 355–60.

126. Young TM, Mathias CJ. The effects of water ingestion on orthostatic hypotension in two groups of chronic autonomic failure: multiple system atrophy and pure autonomic failure. *J Neurol Neurosurg Psychiatry* 2004; **75**: 1737–41.

127. Jankovic J, Gilden JL, Hiner BC *et al.* Neurogenic orthostatic hypotension: a double-blind, placebo-controlled study with midodrine. *Am J Med* 1993; **95**: 38–48.

128. Low PA, Gilden JL, Freeman R, Sheng KN, McElligott MA. Efficacy of midodrine vs placebo in neurogenic orthostatic hypotension. A randomized, double-blind multicenter study. Midodrine Study Group. *JAMA* 1997; **277**: 1046–51.

129. Mathias CJ, Senard JM, Braune S *et al.* L-Threo-dihydroxyphenylserine (L-threo-DOPS; droxidopa) in the management of neurogenic orthostatic hypotension: a multi-national, multi-center, dose-ranging study in multiple system atrophy and pure autonomic failure. *Clin Auton Res* 2001; **11**: 235–42.

130. Kaufmann H, Saadia D, Voustianiouk A *et al.* Norepinephrine precursor therapy in neurogenic orthostatic hypotension. *Circulation* 2003; **108**: 724–8.

131. Alam M, Smith G, Bleasdale-Barr K, Pavitt DV, Mathias CJ. Effects of the peptide release inhibitor, octreotide, on daytime hypotension and on nocturnal hypertension in primary autonomic failure. *J Hypertens* 1995; **13**: 1664–9.

132. Raimbach SJ, Cortelli P, Kooner JS, Bannister R, Bloom SR, Mathias CJ. Prevention of glucose-induced hypotension by the somatostatin analogue octreotide (SMS 201–995) in chronic autonomic failure: haemodynamic and hormonal changes. *Clin Sci.(Lond)* 1989; **77**: 623–8.

133. Beck RO, Betts CD, Fowler CJ. Genitourinary dysfunction in multiple system atrophy: clinical features and treatment in 62 cases. *J Urol* 1994; **151**: 1336–41.

134. Halaska M, Ralph G, Wiedemann A *et al.* Controlled, double-blind, multicentre clinical trial to investigate long-term tolerability and efficacy of trospium chloride in patients with detrusor instability. *World J Urol* 2003; **20**: 392–9.

135. Mathias CJ, Fosbraey P, da Costa DF, Thornley A, Bannister R. The effect of desmopressin on nocturnal polyuria, overnight weight loss, and morning postural hypotension in patients with autonomic failure. *Br Med J (Clin Res Ed)* 1986; **293**: 353–4.

136. Perera R, Isola L, Kaufmann H. Effect of recombinant erythropoietin on anemia and orthostatic hypotension in primary autonomic failure. *Clin Auton Res* 1995; **5**: 211–3.

137. Winkler AS, Marsden J, Parton M, Watkins PJ, Chaudhuri KR. Erythropoietin deficiency and anaemia in multiple system atrophy. *Mov Disord* 2001; **16**: 233–9.

138. Zesiewicz TA, Helal M, Hauser RA. Sildenafil citrate (Viagra) for the treatment of erectile dysfunction in men with Parkinson's disease. *Mov Disord* 2000; **15**: 305–8.

139. Iranzo A, Santamaria J, Tolosa E *et al.* Long-term effect of CPAP in the treatment of nocturnal stridor in multiple system atrophy. *Neurology* 2004; **63**: 930–2.

140. Ghorayeb I, Bioulac B, Tison F. Sleep disorders in multiple system atrophy. *J Neural Transm* 2005; **112**: 1669–75.

141. Nonaka M, Imai T, Shintani T, Kawamata M, Chiba S, Matsumoto H. Non-invasive positive pressure ventilation for laryngeal contraction disorder during sleep in multiple system atrophy. *J Neurol Sci* 2006; **247**: 53–8.

142. Wenning GK, Pramstaller PP, Ransmayr G, Poewe W. Atypical Parkinson syndrome. *Nervenarzt* 1997; **68**: 102–15.

Chapter 2

Progressive supranuclear palsy

Henry Moore, Corneliu Luca and Carlos Singer

History

In 1955, Canadian neurologist J. Clifford Richardson was consulted by a good friend, a 52-year-old business executive, complaining of clumsiness, trouble in seeing and mild forgetfulness. Over the next four years his friend progressively developed an unusual constellation of symptoms including vertical supranuclear ophthalmoplegia, pseudobulbar palsy, dysarthria, dystonic rigidity-in-extension of the neck and mild dementia [1]. In the next few years more patients were identified. By the early 1960s, seven of them had died. Neuropathologists Linnel and Tom at the Banting Institute examined the brains and diagnosed postencephalitic parkinsonism. Richardson disagreed with their conclusion because none of these patients had a history of encephalitis, parkinsonism or oculogyric crises [2].

In 1962, Richardson assisted by John Steele, one of his neurology residents, and Jersy Olszewski, a neuropathologist, reevaluated and reported the pathology of these intriguing cases [2]. In June 1963, at the American Neurological Association meeting in Atlantic City, Richardson presented the first clinical report of the disease. All the reported cases had defects in ocular gaze, "spasticity of the facial musculature" (we suspect dystonia), dysarthria, dysphagia, extensor rigidity of the neck with head retraction and dementia. In a companion report at the meeting of the American Association of Neuropathology, Olszewski described the cardinal neuropathological features of this disease, mainly characterized by the presence of neurofibrillary tangles without senile plaques especially in the brain stem. In April 1964, the report of nine patients, seven of whom had died, was published in the *Archives of Neurology* [1]. The authors suggested a neurodegenerative process. In their 1963 reports, Richardson, Olszewski

and Steel called this condition "heterogeneous system degeneration." In the summer of 1963, Richardson proposed the name progressive supranuclear palsy (PSP). In 1965, the eponym Steele–Richardson–Olszewski syndrome was coined by Andre Barbeau.

Epidemiology

The annual incidence rate of PSP is 5.3 new cases per 100 000 person-years [3]. The prevalence varies from 1 to 6.5 per 100 000 [4]. PSP occurs more often in men, with a mean age at onset of 63 years, 3–5 years later than the typical onset of Parkinson disease (PD). The median survival time is 8.6 years (3–24 years). The mean age of death is 72.3 years (60–89 years). Early bulbar features are associated with 5 years less of life expectancy. The most common cause of death is pneumonia, which is present in 45% of the cases. A recent case–control study performed in France failed to discover any environmental risk factors in patients with PSP compared with controls. However, chronic consumption of *Annona muricata*, a plant that contains acetogenin, a mitochondrial complex I inhibitor, has been associated with development of a PSP-like disease [5].

Clinical variants

PSP is progressive neurological disorder with motor and cognitive components. A number of clinical variants have been described and have been divided into a "classic PSP" variant and a number of other clinical phenotypes grouped as "atypical PSP."

Classic PSP described by Richardson (Richardson syndrome, Steele–Richardson–Olszewski syndrome) accounts for 50% of patients. It is characterized by a symmetric akinetic rigid syndrome, vertical

Uncommon Causes of Movement Disorders, ed. Néstor Gálvez-Jiménez and Paul J. Tuite. Published by Cambridge University Press. © Cambridge University Press 2011.

supranuclear gaze palsy, frontal deficits, prominent postural instability and falls.

PSP–parkinsonism (PSP-P), a second variant is present in 30% of those with PSP. It is characterized by an asymmetric onset of tremor and moderate initial therapeutic response to levodopa. It has less severe and more restricted tau pathology.

Pure akinesia with gait freezing (PAGF), a third presentation of PSP is characterized by early gait disturbances, micrographia, hypophonia and gait freezing.

Other PSP variants include *PSP-corticobasal syndrome (PSP-CBS)* characterized by progressive asymmetric dystonia, apraxia and cortical sensory loss; *PSP-progressive nonfluent aphasia (PSP-PNFA)* characterized by spontaneous nonfluent speech with intact comprehension; and the rarer variants as *PSP with pallido-nigro-luysian atrophy, PSP with frontotemporal dementia, PSP with semantic dementia* and *PSP with cerebellar ataxia.*

Natural history and clinical findings

The variety of clinical manifestations seen in PSP, present challenges to its clinical diagnosis.

The earliest and most disabling symptom of PSP is usually gait and balance impairment, with subsequent unexplained falls and secondary injuries. The average period from the onset of symptoms to the first fall is 16.8 months, as compared to 108 in PD, 42 in multiple system atrophy (MSA), 54 in diffuse Lewy body disease (DLB), and 40.8 in vascular parkinsonism [6]. Using computerized posturography, one study has demonstrated that balance impairment in PSP is different from that PD. In contrast to the short and shuffling steps, stooped posture, narrow base and flexed knees typically seen in PD, PSP patients have a stiff and broad-based gait, with a tendency to have their knees and trunk extended and arms slightly abducted. Instead of turning in bloc, they tend to pivot [7]. The marked instability is a result of visual-vestibular impairment, axial rigidity and bradykinesia [8].

There are several neuro-ophthalmologic abnormalities seen in patients with PSP. The supranuclear ophthalmoplegia (SNO) that defines the disease clinically consists of increasing difficulties in the generation of saccadic and smooth pursuit movements, which tend to follow a sequential involvement of changes in downward vertical then upward vertical and finally horizontal eye movements. Diminished vertical saccades elicited with the optokinetic (OKN) flag may be the earliest oculomotor sign of PSP [9]. The limitations

Table 2.1. Differential diagnosis of supranuclear ophthalmoplegia

PSP
Corticobasal degeneration (CBD)
Dementia with Lewy bodies (DLB)
Postencephalitic parkinsonism
Wernicke encephalopathy
Dorsal midbrain syndrome
Primary pallidal degeneration
Prion disease
Paraneoplastic syndrome
Progressive subcortical gliosis
Niemann–Pick type C
Gaucher disease
Kufor–Rabek syndrome

in generation of these eye movements can be overcome with doll's eyes maneuver. In the late stages of the disease, the SNO may evolve into a nuclear ophthalmoplegia with the doll's eye maneuvers becoming ineffectual.

In spite of its key position as a pivotal sign of the disease, cases of pathologically proven PSP without supranuclear ophthalmoplegia have been described. Moreover, it is important to mention that there are causes of supranuclear ophthalmoplegia other than PSP. See Table 2.1.

PSP patients may complain of blurred vision, diplopia and eye irritation (30%). Square-wave jerks may be seen in PSP but are not specific to the disorder. Other neuro-ophthalmologic manifestations include decrease in blink rate, persistence of ocular fixation, limitation or absence of convergence, internuclear ophthalmoplegia, blepharospasm, apraxia of eyelid opening, eyelid retractions (Cowper's sign) and loss of Bell's phenomenon. Anti-saccades – provoked by instructing the patient to look in the direction opposite to the visual stimulus – are affected and seem to correlate well with frontal lobe dysfunction in PSP. Patients with PSP have a higher percentage of errors in the anti-saccade task compared with patients with PD or other atypical parkinsonian disorders.

The procerus sign consists of a sustained contraction of the procerus muscle [10], which may be associated with a peculiar facial expression (astonished, worried, reptile-like features). The corrugators and orbicularis oculi muscles may also be involved. This sign can be viewed as a form of focal dystonia and it is not a specific finding for PSP, as it can be seen in corticobasal degeneration (CBD), Meige syndrome, and even in healthy people.

Patients with PSP can also present with pseudobulbar symptoms characterized by dysarthria, dysphagia and emotional incontinence. Progressive dysphagia may eventually require feeding tube placement. Speech can be spastic, hypernasal, hypokinetic, ataxic, monotonous, and associated with low-pitch dysarthria. The speech rate can be slow or fast and some patients can have stuttering, palilalia or continuous involuntary vocalizations as moaning.

Dystonia, may be present in 40–60% of the patients at some point of their disease. Blepharospasm is the most common form of dystonia in PSP. It is associated with lid function abnormalities – frequently referred to as apraxia of eyelid opening – which have been related to supranuclear inhibition of the levator palpebrae (apraxia of eyelid opening) or to actual lid freezing [11]. At the level of the neck, dystonia is usually in extension, but neck flexion dystonia, more often associated with MSA, can also be seen in PSP. Distal limb dystonia, sometimes unilateral, may also be seen.

Cognitive dysfunction with relative preservation of the short-term memory is seen in PSP. As the disease progresses, the patients may develop subcortical dementia characterized by cognitive slowing and executive dysfunction.

Patients with PSP may show neuropsychiatric abnormalities such as apathy, disinhibition, dysphoria, anxiety, irritability, difficulties in the recognition of emotion in others, and loss of insight. Similarly to PD, there are cases of impulse control behavior reported in patients with pathologically proven PSP treated with dopamine agonists.

The "applause sign" described by Dubois may be seen in up to 70% of patients with PSP [12]. It is characterized by persistence of clapping after the patient is instructed to clap consecutively three times as quickly as possible [12]. It may be due to basal ganglia failure (inability to stop an automatic activity once it is initiated) or frontal lobe failure (decreased ability to plan a specific program of 3 claps). The "three clap test" correctly identified 81.8% of the patients in a comparison of PSP with frontotemporal dementia and 75% of the patients in a comparison of PSP and PD. Another study found that the specificity of the applause sign is 100% in distinguishing parkinsonian disorders and Huntington disease from normal subjects, but was not specific for PSP [13].

Sleep disturbances can be present in PSP. This includes reduction of REM sleep and sleep spindles, reduction of sleep efficiency, periodic limb movements of sleep (PLMS), sleep disordered breathing and REM behavior disorder (RBD), with the latter as frequent and pronounced as in PD. There is also hypnoagnosia (reduced self-perception of sleep dysfunction), which is not seen in PD [14].

Autonomic dysfunction was studied by autonomic anamnesis and function tests in 32 PSP patients, 26 PD patients and 27 healthy controls. PSP and PD patients presented with significant autonomic dysfunction. The parasympathetic cardiovascular system was involved to a similar extent in PD and PSP patients, whereas sympathetic cardiovascular dysfunction was more frequent and severe in PD patients [15]. In addition, autopsy studies have demonstrated damage to autonomic centers in the lower brain stem in PSP patients.

A clinical rating scale for PSP (PSP-Rating Scale, PSP-RS) has been developed. It evaluates 28 items grouped in six categories: daily activities by history, behavior, bulbar, ocular motor, limb motor and gait/midline. Scores range from 0 to 100. Inter-rater reliability is good, with intra-class correlation coefficient for the overall scale of 0.86 (95% CI 0.65–0.98) [16]. Litvan *et al.* published in 1996 the NINDS-SPSP clinical criteria for diagnosis of PSP with the definitive diagnosis requiring a pathological confirmation [17]. The report included 24 patients with PSP among 105 autopsy-proven cases of several neurodegenerative disorders. This analysis identified vertical supranuclear palsy with downward gaze abnormalities and postural instability with unexplained falls as the best features for predicting the diagnosis [17].

There are other conditions that may cause a PSP phenotype without the pathological findings of PSP and must be excluded before the diagnosis of idiopathic PSP is considered [18]. They include among others: vascular PSP, corticobasal degeneration, dementia of Lewy body, postencephalitic parkinsonism, Whipple disease, Creutzfeldt–Jakob disease and paraneoplastic syndromes. After idiopathic PSP, "vascular" PSP is the second most common cause of PSP syndrome. This condition is characterized by asymmetric and lower-body involvement, cortical and pseudobulbar signs, dementia, bowel and bladder incontinence [19] and MRI evidence of white matter hyperintensities.

Genetics

Progressive supranuclear palsy is predominantly a sporadic disorder. However, the search for genetic factors – be they causative or contributory – is on-going. For example, recent linkage studies in one large Spanish family with PSP have identified a locus on chromosome 1q13.1 [20]. Currently, PSP is recognized as a tauopathy, a disorder with an abnormal intraneuronal accumulation of the tau protein in multiple cortical and subcortical sites. This protein is encoded by the MAPT (microtubule-associated protein tau) gene located on chromosome 17q21. The MAPT connection has been buttressed with cases of familial PSP with autosomal dominant transmission linked to mutations in the MAPT gene.

The MAPT messenger RNA (mRNA) consists of 16 exons (E1–E16). In the adult human brain, six tau isoforms (encompassing between 352 and 441 amino acids) are generated by a mechanism of alternative mRNA splicing. In the healthy human brain, there is a balanced ratio of 3R and 4R isoforms (50%–50%). Splice modifiers acting at the splice donor site of E10 change the isoform ratio in PSP, resulting in an increase in the aggregation-prone 4R tau isoforms [21].

The best-established genetic risk factor for sporadic PSP is the H1 haplotype of the MAPT gene [22,23], while the H2 haplotype is protective. H1 allele increases MAPT transcription and exon 10 splicing. Since the H1 haplotype has a high prevalence among healthy controls, it is considered a predisposing condition only, requiring additional genetic or environmental cofactors to trigger the disease. A more comprehensive genome-wide association study is currently under way. DNA samples from more than 1100 autopsy-confirmed cases of PSP are being studied to find other genetics factors implicated in the disease.

Etiology and pathogenesis

The etiology of PSP is unknown. Genetic predisposition (see the section on genetics) and a limited set of environmental toxins have been identified, but much work is needed in this field. Certain mitochondrial neurotoxins have been described and associated with PSP pathology. The acetogenins, which are highly lipophilic and extremely potent inhibitors of complex I, are contained in plants of the Annonaceae family, in particular *Annona muricata*. Chronic consumption of these plants in Guadeloupe [5], but also in other regions, has been associated with cases with a PSP-like disease. Autopsy performed in three cases confirmed the neuropathological findings of PSP.

The main pathogenic mechanisms involve **oxidative damage**, **mitochondrial dysfunction** and **abnormal protein processing**. The inner membrane of the mitochondria contains the respiratory chain (complex I–V), whose function is to maintain adequate levels of ATP by aerobic oxidative phosphorylation. Mitochondria are the major cellular source of reactive oxygen species, particularly by complex I. Under conditions of excessive production or defective clearance of reactive oxygen species, oxidation of cellular macromolecules including proteins, lipids and DNA occurs that ultimately affects complex I as well as other proteins of the oxidative phosphorylation. The result is bioenergetic deficits with defective complex I activity resulting in more reactive oxygen species generation.

Postmortem immunochemical studies have provided evidence for oxidative stress in PSP brains. Cybrids (cells whose cytoplasm has been hybridized with patient's mitochondria) generated using mitochondria from PSP patients have been shown to have reduced complex I activity, ATP production and oxygen consumption, indicating oxidative damage [24].

(^{18}F)Fluorodeoxyglucose (FDG) positron emission tomography (PET) studies have shown cerebral hypometabolism in patients with PSP. Proton and phosphorus magnetic resonance spectroscopy (^{1}H and ^{31}P MRS) studies showed decreased concentration of high-energy phosphates in basal ganglia and frontal lobes, without *N*-acetylaspartate (NAA) alterations, suggesting that this phenomenon is not secondary to neuronal death but rather to mitochondrial dysfunction [25].

Increased oxidative stress and reactive oxygen species may activate tau-kinases in PSP neurons and glial cells and cause hyperphosphorylation of tau [26]. Hyperphosphorylated tau is more prone to aggregation than dephosphorylated tau. Studies with complex I inhibitors have been found to cause decreased ATP levels, neuronal cell death and somatodendritic redistribution of phosphorylated tau protein from axons to the cell body in primary cultures of fetal rat striatum [27]. This suggests that ATP depletion is the main cause of tau redistribution. In chronic complex I inhibition, the combination of somatodendritic redistribution and tau hyperphosphorylation may result in tau aggregation that may cause further mitochondrial dysfunction.

Progressive supranuclear palsy is not a primary neurotransmitter disease. There is marked reduction in striatal dopamine and choline acetyltransferase activity in patients with PSP. Glutamate has been found to be increased in the striatum, pallidum, nucleus accumbens and occipital and temporal cortex. The significance of any of these neurotransmitter-related findings remains poorly understood.

Pathology

Neuronal cell loss involves both cortical and subcortical structures, in particular the subthalamic nucleus (STN), globus pallidus, superior colliculi, pretectal regions, periaqueductal gray matter, substantia nigra, thalamus, cerebellum, pontine tegmentum, and spinal cord [28]. Microscopically, there are neurofibrillary tangles in neurons, neuropil threads in neuronal processes, coiled bodies in oligodendrocytes (cytosolic), tufted astrocytes in the basal ganglia, amygdala and the motor cortex; and the absence of neuritic plaques.

Patients with the PSP variant of pure akinesia with gait freezing (PAGF) have severe atrophy and neuronal loss only in the globus pallidus, substantia nigra and subthalamic nucleus [29]. In the PSP-CBS and the PSP-PNFA variants a higher amount of cortical PSP pathology has been described, as opposed to subcortical pathology typically seen in typical PSP [30].

Ultrastructurally, tau aggregates present as paired helical filaments and spherical filaments. Biochemical examinations have shown abnormal accumulation of insoluble, hyperphosphorylated specimens of MAPT, with altered ratio of tau isoforms (3R tau and 4R tau) in favor of the 4R tau.

Although PSP is a tauopathy, there is evidence of α-synuclein aggregation in some patients with PSP. It remains unclear whether Lewy bodies in PSP represent the aging process or the coexistence of PD [31].

Diagnostic investigations

The diagnosis of PSP is clinical. Imaging techniques have a complementary value in the diagnosis. Ancillary electrophysiologic studies may add useful information, while CSF biomarkers are still a work-in-progress.

Brain MRI shows generalized and brain stem (particularly midbrain) atrophy. Dorsal midbrain atrophy is a result of degeneration of superior colliculi, and flattening of the third ventricle floor on sagittal MRI images. Warmuth-Metz and colleagues reported a decrease in the anteroposterior diameter of the midbrain. In contrast to PD patients (mean 18.5 mm), PSP patients had a significantly smaller diameter (13.4 mm) on axial T2-weighted MRI [32]. In another study, Oba and colleagues found a decrease in midbrain area on midsagittal MRI. The average midbrain area in patients with PSP was 56 mm², which was significantly smaller than that in patients with PD (103 mm²) or MSA-P (97.2 mm²). The ratio of midbrain area to pons area was found to reliably differentiate these three disorders [33].

On the midsagittal view of the MRI a so called "hummingbird sign" or "penguin sign" has been described [33]. This configuration is the result of atrophy of the most rostral midbrain tegmentum, pontine base and cerebellum, which appear to correlate with the bill, head, body and wing of these birds. This sign is not specific for PSP and can be seen in elderly people with no neurological signs and enlargement of the third ventricle. A "morning glory sign" has been described in PSP. This is a consequence of midbrain atrophy with concavity of the lateral margin of the midbrain tegmentum, resembling the lateral margin of the morning glory flower. The "eye of the tiger sign," typically described in neurodegeneration with brain iron accumulation type 1, has been reported in few patients with PSP.

The value of diffusion-weighted imaging (DWI) and apparent diffusion coefficient (ADC) MRI sequences has been studied in PSP. ADC ratios (rADCs) were significantly increased in putamen, globus pallidus and caudate nucleus in patients with PSP compared with those with PD. Putaminal rADC may discriminate PSP and PD with a sensitivity of 90% and a positive predictive value of 100%. However, DWI failed to discriminate PSP and MSA-parkinsonism subtype (MSA-P) [34].

Diffusion tensor imaging (DTI) and voxel-based morphometry (VBM) are other tools that may be useful in PSP. There is evidence for gray and white matter degeneration even in early stages of PSP [35]. Using VBM, Boxer and colleagues found distinct patterns of atrophy between patients with PSP and CBD. CBD patients had a marked asymmetric (L > R) pattern of atrophy involving the premotor cortex, superior parietal lobe and striatum, whereas PSP patients had atrophy of the midbrain, pons, thalamus and striatum [36].

(¹⁸F)Fluorodeoxyglucose PET studies (FDG-PET) have shown decreased metabolic activity in the caudate, putamen and prefrontal cortex in PSP patients. However, the earliest finding appears to be glucose hypometabolism in the midbrain [37]. With (^{18}F) fluorodopa (F-dopa) PET, uptake of F-dopa is usually reduced in PSP, but may be normal on early stages. This suggests that the parkinsonian findings in early PSP are related to postsynaptic receptor changes rather than loss in presynaptic neurons. In one study, F-dopa uptake was markedly reduced in the caudate as well as the anterior and posterior putamen of PSP patients. In contrast, the uptake is reduced only in the posterior putamen in PD patients [38]. F-dopa PET can differentiate between PD and PSP, but it is less accurate in differentiating PD from MSA [39]. Using ^{123}I β-CIT single-photon emission computed tomography (SPECT), Pirker and colleagues showed a marked reduction of striatal binding in PD, PSP, MSA and CBD; nevertheless the pattern of the abnormality did not allow differentiation between these two disorders [40].

Transcranial ultrasound has also been used in this disorder. A normal echogenic substantia nigra (SN) is a typical finding in transcranial sonography in PSP, as opposed to a hyperechogenic SN which is characteristic of PD.

Sleep studies of PSP patients have shown insomnia, marked reduction in percentage of REM sleep, RBD (as frequent and as pronounced as in PD), PLMS and sleep disordered breathing [14]. Some patients with PSP may present with urinary or fecal incontinence secondary to loss of neurons in the Onuf's nuclei of the S2–S4 segments of the anterior horn of the spinal cord. Anal sphincter EMG is abnormal in 42% of the patients with PSP [41]. Problems with micturition are less common than in MSA, but more common than in PD. Urodynamic studies in PSP have shown detrusor hyperreflexia or dyssynergia.

Several cerebrospinal fluid (CSF) biomarkers have been studied in this condition. They include brain-related proteins (BRPs) present in neurons and glial cells that are released in the CSF after brain tissue damage caused by a variety of neurological diseases. There is evidence of decreased tau 33 kDa/55 kDa ratio in patients with PSP as opposed to other neurodegenerative disorders. One study showed that a decreased CSF tau isoform ratio correlated significantly with brain stem atrophy. The tau isoform ratio was the lowest in PSP with no overlap with any other neurodegenerative diseases [42]. This truncated tau production, which selectively affects brain stem neurons, is being proposed as specific and reliable marker for PSP.

In sequential analyses of CSF axonal and glial markers on PD and atypical parkinsonian disorders, Constantinescu found increased CSF levels of neurofilament light protein (NFL) in patients with PSP, MSA and CBD. NFL is a marker of neuronal damage, and is usually normal in patients with PD. In addition, CSF levels of glial fibrillary acidic protein (GFAP), a protein expressed mainly in fibrillary astrocytes, were similar in all investigated groups. Sequential analyses of CSF NFL and CSF GFAP levels showed relatively stable levels over time in all the investigated parkinsonian disorders, suggesting that the rate of neuronal degeneration is rather constant over time [43].

Management

There is neither a cure nor an effective neuroprotective therapy for PSP. Several pharmacological agents have been tried without success. Levodopa and dopamine agonists can certainly be tried in early stages of the disease. They may produce mild improvement in the parkinsonism, but most of the patients fail to respond to these drugs owing to a marked loss in postsynaptic D2 receptors.

Idazoxan, a potent and selective α2-presynaptic inhibitor that increases norepinephrine transmission, improved motor function in nine PSP patients [44]. These observations have not been replicated.

Anticholinergic drugs should be avoided in PSP patients, as they are particularly sensitive to cholinergic blockade. Donepezil has not been found to be beneficial in a placebo-control trial of 21 patients with PSP with and some have suggested it could worsen motor function [45]. Rivastigmine, an acetylcholinesterase and butyrylcholinesterase inhibitor, was shown to have a slight clinical benefit in cognition in five PSP patients treated for 5 months [46].

Amantadine at 100 mg twice daily was assessed in a retrospective study in patients with MSA and PSP. Six out of 14 PSP patients (42.9%) had some symptomatic improvement, a benefit that may be related to amantadine's NMDA antagonist properties [47].

Zolpidem, a GABA agonist of the benzodiazepine type 1 receptor, has been shown to moderately improve the voluntary saccadic eye movements and motor function in 10 patients with PSP compared with placebo, but the benefits were not sustained [48].

Botulinum toxin may be helpful in treating blepharospasm with or without eye opening apraxia, and other focal dystonias.

A swallowing evaluation is recommended in patients with dysphagia. Evidence of marked dysphagia would require placement of a feeding tube, but there is no evidence that tube feeding prevents aspiration.

Experimental therapies

There are some novel and experimental therapies in PSP. Inhibitors of transglutaminase, an enzyme responsible for cross-linking and stabilization of tau filaments into NFT, may have a neuroprotective effect in the disease. Glycogen synthase kinase 3β (GSK-3β) inhibitors such as valproic acid, which inhibit the abnormal phosphorylation of tau protein, may exert neuroprotective effects [49]. Other kinase inhibitors such as lithium, noscovitine and olomoucine may be useful in PSP. However, a phase II trial with lithium was stopped because of poor tolerability. A new compound, tideglusib (Nypta), is being actively studied in phase II trial. Danuvetide, a medication that produces stabilization of microtubules, is currently being studied in phase II trial.

Coenzyme Q_{10}, a facilitator in the transport of electrons from complexes I and II to complex III, with the potential of restoring the impaired complex I activity in PSP, has been studied in a double-blind phase II trial versus placebo. Twenty-one patients with probable PSP received a dose of CoQ_{10} of 5 mg/kg/day for 6 weeks. Compared with placebo, there was an increased ratio of high-energy metabolites to low-energy metabolites, as measured by ^{31}P and ^{1}H MRS. PSP rating scale and frontal assessment battery (FAB) scores improved significantly in those on active treatment compared with those taking a placebo [50]. A phase III trial is currently under way.

A nutrient cocktail composed of pyruvate (free scavenger), niacinamide (which boosts the mitochondrial cofactor NAD^+) and creatine (a rapidly accessible cellular energy buffer) has been shown to be neuroprotective in various animal models of brain injury or neurodegeneration, and is currently being studied in a phase I trial.

Deep brain stimulation has not been consistently studied in PSP. There is an anecdotal report of a patient with levodopa-responsive parkinsonism, initially diagnosed as PD, who underwent bilateral deep brain stimulation of the subthalamic nucleus for motor fluctuations and dyskinesias with good results. As the disease progressed, the patient met clinical criteria for PSP-P. The benefit obtained from DBS for the parkinsonism was still apparent 4 years later [51].

Conclusions

Progressive supranuclear palsy is a four-repeat tauopathy with multiple clinical phenotypes. It is considered to be a sporadic disorder, although familial cases have been reported. Pathologically, it is defined by accumulation of tau protein in several regions of the brain. The etiology is unknown, but several mechanisms including tau dysfunction, genetic predisposition, oxidative damage, mitochondrial dysfunction, abnormal protein processing and environmental risk factors have been implicated. There are several clinical phenotypes of the disease depending of the levels and topography of tau accumulation. Multiple causes of secondary PSP, including vascular PSP without the typical pathological changes, have been described and must be recognized before making the diagnosis of idiopathic PSP. Multiple diagnostic tools including the development of CSF biomarkers have been proposed, but the diagnosis remains primarily clinical. There is no known curative or neuroprotective therapy for the disease. Novel promising experimental therapies targeting tau and mitochondrial dysfunction are currently being studied.

References

1. Steele JC, Richardson JC, Olszewski J. Progressive supranuclear palsy. A heterogeneous degeneration involving the brain stem, basal ganglia and cerebellum with vertical gaze and pseudobulbar palsy, nuchal dystonia and dementia. *Arch Neurol* 1964; **10**: 333–59.

2. Williams DR, Lees AJ, Wherrett JR, Steele JC. J. Clifford Richardson and 50 years of progressive supranuclear palsy. *Neurology* 2008; **70**(7): 566–73.

3. Bower JH, Maraganore DM, McDonnell SK, Rocca WA. Incidence of progressive supranuclear palsy and multiple system atrophy in Olmsted County, Minnesota, 1976 to 1990. *Neurology* 1997; **49**(5): 1284–8.

4. Nath U, Ben-Shlomo Y, Thomson RG *et al*. The prevalence of progressive supranuclear palsy (Steele–Richardson–Olszewski syndrome) in the UK. *Brain* 2001; **124**(Pt 7): 1438–49.

5. Caparros-Lefebvre D, Elbaz A. Possible relation of atypical parkinsonism in the French West Indies with consumption of tropical plants: a case-control study. Caribbean Parkinsonism Study Group. *Lancet* 1999; **354**(9175): 281–6.

6. Williams DR, Watt HC, Lees AJ. Predictors of falls and fractures in bradykinetic rigid syndromes: a retrospective study. *J Neurol Neurosurg Psychiatry* 2006; **77**(4): 468–73.

7. Ondo W, Warrior D, Overby A *et al*. Computerized posturography analysis of progressive supranuclear

palsy: a case–control comparison with Parkinson's disease and healthy controls. *Arch Neurol* 2000; **57**(10): 1464–69.

8. Jankovic J, Friedman DI, Pirozzolo FJ, McCrary JA. Progressive supranuclear palsy: motor, neurobehavioral, and neuro-ophthalmic findings. *Adv Neurol* 1990; **53**: 293–304.

9. Garbutt S, Riley DE, Kumar AN, Han Y, Harwood MR, Leigh RJ. Abnormalities of optokinetic nystagmus in progressive supranuclear palsy. *J Neurol Neurosurg Psychiatry* 2004; **75**(10): 1386–94.

10. Romano S, Colosimo C. Procerus sign in progressive supranuclear palsy. *Neurology* 2001; **57**(10): 1928.

11. Jankovic J. Apraxia of lid opening. *Mov Disord* 1995; **10**(5): 686–7.

12. Dubois B, Slachevsky A, Pillon B, Beato R, Villalponda JM, Litvan I. "Applause sign" helps to discriminate PSP from FTD and PD. *Neurology* 2005; **64**(12): 2132–3.

13. Wu LJ, Sitburana O, Davidson A, Jankovic J. Applause sign in Parkinsonian disorders and Huntington's disease. *Mov Disord* 2008; **23**(16): 2307–11.

14. Sixel-Doring F, Schweitzer M, Mollenhauer B, Trenkwalder C. Polysomnographic findings, video-based sleep analysis and sleep perception in progressive supranuclear palsy. *Sleep Med* 2009; **10**(4): 407–15.

15. Schmidt C, Herting B, Prieur S *et al.* Autonomic dysfunction in patients with progressive supranuclear palsy. *Mov Disord* 2008; **23**(14): 2083–9.

16. Golbe LI, Ohman-Strickland PA. A clinical rating scale for progressive supranuclear palsy. *Brain* 2007; **130**(Pt 6): 1552–65.

17. Litvan I, Agid Y, Calne D *et al.* Clinical research criteria for the diagnosis of progressive supranuclear palsy (Steele–Richardson–Olszewski syndrome): report of the NINDS-SPSP international workshop. *Neurology* 1996; **47**(1): 1–9.

18. Azher SN, Jankovic J. Clinical aspects of progressive supranuclear palsy. *Handb ClinNeurol* 2008; **89**: 461–73.

19. Winikates J, Jankovic J. Vascular progressive supranuclear palsy. *J Neural Transm Suppl* 1994; **42**: 189–201.

20. Ros R, Gomez Garre P, Hirano M *et al.* Genetic linkage of autosomal dominant progressive supranuclear palsy to 1q31.1. *Ann Neurol* 2005; **57**(5): 634–41.

21. Stamelou M, de Silva R, Arias-Carrion O *et al.* Rational therapeutic approaches to progressive supranuclear palsy. *Brain* 2010; **133**(Pt 6): 1578–90.

22. Higgins JJ, Golbe LI, De Biase A, Jankovic J, Factor SA, Adler RL. An extended 5′-tau susceptibility haplotype in progressive supranuclear palsy. *Neurology* 2000; **55**(9): 1364–7.

23. Melquist S, Craig DW, Huentelman MJ *et al.* Identification of a novel risk locus for progressive supranuclear palsy by a pooled genomewide scan of 500 288 single-nucleotide polymorphisms. *Am J Hum Genet* 2007; **80**(4): 769–78.

24. Albers DS, Beal MF. Mitochondrial dysfunction in progressive supranuclear palsy. *Neurochem Int* 2002; **40**(6): 559–64.

25. Stamelou M, Pilatus U, Reuss A *et al.* In vivo evidence for cerebral depletion in high-energy phosphates in progressive supranuclear palsy. *J Cereb Blood Flow Metab* 2009; **29**(4): 861–70.

26. Ferrer I, Barrachina M, Puig B. Glycogen synthase kinase-3 is associated with neuronal and glial hyperphosphorylated tau deposits in Alzheimer's disease, Pick's disease, progressive supranuclear palsy and corticobasal degeneration. *Acta Neuropathol* 2002; **104**(6): 583–91.

27. Hollerhage M, Matusch A, Champy P *et al.* Natural lipophilic inhibitors of mitochondrial complex I are candidate toxins for sporadic neurodegenerative tau pathologies. *Exp Neurol* 2009; **220**(1): 133–42.

28. Hauw JJ, Daniel SE, Dickson D *et al.* Preliminary NINDS neuropathologic criteria for Steele–Richardson–Olszewski syndrome (progressive supranuclear palsy). *Neurology* 1994; **44**(11): 2015–19.

29. Dickson DW, Ahmed Z, Algom AA, Tsuboi Y, Josephs KA. Neuropathology of variants of progressive supranuclear palsy. *Curr Opin Neurol* 2010; **23**(4): 394–400.

30. Josephs KA, Boeve BF, Duffy JR *et al.* Atypical progressive supranuclear palsy underlying progressive apraxia of speech and nonfluent aphasia. *Neurocase* 2005; **11**(4): 283–96.

31. Mori H, Oda M, Komori T *et al.* Lewy bodies in progressive supranuclear palsy. *Acta Neuropathol* 2002; **104**(3): 273–8.

32. Warmuth-Metz M, Naumann M, Csoti I, Solymosi L. Measurement of the midbrain diameter on routine magnetic resonance imaging: a simple and accurate method of differentiating between Parkinson disease and progressive supranuclear palsy. *Arch Neurol* 2001; **58**(7): 1076–9.

33. Oba H, Yagishita A, Terada H *et al.* New and reliable MRI diagnosis for progressive supranuclear palsy. *Neurology* 2005; **64**(12): 2050–55.

34. Seppi K, Schocke MF, Esterhammer R *et al.* Diffusion-weighted imaging discriminates progressive supranuclear palsy from PD, but not from the parkinson variant of multiple system atrophy. *Neurology* 2003; **60**(6): 922–7.

35. Padovani A, Borroni B, Brambati SM *et al.* Diffusion tensor imaging and voxel based morphometry study in early progressive supranuclear palsy. *J Neurol Neurosurg Psychiatry* 2006; **77**(4): 457–63.

36. Boxer AL, Geschwind MD, Belfor N *et al.* Patterns of brain atrophy that differentiate corticobasal degeneration syndrome from progressive supranuclear palsy. *Arch Neurol* 2006; **63**(1): 81–6.

37. Mishina M, Ishii K, Mitani K *et al.* Midbrain hypometabolism as early diagnostic sign for progressive supranuclear palsy. *Acta Neurol Scand* 2004; **110**(2): 128–35.

38. Brooks DJ, Ibanez V, Sawle GV *et al.* Differing patterns of striatal ^{18}F-dopa uptake in Parkinson's disease, multiple system atrophy, and progressive supranuclear palsy. *Ann Neurol* 1990; **28**(4): 547–55.

39. Burn DJ, Sawle GV, Brooks DJ. Differential diagnosis of Parkinson's disease, multiple system atrophy, and Steele–Richardson–Olszewski syndrome: discriminant analysis of striatal ^{18}F-dopa PET data. *J Neurol Neurosurg Psychiatry* 1994; **57**(3): 278–84.

40. Pirker W, Asenbaum S, Bencsits G *et al.* [^{123}I]beta-CIT SPECT in multiple system atrophy, progressive supranuclear palsy, and corticobasal degeneration. *Mov Disord* 2000; **15**(6): 1158–67.

41. Sakakibara R, Hattori T, Tojo M, Yamanishi T, Yasuda K, Hirayama K. Micturitional disturbance in progressive supranuclear palsy. *J Auton Nerv Syst* 1993; **45**(2): 101–06.

42. Borroni B, Malinverno M, Gardoni F *et al.* Tau forms in CSF as a reliable biomarker for progressive supranuclear palsy. *Neurology* 2008; **71**(22): 1796–803.

43. Constantinescu R, Rosengren L, Johnels B, Zetterberg H, Holmberg B. Consecutive analyses of cerebrospinal fluid axonal and glial markers in Parkinson's disease and atypical Parkinsonian disorders. *Parkinsonism Relat Disord* 2010; **16**(2): 142–45.

44. Ghika J, Tennis M, Hoffman E, Schoenfeld D, Growdon J. Idazoxan treatment in progressive supranuclear palsy. *Neurology* 1991; **41**(7): 986–91.

45. Litvan I, Phipps M, Pharr VL, Hallett M, Grafman J, Salazar A. Randomized placebo-controlled trial of donepezil in patients with progressive supranuclear palsy. *Neurology* 2001; **57**(3): 467–73.

46. Liepelt I, Gaenslen A, Godau J *et al.* Rivastigmine for the treatment of dementia in patients with progressive supranuclear palsy: clinical observations as a basis for power calculations and safety analysis. *Alzheimers Dement* 2010; **6**(1): 70–4.

47. Rajrut AH, Uitti RJ, Fenton ME, George D. Amantadine effectiveness in multiple system atrophy and progressive supranuclear palsy. *Parkinsonism Relat Disord* 1997; **3**(4): 211–14.

48. Daniele A, Moro E, Bentivoglio AR. Zolpidem in progressive supranuclear palsy. *N Engl J Med* 1999; **341**(7): 543–4.

49. Chen G, Huang LD, Jiang YM, Manji HK. The mood-stabilizing agent valproate inhibits the activity of glycogen synthase kinase-3. *J Neurochem* 1999; **72**(3): 1327–30.

50. Stamelou M, Reuss A, Pilatus U *et al.* Short-term effects of coenzyme Q_{10} in progressive supranuclear palsy: a randomized, placebo-controlled trial. *Mov Disord* 2008; **23**(7): 942–9.

51. Bergmann KJ, Salak VL. Subthalamic stimulation improves levodopa responsive symptoms in a case of progressive supranuclear palsy. *Parkinsonism Relat Disord* 2008; **14**(4): 348–52.

Corticobasal degeneration

Pichet Termsarasab and David E. Riley

History

Rebeiz and colleagues first reported clinical and patho-logical findings in three patients with "corticodenta-tonigral degeneration with neuronal achromasia" in 1967 and 1968 [1, 2]. The name derived partly from the finding of numerous large neurons with pale-staining cytoplasm, especially in deep cortical layers, due to loss of Nissl substance, termed "neuronal achromasia." No additional reports of this disease were added until a single clinicopathologic case in 1985 [3]. In 1990, Riley and colleagues published the first clinically diagnosed cases, a total of 15 patients, some with detailed clin-ical descriptions, including two autopsy-verified cases [4]. This report outlined a seemingly characteristic, predominantly motor syndrome that quickly gained widespread recognition.

Over time, however, corticobasal degeneration was found to have considerable heterogeneity [5]. Some patients with clinically diagnosed corticobasal degeneration were proven pathologically to have other diseases, e.g., progressive supranuclear palsy (PSP), Alzheimer disease, Creutzfeldt–Jakob disease (CJD), Pick disease, and other disorders. In addition, patients with pathologically proven corticobasal degeneration showed variant clinical features. The high number of false-positive diagnoses associated with alternate pathologies, and of false-negative diagnoses associated with other clinical presentations, prompted Boeve and colleagues to suggest the term corticobasal syndrome (CBS) for clinical diagnosis and reserve the term cor-ticobasal degeneration (CBD) for pathological diagno-sis [6]. This terminological distinction will be followed in this chapter, although one often sees "corticobasal degeneration" and "cortical-basal ganglionic degener-ation" being used for clinical diagnosis in neurologic practice.

Clinical findings

As indicated in the name "corticobasal syndrome," clinical findings can be grouped into two main categor-ies, those related to cerebral cortical deficits and those related to basal ganglia involvement. A third group con-sists of commonly found features with uncertain local-ization. Most of these disease manifestations appear in a highly asymmetric pattern, developing insidiously and gradually worsening. The typical CBS patient has asymmetric apraxia, akinesia, rigidity, dystonia, and tremor or myoclonus, resulting in the characteristic "stiff, dystonic, jerky, useless hand" [4].

Cerebral cortical manifestations most often encountered are apraxia, cortical sensory loss and the "alien limb" phenomenon. Apraxia is defined as loss of ability to carry out familiar purposeful move-ments in the absence of sensory or motor impairment. Clinically, patients appear not to know "how" to per-form a common task. Apraxia is present in up to 70% of patients [7]. Ideomotor apraxia appears to be the most common apraxia in CBS [8], although limb-kinetic apraxia is the dominant apraxia in some reports [7]. Ideomotor apraxia and limb-kinetic apraxia may be present simultaneously in some patients. Assessment of apraxia may be limited by the presence of dystonia, severe rigidity, akinesia or myoclonus. Thus it may be helpful to evaluate apraxia in the less affected upper limb. Ideational apraxia may be the least common type of apraxia in CBS, but some patients have been known to have buccofacial apraxia.

"Alien limb" phenomenon (ALP) refers to autono-mous activity that is perceived as beyond voluntary control in a body part that feels foreign. The movement is more than simple levitation of the limb. Patients may describe the affected limb as "it" and even remark that it is "uncontrollable" or "having a mind of its own."

Uncommon Causes of Movement Disorders, ed. Néstor Gálvez-Jiménez and Paul J. Tuite. Published by Cambridge University Press. © Cambridge University Press 2011.

ALP is more common in upper rather than lower extremities and is not specific to CBS. There are several types of ALP. Callosal ALP, termed "diagonistic dyspraxia," is characterized by intermanual conflict in which one hand acts at cross-purposes with the other. This is associated with anterior callosal lesions and is rare in CBS. "Magnetic apraxia," or frontal ALP, was initially described by Denny-Brown and is characterized by compulsive reaching, groping and grasping [9]. This is the common type found in CBS. *Mitgehen*, or facilitatory paratonia, has also been described [10]. An example is that when some patients are lightly touched on the tip of their finger, they will involuntarily move their hand so that it stays in contact with examiner's finger.

Cortical sensory loss refers to impaired sensory modalities whose perception relies on cortical integrity, such as joint position sense and two-point discrimination, with preservation of normal primary sensory modalities. Agraphesthesia and astereognosis may also be found in patients with cortical sensory loss.

Other cortical manifestations include language dysfunction and cognitive impairment including dementia. Nonfluent aphasia is common in CBS patients. Graham and colleagues reported that phonologic and spelling impairment were prevalent, even in nonaphasic CBS patients [11]. This reflects overlap between progressive nonfluent aphasia and CBS.

Cognitive impairment has become recognized as an important aspect of CBS. Early reports of CBS discounted the role of dementia, likely because most patients were diagnosed in movement disorder clinics. Grimes and colleagues reported that dementia was the most common presentation in 13 pathologically proven CBD patients [12]. Cognitive dysfunction, ignored in early diagnostic criteria, has been included in recently proposed criteria [6]. However, for research purposes, investigators may exclude subjects who show early cognitive disturbances other than apraxia, or speech or language disorders, in order to prevent contamination from Alzheimer disease and other primary dementias [13]. This approach naturally sacrifices diagnostic sensitivity in favor of specificity.

Cognitive impairment in CBS includes acalculia, frontal dysfunction and nonfluent aphasia [14]. Constructional and visuospatial difficulties may also be found. However, semantic memory functioning appears relatively preserved. Some deficits in drawing, copying and handwriting may be due to limb apraxia. Neuropsychological testing may show moderate global

deterioration, a dysexecutive syndrome, explicit learning deficits without retention difficulties, disorders of dynamic motor execution (temporal organization, bimanual coordination, control and inhibition) and symmetric praxis disorders (posture imitation, symbolic gesture execution and object utilization) [15].

Basal ganglia manifestations of CBS almost always include asymmetric akinesia and rigidity, with the latter often pronounced. Dystonia may be prominent. Typically the upper limb is initially affected and it can progress to the contralateral upper limb or the ipsilateral lower limb in a period of >2 years [6]. In a study by Kompoliti and colleagues, parkinsonian features were present in each of 147 patients [16]. These patients were all recruited from movement disorder clinics. The most common parkinsonian sign was rigidity (92%), followed by bradykinesia (80%), gait disorder (80%) and tremor (55%). Dystonia was found in 71%. Unlike in Parkinson disease, levodopa has little effect on parkinsonian symptoms in CBS. Kompoliti and colleagues reported that 24% of the patients had some degree of clinical improvement after levodopa therapy [16].

Dystonia typically affects one upper limb and hand. In the "dystonic clenched fist," the thumb is flexed and adducted toward the palm with the other fingers flexed and wrapping around it. Over the long run, this can cause abrasion or ulcers in the palm. Dystonia can involve the foot, causing foot inversion and limiting ambulation. Initially, patients may have foot dystonia only during walking or reaching. The dystonia of CBS can be quite painful, usually when it involves the upper limb.

Tremor in CBS is different from that seen in Parkinson disease, and likely is not related to basal ganglia involvement. The tremor is fast (6–8 Hz), irregular and jerky, and typically is produced by sustained posture and action. The irregularity may increase and produce a more jerking appearance, eventually evolving into frank myoclonus. Myoclonus in CBS usually has a distribution in the distal part of the upper limb but can progress proximally. The myoclonus is typically induced by tactile stimulation and action, known as "stimulus-sensitive myoclonus" and "action myoclonus." This may resemble cortical reflex myoclonus. However, electrophysiologic studies have shown enhanced long-loop responses without enlarged somatosensory evoked potentials, distinct from cortical reflex myoclonus [17].

Patients with CBS may have eye movement abnormalities that are sometimes difficult to detect at the bedside. Ocular motility studies in CBS showed preserved horizontal saccade velocity but significantly increased horizontal saccade latency ipsilateral to the more apraxic side [18,19]. In PSP, by contrast, there is marked impairment in saccadic velocity rather than increased latency, and vertical saccades are more impaired than horizontal saccades. However, occasional CBS patients exhibit a supranuclear gaze palsy late in the course of their illness. Eyelid opening/closing apraxia can also be seen in CBS patients, though not as frequently as in PSP.

Psychiatric features also occur in CBS patients. According to Litvan and colleagues, patients with CBS exhibit depression (73%), apathy (40%), irritability (20%) and agitation (20%) [20]. Compared with PSP, depression and irritability of patients with CBS were more frequent and severe. Other psychiatric features found in case reports include visual hallucination [21], and pathological laughter or crying [22].

Other poorly localized symptoms include dysarthria and dysphagia. Dysphagia may lead to percutaneous enteric gastrostomy (PEG) tube placement in late-stage CBS. There are also case reports describing Balint syndrome [23] and visuomotor ataxia [24].

Although there have been several sets of clinical diagnostic criteria for CBS, there are no consensus criteria for the diagnosis. Kumar and colleagues proposed diagnostic criteria in 2002 [13], as did Boeve and colleagues in 2003 [6].

Natural history

Corticobasal degeneration usually has onset in the sixth or seventh decade of life with a range of 45–75 years of age; reports of CBS cases outside of this range lack pathological verification [25]. As mentioned earlier, the course of the disease is insidious. In pathologically confirmed cases, the mean disease duration has been 7.9 years with a range of 2.5–12.5 years [26]. This study also suggested that the early presence of widespread parkinsonism or a frontal lobe syndrome is associated with a shorter survival. Dysphagia develops late in the course and can lead to aspiration pneumonia, which may be the leading cause of death in CBD.

Laboratory investigations

In practice, CBS is a clinical diagnosis. Neuroimaging is usually performed to rule out structural causes and may provide supportive data. Other tests that may provide more information in the diagnosis of CBD are metabolic imaging studies, neuropsychological testing, ocular motility studies and electrophysiologic studies including electroencephalography (EEG), electromyography (EMG) and somatosensory evoked potential (SSEP). However, it remains unclear to what extent these studies improve diagnostic accuracy. The gold standard for diagnosis is still pathological study. Unfortunately, only a small portion of the patients reported in medical literature have had autopsy studies. As mentioned earlier, patients with CBS may reveal other diagnoses at autopsy, which may be helpful in furthering our understanding of heterogeneity of CBS in the future.

Neuroimaging

The most common finding of conventional MRI in CBS patients is asymmetrical cerebral atrophy, predominantly contralateral to the side clinically more affected [27]. Atrophy was demonstrated more severely in the posterior frontal and parietal lobes. Temporal and anterobasal frontal atrophy was frequently observed but was less severe [27]. Atrophy of the cerebral peduncle, ipsilateral to the dominant atrophic cerebral hemisphere, was shown in some patients with contralateral corticospinal tract signs [27]. Hyperintensity in the frontal and/or parietal subcortical white matter may be found on fluid-attenuated inversion recovery (FLAIR) images in some patients [27]. Hyperintense signals on T2-W imaging can be found in some patients. Pathology of these subcortical white matter lesions was believed to be from neuronal degeneration, especially demyelination secondary to axonal loss or change. However, Tokumaru and colleagues found that tauopathy was clearly evident in these areas, reflecting primary degeneration rather than secondary [28]. According to Koyama and colleagues, no signal or volume change in the basal ganglia was observed [27]. Nevertheless, mild atrophy of the lentiform nucleus has been reported elsewhere.

Voxel-based morphometry of MRI, which is a neuroimaging analysis technique that allows investigation of focal differences in brain anatomy, using the approach of so-called statistical parametric mapping, may demonstrate more detail in atrophic patterns and may be useful in differentiation between CBS and other diseases such as PSP, Alzheimer disease and frontotemporal dementia (FTD). CBS is associated with asymmetrical atrophy of the bilateral premotor cortex, superior parietal lobules and striatum, while PSP demonstrates atrophy of the midbrain, pons, thalamus and striatum, with minimal involvement of the frontal cortex. Midbrain atrophy is more pronounced in PSP than in CBS, whereas dorsal frontal and parietal cortices are more atrophied in CBS than in PSP. According to Boxer and colleagues, the degree of atrophy of the midbrain and pontine tegmentum and the left frontal eye field could differentiate the patients in CBS and PSP groups with 93% accuracy [29]. Grossman and colleagues compared atrophic patterns revealed by voxel-based morphometric analyses of MRI between CBS, Alzheimer disease and FTD patients. Relative to FTD, CBS patients have less atrophy in the left anterior temporal and the left anterior cingulate regions but greater atrophy in bilateral temporoparietal regions, including the medial parietal cortex [30]. CBD patients have greater atrophy in bilateral parietal and right frontal and temporal regions compared with Alzheimer disease patients.

Diffusion-weighted brain images may also be helpful in differentiation between CBS and the classical phenotype of PSP (Richardson syndrome) and Parkinson disease (PD) [31]. Putaminal apparent diffusion coefficient (ADC) values in CBS and Richardson syndrome were significantly greater than in PD. The hemispheric symmetry ratio is the ratio of the smaller to the larger median value from histograms of ADC in left and right cerebral hemispheres (1 = perfect symmetry). The hemispheric symmetry ratio in CBS is markedly reduced compared with Richardson syndrome and PD. This ratio differentiates CBS patients from Richardson syndrome and PD patients with a sensitivity and specificity of 100%, according to Rizzo and colleagues [31].

Functional MRI (fMRI) has demonstrated decreased activation of the parietal lobe contralateral to the more affected arm when movements are performed with that hand. Functional MRI can also detect abnormalities in the motor and parietal cortex prior to the development of structural abnormalities and even abnormal single photon-emission computed tomography (SPECT) [32].

Other functional neuroimaging studies, including metabolic imaging, may support the clinical impression of involvement of both the cerebral cortex and the basal ganglia, as well as identifying other involved structures. On SPECT there is asymmetric hypoperfusion in the frontoparietal lobes and the basal ganglia, particularly in the putamen, as well as in the thalamus [27,32]. The side of hypoperfusion is contralateral to the side that is more severely clinically affected.

Magnetic resonance spectroscopy may demonstrate significantly reduced N-acetylaspartate/creatine-phosphocreatine (NAA/Cre) ratio in the centrum semiovale, and significantly reduced N-acetylaspartate/choline (NAA/Cho) ratio in the lentiform nucleus and parietal cortex, contralateral to the most affected side [33,34]. These findings may reflect neuronal damage in CBS.

Positron emission tomography (PET) with ^{18}F-labeled 2-deoxyglucose (FDG) for measuring regional rates of glucose metabolism showed asymmetrically reduced cerebral glucose metabolism in the dorsolateral frontal, medial frontal, inferior parietal, sensorimotor and lateral temporal cortex, as well as in the corpus striatum and the thalamus, in the hemisphere contralateral to the clinically more affected side [35].

[^{11}C](R)-(1-[2-Chlorophenyl]-N-methyl-N-[1-methylpropyl]-3-isoquinoline carboxamide (PK11195), a marker of peripheral benzodiazepine binding sites (PBBS) that are expressed by microglia, can be used to demonstrate the degree and distribution of glial response to the degenerative process. [^{11}C](R)-PK11195 PET revealed significantly increased mean [^{11}C](R)-PK11195 binding in the caudate, putamen, substantia nigra, pons, pre- and postcentral gyrus and the frontal lobe, corresponding to the distribution of neuropathological changes [36].

Striatal fluorodopa uptake may be asymmetrically reduced in the caudate nucleus and putamen [37,38]. PET with tracers of dopamine storage capacity and oxygen metabolism can demonstrate depressed cortical oxygen metabolism in the superior and posterior temporal, parietal and occipital associated cortices, as well as in the posterior frontal lobe.

Dopamine transporter imaging revealed decreased presynaptic dopamine transporter binding in all CBD patients, while D2 receptor binding is frequently preserved [39].

Brain parenchyma sonography (BPS) may have a role in differentiating CBS from PSP. Walter and colleagues have reported that substantia nigra hyperechogenicity can be demonstrated in CBS, as reported earlier as a characteristic BPS finding in idiopathic PD [40].

All neuroimaging studies mentioned above were performed in patients with clinically diagnosed CBS, which, as mentioned earlier, likely would have shown pathological heterogeneity. Few studies have been done in autopsy-proven CBD. Josephs and colleagues reviewed 17 autopsy cases of clinically diagnosed CBS patients [41]. Six of these had autopsy-proven CBD. Neither cortical nor corpus callosum atrophy nor subcortical periventricular white matter changes (SPWM) on MRI were found to be specific to CBD. Similar patterns of regional atrophy and SPWM could be seen in other neurodegenerative diseases such as PSP, CJD and some cases of AD. Tokumaru also studied MRI findings in four CBD patients and compared them with neuropathologically confirmed PSP [28]. In cases with midbrain tegmentum atrophy and signal-intensity changes in the subthalamic nuclei, CBD and PSP are difficult to distinguish by MRI alone.

Routine blood, urine and CSF studies are normal in CBD [4]. Several CSF biomarkers such as tau [42–44], orexin [45] and homovanillic acid [46] have been studied, but results have been variable to date.

Neuropsychological testing

Neuropsychological testing may reveal limb apraxia (usually ideomotor), constructional and visuospatial difficulties, acalculia, frontal dysfunction, and nonfluent aphasia [14]. The limb apraxia can cause deficits in drawing, copying and handwriting. Impairment in episodic memory is generally milder than that seen in Alzheimer disease. Semantic memory functioning appears relatively preserved. Vanvoorst and colleagues evaluated neuropsychological testing in nine CBD cases [47]. Clinically, three were diagnosed with FTD, while the other six were given an assortment of nonspecific diagnoses. Only two were diagnosed with CBS by the time of the last clinical evaluation prior to death. Neuropsychometric testing in these nine patients revealed lower scores than the normative sample in learning, letter and category fluency, verbal comprehension, perceptual organization and cognitive flexibility. Depression may also be a common finding.

Electrophysiology

Corticobasal syndrome has been studied with a multitude of neurophysiologic approaches. Ocular motility study was reviewed with the clinical manifestations. Electroencephalography may be normal in the early stages of CBS. Asymmetric slowing, more so on the hemisphere contralateral to the side more clinically affected, can be found [34].

Surface electromyography may reveal focal reflex myoclonus that is produced by two to four short-duration bursts of muscle contraction (usually less than 50 milliseconds) simultaneously in antagonistic muscle pairs [48]. This muscle contraction, called stimulus-sensitive myoclonus, may easily be induced by tapping of the muscle by the examiner's hand or hammer. Back-averaged electroencephalography showed no jerk-lock cortical discharges [17,48]. Localized distribution with distal predominance of myoclonus and stimulus sensitivity resembles features seen in cortical reflex myoclonus. There are no giant SSEPs, while long-loop reflexes (LLRs) are exaggerated. However, cortical relay time estimated by LLR response latency (N20 latency + latency of evoked motor response) is considered too short for corticocortical transmission, even in the nonmyoclonic arm [48].

Transcranial magnetic stimulation (TMS) shows a significantly shorter post-motor-evoked potential (MEP) silent period and a slightly higher motor threshold in the predominantly affected hand in association with a relatively higher amplitude of MEPs [48]. The shorter post-MEP silent period may mainly reflect the defective central inhibitory processes elicited by magnetic stimuli.

Genetics

On the basis of molecular immunohistochemistry of accumulated intracellular proteins, CBS and PSP are classified as "tauopathies." A tauopathy is characterized pathologically by the presence of excessive tau proteins, which are microtubule-associated proteins. Other examples of tauopathies are Alzheimer disease, argyrophilic grain disease (AGD) and Pick disease (PiD). Human tau is encoded by a gene on chromosome 17q21. In the 11-exon segment, alternative mRNA splicing at exons 2, 3 and 10 generates six different tau isoforms, three of them being three-repeat tau isoforms (3R-tau) and three four-repeat tau isoforms (4R-tau). In normal neurons 3R-tau and 4R-tau occur in roughly equal quantities. In CBD and PSP, 4R-tau predominates, while in AD 3R-tau and 4R-tau are equal, and in PiD 3R-tau predominates [49,50]. Another common property of CBD and PSP is their association with the H1 tau haplotype and H1/H1 homozygosity [51]. Thus it appears that CBD and PSP may have a similar pathogenesis, or may even represent points on a spectrum of the same disease.

Most CBD cases are sporadic. However, there have been rare familial case reports with autosomal dominant inheritance. Mutations in *tau* genes have been reported to be associated with sporadic CBD (e.g., P301L [52], N296N [53] mutations) and familial CBS (P301S [54] and G389R [55] mutations). Case reports have also identified progranulin (*PGRN*) gene mutations in familial CBS cases [56,57]. *Tau* gene mutation is more often associated with the clinicopathological phenotype of frontotemporal dementia with parkinsonism linked to chromosome 17 (FTDP-17), while *PGRN* mutation is associated with the clinicopathological phenotype of frontotemporal lobar degeneration with tau-negative/ubiquitin-positive inclusions (FTLD-U), classified as a TAR-DNA binding protein 43 (TDP43) proteinopathy. Thus, there may be a link between CBD, FTDP-17 and FTDP-U.

Pathology

The pathological heterogeneity of CBS and the clinical heterogeneity of CBD are well recognized [5,58]. It should therefore be kept in mind that clinical characteristics, investigations or treatment described in reports of CBS reflect results from various diseases, not limited to CBD. Pathology is the only acceptable method for diagnosing CBD. Standard neuropathological criteria for CBD were proposed by Dickson and colleagues in 2002 [59].

Gross findings in CBD include asymmetric atrophy, more prominent on the side contralateral to the side of greater clinical involvement. Atrophy is marked in the peri-Rolandic region. The superior frontal gyrus is often more affected than the middle and inferior frontal gyri. The temporal and occipital lobes are often spared. There may be volume loss of subcortical white matter in the affected areas and the corpus callosum is sometimes thin. The other major gross feature of CBD pathology is that the substantia nigra is invariably pale.

One of the most striking low-power microscopic findings is that of large "ballooned" neurons with pale-staining cytoplasm. This led Rebeiz and colleagues to include "neuronal achromasia" in the original name for this disorder [2]. However, this finding is not included in Dickson's core criteria, since ballooned neurons are not specific to CBD, and some CBD cases show sparse or no ballooned neurons [59]. If ballooned neurons are not seen, CBD can be diagnosed if there is evidence of core features mentioned below in typical locations. The main histopathological findings are focal cortical neuronal loss, substantia nigra neuronal loss, and characteristic tau-positive neuronal and glial lesions, in particular astrocytic plaques and threadlike processes in gray and white matter seen in a characteristic distribution [59].

Routine histopathological study shows evidence of neuronal loss and reactive astrogliosis. Ballooned neurons are usually seen in layers III, V and VI of affected cerebral cortices. The cytoplasm of ballooned neurons is eosinophilic. There is cytoplasmic swelling, which sometimes extends to proximal dendrites. There is either superficial or laminar spongiosis. Astrocytosis is also prominent in superficial cortical layers and at the gray–white junction. The substantia nigra reveals neuronal loss. Melanin-containing phagocytes may be seen.

Immunohistochemistry, especially tau immunostaining, yields additional information. Tau immunoreactive lesions are usually more widespread than routine pathology. Most affected neurons have diffuse or granular tau immunoreactivity called pre-tangles. Astrocytic plaques are groups of short threadlike astrocytic processes with tau immunoreactivity in the affected areas of gray and white matter. Coiled bodies – tau-positive argyrophilic inclusions in oligodendroglia – can be seen in CBD. They are bundles of fibrils coiling around nuclei with extensions into proximal neuritis, giving them comma-shaped appearances. Neurofibrillary lesions called "corticobasal bodies" are common and can be seen in melanin-containing neurons in the substantia nigra and locus ceruleus. They have similarities to the globose neurofibrillary tangles found in AD and PSP.

Electron microscopy has shown that twisted filaments in CBD are 24 nm in diameter and have periodicity of 160 nm, compared with filaments in Alzheimer disease which are 22 nm in diameter and have periodicity of 80 nm. The filaments in PSP are straight and have diameters of 15–18 nm. These findings militate against the notion that CBD and PSP share a single disease spectrum.

Management

The management of CBD is usually a disheartening process. No curative treatment has been developed. There is no intervention that will alter the progressive nature of this degenerative disease. Recent management has focused on symptomatic and supportive treatment. Of note, according to a subgroup analysis in a study by Kompoliti and colleagues, there is no significant difference in comparison between autopsy-proven CBD patients ($n = 7$) and non-autopsy-proven CBS patients ($n = 140$) [16].

For motor symptoms, levodopa combined with carbidopa can be used for parkinsonian symptoms, but the degree of improvement is much less than that seen in PD. For this reason, a lack of levodopa response has been mentioned as a supportive feature of CBS. Boeve and colleagues recommended increasing the dose of levodopa to at least 750 mg per day administered on an empty stomach before determining unresponsiveness [60]. According to Kompoliti and colleagues, levodopa combined with carbidopa produced clinical improvement in 26% [16]. Bradykinesia and rigidity improved the most. Side-effects from using levodopa included gastrointestinal complaints (15%), confusion (4%), somnolence (4%), dizziness (4%) and hallucination (2%). Dyskinesia did not occur, even in patients who received high doses of levodopa [16]. Nevertheless, levodopa-induced dyskinesia, even in the absence of clinical benefit, has been reported by Frucht and colleagues in one autopsy-proven CBD patient [61].

Dopamine agonists, selegiline and amantadine have been studied in CBS and have shown little clinical benefit. Kompoliti and colleagues reported clinical improvement of 6%, 10% and 13%, respectively, for these agents [16]. Constraint-induced movement therapy (CIMT), which is therapy using the less affected or unaffected limb to perform activities of daily living (ADLs), has been tried in CBS patients by Boeve and colleagues with variable results [60]. Clonazepam, anticonvulsants and propranolol have been tried for tremor but without significant clinical improvement. Clonazepam can occasionally be used successfully for myoclonus.

For dystonia, in particular "dystonic clenched fist," botulinum toxin can be used with an estimated 67% clinical improvement [16]. In addition, botulinum toxin can relieve pain associated with dystonia. Wrapping gauze or other padding around the thumb may prevent abrasion or ulcer in the palm caused by dystonic flexion of the thumb.

According to Kompoliti and colleagues, there is no effective pharmacological treatment for higher cortical function and depression [16]. However, SSRIs have been used by Boeve and colleagues with some improvement of depression [60]. There have been limited studies, especially open-label studies or controlled trials, regarding pharmacological therapy for higher cortical function impairment in CBS. Most reports are based on the author's own clinical experience.

Riley and colleagues reported no improvement in one patient with severe myoclonus and painful dystonia undergoing stereotactic thalamotomy and right dorsal rhizotomy of C5 to T1 [4]. Data about deep brain stimulation of the subthalamic nucleus or globus pallidus are limited. However, from expert clinical experience, there is no benefit of deep brain stimulation in CBS patients.

Owing to the limited role of pharmacological and surgical treatment in CBS, an interdisciplinary approach including physical therapy, occupational therapy and speech therapy is the mainstay of treatment. Apraxia is one of the factors that limit participation in physical therapy, as is depression.

Dysphagia, which may occur in the late stage of the disease, needs evaluation and supportive measures from a speech therapist. Percutaneous endoscopic gastrostomy may be pursued after discussion with the patient and family. This provides not only necessary nutrition but also reduces the risk of aspiration pneumonia, which may be the leading cause of death in CBS patients.

Psychosocial support to the patient and family is also important. Physicians should not only be focused on neurological problems. One way in which physicians can improve a patient's and a caregiver's quality of life is to take on responsibilities beyond the narrow scope of subspecialty care. This would include treatment of psychiatric issues, filling out various forms and paperwork, assisting with entry into skilled nursing facilities, and conducting surveillance for infection or other complications from immobility. A good relationship between physician and patient as well as family is also important. This will encourage patients to return for further evaluation, enhancing participation in clinical research and eventually allowing for postmortem examination. Since pathology is the only definitive diagnostic tool in CBD, autopsy studies remain a vital conduit to more data about this disease, leading to more effective treatment in the future.

Conclusions

CBS and CBD are heterogeneous disorders, one pathologically and the other clinically. While clearly related, they are equally clearly not joined at the nosological hip. Results from clinical research on CBS patients must be viewed as reflecting a hodge-podge of underlying pathological entities. Nevertheless, CBS is a distinctive syndrome, and identification of affected patients has important implications for CBD. The heterogeneity of CBD has contributed to an absence of consensus clinical diagnostic criteria. Only further study of autopsy-proven CBD patients may allow us to develop consistently predictive antemortem criteria.

CBD and PSP share features, including some aspects of underlying molecular pathophysiology. CBD should benefit from research on PSP, particularly since PSP is more common and more reliably identified clinically.

Further investigation of their molecular biology should reveal how fundamentally similar or dissimilar these two conditions are. Identification of additional genes in which mutations or polymorphisms are associated with these disorders could shed more light on this question.

In terms of treatment, future directions may focus on the concept of underlying proteinopathies. The inclusion of CBD under the larger umbrella of tauopathies may allow us to apply discoveries in this general field to multiple specific disorders. Students of CBS would be well served by keeping abreast of developments pertaining to these related disorders.

References

1. Rebeiz JJ, Kolodny EH, Richardson EP Jr. Corticodentatonigral degeneration with neuronal achromasia: a progressive disorder of late adult life. *Trans Am Neurol Assoc* 1967; **92**: 23–6.

2. Rebeiz JJ, Kolodny EH, Richardson EP Jr. Corticodentatonigral degeneration with neuronal achromasia. *Arch Neurol* 1968; **18**(1): 20–33.

3. Case records of the Massachusetts General Hospital. weekly clinicopathological exercises. case 38–1985. A 66-year-old man with progressive neurologic deterioration. *N Engl J Med* 1985; **313**(12): 739–48.

4. Riley DE, Lang AE, Lewis A *et al.* Cortical-basal ganglionic degeneration. *Neurology* 1990; **40**(8): 1203–12.

5. Boeve BF, Maraganore DM, Parisi JE *et al.* Pathologic heterogeneity in clinically diagnosed corticobasal degeneration. *Neurology* 1999; **53**(4): 795–800.

6. Boeve BF, Lang AE, Litvan I. Corticobasal degeneration and its relationship to progressive supranuclear palsy and frontotemporal dementia. *Ann Neurol* 2003; **54**(Suppl 5): S15–19.

7. Soliveri P, Piacentini S, Girotti F. Limb apraxia in corticobasal degeneration and progressive supranuclear palsy. *Neurology* 2005; **64**(3): 448–53.

8. Leiguarda R, Lees AJ, Merello M, Starkstein S, Marsden CD. The nature of apraxia in corticobasal degeneration. *J Neurol Neurosurg Psychiatry* 1994; **57**(4): 455–9.

9. Denny-Brown D. The nature of apraxia. *J Nerv Ment Dis* 1958; **126**(1): 9–32.

10. Fitzgerald DB, Drago V, Jeong Y, Chang YL, White KD, Heilman KM. Asymmetrical alien hands in corticobasal degeneration. *Mov Disord* 2007; **22**(4): 581–4.

11. Graham NL, Bak T, Patterson K, Hodges JR. Language function and dysfunction in corticobasal degeneration. *Neurology* 2003; **61**(4): 493–9.

12. Grimes DA, Lang AE, Bergeron CB. Dementia as the most common presentation of cortical-basal ganglionic degeneration. *Neurology* 1999; **53**(9): 1969–74.

13. Kumar R, Bergeron C, Pollanen M, Lang AE. Cortical-basal ganglionic degeneration. In: Jankovic J, Tolosa E, eds. *Parkinson's Disease and Movement Disorders.* 3rd ed. Baltimore, MD: William & Wilkins; 1998. 297–316.

14. Graham NL, Bak TH, Hodges JR. Corticobasal degeneration as a cognitive disorder. *Mov Disord* 2003; **18**(11): 1224–32.

15. Pillon B, Blin J, Vidailhet M *et al.* The neuropsychological pattern of corticobasal degeneration: comparison with progressive supranuclear palsy and Alzheimer's disease. *Neurology* 1995; **45**(8): 1477–83.

16. Kompoliti K, Goetz CG, Boeve BF *et al.* Clinical presentation and pharmacological therapy in corticobasal degeneration. *Arch Neurol* 1998; **55**(7): 957–61.

17. Carella F, Ciano C, Panzica F, Scaioli V. Myoclonus in corticobasal degeneration. *Mov Disord* 1997; **12**(4): 598–603.

18. Vidailhet M, Rivaud-Pechoux S. Eye movement disorders in corticobasal degeneration. *Adv Neurol* 2000; **82**: 161–7.

19. Rivaud-Pechoux S, Vidailhet M, Gallouedec G, Litvan I, Gaymard B, Pierrot-Deseilligny C. Longitudinal ocular motor study in corticobasal degeneration and progressive supranuclear palsy. *Neurology* 2000; **54**(5): 1029–32.

20. Litvan I, Cummings JL, Mega M. Neuropsychiatric features of corticobasal degeneration. *J Neurol Neurosurg Psychiatry* 1998; **65**(5): 717–21.

21. Nagaoka K, Ookawa S, Maeda K. A case of corticobasal degeneration presenting with visual hallucination. *Rinsho Shinkeigaku* 2004; **44**(3): 193–7.

22. Thumler BH, Urban PP, Davids E *et al.* Dysarthria and pathological laughter/crying as presenting symptoms of corticobasal-ganglionic degeneration syndrome. *J Neurol* 2003; **250**(9): 1107–8.

23. Mendez MF. Corticobasal ganglionic degeneration with balint's syndrome. *J Neuropsychiatry Clin Neurosci* 2000; **12**(2): 273–5.

24. Okuda B, Kodama N, Tachibana H, Sugita M, Tanaka H. Visuomotor ataxia in corticobasal degeneration. *Mov Disord* 2000; **15**(2): 337–40.

25. DePold Hohler A, Ransom BR, Chun MR, Troster AI, Samii A. The youngest reported case of corticobasal degeneration. *Parkinsonism Relat Disord* 2003; **10**(1): 47–50.

26. Wenning GK, Litvan I, Jankovic J *et al.* Natural history and survival of 14 patients with corticobasal degeneration confirmed at postmortem examination. *J Neurol Neurosurg Psychiatry* 1998; **64**(2): 184–9.

27. Koyama M, Yagishita A, Nakata Y, Hayashi M, Bandoh M, Mizutani T. Imaging of corticobasal degeneration syndrome. *Neuroradiology* 2007; **49**(11): 905–12.

28. Tokumaru AM, Saito Y, Murayama S *et al.* Imaging-pathologic correlation in corticobasal degeneration. *AJNR Am J Neuroradiol* 2009; **30**(10): 1884–92.

29. Boxer AL, Geschwind MD, Belfor N *et al.* Patterns of brain atrophy that differentiate corticobasal degeneration syndrome from progressive supranuclear palsy. *Arch Neurol* 2006; **63**(1): 81–6.

30. Grossman M, McMillan C, Moore P *et al.* What's in a name: voxel-based morphometric analyses of MRI and naming difficulty in Alzheimer's disease, frontotemporal dementia and corticobasal degeneration. *Brain* 2004; **127**(Pt 3): 628–49.

31. Rizzo G, Martinelli P, Manners D *et al.* Diffusion-weighted brain imaging study of patients with clinical diagnosis of corticobasal degeneration, progressive supranuclear palsy and parkinson's disease. *Brain* 2008; **131**(Pt 10): 2690–700.

32. Ukmar M, Moretti R, Torre P, Antonello RM, Longo R, Bava A. Corticobasal degeneration: structural and functional MRI and single-photon emission computed tomography. *Neuroradiology* 2003; **45**(10): 708–12.

33. Tedeschi G, Litvan I, Bonavita S *et al.* Proton magnetic resonance spectroscopic imaging in progressive supranuclear palsy, Parkinson's disease and corticobasal degeneration. *Brain* 1997; **120**(Pt 9): 1541–52.

34. Vion-Dury J, Rochefort N, Michotey P, Planche D, Ceccaldi M. Proton magnetic resonance neurospectroscopy and EEG cartography in corticobasal degeneration: correlations with neuropsychological signs. *J Neurol Neurosurg Psychiatry* 2004; **75**(9): 1352–5.

35. Nagahama Y, Fukuyama H, Turjanski N *et al.* Cerebral glucose metabolism in corticobasal degeneration: comparison with progressive supranuclear palsy and normal controls. *Mov Disord* 1997; **12**(5): 691–6.

36. Gerhard A, Watts J, Trender-Gerhard I *et al.* In vivo imaging of microglial activation with [11C]$_{(R)}$-PK11195 PET in corticobasal degeneration. *Mov Disord* 2004; **19**(10): 1221–6.

37. Nagasawa H, Tanji H, Nomura H *et al.* PET study of cerebral glucose metabolism and fluorodopa uptake in patients with corticobasal degeneration. *J Neurol Sci* 1996; **139**(2): 210–7.

38. Laureys S, Salmon E, Garraux G *et al.* Fluorodopa uptake and glucose metabolism in early stages of corticobasal degeneration. *J Neurol* 1999; **246**(12): 1151–8.

39. Klaffke S, Kuhn AA, Plotkin M *et al.* Dopamine transporters, D2 receptors, and glucose metabolism in corticobasal degeneration. *Mov Disord* 2006; **21**(10): 1724–7.

40. Walter U, Dressler D, Wolters A, Probst T, Grossmann A, Benecke R. Sonographic discrimination of corticobasal degeneration vs progressive supranuclear palsy. *Neurology* 2004; **63**(3): 504–9.

41. Josephs KA, Petersen RC, Knopman DS *et al.* Clinicopathologic analysis of frontotemporal and corticobasal degenerations and PSP. *Neurology* 2006; **66**(1): 41–8.

42. Urakami K, Mori M, Wada K *et al.* A comparison of tau protein in cerebrospinal fluid between corticobasal degeneration and progressive supranuclear palsy. *Neurosci Lett* 1999; **259**(2): 127–9.

43. Urakami K, Wada K, Arai H *et al.* Diagnostic significance of tau protein in cerebrospinal fluid from patients with corticobasal degeneration or progressive supranuclear palsy. *J Neurol Sci* 2001; **183**(1): 95–8.

44. Mitani K, Furiya Y, Uchihara T *et al.* Increased CSF tau protein in corticobasal degeneration. *J Neurol* 1998; **245**(1): 44–6.

45. Yasui K, Inoue Y, Kanbayashi T, Nomura T, Kusumi M, Nakashima K. CSF orexin levels of Parkinson's disease, dementia with lewy bodies, progressive supranuclear palsy and corticobasal degeneration. *J Neurol Sci* 2006; **250**(1–2): 120–3.

46. Kanemaru K, Mitani K, Yamanouchi H. Cerebrospinal fluid homovanillic acid levels are not reduced in early corticobasal degeneration. *Neurosci Lett* 1998; **245**(2): 121–2.

47. Vanvoorst WA, Greenaway MC, Boeve BF *et al.* Neuropsychological findings in clinically atypical autopsy confirmed corticobasal degeneration and progressive supranuclear palsy. *Parkinsonism Relat Disord* 2008; **14**(4): 376–8.

48. Lu CS, Ikeda A, Terada K *et al.* Electrophysiological studies of early stage corticobasal degeneration. *Mov Disord* 1998; **13**(1): 140–6.

49. Katsuse O, Iseki E, Arai T *et al.* 4-repeat tauopathy sharing pathological and biochemical features of corticobasal degeneration and progressive supranuclear palsy. *Acta Neuropathol* 2003; **106**(3): 251–60.

50. Buee L, Delacourte A. Comparative biochemistry of tau in progressive supranuclear palsy, corticobasal degeneration, FTDP-17 and Pick's disease. *Brain Pathol* 1999; **9**(4): 681–93.

51. Houlden H, Baker M, Morris HR *et al.* Corticobasal degeneration and progressive supranuclear palsy share a common tau haplotype. *Neurology* 2001; **56**(12): 1702–6.

52. Mirra SS, Murrell JR, Gearing M *et al.* Tau pathology in a family with dementia and a P301L mutation in tau. *J Neuropathol Exp Neurol* 1999; **58**(4): 335–45.

53. Spillantini MG, Yoshida H, Rizzini C *et al.* A novel tau mutation (N296N) in familial dementia with swollen achromatic neurons and corticobasal inclusion bodies. *Ann Neurol* 2000; **48**(6): 939–43.

54. Bugiani O, Murrell JR, Giaccone G *et al.* Frontotemporal dementia and corticobasal degeneration in a family with a P301S mutation in tau. *J Neuropathol Exp Neurol* 1999; **58**(6): 667–77.

55. Rossi G, Marelli C, Farina L *et al.* The G389R mutation in the MAPT gene presenting as sporadic corticobasal syndrome. *Mov Disord* 2008; **23**(6): 892–5.

56. Masellis M, Momeni P, Meschino W *et al.* Novel splicing mutation in the progranulin gene causing familial corticobasal syndrome. *Brain* 2006; **129**(Pt 11): 3115–23.

57. Spina S, Murrell JR, Huey ED *et al.* Corticobasal syndrome associated with the A9D progranulin mutation. *J Neuropathol Exp Neurol* 2007; **66**(10): 892–900.

58. Schneider JA, Watts RL, Gearing M, Brewer RP, Mirra SS. Corticobasal degeneration: Neuropathologic and clinical heterogeneity. *Neurology* 1997; **48**(4): 959–69.

59. Dickson DW, Bergeron C, Chin SS *et al.* Office of rare diseases neuropathologic criteria for corticobasal degeneration. *J Neuropathol Exp Neurol* 2002; **61**(11): 935–46.

60. Boeve BF, Josephs KA, Drubach DA. Current and future management of the corticobasal syndrome and corticobasal degeneration. *Handb Clin Neurol* 2008; **89**: 533–48.

61. Frucht S, Fahn S, Chin S, Dhawan V, Eidelberg D. Levodopa-induced dyskinesias in autopsy-proven cortical-basal ganglionic degeneration. *Mov Disord* 2000; **15**(2): 340–3.

The apraxias in movement disorders

Roneil Malkani and Cindy Zadikoff

Introduction

In 1900 Hugo Liepmann first described apraxia as the inability to perform purposeful skilled movements in the absence of elementary motor deficits, abnormality of sensation, or impaired comprehension or memory [1]. He noted that a patient may substitute the requested action with an incorrect action, fragment and spatially displace the movements, or perseverate. Liepmann and Maas (1907) postulated that the left hemisphere incorporates not only language but also motor engrams that control purposeful, skilled movement [2]. Liepmann later distinguished two stages of praxis [3]. First, the plan or ideation of movement must be evoked, and then the appropriate motor engrams must be decoded for action execution.

Since those first descriptions, much work has been done to try to further our understanding of praxis and apraxia. The current models of limb praxis, similar to that suggested by Liepmann, involve both conception and production areas [4]. The dominant parietal lobe stores motor engrams for praxis conception, and the dorsal, or parietofrontal, system serves as the production system [5, 6]. The latter can be further divided into a medial system that plays a role in movement preparation and the selection of necessary parameters of movement (e.g., amplitude and velocity) and a lateral system that contributes to temporal perceptions through time-dependent attention and working memory.

Many studies have confirmed the dominance of the left hemisphere in praxis; however, there is some bilateral representation of praxis function, which is why there appears to be sparing of certain left-hand praxis functions after callosal or left hemisphere lesions [7–9]. Moreover, even in the dominant hemisphere the type of apraxia seen varies depending on whether the "lesions" are anterior or posterior, and thus appear to rest upon which neural networks are ultimately disrupted.

It is now clear that there are several types of apraxia based on both the types of errors made (e.g., "temporal errors" in which there is impaired timing and sequencing but the overall content of the movement is recognizable; "spatial errors" in which there is abnormal amplitude or body-part-as-object substitution; and "content errors") and the means by which they are elicited [10]. In this chapter we will begin with a discussion on the basic types of apraxia and then focus on apraxia as it relates to diseases of the basal ganglia.

Currently the major types of apraxia include ideational apraxia, ideomotor apraxia and limb kinetic apraxia (see Table 4.1). There are also more specialized types of apraxia, such as dressing apraxia and apraxia of speech, which will not be covered in this chapter, and several other types that perhaps are incorrectly referred to as apraxia, such as apraxia of eyelid opening (AEO), oculomotor apraxia (OMA), and gait apraxia. These will be briefly addressed as they can be seen in the context of several movement disorders.

Ideational apraxia (IA) is the failure to conceive or formulate an action spontaneously or to command ("what to do"). This results in content errors (e.g., making a pounding motion when using a screwdriver), tool selection errors (e.g., being unable to choose a pen to write a letter), and gesture discrimination errors (e.g., being unable to recognize a well-performed from a poorly performed coin-flip) [11–14]. Additionally, patients with IA have difficulty performing a multiple step task due to errors such as perseveration. While no one anatomical area has been identified, typically lesions in the dominant left hemisphere, including parieto-occipital and parietotemporal regions, are thought to cause this type of apraxia, although left frontal lesions have been described as well [11].

Ideomotor apraxia (IMA) refers to the inability to execute a learned action causing impairment in timing,

Uncommon Causes of Movement Disorders, ed. Néstor Gálvez-Jiménez and Paul J. Tuite. Published by Cambridge University Press. © Cambridge University Press 2011.

Table 4.1. Overview of the types of apraxias.

Type	Definition	Clinical testing	Error types	Anatomy
Ideational apraxia	Patient does not know what to do Impaired ability to recognize and discriminate correct actions [3]	Gesture discrimination tasks Tool selection tasks Actual tool use Multiple step tasks[10, 12, 13]	Content errors Tool-action selection errors Perseverations Impairment in carrying out sequences of actions requiring use of various objects in the correct order	Thought to involve left parieto-occipital and parietotemporal regions[3] Can involve left frontal, frontotemporal, and temporal regions +/− subcortical involvement [11]
Ideomotor apraxia	Disorder of goal-directed movement Patient knows what to do but not how to do it [12]	Pantomime to use tool results in incorrect but recognizable action Improves on imitation and actual tool use Transitive gestures are affected more than intransitive gestures Voluntary automatic dissociation is present (more apparent in clinical setting than everyday life) [10]	Spatial errors (abnormal amplitude, abnormal orientation, or body-part-as-object substitution) Temporal errors (irregular timing or abnormal sequencing)	Multiple areas in the dominant hemisphere; parietal and frontal association areas and the white matter bundles connecting them Less commonly PMC, SMA, basal ganglia, and thalamus Unilateral dominant lesions cause bilateral deficits, more severe contralaterally
Limb-kinetic apraxia	Loss of hand and finger dexterity due to inability to connect or isolate individual movements	All movements are affected: symbolic and nonsymbolic gestures, transitive (i.e., using instruments) and intransitive (i.e., communicative gestures) Mainly distal in finger and hand No voluntary automatic dissociation	Coarse, awkward, and mutilated motions	Contralateral PMC has been implicated [20]

Abbreviations: PMC = premotor cortex; SMA = supplementary motor area.

sequencing and spatial organization of gestural movements [12]. Examples of these types of errors include abnormal orientation of body part when performing the action (e.g., when patients pantomime brushing their hair, they hold their fists tightly with no space for holding the imagined object) or body-part-as-object substitution (e.g., they use their fingers to comb their hair as opposed to pretending to hold a hairbrush). As opposed to patients with ideational apraxia, in IMA patients know "what to do" but not "how to do" it. Patients do not typically complain of this type of apraxia because it improves with normal contextual cues (e.g., they cannot pantomime the ability to use a tool, but they can imitate the movement and when given the object they can perform the task appropriately). Heilman and Rothi in 1982 proposed that there are two types of ideomotor apraxia based on location of the lesion [6, 15]. The left parietal cortex contains the proposed visuokinesthetic motor engrams. Dysfunction in this location causes the first type in which there is disruption of input processing as well as performance deficits, resulting in an inability to discriminate correct from incorrect gesturing. The second type is due to a lesion anterior to the supramarginal gyrus, which disconnects the stored motor engrams from the pre-motor and motor areas, sparing gesture discrimination between well- and poorly performed acts and resulting in an inability to pantomime or imitate. Depending on where the lesion is, this could result in either ipsilateral or bilateral apraxia.

Orofacial apraxia (OFA), a type of IMA, is the inability to imitate or perform volitional movements to command despite preservation of automatic facial movements. Testing includes orofacial gestures that may involve a single or multiple steps, may be meaning-ful or meaningless, or may involve objects. Examples include "puff out your cheeks," "stick out your tongue then bite your lower lip," or "suck on a straw." Patients with OFA may make spatial errors or be unable to cor-rectly perform a sequence of gestures. A case series reported by Pramstaller and Marsden suggests that the pathway for orofacial praxis may be parallel to but sep-arate from that for limb praxis. Lesions causing OFA involve the inferior frontal gyrus, perisylvian central area, insula, and striatum [16].

Limb kinetic apraxia (LKA) is a less studied and, until recently, controversial type of apraxia. Movements are coarse, awkward and mutilated, and the motion becomes amorphous and contaminated by extraneous movements. As opposed to IMA, which is often bilateral but asymmetric, LKA is usually uni-lateral and confined to the limb contralateral to the lesion, often affecting fine manipulation of finger and hand movements more so than proximal movements. IMA causes transitive movements to be more impaired than intransitive movements, whereas LKA affects all types of movements equally [17, 18]. Also in contradis-tinction to IMA, patients complain about this because it interferes with activities of daily living. It is thought that dysfunction of the premotor cortex causes LKA [17]. The results of a study by Blondel et al. and clin-icopathological evidence in five patients examined by Tsuchiya et al. also support this hypothesis [4, 12, 19, 20].

Multiple types of apraxia can exist within the same individual. Certain features of each do allow distinc-tion between these entities even within a single person. For example, IMA and LKA can be distinguished by the distribution of symptoms, i.e., symmetric or asym-metric and distal or proximal. Furthermore, the types of errors are different. In LKA there are coarse and "awk-ward" errors, but IMA produces spatial and sequenc-ing errors. Thus, in testing praxis, one must look for lateralization depending on handedness, the type of movements being tested, and the pathway though which the movement is evoked. It is also important to test several types of movements under different sce-narios (i.e., pantomime, imitation, and actual tool use). Testing should include both transitive and intransitive gestures. The former includes tool use ("use a ham-mer" or "use a screwdriver"), while the latter does not involve tool use and can be meaningless ("touch your nose") or meaningful ("wave goodbye" or "hitchhike"). Conveyance of these gestures requires both conception and proper execution. It is important to keep in mind that in pantomiming, gestures are taken out of context and as a result are unfamiliar and "abstract"[21].

The role of the basal ganglia in praxis

Apraxia can be seen in a number of diseases of the basal ganglia (BG) and so it stands to reason that the BG are involved in praxis production; thus, dysfunction of the BG could lead to apraxia (Table 4.2). Alexander et al. proposed the existence of five parallel circuits involv-ing the BG and cortex [22]. In the motor circuit, which involves praxis, the putamen is the center of the circuit. It receives somatotopically organized input from the motor and sensory cortex as well as area 6, including the premotor area and the supplementary motor area (SMA). The putamen then projects in a topographic-ally organized manner to the ventrolateral globus pal-lidus (GP) and the substantia nigra. This part of the GP projects to thalamus and back to the SMA. The BG may be activated in selecting motor programs and inhib-iting competing ones[23]. It may also participate in kinematic parameters of arm movement. For example, there are specific neurons in the caudate nucleus that discharge in relation to the direction and amplitude of movement, and there are pallidal neurons that are more complex and are influenced by context and degree of movement difficulty[24].

Various methods have been used to study the role of the BG in praxis, including imaging studies. Jueptner and Weiller examined the role of the BG and cerebellum in the control of movements using PET during different tasks [25]. Movement selection, new learned movements and over-learned movements all activated various parts of the BG and cortex. The cere-bellum was not activated when subjects made new decisions, attended to actions, or selected movements, such as with line generation. However the neocer-ebellum was engaged during line retracing, suggest-ing that the cerebellum is involved in monitoring and optimizing the movement and the outcome (afferent/

Table 4.2. Comparison of limb apraxia in various movement disorders.

	CBD	PSP	PD	MSA	DLB	HD
IMA	Common	Common	Uncommon	Rare	Not formally studied	Present
LKA	Common	Uncommon	Uncommon	Not present	Not present	Not present
IA	Present	Uncommon	Not present	Not present	Present later in disease course	Not present

Abbreviations: IMA = ideomotor apraxia; LKA = limb kinetic apraxia; IA = ideational apraxia; CBD = corticobasal degeneration; PSP = progressive supranuclear palsy; PD = Parkinson's disease; MSA = multiple systems atrophy; DLB = dementia with Lewy bodies; AD = Alzheimer's disease; HD = Huntington's disease

sensory component), whereas BG is concerned with movement and muscle selection (efferent/motor component).

In 1996 Pramstaller and Marsden examined 82 cases of apraxia due to deep lesions [16]. Rarely were there isolated BG lesions, but when they occurred they involved the left putamen or thalamus. Most of these patients had large lesions, and it is the additional involvement of the white matter tracts passing near the BG that often caused apraxia. Thus, while the BG is involved in praxis production, it seems unlikely that lesions of the BG alone cause apraxia. Rather, the BG likely alters the expression of apraxia [26].

There are two types of apraxias involving the eyes that are possibly misnomers and do not represent "true apraxias"; however, as they are seen in the context of several movement disorders they will be discussed briefly below.

Apraxia of eyelid opening

Apraxia of eyelid opening was initially described by Goldstein and Cogan in 1965 as a difficulty in initiating the act of eyelid opening [27]. Lepore and Duvoisin described this phenomenon in six patients in whom the eyelids would remain shut until the upper lids slowly elevated spontaneously. These patients would often vigorously contract the frontalis muscle to no avail, despite the absence of ongoing orbicularis oculi contraction [28]. AEO likely represents a form of dystonia or levator palpebrae inhibition rather than apraxia. Neither cause is consistent with the current concepts of limb apraxia. Krack and Marion refer to AEO as "focal eyelid dystonia" given that it has spontaneous triggers, improves with sensory tricks, and responds to botulinum toxin injection. Many of the triggers and sensory tricks are the same as those noted in blepharospasm.

Their series included two patients with parkinsonism, in which both had dystonia preceding the onset of parkinsonism [29]. However, dystonia may not account for all cases of AEO. Inappropriate levator inhibition may also play a role in the inability to initiate eye opening in some patients. Arimideh *et al.* reported a patient with isolated levator inhibition who did not have ongoing spasms of the eyelids but had frequent involuntary drooping of the lids. Electromyography showed no dystonic activity of the orbicularis oculi but did show frequent episodes of inhibition of levator palpebrae activity [30].

AEO is seen in a variety of disorders, most commonly blepharospasm, but also progressive supranuclear palsy (PSP), Parkinson disease (PD), corticobasal degeneration (CBD), spinocerebellar ataxia type 2, spinocerebellar ataxia type 3, Osler–Rendu–Weber disease, and neurodegeneration with brain iron accumulation [29, 31–34]. AEO has also been noted in 5–30% of patients with PD after implantation of deep brain stimulation electrodes in the subthalamic nucleus. Increasing the stimulation frequency has been reported to improve AEO in this setting [35, 36]. AEO typically responds to injection of botulinum toxin, particularly when it is injected toward the palpebral rather than the orbital part of orbicularis oculi, regardless of etiology [29, 32].

Oculomotor apraxia

Eye movement abnormalities that have been termed oculomotor apraxia (OMA) have been seen in a group of movement disorders. OMA was originally described by Cogan as a congenital syndrome in which the eyes could not be rotated in the desired direction intentionally but full eye movement could be executed at random [37]. In a subsequent case series by Cogan and Adams, two patients with previously normal eye movements developed the inability to move the eyes to command or stimulation despite normal random and vestibular eye movements. One such case was also associated with limb IMA and OFA [38].

Patients with oculomotor apraxia use head thrusts to direct gaze to a particular target. The primary difficulty is in saccade initiation, but there is also impaired cancellation of the vestibulo-ocular response. As a result, a patient can move the head toward the target but overshoots it.

Similar eye movement abnormalities, though not exactly as described by Cogan, have been seen in corticobasal degeneration (CBD). In Cogan's initial description, only horizontal eye movements were affected [37,38]. In CBD, horizontal and vertical eye movements are both affected, and typically the saccade latency rather than the velocity is impaired. Voluntary initiation of horizontal saccades may be delayed or even absent but may improve if the patient is given an object to look at. Eye blinking and head movements may be used to help initiate gaze shifts [39]. Rivaud-Pechoux *et al.* suggested that these eye abnormalities may distinguish CBD from PSP, in which vertical saccade velocity – not latency as in CBD – is impaired [40].

There is a group of inherited degenerative ataxias with childhood age of onset that involve OMA, including ataxia with oculomotor apraxia type 1 (AOA1), ataxia with oculomotor apraxia type 2 (AOA2), and ataxia telangiectasia. All are autosomal recessive disorders, and their gene products are involved in DNA repair [41]. Both horizontal and vertical eye movements are affected in these disorders. AOA1 is a disorder with childhood onset of ataxia and OMA, and may include sensorimotor neuropathy, chorea, cognitive decline and hypoalbuminemia [41,42]. AOA2 is a similar disorder with onset in adolescence, but OMA occurs in just over half of patients [43]. Both AOA1 and AOA2 involve extremely hypometric saccades as well as square-wave jerks [42]. Ataxia telangiectasia is also associated with OMA. Two studies have shown prolonged vertical and horizontal saccade latencies and hypometric saccades, and in one study 30% of patients had head thrusts [44].

There is controversy regarding whether OMA is actually an apraxia. Vidailhet and Rivaud-Pechoux showed a correlation between apraxia scores and saccade latency, suggesting this ocular manifestation as an apraxia [45]. However, Harris *et al.* have proposed that this dysfunction should instead be called "saccadic failure" on the basis of the suggested mechanism underlying the oculomotor abnormalities [41, 44, 46]. Furthermore, under its strictest definition, apraxia is the inability to perform a learned or skilled motor act, and saccade initiation is neither a learned nor a skilled activity. Additionally, dysfunction in the mechanisms of saccades as mentioned above do not fit with the models of IA, IMA, or LKA discussed. We therefore agree that OMA is a misnomer and that "saccadic failure" is a more appropriate term [46].

Gait apraxia

The term gait apraxia is perhaps another misnomer. It is different from leg apraxia, and often they do not coexist. Leg apraxia can be tested by similar means as the arm (e.g., kick a ball, stub out a cigarette) but it is much less frequently studied than upper extremity apraxia, partly because of lack of standardized testing and because fewer movements and less complex tasks can be tested [26].

Gait apraxia, on the other hand, has received considerable attention in the literature. The term is often used in conjunction with a group of similar gait disorders such as cautious gait, gait ignition failure, frontal lobe gait, subcortical disequilibrium, and frontal disequilibrium [47, 48]. Classification and terminology are often confusing, and the described syndromes have overlapping features. Nutt *et al.* grouped these disorders as higher-level gait disorders and rejected the term "gait apraxia"[48]. Patients with bilateral apraxia or sitting apraxia may have normal gait, and those with "gait apraxia" may not have limb apraxia [5, 49]. Again, under its strictest definition, apraxia is the inability to perform "skilled or learned motor acts." Like OMA as noted above, locomotion is not a consciously learned action; rather, it is a repetitive motor pattern involving spinal cord generators and modified by brain stem and cortex [50]. Since walking is a more "hard-wired" action, one could argue that "gait apraxia" cannot exist. With better understanding of the underlying anatomy and physiology of these gait disorders, perhaps a uniform and accepted nomenclature can be devised and current confusion eliminated [26].

Corticobasal degeneration

Corticobasal degeneration (CBD) is a rare parkinsonian disorder characterized by unilateral parkinsonism, apraxia, cortical sensory abnormalities, alien limb phenomenon, and sometimes parietal dysfunction later in the disease [51]. Because the majority of studies discussed below have referred to "corticobasal degeneration," we will use that terminology. However, it has become increasingly clear from clinicopathological studies that a variety of diseases can result in the clinical syndrome ascribed to corticobasal degeneration, highlighting the notion that it is the distribution of pathology, rather than the pathological substrate, that results in the syndrome described above. As such, it is more appropriate to refer to corticobasal syndrome, with the specific disease entity based on pathological confirmation [52]. Furthermore, because apraxia is considered a hallmark of CBD and is a component of all proposed diagnostic criteria, this serves an source of clinical bias [51]. As such, a high proportion of patients are diagnosed clinically with CBD because they have apraxia [26].

In "classic" CBD, IMA and LKA have most commonly been identified, although IA can also be seen. IMA is usually bilateral, but asymmetric and is best assessed in the less affected (i.e., less bradykinetic, dystonic, rigid) limb. Leiguarda et al. studied the less affected limb in 14 patients with clinically diagnosed CBD [12]. Eleven had IMA that was worse with transitive than intransitive actions, and most made more spatial errors than sequencing or timing errors. Three of these subjects also made errors such as mislocations, misuse, absent or unrecognizable responses, and gesture recognition deficits suggestive of coexisting IA. Alien limb behavior was found only in patients with IMA. The severity of both IMA and IA significantly correlated with worse cognitive scores. Ideomotor apraxia correlated with tasks sensitive to frontal lobe dysfunction, whereas IA correlated with the presence of primitive reflexes. Several other studies have also observed IMA in patients with CBD. While these patients made errors on gesture to command or imitation, most had preserved gesture recognition [19,53].

Imaging studies have been used to correlate apraxia in CBD with structural abnormalities. The study by Soliveri et al. showed that patients with CBD more frequently had significant IMA and more frequently had asymmetric frontoparietal atrophy than patients with PSP [54]. Using diffusion tensor imaging and voxel-based morphometry, Borroni et al. examined 20 CBD patients with IMA and LKA. Compared with controls, the patients with CBD had reduced fractional anisotropy on diffusion tensor imaging in the long frontoparietal connecting tracts, intraparietal association fibers, corpus callosum, and sensorimotor projections of the

cortical hand areas. Voxel-based morphometry showed reduced gray matter in the left hemisphere, including inferior frontal and premotor cortices, parietal operculum, superior temporal gyrus, hippocampus, right cerebellum and bilateral pulvinar nuclei. Total apraxia scores on the De Renzi apraxia battery correlated with atrophy of the parietal operculum bilaterally and fractional anisotropy in the left dorsolateral parietofrontal association fibers. There was also a correlation between the simple gesture subscore and reduced fractional anisotropy in hand sensorimotor connecting fibers bilaterally [55].

Functional brain imaging has also been used to try to understand the networks involved in limb apraxia in CBD. One study by Sawle et al. examined six CBD patients using $^{15}O_2$-PET. The results showed decreased metabolism in the frontoparietal region, particularly the superior prefrontal cortex and the lateral and mesial premotor areas, suggesting that dysfunction of these areas may account for many of the errors seen in IMA [56]. Using FDG-PET, Eidelberg showed that in comparison with controls and patients with PD, five CBD patients had reduced glucose metabolism globally but asymmetrically in the inferior parietal, medial temporal and thalamic regions [57]. Other studies have confirmed hypometabolism on FDG-PET in these areas, including the frontal and sensorimotor areas, with the more affected hemisphere contralateral to the more affected limb [58]. Additionally, ^{99m}Tc-D,L-hexamethylpropylene amine oxime brain perfusion SPECT studies have shown reduced regional cerebral blood flow in the posterior frontal lobe, parietal lobe, caudate nucleus, putamen and thalamus in the more affected hemisphere (contralateral to the more affected limb) when compared with controls [59]. It is important to note, however, that most patients in these imaging studies had other deficits, including dystonia and rigidity, and that most of these functional imaging studies were done in the resting state and not while the patient was undergoing tests of praxis. Thus, one cannot be certain about the relationship between the metabolic findings and the presence of apraxia [26].

Recently there has been a renewed interest in LKA in patients with CBD. LKA is the most "motor" of the apraxias and can be the most difficult to distinguish from more elemental deficits such as rigidity, weakness or dystonia, which is one reason why it has been controversial and largely neglected. As mentioned earlier, LKA and IMA can be seen in the same limb; however, there are a number of features described above that can help distinguish these entities in an individual. Leiguarda *et al.* studied apraxia with tool selection tests, transcranial magnetic stimulation (TMS), and three-dimensional motor analysis in patients with CBD, PD without apraxia, and controls [17]. They found that all subjects with CBD had slow, coarse and awkward movements with a lack of interdigital coordination that did not appear to be explained by bradykinesia and was felt to represent LKA. Of note, moderate to severe IMA was found in all CBD patients, particularly if the dominant hemisphere was involved. TMS showed a shorter cortical silent period only on the more affected hemisphere of the apraxic patients compared with controls and patients with PD, suggesting that a disruption of intracortical inhibitory mechanism may play a role in the genesis of LKA or IMA.

Orofacial apraxia has also been reported in patients with CBD. This type of apraxia has not been studied in depth and it is likely underreported. Both Pillon *et al.* and Frattali and Sonies reported that most patients with CBD had OFA [60, 61] These findings were confirmed by Ozsancak, who distinguished CBD from multiple systems atrophy (MSA), PD and PSP, in part on the basis of the presence of OFA [62]. The CBD patients made significantly more sequential errors (e.g., "blow up your cheeks then bite your lower lip") than the others [12, 62]. However, Leiguarda *et al.* reported that 10 out of 12 patients with PSP they studied did have OFA, so it may not distinguish PSP from CBD [63].

Progressive supranuclear palsy

Compared with the other diseases discussed, progressive supranuclear palsy (PSP) is the one that can often be the most challenging to distinguish from CBD, especially in the absence of a vertical supranuclear gaze palsy suggesting PSP or lateralizing signs suggesting CBD.

Patients with PSP may develop IMA with spared gesture recognition. Leiguarda *et al.* found that 8 out of 12 patients with PSP assessed with a comprehensive apraxia battery had bilateral IMA [63]. Gesture discrimination was spared in all the patients, but two of them who also had significant cognitive impairment had difficulty with multiple-step tasks, suggesting IA as well. Other studies have also confirmed these findings [18, 64]. In one such study examining IMA in PSP compared with CBD, both groups demonstrated apraxia, although it seemed to be worse in CBD patients [18]. While transitive tasks were more affected than intransitive tasks in both groups, this difference

was more prominent in PSP. Interestingly, the authors also reported that in CBD distal movements were more affected than proximal movements. While it is possible that this difference might distinguish IMA in PSP from CBD, this finding may have been due to coexistence of LKA in the CBD patients [22, 25].

In PSP, more severe apraxia has been shown to correlate with worse scores on the mini-mental status exam, frontal lobe dysfunction and other cognitive tasks [63, 65]. Soliveri *et al.* found that demented PSP patients were more apraxic that nondemented patients and had more problems with complex than with simple tasks [65]. These findings suggest that apraxia in PSP is due to dysfunction in the anterior cortical structures, such as the prefrontal cortex, when severe enough to cause cognitive dysfunction.

Parkinson disease

Ideomotor apraxia (IMA) has been noted in patients with PD to a lesser extent than in patients with PSP and CBD. In 1986, Goldenberg examined 42 patients with PD and found evidence of IMA [66]. The deficits were primarily in whole limb movement sequences (e.g., "make a fist beside the head then extend the arm and form a ring with the thumb and middle finger"). Total apraxia scores correlated with tests of visuospatial ability. Leiguarda *et al.* administered a comprehensive apraxia battery to 45 subjects with PD, and 12 of them exhibited bilateral IMA for transitive movements but not intransitive movements. Movement discrimination and comprehension were spared [63]. In this same study, apraxia scores did not correlate with disease duration, Hoehn and Yahr stage, or Unified Parkinson's Disease Rating Scale, but there was a correlation between IMA and body bradykinesia, frontal lobe dysfunction and depression. In another study by Monza *et al.*, 7 out of 14 patients administered an apraxia battery testing gesture production had borderline apraxia scores. None of them scored in the apraxic range [67]. Simple tapping was no different from controls, but patients with PD had more difficulty with sequential tapping. Therefore, bradykinesia alone cannot account for sequence errors, suggesting that these errors may be due to IMA.

There has been recent focus on studying LKA in patients with PD. On comparison of finger tapping and coin rotation, Quencer *et al.* found no difference in finger tapping between PD in the "on" state versus controls, but those with PD had significantly slower coin rotation [68]. Gebhardt *et al.* conducted a similar study that showed a significant improvement in finger tapping between "on" and "off" states in PD patients but only a modest improvement in coin rotation [69]. The authors conclude that because finger tapping improved in the "on" state whereas coin rotation did not, the disability with coin rotation cannot be explained by bradykinesia and thus must represent LKA, possibly due to interruption of transmission between time- and space-representation of skilled movement and target areas of motor cortex secondary to basal ganglia dysfunction [69]. While one cannot disagree that patients did worse with the coin rotation task than the finger-tapping task, coin rotation is a much more complex task and so their conclusion that impairment seen in coin rotation is caused by LKA can be debated [70].

Multiple system atrophy

Relatively little has been published about apraxia in multiple system atrophy (MSA). In a study by Leiguarda *et al.*, 10 patients with MSA were tested with a comprehensive apraxia battery but none of them had IMA [63]. In a kinematic analysis, MSA patients had an abnormal orientation of movement axis when asked to pretend to cut a loaf of bread, but this was less severe than in patients with PD or PSP [71]. Moreover, Monza *et al.* found IMA in 2/19 patients and an additional 4/19 had scores suggestive of "borderline apraxia" based on the De Renzi test [67]. Most errors were due to "clumsiness" (i.e., delay or inability to initiate gestures, reduced amplitude of movement, and perplexity in executing gestures) and sequencing errors. Gesture recognition was spared. Executive dysfunction was present in the majority of these patients, suggesting that perhaps in most patients with MSA it is the relative lack of cognitive impairment that spares the praxis system. Finally, Ozsancak *et al.* did not find OFA in any of eight MSA patients evaluated, and there have been no reports of LKA in MSA [62].

Dementia with Lewy bodies

There have been no reports of IMA in patients with dementia with Lewy bodies (DLB), but there are a few studies on constructional apraxia. Constructional apraxia – the inability to reproduce visually presented objects or arrange component elements in the correct spatial relationships in the absence of visual and motor impairment – has previously been shown to be more often impaired in patients with DLB than in those with Alzheimer dementia (AD) [72, 73] Cormack *et al.*

studied constructional apraxia with pentagon drawing in patients with Parkinson disease dementia (PDD), DLB and AD. Patients with DLB did worse than patients with AD and PD, but could not be distinguished from patients with PDD. Constructional apraxia correlated with global cognitive dysfunction in PDD and AD but not in DLB, suggesting there is dissociation of constructional ability from global cognitive abilities in patients with DLB [73].

Huntington disease

Shelton *et al.* reported that three out of nine Huntington disease (HD) patients they studied had IMA on the basis of an apraxia battery including gesture discrimination, imitation and actual object use. An additional four patients made at least two apraxic errors, most commonly spatial errors such as body-part-as-object substitution [74]. In these patients movement discrimination was spared, suggesting an anterior type of apraxia. This is consistent with frontal lobe dysfunction, which is further supported by the early cognitive deficits in HD, such as decreased concentration, apathy and impaired executive dysfunction, all of which also suggest abnormalities of frontal lobe function. Hamilton *et al.* also studied praxis in a group of HD patients in 2003 [75]. They found that 35% of the 20 patients studied had IMA, which was worse with transitive than with intransitive movements. These findings were confirmed in another study in which 41 HD patients were examined. Patients with HD scored worse than controls, and 80% of patients with stage 4 disease had apraxia [76]. In all these studies, apraxia scores correlated with disease duration and severity but not with cognitive impairment. In the only study to compare CAG repeats with severity of apraxia, apraxia scores were not correlated with the number of CAG repeats.

Summary

Praxis involves comprehension of desired movement and sequencing as well as execution of the appropriate motor program and inhibition of inappropriate ones. The left hemisphere is dominant in praxis but there is some bilateral representation. Apraxia results from dysfunction in parietal cortex or frontal areas (e.g., SMA and PMC), or a disconnection between them. The BG appears to be important in the selection of motor programs and inhibition of competing programs and participates in kinematic parameters of movement.

There are several types of apraxia, including IA, IMA and LKA, that are seen with degenerative movement disorders, particularly in association with cognitive dysfunction. Because IMA improves when given the actual tool to use, it causes little to no disability. On the other hand, LKA results in loss of control in fine finger movements, and IA leads to poor gesture recognition that does not improve with tool use; thus, these latter types of apraxia can result in significant disability. It is important to recognize that more that one type of apraxia may coexist in the same patient. Additionally, the term "apraxia" is misapplied to some motor disturbances that are seen in some movement disorders. Further studies are needed to clarify the cause of these motor disturbances and answer the many questions that remain when examining apraxia in patients with movement disorders. Only then will it be possible to begin to understand the complex neural network involved in praxis in these movement disorders.

References

1. Liepmann H. Das Krankheitsbild der Apraxie ("motorischen asymbolie"). Aufgrund eines Falles von einseitger Apraxie. Berlin: Verlag von S Karger; 1900.

2. Liepmann H, Maas O. Fall von linksseitiger Agraphie und Apraxie bei rechtsseitiger Lahmung. *J Psychol Neurol* 1907; **10**: 214–27.

3. Liepmann H. Apraxie. *Ergebn ges Med* 1920; **1**: 516–43.

4. Roy EA, Square PA. Common considerations in the study of limb, verbal and oral apraxia. In: Roy EA, ed. *Neuropsychological Studies of Apraxia and Related Disorders*. Amsterdam: North-Holland; 1985: 111–61.

5. Geschwind N. The apraxias: neural mechanisms of disorders of learned movement. *Am Sci* 1975; **63**(2): 188–95.

6. Heilman KM, Rothi LJ, Valenstein E. Two forms of ideomotor apraxia. *Neurology* 1982; **32**(4): 342–6.

7. Basso A, Luzzatti C, Spinnler H. Is ideomotor apraxia the outcome of damage to well-defined regions of the left hemisphere? Neuropsychological study of CAT correlation. *J Neurol Neurosurg Psychiatry* 1980; **43**(2): 118–26.

8. De Renzi E, Motti F, Nichelli P. Imitating gestures. A quantitative approach to ideomotor apraxia. *Arch Neurol* 1980; **37**(1): 6–10.

9. Geschwind N, Kaplan E. A human cerebral deconnection syndrome. A preliminary report. *Neurology* 1962; **12**: 675–85.

10. Rothi LG, Mack L, Verfaellie M *et al*. Ideomotor apraxia: error pattern analysis. *Aphasiology* 1988; **2**: 381–8.

11. Heilman KM, Maher LM, Greenwald ML *et al*. Conceptual apraxia from lateralized lesions. *Neurology* 1997; **49**(2): 457–64.

12. Leiguarda R, Merello M, Balej J. Apraxia in corticobasal degeneration. *Adv Neurol* 2000; **82**: 103–21.

13. Ochipa C, Rothi LJ, Heilman KM. Conduction apraxia. *J Neurol Neurosurg Psychiatry* 1994; **57**(10): 1241–4.

14. Rothi LJ, Heilman KM, Watson RT. Pantomime comprehension and ideomotor apraxia. *J Neurol Neurosurg Psychiatry* 1985; **48**(3): 207–10.

15. Heilman K, Rothi LJG. Apraxia. In: Heilman K, Valenstein, E eds. *Clinical Neuropsychology*. 2nd ed. New York: Oxford University Press; 1985: 131–50.

16. Pramstaller PP, Marsden CD. The basal ganglia and apraxia. *Brain* 1996; **119**(Pt 1): 319–40.

17. Leiguarda RC, Merello M, Nouzeilles MI *et al*. Limb-kinetic apraxia in corticobasal degeneration: clinical and kinematic features. *Mov Disord* 2003; **18**(1): 49–59.

18. Pharr V, Uttl B, Stark M *et al*. Comparison of apraxia in corticobasal degeneration and progressive supranuclear palsy. *Neurology* 2001; **56**(7): 957–63.

19. Blondel A, Eustache F, Schaeffer S *et al*. [Clinical and cognitive study of apraxia in cortico-basal atrophy. A selective disorder of the production system]. *Rev Neurol (Paris)* 1997; **153**(12): 737–47.

20. Tsuchiya K, Ikeda K, Uchihara T *et al*. Distribution of cerebral cortical lesions in corticobasal degeneration: a clinicopathological study of five autopsy cases in Japan. *Acta Neuropathol* 1997; **94**(5): 416–24.

21. Rapcsak SZ, Ochipa C, Beeson PM *et al*. Praxis and the right hemisphere. *Brain Cogn* 1993; **23**(2): 181–202.

22. Alexander GE, DeLong MR, Strick PL. Parallel organization of functionally segregated circuits linking basal ganglia and cortex. *Annu Rev Neurosci* 1986; **9**: 357–81.

23. Leiguarda R. Limb apraxia: cortical or subcortical. *Neuroimage* 2001; **14**(1 Pt 2): S137–41.

24. Kermadi I, Joseph JP. Activity in the caudate nucleus of monkey during spatial sequencing. *J Neurophysiol* 1995; **74**(3): 911–33.

25. Jueptner M, Weiller C. A review of differences between basal ganglia and cerebellar control of movements as revealed by functional imaging studies. *Brain* 1998; **121**(Pt 8): 1437–49.

26. Zadikoff C, Lang AE. Apraxia in movement disorders. *Brain* 2005; **128**(Pt 7): 1480–97.

27. Goldstein JE, Cogan DG. Apraxia of lid opening. *Arch Ophthalmol* 1965; **73**: 155–9.

28. Lepore FE, Duvoisin RC. "Apraxia" of eyelid opening: an involuntary levator inhibition. *Neurology* 1985; **35**(3): 423–7.

29. Krack P, Marion MH. "Apraxia of lid opening," a focal eyelid dystonia: clinical study of 32 patients. *Mov Disord* 1994; **9**(6): 610–5.

30. Aramideh M, Ongerboer de Visser BW, Koelman JH et al. Clinical and electromyographic features of levator palpebrae superioris muscle dysfunction in involuntary eyelid closure. *Mov Disord* 1994; **9**(4): 395–402.

31. Jankovic J, Friedman DI, Pirozzolo FJ et al. Progressive supranuclear palsy: motor, neurobehavioral, and neuro-ophthalmic findings. *Adv Neurol* 1990; **53**: 293–304.

32. Kanazawa M, Shimohata T, Sato M et al. Botulinum toxin A injections improve apraxia of eyelid opening without overt blepharospasm associated with neurodegenerative diseases. *Mov Disord* 2007; **22**(4): 597–8.

33. Sachin S, Goyal V, Singh S et al. Clinical spectrum of Hallervorden–Spatz syndrome in India. *J Clin Neurosci* 2009; **16**(2): 253–8.

34. Sepe-Monti M, Giubilei F, Marchione F et al. Apraxia of eyelid opening in a case of atypical corticobasal degeneration. *J Neural Transm* 2003; **110**(10): 1145–8.

35. Gervais-Bernard H, Xie-Brustolin J, Mertens P et al. Bilateral subthalamic nucleus stimulation in advanced Parkinson's disease: five year follow-up. *J Neurol* 2009; **256**(2): 225–33.

36. Strecker K, Meixensberger J, Schwarz J et al. Increase of frequency in deep brain stimulation relieves apraxia of eyelid opening in patients with Parkinson's disease: case report. *Neurosurgery* 2008; **63**(6): E1204; discussion E04.

37. Cogan DG. A type of congenital ocular motor apraxia presenting jerky head movements. *Am J Ophthalmol* 1953; **36**(4): 433–41.

38. Cogan DG, Adams RD. A type of paralysis of conjugate gaze (ocular motor apraxia). *AMA Arch Ophthalmol* 1953; **50**(4): 434–42.

39. Lang AE, Riley DE, Bergeron C. Cortical-basal ganglionic degeneration. In: Calne DB, ed. *Neurodegenerative Diseases*. Philadelphia: W.B. Saunders; 1994; 977–94.

40. Rivaud-Pechoux S, Vidailhet M, Gallouedec G et al. Longitudinal ocular motor study in corticobasal degeneration and progressive supranuclear palsy. *Neurology* 2000; **54**(5): 1029–32.

41. Onodera O. Spinocerebellar ataxia with ocular motor apraxia and DNA repair. *Neuropathology* 2006; **26**(4): 361–7.

42. Le Ber I, Moreira MC, Rivaud-Pechoux S et al. Cerebellar ataxia with oculomotor apraxia type 1: clinical and genetic studies. *Brain* 2003; **126**(Pt 12): 2761–72.

43. Anheim M, Monga B, Fleury M et al. Ataxia with oculomotor apraxia type 2: clinical, biological and genotype/phenotype correlation study of a cohort of 90 patients. *Brain* 2009; **132**(Pt 10): 2688–98.

44. Lewis RF, Lederman HM, Crawford TO. Ocular motor abnormalities in ataxia telangiectasia. *Ann Neurol* 1999; **46**(3): 287–95.

45. Vidailhet M, Rivaud-Pechoux S. Eye movement disorders in corticobasal degeneration. *Adv Neurol* 2000; **82**: 161–7.

46. Harris CM, Shawkat F, Russell-Eggitt I et al. Intermittent horizontal saccade failure ('ocular motor apraxia') in children. *Br J Ophthalmol* 1996; **80**(2): 151–8.

47. Liston R, Mickelborough J, Bene J et al. A new classification of higher level gait disorders in patients with cerebral multi-infarct states. *Age Ageing* 2003; **32**(3): 252–8.

48. Nutt JG, Marsden CD, Thompson PD. Human walking and higher-level gait disorders, particularly in the elderly. *Neurology* 1993; **43**(2): 268–79.

49. Kremer M. Sitting, standing, and walking. *Br Med J* 1958; **2**(5088): 63–8.

50. Shik ML, Orlovsky GN. Neurophysiology of locomotor automatism. *Physiol Rev* 1976; **56**(3): 465–501.

51. Litvan I, Bhatia KP, Burn DJ et al. Movement Disorders Society Scientific Issues Committee report: SIC Task Force appraisal of clinical diagnostic criteria for Parkinsonian disorders. *Mov Disord* 2003; **18**(5): 467–86.

52. Boeve BF, Lang AE, Litvan I. Corticobasal degeneration and its relationship to progressive supranuclear palsy and frontotemporal dementia. *Ann Neurol* 2003; **54**(Suppl 5): S15–9.

53. Pillon B, Dubois B, Agid Y. Cognitive deficits in non-Alzheimer's degenerative diseases. *J Neural Transm Suppl* 1996; **47**: 61–71.

54. Soliveri P, Monza D, Paridi D et al. Cognitive and magnetic resonance imaging aspects of corticobasal degeneration and progressive supranuclear palsy. *Neurology* 1999; **53**(3): 502–7.

55. Borroni B, Garibotto V, Agosti C et al. White matter changes in corticobasal degeneration syndrome and correlation with limb apraxia. *Arch Neurol* 2008; **65**(6): 796–801.

56. Sawle GV, Brooks DJ, Marsden CD et al. Corticobasal degeneration. A unique pattern of regional cortical oxygen hypometabolism and striatal fluorodopa uptake demonstrated by positron emission tomography. *Brain* 1991; **114**(Pt 1B): 541–56.

57. Eidelberg D, Dhawan V, Moeller JR et al. The metabolic landscape of cortico-basal ganglionic degeneration: regional asymmetries studied with positron emission tomography. *J Neurol Neurosurg Psychiatry* 1991; **54**(10): 856–62.

58. Blin J, Vidailhet MJ, Pillon B et al. Corticobasal degeneration: decreased and asymmetrical glucose consumption as studied with PET. *Mov Disord* 1992; **7**(4): 348–54.

59. Markus HS, Lees AJ, Lennox G et al. Patterns of regional cerebral blood flow in corticobasal degeneration studied using HMPAO SPECT; comparison with Parkinson's disease and normal controls. *Mov Disord* 1995; **10**(2): 179–87.

60. Frattali CM, Sonies BC. Speech and swallowing disturbances in corticobasal degeneration. *Adv Neurol* 2000; **82**: 153–60.

61. Pillon B, Blin J, Vidailhet M *et al*. The neuropsychological pattern of corticobasal degeneration: comparison with progressive supranuclear palsy and Alzheimer's disease. *Neurology* 1995; **45**(8): 1477–83.

62. Ozsancak C, Auzou P, Dujardin K *et al*. Orofacial apraxia in corticobasal degeneration, progressive supranuclear palsy, multiple system atrophy and Parkinson's disease. *J Neurol* 2004; **251**(11): 1317–23.

63. Leiguarda RC, Pramstaller PP, Merello M *et al*. Apraxia in Parkinson's disease, progressive supranuclear palsy, multiple system atrophy and neuroleptic-induced parkinsonism. *Brain* 1997; **120** (Pt 1): 75–90.

64. Soliveri P, Piacentini S, Paridi D *et al*. Distal-proximal differences in limb apraxia in corticobasal degeneration but not progressive supranuclear palsy. *Neurol Sci* 2003; **24**(3): 213–4.

65. Soliveri P, Piacentini S, Girotti F. Limb apraxia and cognitive impairment in progressive supranuclear palsy. *Neurocase* 2005; **11**(4): 263–7.

66. Goldenberg G, Wimmer A, Auff E *et al*. Impairment of motor planning in patients with Parkinson's disease: evidence from ideomotor apraxia testing. *J Neurol Neurosurg Psychiatry* 1986; **49**(11): 1266–72.

67. Monza D, Soliveri P, Radice D *et al*. Cognitive dysfunction and impaired organization of complex motility in degenerative parkinsonian syndromes. *Arch Neurol* 1998; **55**(3): 372–8.

68. Quencer K, Okun MS, Crucian G *et al*. Limb-kinetic apraxia in Parkinson disease. *Neurology* 2007; **68**(2): 150–1.

69. Gebhardt A, Vanbellingen T, Baronti F *et al*. Poor dopaminergic response of impaired dexterity in Parkinson's disease: bradykinesia or limb kinetic apraxia? *Mov Disord* 2008; **23**(12): 1701–6.

70. Landau WM, Mink JW. Is decreased dexterity in Parkinson disease due to apraxia? *Neurology* 2007; **68**(2): 90–1.

71. Leiguarda R, Merello M, Balej J *et al*. Disruption of spatial organization and interjoint coordination in Parkinson's disease, progressive supranuclear palsy, and multiple system atrophy. *Mov Disord* 2000; **15**(4): 627–40.

72. Ala TA, Hughes LF, Kyrouac GA *et al*. Pentagon copying is more impaired in dementia with Lewy bodies than in Alzheimer's disease. *J Neurol Neurosurg Psychiatry* 2001; **70**(4): 483–8.

73. Cormack F, Aarsland D, Ballard C *et al*. Pentagon drawing and neuropsychological performance in Dementia with Lewy Bodies, Alzheimer's disease, Parkinson's disease and Parkinson's disease with dementia. *Int J Geriatr Psychiatry* 2004; **19**(4): 371–7.

74. Shelton PA, Knopman DS. Ideomotor apraxia in Huntington's disease. *Arch Neurol* 1991; **48**(1): 35–41.

75. Hamilton JM, Haaland KY, Adair JC *et al*. Ideomotor limb apraxia in Huntington's disease: implications for corticostriate involvement. *Neuropsychologia* 2003; **41**(5): 614–21.

76. Hodl AK, Hodl E, Otti DV *et al*. Ideomotor limb apraxia in Huntington's disease: a case-control study. *J Neurol* 2008; **255**(3): 331–9.

Wilson disease

Neeraj Kumar

Wilson disease (WD) is a rare autosomal recessive disorder of copper metabolism that results in copper accumulation and multiorgan damage. The brain and liver are preferentially affected. Prompt institution of treatment is essential for a favorable outcome. Untreated disease is likely fatal. This chapter reviews the clinical presentation, diagnosis and management of WD. The emphasis is on neurologic aspects of the disease. Several recent review articles provide detailed bibliographies for the interested reader [1–10].

The worldwide prevalence of WD ranges from 1 in 5000 to 1 in 30 000, the carrier frequency is 1 in 90, and the incidence ranges from 15 to 30 per million [11]. Wilson disease is more prevalent in those populations in which consanguineous marriage is common. Particularly high prevalence and incidence have been noted in East Asia, Sardinia, Greece and Italy.

History

Wilson disease was first described in 1912 by the American-born British neurologist Samuel Alexander Kinnier Wilson [12]. He described it as a rare, familial, progressive, fatal disease characterized by neurologic deficits and liver cirrhosis. Figure 5.1 is from the original manuscript and shows the appearance of the face and hand in an afflicted patient (Figure 5.1a) and cystic changes in the basal ganglia in the brain of another patient (Figure 5.1b). Table 5.1 notes some landmark historical developments in our understanding of WD. For additional details the reader is directed to a recent comprehensive review on the history of WD [13]. Other terms that have been used to describe the disease over the decades have included Westphal–Strümpell pseudosclerosis, cerebral pseudosclerosis, hepatocerebral degeneration, hepatolenticular degeneration, neurohepatic degeneration and hepatocerebral dystrophy.

Genetics

Wilson disease is caused by mutations in the gene coding for a metal-transporting P-type ATPase (*ATP7B*) [14–17]. The gene is located on chromosome 13. The WD protein is a late endosome-associated membrane protein that binds copper in its large N-terminal domain and then translocates it to the endosomal lumen, ultimately delivering excess copper to biliary canaliculi for excretion. The WD protein is also responsible for incorporation of copper into apoceruloplasmin. Approximately 300 mutations have been identified in the WD gene and many more are likely to exist [18]. A majority of affected individuals are compound heterozygotes. In most ethnic groups a small number of mutations are prevalent in addition to other more rare mutations. Two commonly observed mutations among Europeans and North Americans are *His1069Gln* and *Gly1267Arg*. Deletions, insertions, splice site mutations, missense and nonsense mutations have all been identified; missense mutations are most frequent. Nonsense mutations and frameshift deletions cause a truncation of the translated protein and may result in a more severe form of the disease [19]. The same mutation may be associated with different phenotypes. This suggests the presence of additional modifying factors. The phenotype can be modulated by modifier genes such as *ATOX1* and *COMMD1* (originally called *MURR1*). Patients with apoE epsilon 3/3 genotype have a delayed onset of symptoms compared with all other apoE genotypes [20].

Pathophysiology

Copper absorbed by the intestinal cells is stored in the enterocytes (bound to metallothionein) in a nontoxic form (Figure 5.2). It is delivered into the circulation by the copper transporting protein ATP7A. Copper complexed to albumin reaches the liver. Figure 5.3

Uncommon Causes of Movement Disorders, ed. Néstor Gálvez-Jiménez and Paul J. Tuite. Published by Cambridge University Press. © Cambridge University Press 2011.

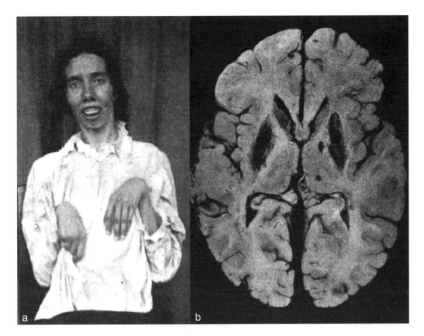

Figure 5.1. Two illustrations from S.A.K. Wilson's original 1912 monograph. (a) One of the original patients described. Note the hand dystonia, open mouth and vacant expression. The patient is grasping her nightdress in order to keep her right hand steady, likely because of a coexisting tremor. (b) Axial brain section through the hemispheres in a patient with WD from one of the original patients described. Note the cavitary changes in the basal ganglia. (Reproduced from reference 12.)

Table 5.1. Landmark historical developments in WD.

1902	Description of corneal pigment rings in a patient with "pseudosclerosis" by Kayser (later called K-F ring) (Additional descriptions provided by Fleischer in 1903 and 1912)
1912	Wilson's original description of "a familial nervous disease associated with cirrhosis of the liver"[12]
1912	Hall suggests an autosomal recessive inheritance pattern
1913	Rumpel identifies excess copper in the liver of a patient dying with WD
1922	Siemerling and Oloff describe the association of K-F rings and sunflower cataracts and note similarity of the cataracts to those produced by a copper-containing foreign body in the eye
1934	Gerlach and Rohrschneider confirm the presence of excess copper in the K-F ring
1948	Mandelbrote and Cumings demonstrate disturbance of copper metabolism in WD, Cumings suggests that treatment with dimercaprol (BAL) might be beneficial
1951	Cumings and Denny Brown and Porter show efficacy of BAL in WD
1952	Scheinberg and Gitlin, and Bearn and Kunkel independently reported on ceruloplasmin deficiency in WD
1956	Walshe introduces penicillamine as a treatment in WD
1961	Schouwink shows that zinc salts block copper absorption in the gut and could be of value in the treatment in WD (This is pursued further as a treatment in WD by Hoogenraad in 1979 and by Brewer in 1983)
1969	Walshe reports on trientine as an alternative to penicillamine in WD treatment
1974	Frommer demonstrates impaired biliary excretion of copper in WD
1982	Starzl report on the first liver transplantation in WD
1984	Walshe reports on tetrathiomolybdate as a therapeutic option in WD (This is pursued further by Brewer in 1991)
1993	Three separate groups report on identification of the WD gene [14–16]

Reproduced with permission from reference 13.
Abbreviations: BAL, Bristish anti-Lewisite; K-F, Kayser–Fleischer; WD, Wilson disease.

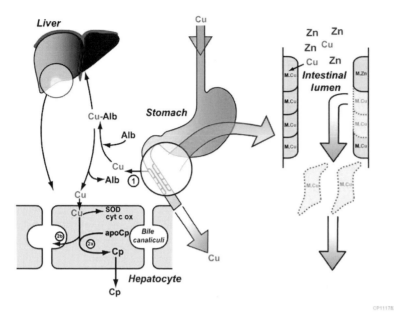

Figure 5.2. **Mechanism of action of zinc in reducing copper absorption and sites of defect in copper deficiency**. Excretion of copper into the gastrointestinal tract is the major pathway that regulates copper homeostasis and prevents deficiency or toxicity. The zinc-induced inhibition of copper absorption could be the result of competition for a common transporter or a consequence of induction of metallothionein in enterocytes. Metallothionein has a higher binding affinity for copper than for zinc. Copper is retained within the enterocytes and lost as the intestinal cells are sloughed off. Failure to mobilize absorbed copper from intestinal cells forms the basis of Menkes disease (1). In Wilson disease there is decreased incorporation of copper into ceruloplasmin (2a) and impaired biliary excretion of copper (2b). *Abbreviations*: Cu, copper; Zn, zinc; Cp, ceruloplasmin; M, metallothionein; alb, albumin; SOD, superoxide dismutase; cyt c ox, cytochrome *c* oxidase. (Reproduced from reference 82.) (See the color plate section for a color version of this figure.)

is a schematic representation of copper metabolism in the hepatocyte. Impaired function of ATP7B (the WD protein) leads to decreased hepatocellular excretion of copper into bile with subsequent hepatocellular copper accumulation and injury. Additionally, the defective ATP7B protein likely fails to incorporate copper into apoceruloplasmin. This results in secretion of apoceruloplasmin instead of holoceruloplasmin. Apoceruloplasmin has a shorter half-life than holoceruloplasmin and is rapidly metabolized. A reduced serum ceruloplasmin level results. Urinary copper excretion increases in WD, but this increase is unable to compensate for the defect in biliary copper excretion. When hepatic storage capacity is exceeded, copper is released into the blood and is deposited in other organs such as brain, cornea, kidney and bones. There is an increase in the circulating free copper which is toxic. Copper elevation causes a reduction in the protein X-linked inhibitor of apoptosis (XIAP), which causes caspase 3-initiated apoptosis and cell death [21].

The primary cerebral pathology is in the basal ganglia. Copper deposition causes a brownish discoloration

of the lenticular nuclei. Additional sites of involvement are the thalamus, brain stem, cerebellum and cerebral cortex. With disease progression there is necrosis and gliosis. Cystic changes in the basal ganglia (Figure 5.1b) are a characteristic finding.

Clinical findings

The initial presentation of WD is neurologic, hepatic and psychiatric in approximately 40%, 40% and 20% of cases respectively. WD presents with liver disease more often in children and young adults than in older individuals. Any patient younger than 50 years with unexplained liver disease should be screened for WD. Patients who present with neurologic disease generally do so in the second and third decades. Most patients with neurologic involvement have liver disease at the time of presentation but they are not symptomatic from their liver disease. The possibility of WD should be considered in any young patient with a movement disorder. Presentation with neurologic disease as late as the eighth decade has also been reported [22]. Clinical manifestations of copper excess are relatively rare in the preschool age, probably because copper accumulation

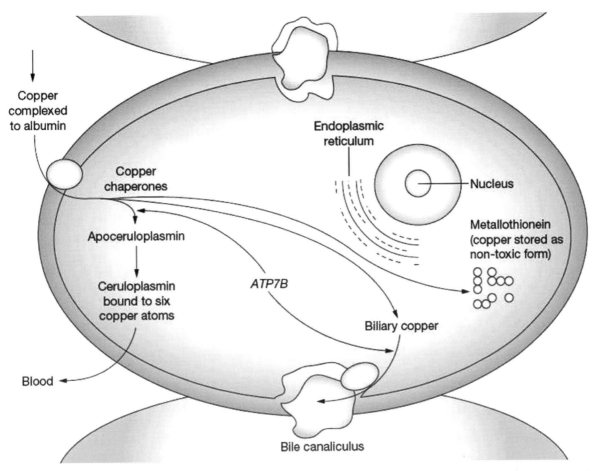

Figure 5.3. Schematic representation of copper metabolism within a liver cell. Copper absorbed by the intestinal cells is complexed to albumin and reaches the liver. In the hepatocyte the chaperone protein ATOX1 directs copper to its binding targets. Some copper is bound to metallothionein in a nontoxic form. ATP7B (the WD protein) mediates the incorporation of six copper molecules into apoceruloplasmin, forming ceruloplasmin. Ceruloplasmin is an α2-globulin glycoprotein with oxidase activity. It is the principal copper-carrying protein in the body. Under conditions of excess copper, ATP7B redistributes to the cytoplasmic vesicles where it transports excess copper across the hepatocyte apical membrane into the biliary canaliculi for excretion. *Abbreviation: ATP7B*, Wilson disease gene. (Reproduced with permission from reference 5.)

takes time to develop. Many atypical presentations are recognized (Table 5.2).

The most common mode of hepatic presentation in WD is progressive cirrhosis. In some cases incidental detection of hepatomegaly, splenomegaly due to portal hypertension, or elevated serum aminotransferases may be the only abnormality. Hepatic presentations also include acute hepatitis, recurrent hepatitis, chronic active hepatitis, fulminant hepatitis, or liver failure. Viral hepatitis or autoimmune hepatitis are frequently entertained differential diagnoses. Five percent of all cases of acute liver failure are due to WD [23]. This mode of presentation has a high mortality. Hemolysis induced by copper released from necrotic hepatocytes

may complicate acute liver disease. Associated renal failure may be present.

Three main neurological phenotypes are recognized: (1) a parkinsonian syndrome, (2) generalized dystonia, (3) postural and intention tremor with ataxia and dysarthria ("pseudosclerosis"). The onset is generally subacute or chronic. Rarely acute onset generalized severe dystonia (status dystonicus) or chorea or tremor may be seen [24]. The most frequent presenting neurologic manifestation of WD is tremors. The tremor may be resting, postural, or kinetic. A proximal, slow, high-amplitude upper extremity tremor is the classic finding. It may take on a coarse, "wing-beating" appearance. Tremor in WD may also be distal and small in

Table 5.2. Clinical manifestations of Wilson disease.

Neurological	*Classic manifestations*: tremor (any type), parkinsonian syndrome, dystonia, cerebellar syndrome, dysarthria *Other manifestations*: gait disturbance, pseudobulbar palsy, abnormalities in extraocular movements (slow horizontal saccades, upgaze restriction, impaired convergence), autonomic dysfunction, olfactory dysfunction, cognitive difficulties *Rare*: chorea, hemichorea, tics, myoclonus, athetosis, seizures, eyelid apraxia, ophthalmoplegia, pyramidal tract involvement, altered rapid eye movement sleep, cramps, writer's cramp, hypersomnia, and priapism *Reported*: "whispering dysphonia" [26], inspiratory laugh [27], presentation with a respiratory dyskinesia related cough [28], painless variant of painful legs and moving toes [30], isolated tongue protrusion movements [31], peripheral neuropathy [34] *Not affected*: vision, sensation
Hepatic	Progressive cirrhosis (compensated or decompensated), incidental detection of hepatomegaly/splenomegaly/serum aminotransferases, fulminant hepatic failure (with or without hemolysis/ renal failure), hepatitis (acute, recurrent, chronic active, fulminant) *Rare*: hepatoma or hepatocellular carcinoma
Psychiatric	Depression, anxiety, phobias, personality or behavior change: inattention, hyperactivity, impulsivity, obsessions, compulsions Coordination difficulty and deterioration in school work *Rare*: psychosis, schizophrenia, antisocial or criminal behaviors, sexual preoccupation, disinhibition
Hematology	Hemolytic anemia, thrombocytopenia *Rare*: WD in a patient with the anti-phospholipid antibody syndrome
Ophthalmic	K-F rings, sunflower cataracts *Rare*: night blindness, optic neuritis, optic disc pallor, exotropic strabismus
Renal (rare)	Renal tubular dysfunction (hypercalciuria, hyperphosphaturia, aminoaciduria), nephrocalcinosis, hypokalemia with muscle weakness with or without respiratory paralysis (possibly due to renal tubular dysfunction)
Cardiac (rare)	Cardiomyopathy, congestive hear failure, arrhythmias
Endocrine (rare)	Hypoparathyroidism, glucose intolerance, hypoglycemia
Musculoskeletal (rare)	Osteoporosis, osteomalacia, rickets, osteochondritis, osteoarthritis, osteochondritis dissecans, chondrocalcinosis, spontaneous fractures, vertebral column abnormalities, subchondral cyst formation, azure lunulae of fingernails
Gynecologic (rare)	Infertility, menstrual irregularity, delayed puberty, gynecomastia, repeated miscarriages
Dermatologic (rare)	Leg hyperpigmentation (misinterpreted as Addison disease)

amplitude. Head titubation may be present. Dystonia is seen in nearly 40% of cases with a neurologic presentation and may involve the tongue, face, jaw, pharynx, neck, trunk and limbs [25]. Dystonia of the face and jaw may result in a stiff face with gaping mouth ("vacuous smile," "risus sardonicus") (Figure 5.1a), drooling, and dysarthria. The dysarthria seen in WD may have extrapyramidal or cerebellar or infrequently pyramidal features. Rarely patients can become anarthric and mute. A "whispering dysphonia" has been described in WD [26]. Also described is an unusual laugh in which

most of the sound is generated during inspiration [27]. An unusual cough due to respiratory dyskinesia has been reported as a presenting symptom [28]. Chorea, tics, athetosis and myoclonus are unusual. Generalized myoclonus associated with extensive white matter lesions has been described [29]. Early pseudobulbar features are common. Cerebellar dysfunction develops in approximately 25% of patients with neurologic WD. It is unusual for WD to present as a gait disorder. A painless variant of painful legs and moving toes has been reported in WD [30]. Isolated tongue protrusion movements may occur [31]. Abnormalities in extraocular movements such as slow horizontal saccades, upgaze restriction, impaired convergence and rarely eyelid apraxia or ophthalmoplegia may be seen. Seizures are infrequent [32]. Status epilepticus is rare. Autonomic dysfunction has been reported in nearly a third of cases with neurologic WD [33]. A peripheral neuropathy may also be seen and is rarely the presenting manifestation [34]. Olfactory dysfunction may be present in patients with neurologic WD; the same may parallel the severity of neurologic disease [35]. Vision and sensation are not affected. Paralysis does not occur. Pyramidal tract involvement is rare. Other reported manifestations include altered rapid eye movement sleep, hypersomnia, cramps, writer's cramp and priapism. Cognitive difficulties include frontal-executive dysfunction, difficulty with visuospatial processing, impaired memory and pseudobulbar emotional affect [36]. Cognitive impairment is often more apparent than real. Many individuals with neurologic or psychiatric disease have cirrhosis but are not symptomatic from their liver disease. In the presence of advanced liver disease, the neurologic manifestations may be mistaken for hepatic encephalopathy.

Psychiatric symptoms may predominate or antedate the neurologic symptoms [37, 38]. Psychiatric manifestations appear at some point in the course of the disease in most patients with neurologic WD. Wilson disease should be considered with unexplained psychiatric symptoms in young individuals, particularly if accompanied by neurologic or hepatic dysfunction. The most common psychiatric manifestations of WD include personality or behavior changes and mood disturbances, most commonly depression. Psychosis is rare, Antisocial or criminal behavior and sexual preoccupation and disinhibition have been reported. Other psychiatric manifestations include anxiety, phobias, attention deficit hyperactivity disorder, impulsivity, delusions, obsessive compulsive behavior, schizophrenia and manic-depressive psychosis. In the pediatric age group the manifestations are often subtle and may include coordination difficulty and deterioration in schoolwork.

Copper accumulation in the Descemet's membrane in the limbic area of the cornea (Kayser–Fleischer ring or K-F ring) is frequently seen in patients with WD, particularly so in those who have neurologic manifestations (Figure 5.4). Excess copper is uniformly distributed throughout the inner surface of the cornea. Sulfur–copper complexes are found only in the

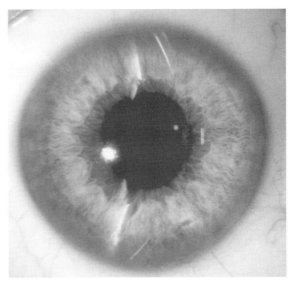

Figure 5.4. Kayser–Fleischer ring. The Kayser–Fleischer ring is due to copper accumulation in the Descemet's membrane in the limbic area of the cornea. It is frequently seen in patients with WD, particularly so in those who have neurologic manifestations. The ring is frequently not seen in those with only hepatic involvement. (See the color plate section for a color version of this figure.)

Descemet's membrane and account for the visible ring [39]. The color of the ring can be gold, brown, or green. It can be difficult to see in individuals with brown irises and is best visualized by slit lamp. Ring formation is first evident in the superior aspect of the cornea, then the inferior aspect, followed by the medial and lateral aspects. The pigment first appears in the periphery of the cornea at the limbus and then spreads centrally. The ring is frequently not seen in asymptomatic siblings and in those with only hepatic involvement (particularly children) [40]. Rarely patients with neurologic WD may not have the K-F rings [40, 41]. K-F rings are generally bilateral; unilateral formation has been reported [42]. The ring is not pathognomonic of WD and may be rarely seen in other cases of cholestatic liver disease. The K-F ring can disappear with therapy. Copper deposits in the lens are a rare occurrence and may also be seen on slit-lamp examination. They assume a sunburst or sunflower appearance (sunflower cataract) with a central disc and radiating petal-like spokes [39] and these too may also normalize with effective therapy.

Investigations

Patients with WD may show laboratory evidence of hepatic, hematologic, or renal derangement. These tests, in particular pattern of derangement in liver enzymes in patients presenting with hepatic failure, are suggestive but lack diagnostic specificity. Liver histology findings are also nonspecific. Absence of the "second peak" in the radio-copper test had been used for the diagnosis of WD. Significant overlap between affected patients and heterozygotes and technical challenges have resulted in abandonment of the test. A combination of clinical findings and biochemical testing is necessary to establish a diagnosis of WD. The laboratory hallmarks of WD include a low serum ceruloplasmin and an elevated urine 24-hour copper excretion. Hepatic copper is frequently elevated. These tests, along with genetic testing and MRI are the primary diagnostic modalities. There is no single ideal test (Table 5.3).

Serum ceruloplasmin is frequently reduced in WD; a commonly cited value is less than 20 mg/dl. However, the cut off level and normal ceruloplasmin range is dependent on the assay used (enzymatic or immunologic) and varies considerably among different laboratories. Immunologic assays are easier to perform and standardize but overestimate ceruloplasmin concentrations since they do not discriminate between apoceruloplasmin and holoceruloplasmin. Serum ceruloplasmin may be normal in 15%–25% of patients with WD, particularly so with a hepatic presentation [40]. A normal ceruloplasmin level cannot exclude the diagnosis of WD. Ceruloplasmin levels tend to be lower in patients with K-F rings or neurologic disease, and higher in patients with a hepatic presentation of WD. Approximately 10–20% of heterozygotes have decreased level of serum ceruloplasmin [43]. A low ceruloplasmin can also be seen in chronic or fulminant liver disease, in copper deficiency of various causes, and with renal or enteric protein loss. Ceruloplasmin is absent in aceruloplasminemia (a disorder of iron metabolism). Serum ceruloplasmin is low in carriers of aceruloplasminemia. A low level of ceruloplasmin is therefore not sufficient to make the diagnosis of WD. A subnormal ceruloplasmin in fact has a very low positive predictive value for WD [43]. Serum ceruloplasmin concentration is age-dependent. It can be low in normal neonates, rises to adult levels in the first year, further increases to its maximum at 2–3 years of age, and then falls until 12 years of age when it reaches adult levels. Ceruloplasmin is also an acute-phase reactant and its levels increases with inflammation, infection, trauma, hepatitis, estrogen supplementation, steroid use and pregnancy.

Most of the copper in serum is bound to ceruloplasmin; less than 5% circulates as free copper. Normal serum copper ranges from 75 to 145 µg/dl. Serum copper in WD is frequently less than 100 µg/dl. This simply reflects reduced ceruloplasmin. Hemolysis associated with liver disease may result in substantially elevated serum copper levels. In acute fulminant hepatic failure due to WD, serum copper levels may be markedly elevated owing to sudden copper release from tissue stores. Normal or elevated serum copper in association with decreased ceruloplasmin indicates increase in non-ceruloplasmin-bound copper. Normal values of non-ceruloplasmin (free) copper range from 8 to 12 µg/dl. This nonceruloplasmin-bound copper is over 25 µg/dl in most untreated patients with WD. It is also elevated in acute liver failure of any cause, chronic cholestasis, and copper poisoning. Direct measurements of free copper concentration is not routinely available [44]. The free serum copper can be calculated by subtracting three times the ceruloplasmin level (mg/dl) from the total serum copper (µg/dl) [5]. The non-ceruloplasmin-bound copper concentration is useful in monitoring therapy and values <5 µg/dl in combination with low 24-hour urinary copper excretion may indicate systemic copper depletion that may rarely occur with prolonged therapy. This measurement is also valuable in cases in which falsely high levels of serum ceruloplasmin are suspected, and when a measurement of urinary copper is difficult to obtain.

Urinary copper excretion reflects the amount of non-ceruloplasmin-bound copper in the circulation. Twenty-four-hour urinary copper excretion is frequently increased in patients with WD (generally over 100 µg). Twenty-four-hour urinary copper excretion may be less than 100 µg at presentation in approximately 10–20% of patients diagnosed with WD [40]. Despite this limitation it is perhaps the best available screening test. It may be elevated in other cholestatic disorders also. Intermediate levels of urinary copper excretion may be seen in heterozygote and presymptomatic individuals. Incorrect collection and copper contamination are common sources of error. Copper-free jugs should be used for collection. Samples from children may show reduced urinary copper excretion because of difficulties with sample collection. Urinary copper excretion may not be elevated in neonates with low body copper load. Even after administration of penicillamine, 24-hour urinary copper is not consistently elevated in WD [45]. Further, this provocation test has only been standardized in a pediatric population.

Normal liver copper concentrations rarely exceed 50 µg/g dry weight of liver. In about 80% of patients with

Table 5.3. Laboratory diagnosis of Wilson disease (WD).

Parameter	Normal	Causes of increase	Causes of decrease	Additional comments
Serum ceruloplasmin (Reduced in WD, often <20 mg/dl)	20–40 mg/dl (varies among different laboratories, depends on method employed)	Infection Inflammation Trauma Hepatitis Estrogen supplementation Steroid use Pregnancy	WD Approximately 20% of WD heterozygotes Chronic or fulminant liver disease Renal or enteric protein loss Copper deficiency (gastric surgery, malabsorption zinc ingestion) Aceruloplasminemia Aceruloplasminemia (or carrier state) Neonates	Normal in approximately 20% of WD patients, particularly with hepatic presentation Ceruloplasmin is an acute-phase reactant
Serum copper (Reduced in WD, often <100 µg/dl)	75–145 µg/dl	Acute liver disease with or without hemolysis Copper poisoning	WD Copper deficiency Cirrhosis	Generally parallels ceruloplasmin Useful for calculating non-ceruloplasmin-bound (free) serum copper
Urinary 24-hour copper excretion (Elevated in WD, often >100 µg)	15–60 µg	WD WD heterozygotes and presymptomatic WD (intermediate values) Liver failure Chronic cholestasis Chelators	Copper deficiency	<100 µg/24 h in 10–20% of WD False-negative in presymptomatic cases Care with contamination and incomplete collection Provocative chelation of limited utility
Liver copper (Elevated in WD, often >250 µg/g dry weight)	<50 µg/g dry weight	WD WD heterozygotes and presymptomatic WD (intermediate values) Chronic cholestasis Copper toxicosis	Fulminant liver disease Cirrhosis	False-negative in WD with insufficient tissue and sampling errors Can rarely be <50 µg/g dry weight in WD Care with contamination

WD the value is over 250 µg/g dry tissue [46]. Hepatic copper elevations are also seen in asymptomatic individuals with WD. Hepatic copper concentration in heterozygotes is frequently elevated above normal but does not exceed 250 µg/g dry weight. Other instances of elevated liver copper levels are found in patients with chronic cholestasis, in neonates and young children, in subjects with exogenous copper overload, and in idiopathic copper toxicosis syndromes such as Indian childhood cirrhosis. Hepatic copper may be <50 µg/g in 3.5% of WD cases [46]. Low hepatic copper values may be seen in WD with advanced cirrhosis. The cirrhotic liver may have significant regional differences in hepatic copper distribution and sampling error may be

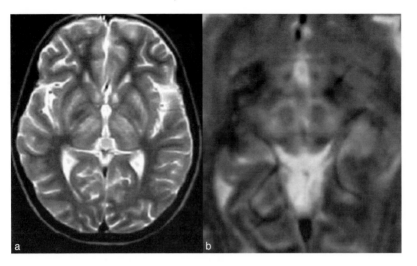

Figure 5.5. Brain MRI in Wilson disease. (a) Axial T2-weighted MRI of a patient with WD showing bilateral basal ganglia and thalamic hyperintensity. (b) Axial T2-weighted MRI of a patient with WD showing "face of the giant panda" sign. (Reproduced with permission from reference 48.)

responsible for normal or borderline values of hepatic copper content. Contamination, particularly in block specimens, may result in falsely elevated hepatic copper values. Despite this limitation determination of hepatic copper is perhaps the best available biochemical test, though it is invasive and is not required in all cases. Its use should be reserved for those cases where simpler approaches have not provided a definitive diagnosis. Further, it is generally not required in patients with neurologic disease as other tests can provide the diagnosis. Its utility is primarily in patients who present with hepatic dysfunction as in these cases the copper has not been discharged to other tissues.

Brain CT is relatively insensitive for the diagnosis of WD. It may reveal hypodensities and atrophy involving the basal ganglia, brain stem, cerebellum and cerebral cortex [47]. Brain MRI abnormalities are seen in nearly all patients with neurological WD [48]. T2-weighted sequences show increased T2 signal in the caudate, putamen, thalamus, midbrain (including substantia nigra pars compacta), periaqueductal gray, pontine tegmentum, medulla, vermis and dentate nuclei [5, 48]. Putaminal lesions with a bilateral, symmetric, concentric-laminar T2 hyperintensity are a characteristic finding. Also reported is increased T2 signal involving the subcortical white matter and cortex [48, 49]. A leukoencephalopathy may be more common in patients of Asian descent [50]. Extensive white matter changes and severe atrophy may be poor prognostic factors [51]. T2-weighted sequences may show midbrain changes that have been referred to as "face of the giant panda" or pontine tegmentum changes that have been referred to as "face of the miniature panda" or both ("double panda sign" or "faces

of the giant panda and her cub") [52–54]. "Face of the giant panda" refers to the appearance that results from hyperintensity of the mesencephalon with sparing of the red nuclei and lateral aspect of the substantia nigra (Figure 5.5). Also reported is the "bright claustrum" sign [55]. These imaging signs are relatively rare. T2-weighted images may also show basal ganglia hypointensity due to deposition of iron in exchange for copper following chelation. On T1-weighted sequences MRI may reveal basal ganglia hypointensities. T1-weighted pallidal hyperintensity may also be seen [48]. This indicates underlying liver disease and may be due to portosystemic shunting and manganese deposition. With disease progression a restricted diffusion pattern involving the basal ganglia may be replaced by increased diffusion [56]. Signal abnormalities vary with stage of the disease and may be reversible with therapy in the early stages.

Magnetic resonance spectroscopy (MRS) in WD may show evidence of neuronal loss (reduction in the *N*-acetylaspartate:creatine and choline:creatine ratios) [57, 58]. Creatine is relatively stable as it is present in glial cells, which are less affected in WD. MRS may also show decreased levels of myo-inositol in patients with portosystemic shunting [57]. MRS may have some utility in monitoring treatment efficacy in WD [59]. Single-photon emission computed tomography (SPECT) imaging has shown evidence of presynaptic dopaminergic damage [60]. SPECT scans have shown a decrease in dopamine transporter function and in D2 receptors in the striatum. Positron emission tomography (PET) using (^{18}F)fluorodopa shows reduced uptake in the striatum indicating loss of the dopaminergic nigrostriatal pathway [61]. Transcranial sonography may show lenticular hyperechogenicity [62]. The same may also be seen in asymptomatic individuals with WD. It has been suggested that this correlates with disease severity and may be useful for disease monitoring.

ATP7B is a relatively large gene (approximately 80 kb in size) and comprises 21 exons [17]. The large number of mutations reported in the WD gene and the presence of regulatory mutations in noncoding regions, had made commercial genetic testing impractical. The advent of high-throughput methodologies has changed the mutation identification paradigm. Molecular testing can be a valuable tool in the work-up of a suspected patient, particularly so when routine testing is equivocal. The presence of two mutations (one per allele) can confirm the diagnosis. While there are several mutations that occur at an appreciable frequency in specific ethnic groups, the vast majority of patients are compound heterozygous for one common mutation and one rare mutation. Given this, the preferred approach is direct DNA sequencing. In this method, the entire coding region of the gene is sequenced without prior selection of candidate exons. Furthermore, once mutations are identified in the index patient, asymptomatic relatives can be screened for carrier status by direct mutation analysis of the known familial mutations. Haplotype analysis of markers around the *ATP7B* gene may have a role in sibling screening when it has not been possible to detect both mutations in the index patient by mutation analysis or direct DNA sequencing.

All first-degree relatives of known patients should be screened for WD. Laboratory abnormalities or clinical signs may indicate need for prophylactic treatment. In some cases a liver biopsy or molecular genetic testing may be required.

Treatment

The treatment of WD is directed at restoring and maintaining copper balance. A lifelong commitment to treatment is required. Limitation of dietary copper intake is desirable but is generally ineffective. Pharmacological management is necessary (Table 5.4). Pharmacologic treatment is based on the use of chelators to promote copper excretion or of zinc to reduce copper absorption, or both. The initial treatment of symptomatic patients is with chelating agents such as penicillamine or trientine. Some reports suggest that primary treatment with zinc alone may be adequate in some patients. In the maintenance phase (typically 2–6 months after initiation of therapy), the dose of these chelating agents is reduced. Alternatively, the chelators are replaced by

zinc or zinc is added to prevent further copper absorption. The potential role of combination therapy of zinc in conjunction with, but temporally separated from, a chelator such as trientine or penicillamine or tetrathiomolybdate has theoretical appeal but few studies are available [63, 64]. Asymptomatic patients are treated with maintenance doses of chelators or zinc from the outset. The definitive treatment is liver transplantation. Transplantation is considered in patients refractory to medical treatment and is often required in patients who present with fulminant hepatic failure. Its potential role in patients with neurologic disease is encouraging but awaits further studies. The severity of the disease at the time of initiation of treatment determines the level of disability. Complete recovery can be expected with timely intervention. Residual dysarthria and mild dystonia are common neurologic sequelae.

Penicillamine has a free sulfhydryl group that functions as the copper-chelating moiety. It reduces copper bound to protein, which in turn decreases affinity of the protein to copper and permits binding of copper to penicillamine. It may also act by inducing metallothionein in individuals with WD. By promoting metallothionein synthesis, it detoxifies tissue copper. Copper chelation with penicillamine is an effective therapy for WD [65]. It is started in a dose of 250–500 mg/day and increased by 250 mg every 4–7 days to a target dose of 1–2 g/day in two to four divided doses. Initial neurologic deterioration may occur. There are no data to confirm that a gradual titration decreases the risk of initial neurologic deterioration. Penicillamine should be given 1 hour before or 2 hours after meals. Penicillamine is a pyridoxine antagonist. Vitamin B_6 supplementation in a dose of 25–50 mg/week is often recommended. Currently, however, penicillamine is synthesized and the racemic mixtures that interfered with pyridoxine action are no longer used. There is no consensus on the continued need for pyridoxine supplementation. The copper mobilized by penicillamine is then excreted in the urine. It takes weeks (often 2–6 months) before clinical improvement is evident and improvement may continue over 1–2 years. Psychiatric manifestations improve less consistently than neurologic disease. Initially there is significant cupruresis. Subsequently copper excretion decreases to around 0.5 mg/day. Serum ceruloplasmin tends to decrease after initiation of treatment. It may increase with recovery of synthetic liver function. With established clinical and biochemical benefit, the dose of penicillamine

Table 5.4. Treatment of Wilson disease.

	Mechanism of action	Dose	Side-effects	Additional comments
Penicillamine 250 mg capsule 250 mg tablet	Chelation of copper	*Initial*: 1000–2000 mg/day *Maintenance*: 500–1000 mg/day	*Early*: leukopenia, eosinophilia, thrombocytopenia, fever, cutaneous, lymphadenopathy, proteinuria *Late*: nephrotoxicity, lupuslike, polyarthritis, Goodpasture syndrome, myasthenia gravis-like, polymyositis, bone marrow suppression, loss of taste, IgA depression, serous retinitis, hepatotoxicity, dermatologic toxicities	On empty stomach, 2–4 divided doses a day Initial neurologic deterioration Monitoring: cell blood count, liver enzymes, serum copper and ceruloplasmin, 24-hour urine copper Target 24-hour urinary copper: 200–500 µg
Trientine 250 mg capsule	Chelation of copper	*Initial*: 750–2000 mg/day *Maintenance*: 750–1000 mg/day	Sideroblastic anemia, pancytopenia Lupus nephritis Copper deficiency (rare)	On empty stomach, 2–3 divided doses Target 24-hour urinary copper: 200–500 µg
Zinc Zinc-220 capsule (220 mg of zinc sulfate containing 50 mg of elemental zinc) Many other formulations	Decrease copper absorption	*Initial*: 150 mg elemental zinc/day *Maintenance*: 75–100 mg elemental zinc/day	Gastrointestinal distress Copper deficiency (rare)	On empty stomach, 2–3 divided doses a day Target 24-hour urinary copper: <75 µg Target 24-hour urinary zinc: >2000 µg
Tetrathiomolybdate Investigational drug	Decrease copper absorption and chelation	*Initial*: 20 mg three times a day with meals and 20 mg three times a day between meals (Not intended for long-term use)	Bone marrow suppression Aminotransferase elevation Copper deficiency (rare)	With and between meals, 6 divided doses Initial neurologic deterioration is rare and may relate to rapid dose escalation

For all treatment modalities the target non-ceruloplasmin-bound copper is 5–15 µg/day.

can be reduced to 500–1000 mg/day in two divided doses. Zinc can be added and is given on an empty stomach, temporally separated from penicillamine. With maintenance therapy, 24-hour urinary copper excretion should be in the range 200–500 µg/day and non-ceruloplasmin-bound copper should normalize; a suggested target is between 5 and 15 µg/dl. An increase in receding or stable 24-hour urinary copper excretion may indicate suboptimal compliance. A serum non-ceruloplasmin-bound copper level below 5 µg/dl may suggest overtreatment. During penicillamine administration, clinical, hematologic, biochemical (transaminases, serum ceruloplasmin and copper) and urinary (protein and 24-hour copper) parameters are monitored periodically (weekly for the first month, monthly for the next 6 months, and 6-monthly thereafter). Significant toxicity including acute neurologic deterioration following initiation of therapy has raised some skepticism about penicillamine being the first-line agent [66–68]. The neurologic deterioration can be severe; in one patient it resulted in severe dystonia (status dystonicus) and death [25]. Worsening of neurologic symptoms during the initial treatment phase is generally seen after 6 weeks but may be seen from 2 weeks to 12 months. Following initial deterioration, patients may not return to their baseline level of functioning. When neurologic deterioration is present, the drug can be withdrawn and reintroduced in a smaller dose with a slower titration with or without steroid cover. If neurologic deterioration recurs, the medication should be withdrawn and replaced by other chelators or zinc alone. Severe side-effects requiring drug discontinuation occur in 10–30% of patients. Immune-mediated side-effects generally occur within the first 3 weeks and if they are present prompt cessation of therapy is required. These include leukopenia, eosinophilia, thrombocytopenia, fever and cutaneous eruptions, lymphadenopathy and proteinuria. Late reactions include nephrotoxicity (nephrotic syndrome), lupus-like syndrome, polyarthritis, Goodpasture syndrome, myasthenia gravis-like syndrome, polymyositis, bone marrow suppression, loss of taste, immunoglobulin A depression, serous retinitis (retinal hemorrhages), hepatotoxicity and a spectrum of dermatologic toxicities (aphthous stomatitis, elastosis perforans serpiginosa, progeriatric changes). Penicillamine dermatopathy refers to a brownish skin discoloration and is due to recurrent subcutaneous bleeding during incidental trauma [69]. There is damage of collagen and elastin, which causes weakness of subcutaneous tissue so that slight trauma causes bleeding, leaving brown papules with wrinkling and thinning of the skin. Also reported is hypothyroidism in children and in infants born to a mother on penicillamine treatment for WD [70].

Trientine (triethylenetetramine) has a similar mechanism of action to that of penicillamine. It is less potent and the initial deterioration is of less concern [63, 67]. It is considered by many as the initial therapy of choice, even with decompensated liver disease. It is often used in patients intolerant to penicillamine.

The usual dose is 750–2000 mg/day in two or three divided doses on an empty stomach. Lower doses (750 or 1000 mg/day) are used for maintenance therapy. The targeted 24-hour urinary copper excretion should be in the range 200–500 μg/day and non-ceruloplasmin-bound copper should normalize. Sideroblastic anemia is a major adverse effect. Pancytopenia and lupus nephritis have been reported rarely. Copper deficiency induced by trientine may result in iron overload in livers of patients with WD, similar to that observed for penicillamine [71].

Zinc induces metallothionein formation in the intestinal enterocyte. The increased metallothionein binds copper preferentially and traps it within the intestinal mucosal cells. These cells are eventually sloughed off and excreted in the feces. Since copper also enters the gastrointestinal tract from saliva and gastric secretions, zinc can remove stored copper and generate a negative copper balance [72]. Zinc may also act by inducing levels of hepatocellular metallothionein [73]. Zinc has assumed an increasingly important role in the management of WD [72, 74]. It has a role in chronic maintenance therapy following initial therapy with more potent decoppering agents and for management of WD in pregnancy and in children. More recently, zinc monotherapy has been proposed as initial therapy, particularly so for mild cases. Owing to the slow response it is not the preferred agent for initial therapy in severe cases. It has a role in the life-long management of preclinical WD. Zinc is administered as acetate, sulfate, or gluconate. Acetate may cause the least gastrointestinal distress and gluconate may be more tolerable than sulfate. Zinc sulfate (25–50 mg three times a day at least 1 hour apart from meals) may help maintain a neutral or even negative copper balance. Neurologic deterioration is uncommon. Urinary copper excretion should be less than 75 μg per 24 hours on stable treatment. A 24-hour urinary zinc excretion of less than 2 mg indicates inadequate compliance. In a patient on zinc maintenance therapy, a 24-hour urinary copper below 35 μg may indicate copper deficiency due to overtreatment. Additionally, non-ceruloplasmin-bound copper should normalize with effective treatment. Rarely, overtreatment of WD with zinc may cause hematologic manifestations of copper deficiency or a copper deficiency-related axonal sensorimotor peripheral neuropathy [75].

Ammonium tetrathiomolybdate has a unique dual mechanism of action. It limits gastrointestinal absorption of copper by forming a nonabsorbable tripartite complex with copper and albumin within the gut lumen. Formation of the same complex in the bloodstream prevents cellular uptake of free copper. This dual mechanism of action necessitates a complicated dosing regimen: ammonium tetrathiomolybdate binds copper in the gut when given with food and is best absorbed into the bloodstream when given on an empty stomach. It has been used in a dose of 60–180 mg/day. A typical regimen is 20 mg given six times a day: three times a day with meals and three times a day between meals. With time, tissue stores become depleted. Initial worsening of neurologic symptoms is rare and may relate to rapid dose escalation [64, 76]. A rapid reduction in circulating non-ceruloplasmin-bound copper occurs during the first 8 weeks of therapy [64, 76, 77]. Rarely, copper depletion and cytopenias, reversible bone marrow suppression, or aminotransferase elevation may complicate ammonium tetrathiomolybdate therapy. It is not intended for long-term treatment. The initial 8 weeks of therapy is followed by long-term maintenance therapy with zinc. Neurologic recovery is often delayed and may occur over the first few years. Ammonium tetrathiomolybdate has not been approved by the FDA and has limited availability.

The mortality rate with medical treatment in patients with WD who develop fulminant hepatic failure is close to 100%. Hepatic transplantation is curative in such individuals. Treatments such as plasmapheresis and hemofiltration may help bridge the patients to transplantation. Orthotopic liver transplantation only partially corrects the underlying metabolic defect and converts the copper kinetics from that characteristic of an individual affected with a homozygous disease to that of an individual who is an obligate heterozygote, thereby resulting in a phenotypic cure. Living donor liver transplantation has also been successfully employed in WD [78]. Copper metabolism may be suboptimal if the donor was a WD carrier. The role of liver transplantation in the management of patients with neurologic WD in the absence of hepatic insufficiency is encouraging but still uncertain [79, 80]. Patients with neuropsychiatric and hepatic dysfunction have a lower survival than those with hepatic dysfunction alone. Many of these patients can be managed with chelation therapy. There are reports of patients who have shown no neurologic improvement or neurologic worsening, as well as reports of patients with neurologic improvement with or without coexisting hepatic disease.

Although penicillamine and trientine are potentially teratogenic, the available information is not sufficient to warrant discontinuation of treatment with these agents during pregnancy. Their use through pregnancy has been associated with a satisfactory outcome, but dose reduction of 25–50% is required. The dosage of zinc salts is maintained without change in pregnancy. Abrupt cessation of the drug can be fatal. With adequate decoppering, maintenance with zinc alone can suffice. Therapy with British anti-Lewisite (BAL) is rarely employed but may have been life-saving in some cases. BAL is not suitable for chronic therapy. Symptomatic treatment with antidystonia drugs such as levodopa, dopamine agonists, tizanidine, baclofen, benzodiazepines and anticholinergics may be beneficial. Botulinum toxin injection can be used in focal limb dystonia. Often more than one antiepileptic drug is required for seizure control. Atypical neuroleptics are used to manage psychiatric disturbance. Hepatic encephalopathy is managed with protein restriction and lactulose.

Conclusion

Advances in genetic testing technology have permitted easier identification of affected alleles. Molecular diagnosis and use of genetic testing in screening of first-degree relatives will likely find wider use. Continued compilation of results of mutation analysis (www.wilsondisease.med.ualberta.ca/database.asp) will permit separation of function-altering mutations from incidental polymorphisms. Population screening using techniques such as immunoassay for urinary ceruloplasmin or ceruloplasmin detection in protein eluted from stored blood spots may find a role in newborn screening. Tetrathiomolybdate may be an additional therapeutic option in patients with a neurological presentation. Living donor liver transplantation holds promise. Liver transplantation for a primary neurologic indication needs further studies. Experimental models for hepatocyte transplant and gene therapy are additional areas of active research. These future directions are discussed in a recent review [81].

References

1. Ferenci P, Caca K, Loudianos G et al. Diagnosis and phenotypic classification of Wilson disease. *Liver Int* 2003; **23**: 139–42.

2. El-Youssef M. Wilson disease. *Mayo Clin Proc* 2003; **78**: 1126–36.

3. Prashanth LK, Taly AB, Sinha S, Arunodaya GR, Swamy HS. Wilson's disease: diagnostic errors and clinical implications. *J Neurol Neurosurg Psychiatry* 2004; **75**: 907–9.

4. Brewer GJ, Askari FK. Wilson's disease: clinical management and therapy. *J Hepatol* 2005; **42**(Suppl 1): S13–21.

5. Das SK, Ray K. Wilson's disease: an update. *Nat Clin Pract Neurol* 2006; **2**: 482–93.

6. Ala A, Walker AP, Ashkan K, Dooley JS, Schilsky ML. Wilson's disease. *Lancet* 2007; **369**: 397–408.

7. Pfeiffer RF. Wilson's disease. *Semin Neurol* 2007; **27**: 123–32.

8. Taly AB, Meenakshi-Sundaram S, Sinha S, Swamy HS, Arunodaya GR. Wilson disease: description of 282 patients evaluated over 3 decades. *Medicine (Baltimore)* 2007; **86**: 112–21.

9. Merle U, Schaefer M, Ferenci P, Stremmel W. Clinical presentation, diagnosis and long-term outcome of Wilson's disease: a cohort study. *Gut* 2007; **56**: 115–20.

10. Roberts EA, Schilsky ML, American Association for Study of Liver Diseases (AASLD). Diagnosis and treatment of Wilson disease: an update. *Hepatology* 2008; **47**: 2089–111.

11. Scheinberg IH, Sternlieb I. Wilson's disease. *Major Probl Intern Med* 1984; **23**: 1–24.

12. Wilson SAK. Progressive lenticular degeneration: a familial nervous disease associated with cirrhosis of the liver. *Brain* 1912; **34**: 295–509.

13. Walshe JM. History of Wilson's disease: 1912 to 2000. *Mov Disord* 2006; **21**: 142–7.

14. Tanzi RE, Petrukhin K, Chernov I *et al.* The Wilson disease gene is a copper transporting ATPase with homology to the Menkes disease gene. *Nat Genet* 1993; **5**: 344–50.

15. Bull PC, Thomas GR, Rommens JM, Forbes JR, Cox DW. The Wilson disease gene is a putative copper transporting P-type ATPase similar to the Menkes gene. *Nat Genet* 1993; **5**: 327–37.

16. Yamaguchi Y, Heiny ME, Gitlin JD. Isolation and characterization of a human liver cDNA as a candidate gene for Wilson disease. *Biochem Biophys Res Commun* 1993; **197**: 271–7.

17. Petrukhin K, Fischer SG, Pirastu M *et al.* Mapping, cloning and genetic characterization of the region containing the Wilson disease gene. *Nat Genet* 1993; **5**: 338–43.

18. Cox DW, Prat L, Walshe JM, Heathcote J, Gaffney D. Twenty-four novel mutations in Wilson disease patients of predominantly European ancestry. *Hum Mutat* 2005; **26**: 280.

19. Gromadzka G, Schmidt HH, Genschel J *et al.* Frameshift and nonsense mutations in the gene for ATPase7B are associated with severe impairment of copper metabolism and with an early clinical manifestation of Wilson's disease. *Clin Genet* 2005; **68**: 524–32.

20. Schiefermeier M, Kollegger H, Madl C *et al.* The impact of apolipoprotein E genotypes on age at onset of symptoms and phenotypic expression in Wilson's disease. *Brain* 2000; **123**(Pt 3): 585–90.

21. Mufti AR, Burstein E, Csomos RA *et al.* XIAP Is a copper binding protein deregulated in Wilson's disease and other copper toxicosis disorders. *Mol Cell* 2006; **17**(21): 775–85.

22. Ala A, Borjigin J, Rochwarger A, Schilsky M. Wilson disease in septuagenarian siblings: raising the bar for diagnosis. *Hepatology* 2005; **41**: 668–70.

23. Schilsky ML, Fink S. Inherited metabolic liver disease. *Curr Opin Gastroenterol* 2006; **22**: 215–22.

24. Poston KL, Frucht SJ. Movement disorder emergencies. *J Neurol* 2008; **255**(Suppl 4): 2–13.

25. Svetel M, Kozic D, Stefanova E, Semnic R, Dragasevic N, Kostic VS. Dystonia in Wilson's disease. *Mov Disord* 2001; **16**: 719–23.

26. Parker N. Hereditary whispering dysphonia. *J Neurol Neurosurg Psychiatry* 1985; **48**: 218–24.

27. Cartwright GE. Diagnosis of treatable Wilson's disease. *N Engl J Med* 1978; **298**: 1347–50.

28. Crone NE, Jinnah HA, Reich SG. Wilson's disease presenting with an unusual cough. *Mov Disord* 2005; **20**: 891–3.

29. Barbosa ER, Silveira-Moriyama L, Machado AC, Bacheschi LA, Rosemberg S, Scaff M. Wilson's disease with myoclonus and white matter lesions. *Parkinsonism Relat Disord* 2007; **13**: 185–8.

30. Papapetropoulos S, Singer C. Painless legs moving toes in a patient with Wilson's disease. *Mov Disord* 2006; **21**: 579–80.

31. Kumar TS, Moses PD. Isolated tongue involvement – an unusual presentation of Wilson's disease. *J Postgrad Med* 2005; **51**: 337.

32. Dening TR, Berrios GE, Walshe JM. Wilson's disease and epilepsy. *Brain* 1988; **111**(Pt 5): 1139–55.

33. Meenakshi-Sundaram S, Taly AB, Kamath V, Arunodaya GR, Rao S, Swamy HS. Autonomic dysfunction in Wilson's disease – a clinical and electrophysiological study. *Clin Auton Res* 2002; **12**: 185–9.

34. Jung KH, Ahn TB, Jeon BS. Wilson disease with an initial manifestation of polyneuropathy. *Arch Neurol* 2005; **62**: 1628–31.

35. Mueller A, Reuner U, Landis B, Kitzler H, Reichmann H, Hummel T. Extrapyramidal symptoms in Wilson's disease are associated with olfactory dysfunction. *Mov Disord* 2006; **21**: 1311–6.

36. Seniow J, Bak T, Gajda J, Poniatowska R, Czlonkowska A. Cognitive functioning in neurologically symptomatic

and asymptomatic forms of Wilson's disease. *Mov Disord* 2002; **17**: 1077–83.

37. Dening TR. The neuropsychiatry of Wilson's disease: a review. *Int J Psychiatry Med* 1991; **21**: 135–48.

38. Lin JJ, Lin KL, Wang HS, Wong MC. Psychological presentations without hepatic involvement in Wilson disease. *Pediatr Neurol* 2006; **35**: 284–6.

39. Wiebers DO, Hollenhorst RW, Goldstein NP. The ophthalmologic manifestations of Wilson's disease. *Mayo Clin Proc* 1977; **52**: 409–16.

40. Steindl P, Ferenci P, Dienes HP *et al*. Wilson's disease in patients presenting with liver disease: a diagnostic challenge. *Gastroenterology* 1997; **113**: 212–8.

41. Demirkiran M, Jankovic J, Lewis RA, Cox DW. Neurologic presentation of Wilson disease without Kayser–Fleischer rings. *Neurology* 1996; **46**: 1040–3.

42. Innes JR, Strachan IM, Triger DR. Unilateral Kayser–Fleischer ring. *Br J Ophthalmol* 1986; **70**: 469–70.

43. Cauza E, Maier-Dobersberger T, Polli C, Kaserer K, Kramer L, Ferenci P. Screening for Wilson's disease in patients with liver diseases by serum ceruloplasmin. *J Hepatol* 1997; **27**: 358–62.

44. McMillin GA, Travis JJ, Hunt JW. Direct measurement of free copper in serum or plasma ultrafiltrate. *Am J Clin Pathol* 2009; **131**: 160–5.

45. Martins da Costa C, Baldwin D, Portmann B, Lolin Y, Mowat AP, Mieli-Vergani G. Value of urinary copper excretion after penicillamine challenge in the diagnosis of Wilson's disease. *Hepatology* 1992; **15**: 609–15.

46. Ferenci P, Steindl-Munda P, Vogel W *et al*. Diagnostic value of quantitative hepatic copper determination in patients with Wilson's disease. *Clin Gastroenterol Hepatol* 2005; **3**: 811–8.

47. Williams FJ, Walshe JM. Wilson's disease. An analysis of the cranial computerized tomographic appearances found in 60 patients and the changes in response to treatment with chelating agents. *Brain* 1981; **104**(Pt 4): 735–52.

48. Sinha S, Taly AB, Ravishankar S *et al*. Wilson's disease: cranial MRI observations and clinical correlation. *Neuroradiology* 2006; **48**: 613–21.

49. Hedera P, Brewer GJ, Fink JK. White matter changes in Wilson disease. *Arch Neurol* 2002; **59**: 866–7.

50. Yoshii F, Takahashi W, Shinohara Y. A Wilson's disease patient with prominent cerebral white matter lesions: five-year follow-up by MRI. *Eur Neurol* 1996; **36**: 392–3.

51. Sinha S, Taly AB, Prashanth LK, Ravishankar S, Arunodaya GR, Vasudev MK. Sequential MRI changes in Wilson's disease with de-coppering therapy: a study of 50 patients. *Br J Radiol* 2007; **80**: 744–9.

52. Giagheddu M, Tamburini G, Piga M *et al*. Comparison of MRI, EEG, EPs and ECD-SPECT in Wilson's disease. *Acta Neurol Scand* 2001; **103**: 71–81.

53. Jacobs DA, Markowitz CE, Liebeskind DS, Galetta SL. The "double panda sign" in Wilson's disease. *Neurology* 2003; **61**: 969.

54. Liebeskind DS, Wong S, Hamilton RH. Faces of the giant panda and her cub: MRI correlates of Wilson's disease. *J Neurol Neurosurg Psychiatry* 2003; **74**: 682.

55. Sener RN. The claustrum on MRI: normal anatomy, and the bright claustrum as a new sign in Wilson's disease. *Pediatr Radiol* 1993; **23**: 594–6.

56. Sener RN. Diffusion MR imaging changes associated with Wilson disease. *AJNR Am J Neuroradiol* 2003; **24**: 965–7.

57. Van Den Heuvel AG, Van der Grond J, Van Rooij LG, Van Wassenaer-van Hall HN, Hoogenraad TU, Mali WP. Differentiation between portal-systemic encephalopathy and neurodegenerative disorders in patients with Wilson disease: H-1 MR spectroscopy. *Radiology* 1997; **203**: 539–43.

58. Lucato LT, Otaduy MC, Barbosa ER *et al*. Proton MR spectroscopy in Wilson disease: analysis of 36 cases. *AJNR Am J Neuroradiol* 2005; **26**: 1066–71.

59. Tarnacka B, Szeszkowski W, Golebiowski M, Czlonkowska A. MR spectroscopy in monitoring the treatment of Wilson's disease patients. *Mov Disord* 2008; **23**: 1560–6.

60. Jeon B, Kim JM, Jeong JM *et al*. Dopamine transporter imaging with [^{123}I]-beta-CIT demonstrates presynaptic nigrostriatal dopaminergic damage in Wilson's disease. *J Neurol Neurosurg Psychiatry* 1998; **65**: 60–4.

61. Snow BJ, Bhatt M, Martin WR, Li D, Calne DB. The nigrostriatal dopaminergic pathway in Wilson's disease studied with positron emission tomography. *J Neurol Neurosurg Psychiatry* 1991; **54**: 12–7.

62. Walter U, Krolikowski K, Tarnacka B, Benecke R, Czlonkowska A, Dressler D. Sonographic detection of basal ganglia lesions in asymptomatic and symptomatic Wilson disease. *Neurology* 2005; **64**: 1726–32.

63. Askari FK, Greenson J, Dick RD, Johnson VD, Brewer GJ. Treatment of Wilson's disease with zinc. XVIII. Initial treatment of the hepatic decompensation presentation with trientine and zinc. *J Lab Clin Med* 2003; **142**: 385–90.

64. Brewer GJ, Askari F, Lorincz MT *et al*. Treatment of Wilson disease with ammonium tetrathiomolybdate: IV. Comparison of tetrathiomolybdate and trientine in a double-blind study of treatment of the neurologic presentation of Wilson disease. *Arch Neurol* 2006; **63**: 521–7.

65. Walshe JM. Penicillamine: the treatment of first choice for patients with Wilson's disease. *Mov Disord* 1999; **14**: 545–50.

66. Brewer GJ, Terry CA, Aisen AM, Hill GM. Worsening of neurologic syndrome in patients with Wilson's dis-

ease with initial penicillamine therapy. *Arch Neurol* 1987; **44**(5): 490–3.

67. Brewer GJ. Penicillamine should not be used as initial therapy in Wilson's disease. *Mov Disord* 1999; **14**: 551–4.

68. LeWitt PA. Penicillamine as a controversial treatment for Wilson's disease. *Mov Disord* 1999; **14**: 555–6.

69. Sternlieb I, Fisher M, Scheinberg IH. Penicillamine-induced skin lesions. *J Rheumatol Suppl* 1981; **7**: 149–54.

70. Hanukoglu A, Curiel B, Berkowitz D, Levine A, Sack J, Lorberboym M. Hypothyroidism and dyshormonogenesis induced by D-penicillamine in children with Wilson's disease and healthy infants born to a mother with Wilson's disease. *J Pediatr* 2008; **153**: 864–6.

71. Shiono Y, Wakusawa S, Hayashi H *et al.* Iron accumulation in the liver of male patients with Wilson's disease. *Am J Gastroenterol* 2001; **96**: 3147–51.

72. Brewer GJ, Hill GM, Prasad AS, Cossack ZT, Rabbani P. Oral zinc therapy for Wilson's disease. *Ann Intern Med* 1983; **99**: 314–9.

73. Schilsky ML, Blank RR, Czaja MJ *et al.* Hepatocellular copper toxicity and its attenuation by zinc. *J Clin Invest* 1989; **84**: 1562–8.

74. Hoogenraad TU, Van Hattum J, Van den Hamer CJ. Management of Wilson's disease with zinc sulphate. Experience in a series of 27 patients. *J Neurol Sci* 1987; **77**(2–3): 137–46.

75. Foubert-Samier A, Kazadi A, Rouanet M *et al.* Axonal sensory motor neuropathy in copper-deficient Wilson's disease. *Muscle Nerve* 2009; **40**: 294–6.

76. Brewer GJ, Hedera P, Kluin KJ *et al.* Treatment of Wilson disease with ammonium tetrathiomolybdate: III. Initial therapy in a total of 55 neurologically affected patients and follow-up with zinc therapy. *Arch Neurol* 2003; **60**: 379–85.

77. Brewer GJ, Askari F, Dick RB *et al.* Treatment of Wilson's disease with tetrathiomolybdate: V. Control of free copper by tetrathiomolybdate and a comparison with trientine. Translational Research: *J Lab Clin Med* 2009; **154**: 70–7.

78. Tamura S, Sugawara Y, Kishi Y, Akamatsu N, Kaneko J, Makuuchi M. Living-related liver transplantation for Wilson's disease. *Clin Transplant* 2005; **19**: 483–6.

79. Schumacher G, Platz KP, Mueller AR *et al.* Liver transplantation in neurologic Wilson's disease. *Transplant Proc* 2001; **33**(1–2): 1518–9.

80. Medici V, Mirante VG, Fassati LR *et al.* Liver transplantation for Wilson's disease: The burden of neurological and psychiatric disorders. *Liver Transpl* 2005; **11**: 1056–63.

81. Schilsky ML. Wilson disease: current status and the future. *Biochimie* 2009; **91**: 1278–81.

82. Kumar N. Copper deficiency myelopathy: human swayback. *Mayo Clin Proc* 2006; **81**: 1371–84.

Neurodegeneration with brain iron accumulation

Paul J. Tuite and Matthew Bower

Introduction

Disruption of iron homeostasis and abnormal deposition of iron in brain structures appear to be common features in neurodegenerative conditions such as Parkinson disease, Alzheimer disease, and Friedreich ataxia. Less common conditions such as pantothenate kinase associated neurodegeneration (PKAN) and infantile neuroaxonal dystrophy (INAD) are also accompanied by iron deposition and have been classified as having neurodegeneration with brain iron accumulation (NBIA). NBIA includes a broad range of phenotypes with age of onset ranging from infancy to adulthood. In spite of the varied clinical presentations, these conditions are all characterized by abnormal deposition of iron in the basal ganglia. While most of these conditions are associated with autosomal recessive inheritance, at least one NBIA disorder is inherited in an autosomal dominant pattern.

History

Of NBIA disorders, the best known is NBIA-1/PKAN, which has been previously known as Hallervorden–Spatz disease (HSD)/Hallervorden–Spatz syndrome (HSS). Because of concerns about the use of brains from Nazi German concentration camps that were knowingly studied by Dr. Julius Hallervorden on the condition that bears his name, most have tried to eliminate the terms HSS or HSD. As for Dr. Hugo Spatz, who was mentor to Hallervorden, the jury is out as to his complicity. As a result, alternative names have been recommended to replace the terms HSD/HSS.

Terminology

The term neurodegeneration with brain iron accumulation (NBIA) encompasses a heterogeneous group of conditions. In an effort to clarify the similarities and/or differences between these conditions, several terminologies have been employed depending upon whether one is trying to distinguish these conditions on the basis of clinical features, genetic etiology, imaging characteristics or postmortem pathology. Most NBIA disorders were originally described by their clinical presentation. The discovery of mutations in the *PANK2* and *PLA2G6* genes in some individuals with NBIA has helped advance research, but has also confused matters as many distinct clinical entities actually share common genetic etiologies. Some have proposed that specific clinical descriptions be replaced by genetic terms such as PKAN and PLAN to denote a relationship to mutations in the *PANK2* and *PLA2G6* genes, respectively [1,2]. The pathological terms NBIA-1 and NBIA-2 have also been increasingly used to describe NBIA disorders related to mutations in the *PANK2* and *PLA2G6* genes, respectively.

Because each type of taxonomy (genetic, clinical, and pathological) has its own utility, it is possible that these three overlapping sets of nomenclature will continue to be used somewhat interchangeably. Unfortunately for patients and clinicians, this may lead to confusion in understanding a condition and in reviewing medical literature. Table 6.1 correlates clinical, genetic, and pathological terms. In some cases, such as with HSS/HSD, the term may be encountered in some publications, but is no longer used clinically. In other cases distinct clinical syndromes, such as INAD, atypical NAD and Karak syndrome, are now grouped under a common term: PLAN. Likewise these conditions share the same online Mendelian inheritance in man (OMIM) catalog number, which is based on sharing the same causative gene.

Uncommon Causes of Movement Disorders, ed. Néstor Gálvez-Jiménez and Paul J. Tuite. Published by Cambridge University Press. © Cambridge University Press 2011.

Table 6.1. NBIA nomenclature.

Clinical syndrome	Causative gene	Pathological term
PKAN (OMIM 234200)	*PANK2* (OMIM 606157)	NBIA-1 (OMIM 234200)
HSS/HSD (OMIM 234200)	*PANK2* (OMIM 606157)	NBIA-1 (OMIM 234200)
HARP (OMIM 607236)	*PANK2* (OMIM 606157)	NBIA-1 (OMIM 234200)
PLAN (OMIM 256600)	*PLA2G6* (OMIM 603604)	NBIA-2 (OMIM 610217)
INAD/NAD (OMIM 256600)	*PLA2G6* (OMIM 603604)	NBIA-2 (OMIM 610217)
Karak syndrome (OMIM 608395)	*PLA2G6* (OMIM 603604)	NBIA-2 (OMIM 610217)
Dystonia-Parkinsonism (PARK14)	*PLA2G6* (OMIM 603604)	None
Neuroferritinopathy (OMIM 606159)	*FTL* (OMIM 134790)	None
Aceruloplasminemia (OMIM 604290)	*CP* (OMIM 117700)	None

OMIM, Online Mendelian Inheritance in Man; FTL, ferritin light chain; PKAN, pantothenate kinase associated neurodegeneration.

Table 6.2. Clinical features of NBIA-1/PKAN.

	Classic	Atypical
Onset	First decade	Second or third decade
Progression of symptoms	Loss of ambulation 10 years after onset	Loss of ambulation 15–40 years after onset
Clinical findings	Gait, dystonia, chorea, CST, retinitis pigmentosa, optic atrophy (rare)	Speech, dystonia, rigidity, depression, OCD, personality changes
MRI	EOTS	EOTS

Primary data presented in reference [61]
CST, corticospinal tract findings, e.g., hyperreflexia, spasticity, up-going toe signs, etc.; OCD, obsessive compulsive disorder; EOTS, eye of the tiger sign (discussed in the neuroimaging section).

PKAN/NBIA1

Clinical findings/diagnostic criteria

There are two large clinical series [1,3] that outline the major clinical features of those with NBIA-1 and *PANK2* mutations, i.e., those with PKAN. Typically most individuals with PKAN have a classic course (see Table 6.2) with onset before the age of 6 years and rapid progression. In contrast, those with the atypical form generally have a later onset at 13–14 years of age and there is slower progression. Nonetheless, the age of onset and course of disease are not invariant.

Classic PKAN

With classic PKAN individuals often first develop dysarthria, rigidity and dystonia that affects gait. Later, individuals may manifest spasticity, hyperreflexia and extensor toe signs (see Table 6.2) [4]. Cognitive

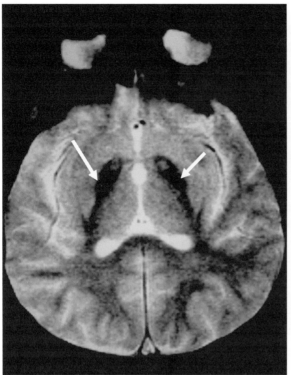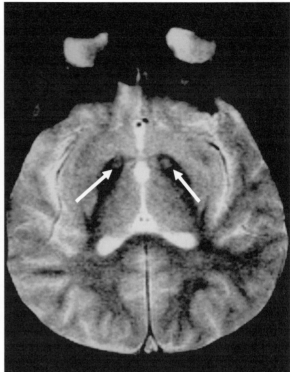

Figure 6.1. Eye of the tiger sign. Arrows in the image on the left identify the area of pallidal hypointensity. The arrows in the image on the right identify the classic central area of pallidal hyperintensity that is characteristic of the eye of the tiger sign.

changes occur and the severity correlates with the degree of motor impairment. Occasionally, presentation with features of attention deficit hyperactivity disorder, clumsiness or developmental delay (usually motor but it can be global) has been noted [4]. Retinal degeneration is a classic feature but may not be present on routine eye examination. Electroretinographic studies may be useful in this regard [4]. Chorea/dyskinesia, myoclonus, seizures and optic atrophy have all been reported [3,5,6].

Some state that all symptomatic individuals with PKAN should have the "eye of the tiger sign" (EOTS) on MRI imaging (Figure 6.1), but this sign is not necessarily pathognomonic of PKAN as it can be seen in other conditions [7–10]

Atypical PKAN

Atypical PKAN initially manifests with speech changes, gait difficulties, tics and psychiatric features, e.g., depression, emotional lability, obsessive-compulsive features and violent tendencies [4]. The degree of severity of motor difficulties is less than with the classic form, as is the rate of progression [1,4]. After 15–40

years of symptoms, affected individuals with atypical PKAN may lose the ability to ambulate [1,4].

Of course there are also rare presentations: late-onset with parkinsonism [11], pure akinesia without dementia presenting with a relatively indolent course [12], and choreoathetoid [13].

Natural history

Rates of change are variable in both classic and atypical PKAN [1]. Some individuals experience rapid clinical deterioration, which may stabilize and then be followed by another cycle of worsened function.

Neuroimaging

Magnetic resonance imaging is useful in evaluating individuals suspected to have NBIA-1/PKAN (see Table 6.3) [8]. T2-weighted MRI methods are sensitive in detecting iron, which may increase with age and/or disease duration [8]. Increasing iron appears as pallidal hypointensity, which is a nonspecific finding. Beta-thalassemia major, HIV and Wilson disease have also been associated with gradient echo (T2*) hypointensity

Table 6.3. MRI neuroimaging features of NBIA.

Finding	PKAN/ NBIA-1	PLAN/ NBIA-2	Neuroferritinopathy	Aceruloplasminemia
EOTS	++	−	+/−	−
Hypointense globus pallidus	++	++	++	++
Central hyperintensity globus pallidus	++	−	+/−	−
Hypointense substantia nigra	+/−	++	++	++
Hypointense dentate nucleus	+/−	+/−	++	++
Hypointense caudate	−	−	+/−	++
Hypointense putamen	−	−	++	++
Hypointense thalamus	−	−	+/−	++
Cavitation of basal ganglia	−	−	+/−	−
Cerebellar abnormalities	−	++ Atrophy	−	+/− Dentate hypointensity
Cerebral abnormalities	−	−	−	++

Primary data presented in reference 8.
++ = finding is present in most cases; +/− = finding is common, but not universally present; − = finding has rarely, if ever, been reported.

of the pallidum, caudate and putamen [8]. T2* is preferred over fast spin echo (FSE) owing to its better sensitivity in detecting iron [8]. Additional methods are being developed such as susceptibility-weighted imaging (SWI) and spin-lock (i.e., T2rho), which are also likely to appreciate changes in iron.

The EOTS is composed of a central hyperintensity on T2-weighted imaging, which has been ascribed to gliosis, increased water content, neuronal loss and changes in the neuropil [3,10]. The central hyperintensity is surrounded by pallidal hypointensity, which has been attributed to the presence of iron. Typically the T2-weighted pallidal hyperintensity appears to precede the development of pallidal hypointensity [14]. Additionally, MRI changes may pre-date onset of symptoms or they may appear after clinical decline [15]. Several factors may influence whether the EOTS is observed on MRI, including the strength of the magnet (should be >0.5 tesla), the experience of the individual

interpreting the images, the age of the affected individual and the disease duration [4].

The discovery of the EOTS should prompt the clinician to consider evaluating for a *PANK2* mutation. In some case series, the presence of the EOTS was highly predictive of the presence of *PANK2* mutations [1]. However, the EOTS is supportive but not specific for those with a *PANK2* mutation [9,16]. The EOTS has been reported on at least one occasion in the following conditions: corticobasal degeneration/ syndrome[17], neuroferritinopathy [8], multiple system atrophy [18], progressive supranuclear palsy [7], young-onset levodopa-responsive parkinsonism [19], learning disability with decline in cognitive and motor function [7] and Karak syndrome[20], and even in an asymptomatic individual [7]. It should be noted that the majority of individuals with EOTS have only been clinically defined without pathological confirmation; thus a greater understanding is

Table 6.4. Serum laboratory measures and NBIA conditions.

	PANK2/PKAN	PLAN	Aceruloplasminemia	Neuroferritinopathy
Ceruloplasmin	Normal	Normal	Absent[a]	Normal
Copper	Normal	Normal	Low	Normal
Ferritin	Normal	Normal	High	Low[b]
Iron	Normal	Normal	Normal	Normal

[a] Rare cases reported where ceruloplasmin is present, but lacks ferroxidase activity.
[b] May be normal in premenopausal women.

still needed as to the specificity of the EOTS sign for PKAN disorders.

In addition to the EOTS finding on MRI, affected individuals will often show evidence of iron deposition in the substantia nigra. A minority of individuals also have hypointensity of the dentate nucleus [8]. In order to differentiate between the various forms of NBIA, one group recommends careful evaluation for iron deposition in the following brain structures: globus pallidus, substantia nigra, dentate nucleus, cerebral cortex, putamen, caudate, and thalamus [8].

The utility of MRI in tracking disease progression is uncertain. Some suggest that once a diagnosis of NBIA is made with the assistance of MRI, additional MRI studies may not be helpful [4]. Novel MRI methods such as diffusion-tensor imaging, spin-lock, and high-field structural and spectroscopic imaging may provide greater abilities to monitor disease progression and aid in monitoring experimental treatments.

While MRI features may be helpful in establishing a clinical diagnosis, there is significant overlap among the NBIA disorders. Therefore, the radiographic presentation should be considered in the context of the history, clinical examination and relevant laboratory evaluations [8].

Laboratory investigations

Additional clinical investigations that may be performed to evaluate individuals with suspected NBIA may include serum ceruloplasmin, copper, ferritin and iron levels (Table 6.4).

Genetics

Mutations in the *PANK2* gene, which was first described in 2001 [21], are estimated to account for about half of individuals with NBIA [4]. Rough estimates indicate that the disease frequency in the general population is approximately 1–3/1 000 000. A carrier frequency of 1:275–1:500 has been estimated, but this is based upon

estimated disease frequency [22]. Given the rarity of these conditions and the varied clinical presentations, these numbers should be viewed as estimates.

Normal function of gene

The *PANK2* gene is located on chromosome 20p13-p12.3, and consists of 6 exons, the first of which is non-coding. *PANK2* encodes the pantothenate kinase 2 enzyme, which is a key regulator of coenzyme A (CoA) biosynthesis. Panthothenate kinase metabolizes vitamin B_5 (pantothenic acid), which ultimately leads to CoA production. The *PANK2* gene appears to have two possible initiation codons, only one of which leads to the presence of a mitochondrial targeting sequence in the mature protein. The use of both initiation codons may explain the distribution of PANK2 protein in both the mitochondria and cytoplasm [23].

Suspected consequence of mutations

Mutations in the *PANK2* gene have been hypothesized to cause disease through one of two mechanisms. Because *PANK2* deficiency is predicted to result in mitochondrial CoA deficiency, some have postulated that *PANK2* mutations may exert their influence through oxidative stress in high-energy tissues such as the basal ganglia and retina. Alternatively, the accumulation of the substrate cysteine may play a critical role as cysteine undergoes auto-oxidation in the presence of free iron, generating toxic free radicals. It is possible that both processes contribute to the pathology seen in PKAN.

Genotype–phenotype correlation

Genotype–phenotype information is limited in PKAN. In general, individuals with two null mutations (nonsense or frameshift mutations) demonstrate the classic PKAN phenotype. Individuals with atypical PKAN generally have at least one (and most commonly have two) missense mutations in the *PANK2* gene. It is not clear whether these missense mutations encode proteins with some residual function, or whether the mutations can complement one another at the protein level to provide some minimal level of function [24].

The term HARP syndrome was initially used to describe individuals in two families with the combination of hypoprebetalipoproteinemia, acanthocytosis, retinitis pigmentosa and pallidal degeneration. The clinical and pathological overlap with PKAN led to the discovery that HARP is allelic with PKAN. Mutations identified in two families with HARP syndrome have all localized in the same region of the *PANK2* gene (exons 4 and 5) [25,26]. It is unclear whether this is coincidental or whether mutations in this region have a specific effect on serum lipids. It has also been suggested that the serum lipid abnormalities may have been a coincidental finding in these families and are unrelated to the *PANK2* mutations [24].

Gene testing

At the time of this publication, two laboratories in the United States and several European laboratories are offering full sequencing of the coding region of the *PANK2* gene. Sequence analysis will identify point mutations and small-scale deletions or duplications within the coding regions of the *PANK2* gene. This type of analysis will not identify mutations that reside in other regions of the gene (promoters, enhancers, or deep intronic regions). In addition, sequence analysis cannot identify large deletions or duplications.

Some have estimated that 97% of individuals with the classic EOTS MRI sign will have at least one mutation identified by sequencing of the *PANK2* gene [4]. In most cases, two mutations are identified. However, a subset of patients (~10%) have only one identifiable *PANK2* mutation. Recent studies have suggested that about 25% of these individuals with a single mutation may harbor a large-scale deletion or duplication involving the *PANK2* gene. As sequencing will not detect these deletions, other technology such as quantitative real-time polymerase chain reaction (PCR) must be employed [27]. The presence of either one or two mutations in the *PANK2* gene, in the context of the EOTS, is considered consistent with a diagnosis of PKAN. Individuals with only one mutation are presumed to carry a second mutation that cannot be identified by current technology.

If two clearly pathogenic mutations are identified, carrier testing and prenatal testing may be available to families. Carrier and prenatal testing requests should always be discussed with a laboratory director before being offered. This type of testing is often approved on a case-by-case basis after discussion with the laboratory.

Pathology

Grossly the brain is atrophic and there is a yellowish-brownish discoloration of the pallidum. Microscopically, there is iron deposition, neuronal loss, gliosis, and axonal spheroids in the medial pallidum and substantia nigra pars reticulata [3,6,11]. Iron is often present as well in the red nucleus and dentate nucleus, and axonal spheroids may be present in the nuclei of the posterior columns [3]. Involvement of other areas have included muscle pathology (myeloid structures, sense bodies and fiber splitting) [28], liver and pituitary changes[29] and sea-blue histiocytes and osmiophilic inclusions on bone marrow biopsy [6,30].

Management

There is no disease-modifying treatment. Nonetheless, it is expected that novel therapies will be developed to address the related pathogenic mechanisms of disease. To date there has not been published a clinical trial for the treatment of NBIA/PKAN, partly owing to the relative rarity of the condition. Nonetheless, a trial of the iron chelator deferiprone is reportedly underway in Italy [4]. The scientific rationale to this approach is that iron chelation may lessen iron catalysis of excess cysteine into free radicals, i.e., it could reduce oxidative stress [4]. There are as well a few case reports suggesting that such a treatment may be helpful in non-PKAN forms of NBIA. A single case showed that oral deferiprone at 15 mg/kg twice daily for 6 to 8 months provided clinical benefit in a 61-year-old woman with oral and appendicular chorea, bradykinesia, blepharospasm, postural instability, cognitive decline and wide-based gait [31]. The brain MRI that showed evidence of iron deposition without EOTS prior to treatment improved as the individual responded to treatment. Another report stated that an individual with aceruloplasminemia (without iron deposition noted on brain MRI) treated with the iron chelator deferasirox at 1000 mg daily improved in function [32].

Since there is no proven-disease modifying treatment, management of NBIA is primarily symptomatic with treatments focused on alleviating dystonia and spasticity. Anticholinergic agents, such as trihexyphenidyl and benztropine, may be helpful in lessening dystonia; whereas oral and/or intrathecal baclofen (ITB) and oral tizanidine may reduce spasticity. The data supporting the efficacy of ITB are sparse for NBIA [33]. Others have employed lesion-based brain surgery or deep brain stimulation (DBS) to ameliorate symptoms [34, 35]. An international study of DBS for NBIA is underway [4].

An assortment of secondary issues can occur in NBIA owing to the progressive dystonia and spasticity and resultant wheelchair-bound state. One particular problem is that dystonia may accelerate arthritis of the neck, which can result in the development of a cervical myelopathy [36]. Thus careful monitoring for abrupt changes in function is needed, and if appropriate repeat MRI imaging along with surgical intervention may be needed. More commonly, affected individuals develop swallowing impairment with associated weight loss, prompting consideration for feeding tube placement. Other concerns include the need for an aggressive bowel regimen to manage constipation, treatment strategies to prevent skin breakdown and deep venous thrombosis, and management of urinary incontinence.

PLAN/NBIA-2

NBIA-2 is transmitted in an autosomal recessive fashion and it associated with mutations in the *PLA2G6* gene. The genetic term PLAN has been proposed to encompass NBIA disorders associated with mutations in the *PLA2G6* gene [37,38]. The clinical entities associated with PLAN are quite heterogeneous and include neuroaxonal dystrophy (NAD), infantile NAD (INAD), Karak syndrome, and one type of dystonia-parkinsonism. Mutations in the *PLA2G6* gene are the second most common cause of NBIA after *PANK2*.

Clinical presentation

Classic INAD begins before 3 years of life with motor and cognitive regression, hypotonia, as well as progressive paraplegia, bulbar dysfunction, cerebellar features, cerebellar atrophy on brain MRI, blindness with optic atrophy, denervation atrophy on electromyography and dystrophic axons on sural nerve biopsy [2]. Based on its name, INAD has been associated with nerve pathology, but this may not always be demonstrated on electromyographic studies or sural nerve biopsy, making the diagnosis difficult on clinical grounds [2]. Some accept the presence of dystrophic axons from other

tissues biopsied such as the conjunctiva, skin, muscle or rectum with additional microscopic features [37].

Several other clinical phenotypes have been reported in conjunction with mutations in the *PLA2G6* gene.

- Atypical NAD is characterized by a later age of onset (average 4.4 years) and a slower clinical course. Atypical NAD shares the primary features of ataxia, gait instability but differs from INAD in that speech delays and diminished social interactions may be prominent [4].
- Karak syndrome, which is a degenerative cerebellar and basal ganglia disorder, has been described in two Jordanian Arab brothers from the town of Karak. The brothers presented with ataxia, dystonia, spasticity and intellectual decline. The authors reported the presence of the EOTS on brain MRI [20]. A homozygous p.R632W mutation in the *PLA2G6* gene was identified in both affected siblings. Karak syndrome is now considered part of the PLAN spectrum of disorders.
- Two consanguineous families with adult-onset dystonia-parkinsonism have been described in conjunction with homozygous mutations in the *PLA2G6* gene. The affected individuals did not have typical iron-laden MRI changes [39,40]. The *PLA2G6* gene has now been allocated the PARK14 designation, demonstrating an unexpected overlap between NBIA and the common clinical entity of Parkinson disease [41].

Neuroimaging

Upon review of MRIs for individuals with PLAN, there may be pallidal and nigral iron deposition and cerebellar atrophy [2]. Hypointensity of the dentate nuclei is sometimes observed [8].

Genetics

PLA2G6 mutation analysis should be considered for individuals with rapid motor and cognitive decline accompanied by dystonia and without epilepsy or dysmorphic features in children with an INAD presentation [2]. Gene testing with sequencing of the exons and adjacent intronic regions is clinically available in the United States and Europe. This testing identifies ~85% of mutations in the *PLA2G6* gene. Approximately 10% of mutation-positive individuals have only one identifiable mutation [4]. These individuals may harbor large duplications or deletions that cannot be detected by standard sequencing tests [27]. Testing for these large rearrangements is now clinically available using a technique called multiplex ligation-dependent probe amplification (MLPA).

The original study identifying mutations in the PLA2G6 gene included five individuals with pathological evidence for INAD, but with no mutations in the PLA2G6 gene [37]. Linkage data in this study supported the existence of at least one additional genetic locus associated with the INAD phenotype [37]. To date, a specific gene has not been identified at this locus.

Management

Disease-modifying treatments such as iron chelation remain unproven but of interest. Symptomatic therapies may be directed at management of seizures, spasticity, abnormal movements, drooling, constipation, swallowing dysfunction and neuropsychiatric problems. Involvement with physical, speech and occupational therapy will be helpful. Patients may ultimately need gastric feeding tubes placed to maintain nutrition, as well as a tracheostomy. Hearing and vision assessments may be helpful in assessing nonverbal individuals.

Neuroferritinopathy

Neuroferritinopathy was first reported in a large English family by Curtis et al. [42]. Neuroferritinopathy is an exceedingly rare condition with only 50 affected individuals reported worldwide [43]. The autosomal dominant pattern of inheritance is unique among the NBIA disorders.

Clinical presentation

Neuroferritinopathy typically presents in adult life around 40 years of age with dystonia or chorea; though rarely individuals may manifest parkinsonism or ataxia [44]. The presence of adult-onset chorea in conjunction with autosomal dominant inheritance is reminiscent of the clinical presentation of Huntington disease. However, these two conditions are readily distinguished by MRI findings (see below). The dystonia usually involves orofacial musculature and it may be brought on with speaking, i.e., action dystonia. Some individuals experience orolingual dyskinesias and frontalis muscle overactivity. At times the movements begin focally and then generalize; sometimes there is asymmetry with regard to the severity of the movements that persists as the disease evolves. Cognitive and

behavioral changes may also develop. One juvenile-onset case has been reported with mental retardation, psychosis, ataxia, bradykinesia and plantar extensor responses [45].

Laboratory investigations

Serum ferritin may be low, but this is not always the case [46]. No specific cut-off has been established.

Neuroimaging

MRI may show cavitation of the basal ganglia [42]. Use of iron-sensitive T2* MRI methods may demonstrate hypointensity of the dentate nucleus, cerebral cortex, substantia nigra, putamen, caudate, or thalamus [8].

Genetics

The association between neurodegeneration and mutations in the gene for the ferritin light polypeptide (FTL) (OMIM 134790) was first reported by Curtis et al. [42]. They identified a frameshift mutation in the FTL gene in one large family and five unrelated individuals from Northern England. Additional analyses demonstrated that all affected individuals shared a common haplotype; suggesting a shared ancestor.

To date, approximately 50 individuals have been identified worldwide with neuroferritinopathy. The majority of these individuals share the common mutation identified by Curtis et al. Sequencing for mutations in the FTL gene is clinically available. The FTL gene is located on chromosome 19q13.3-q13.4. The gene has four exons and encodes the ferritin light-chain polypeptide. Ferritin heavy and light chains form functional ferritin molecules that are capable of both the transport and detoxification of iron molecules. The majority of mutations reported to date (5/6) are frameshift mutations in exon 4 that result in an elongated ferritin light-chain protein. These mutations are predicted to disrupt the iron storage function of ferritin [47]. Mutations in the same gene have been associated with hyperferritinemia-cataract syndrome (OMIM 600886), which is an autosomal dominant condition with elevated ferritin and cataracts.

Pathology

On gross pathological examination, there may be evidence of cystic degeneration of the globus pallidus and other basal ganglia structures. Histopathology may show reddish discoloration of the basal ganglia, iron/

ferritin-positive spherical inclusions in the globus pallidum, and neuroaxonal spheroids [42].

Management

Although it may be seem reasonable to employ antioxidant and iron-modulating therapies, there are limited data as to their efficacy. Current treatments under evaluation include venesection, iron chelation and coenzyme Q_{10} therapy [48,49]. Symptomatic therapies for abnormal movements may be helpful. Clinicians have used a spectrum of agents starting with levodopa compounds and including anticholinergics, benzodiazepines, dopamine depletors (e.g., tetrabenazine) and possibly antipsychotics, all with limited benefit [50]. Botulinum toxin injection could be employed for treatment of focal dystonia. Ancillary services such as physical, occupational and speech therapy may be useful in addressing limitations in activities in daily living.

Aceruloplasminemia

Aceruloplasminemia is a rare autosomal recessive NBIA disorder caused by mutations in the ceruloplasmin (Cp) gene (*CP*) with resultant alterations in copper and iron metabolism. Aceruloplasminemia has been primarily described in individuals of Japanese ancestry, though it has been reported in other ethnicities.

Clinical presentation

McNeill *et al.* reviewed the clinical presentation of all 32 published cases and one unpublished case of aceruloplasminemia [51]. Retinal degeneration, diabetes mellitus, anemia and neurological manifestations are the most common features. Neurological findings include, in decreasing frequency: cerebellar ataxia (dysarthria, gait and limb ataxia, and nystagmus), involuntary movements (craniofacial dystonia, tremor, chorea, and parkinsonism), and cognitive impairment (including dementia) [52]. The age of onset is usually between 25 and 60 years of age, but presentation in the second decade has been reported.

Neuroimaging

An iron sensitive MRI T2* sequence typically demonstrates hypointensity of the globus pallidum, dentate nucleus, substantia nigra, putamen, caudate and thalamus. There is generally no cavitation of the basal ganglia, which is a feature commonly seen with neuroferritinopathy [8]. In addition to abnormal iron deposition in the central nervous system, affected individuals generally display increased iron in the liver, which is detectable by T2-weighted MRI studies.

Genetics

Mutations in the *CP* gene were first identified by Harris *et al.* [53]. The *CP* gene encodes the Cp precursor protein. Alternative splicing of the transcript results in the two main forms of Cp protein. The secreted form is produced in the liver, whereas the globus pallidus internus form is expressed primarily in astrocytes and plays a role in brain iron homeostasis. An assortment of mutations have been discovered, some of which result in deficiency of Cp in the blood whereas other have been associated with normal Cp blood levels but absent ferroxidase activity. Clinical testing for mutations in the *CP* gene is not currently available. Carrier and prenatal testing may be available to families that have mutations identified in a research laboratory.

Aceruloplasminemia has been classically described as an autosomal recessive disorder. Clinical findings have not been reported in heterozygous (carrier) parents or siblings of affected individuals. Symptoms have been reported in five heterozygous probands, but it is not clear whether these individuals are manifesting heterozygotes or whether they harbor second mutations that were not detected [51].

Laboratory investigations

Serum ceruloplasmin is typically absent, i.e., not detectable by western blot (normal 21–36 mg/dl) [54]. Additional tests demonstrate low serum copper (<10 µg/dl [normal 70–125 µg/dl]), low serum iron (<45 µg/dl [normal males 60–180 µg/dl; normal females 10–140 µg/dl]), high serum ferritin (850–4000 ng/dl [normal males 45–200 ng/ml; normal females 30–100 ng/ml]), and usually absent plasma ceruloplasmin ferroxidase activity (normal 500–680 U/l). In atypical cases serum ceruloplasmin levels may be normal but ceruloplasmin ferroxidase activity is lacking [55]. Abdominal MRI may be done to evaluate for the presence of iron. Hepatic iron and copper concentrations are increased, as measured by liver biopsy and quantified in µmol/g dry weight [54].

Fluorescein angiography may be performed to evaluate retinal abnormalities and distinguish them from diabetic retinopathy [56].

Pathology

Pathological examination reveals abnormal deposition of iron in the liver, islet beta cells, basal ganglia, and to a lesser degree, cerebral cortex and the cerebellum. Astrocytic deformity and globular structures appear to be characteristic neuropathological findings [57].

Management

There is no curative treatment at the present. It is hoped that gene therapies may be useful in the future. Presently treatment is primarily symptomatic, though it may be possible to reduce brain and liver iron burden and thereby alter the course of disease. Thus, iron chelating agents such as deferoxamine (also known as desferrioxamine, desferoxamine, DFO or DFOA) have been employed [58]. Some recommend the use of IV DFO along with fresh-frozen human plasma (FFP) to decrease liver iron [54,59]. Repetitive treatment with FFP may prove useful in improving or stabilizing neurological features. Others use vitamin E and/or zinc to prevent liver and pancreatic injury [60].

Conclusion

Disorders of neurodegeneration with brain iron accumulation (NBIA) share the common feature of iron deposition in the basal ganglia. In spite of this shared finding, the clinical spectrum is quite diverse. This chapter summarizes what is known about NBIA disorders at the time of this publication. Given the rapid pace of genetic discovery and development of novel MRI techniques, it is likely that clinicians will need to familiarize themselves with the latest in diagnosis and/or treatment of these conditions. Future research will be needed to sort out the question whether the iron deposition causes neurodegeneration in NBIA disorders or whether this represents an incidental finding. The question whether common variations or carrier status for rare mutations in NBIA genes could confer risk for more common neurodegenerative conditions, such as Parkinson disease and Alzheimer disease, remains to be answered. While the NBIA disorders are quite rare, understanding the pathological phenomenon of brain iron deposition may provide insight into the pathophysiology of common neurological diseases.

References

1. Hayflick SJ, Westaway SK, Levinson B *et al.* Genetic, clinical, and radiographic delineation of Hallervorden–Spatz syndrome. *N Engl J Med* 2003; **348**(1): 33–40.

2. Kurian MA, Morgan NV, MacPherson L *et al.* Phenotypic spectrum of neurodegeneration associated with mutations in the PLA2G6 gene (PLAN). *Neurology* 2008; **70**(18): 1623–9.

3. Dooling EC, Schoene WC, Richardson EP Jr. Hallervorden–Spatz syndrome. *Arch Neurol* 1974; **30**(1): 70–83.

4. Gregory A, Polster BJ, Hayflick SJ. Clinical and genetic delineation of neurodegeneration with brain iron accumulation. *J Med Genet* 2009; **46**(2): 73–80.

5. Tripathi RC, Tripathi BJ, Bauserman SC, Park JK. Clinicopathologic correlation and pathogenesis of ocular and central nervous system manifestations in Hallervorden–Spatz syndrome. *Acta Neuropathol* 1992; **83**(2): 113–19.

6. Swaiman KF. Hallervorden–Spatz syndrome and brain iron metabolism. *Arch Neurol* 1991; **48**(12): 1285–93.

7. Kumar N, Boes CJ, Babovic-Vuksanovic D, Boeve BF. The "eye-of-the-tiger" sign is not pathognomonic of the PANK2 mutation. *Arch Neurol* 2006; **63**(2): 292–3.

8. McNeill A, Birchall D, Hayflick SJ *et al.* T2* and FSE MRI distinguishes four subtypes of neurodegeneration with brain iron accumulation. *Neurology* 2008; **70**(18): 1614–19.

9. Baumeister FA, Auer DP, Hortnagel K, Freisinger P, Meitinger T. The eye of the tiger sign is not a reliable disease marker for Hallervorden–Spatz syndrome. *Neuropediatrics* 2005; **36**(3): 221–2.

10. Savoiardo M, Halliday WC, Nardocci N *et al.* Hallervorden–Spatz disease: MR and pathologic findings. *AJNR Am J Neuroradiol* 1993; **14**(1): 155–62.

11. Halliday W. The nosology of Hallervorden–Spatz disease. *J Neurol Sci* 1995; **134**(Suppl): 84–91.

12. Molinuevo JL, Marti MJ, Blesa R, Tolosa E. Pure akinesia: an unusual phenotype of Hallervorden–Spatz syndrome. *Mov Disord* 2003; **18**(11): 1351–3.

13. Grimes DA, Lang AE, Bergeron C. Late adult onset chorea with typical pathology of Hallervorden-Spatz syndrome. *J Neurol Neurosurg Psychiatry* 2000; **69**(3): 392–5.

14. Hayflick SJ, Hartman M, Coryell J, Gitschier J, Rowley H. Brain MRI in neurodegeneration with brain iron accumulation with and without PANK2 mutations. *Am J Neuroradiol* 2006; **27**(6): 1230–3.

15. Hayflick SJ, Penzien JM, Michl W, Sharif UM, Rosman NP, Wheeler PG. Cranial MRI changes may precede symptoms in Hallervorden–Spatz syndrome. *Pediatr Neurol* 2001; **25**(2): 166–169.

16. Valentino P, Annesi G, Ciro Candiano IC *et al.* Genetic heterogeneity in patients with pantothenate kinase-associated neurodegeneration and classic magnetic resonance imaging eye-of-the-tiger pattern. *Mov Disord* 2006; **21**(2): 252–4.

17. Molinuevo JL, Munoz E, Valldeoriola F, Tolosa E. The eye of the tiger sign in cortical-basal ganglionic degeneration. *Mov Disord* 1999; **14**(1): 169–71.

18. Strecker K, Hesse S, Wegner F, Sabri O, Schwarz J, Schneider JP. Eye of the tiger sign in multiple system atrophy. *Eur J Neurol* 2007; **14**(11): e1–e2.

19. Barbosa ER, Bittar MS, Bacheschi LA, Comerlatti LR, Scaff M. Precocious Parkinson's disease associated with "eye-of-the-tiger" type pallidal lesions. *Arq Neuropsiquiatr* 1995; **53**(2): 294–7.

20. Mubaidin A, Roberts E, Hampshire D *et al.* Karak syndrome: a novel degenerative disorder of the basal ganglia and cerebellum. *J Med Genet* 2003; **40**(7): 543–6.

21. Zhou B, Westaway SK, Levinson B, Johnson MA, Gitschier J, Hayflick SJ. A novel pantothenate kinase gene (PANK2) is defective in Hallervorden–Spatz syndrome. *Nat Genet* 2001; **28**(4): 345–349.

22. Gregory A, Hayflick SJ. Panthothenate kinase-associated neurodegeneration. Available at: www.genetests. org. Initial Posting: August 13, 2002; Last Update: March 23, 2010. (Accessed January 3, 2011).

23. Johnson MA, Kuo YM, Westaway SK *et al.* Mitochondrial localization of human PANK2 and hypotheses of secondary iron accumulation in pantothenate kinase-associated neurodegeneration. *Ann NY Acad Sci* 2004; **1012**: 282–8.

24. Hayflick SJ. Unraveling the Hallervorden–Spatz syndrome: pantothenate kinase-associated neurodegeneration is the name. *Curr Opin Pediatr* 2003; **15**(6): 572–7.

25. Houlden H, Lincoln S, Farrer M, Cleland PG, Hardy J, Orrell RW. Compound heterozygous PANK2 mutations confirm HARP and Hallervorden–Spatz syndromes are allelic. *Neurology* 2003; **61**(10): 1423–6.

26. Ching KH, Westaway SK, Gitschier J, Higgins JJ, Hayflick SJ. HARP syndrome is allelic with panthothenate kinase-associated neurodegeneration. *Neurology* 2002; **58**(11): 1673–4.

27. Haverfield EV, Dempsey MA, Gregory A, Westaway SK, Hayflick SJ, Das S. Intragenic deletion and duplication analysis of PANK2 and PLA2G6 genes in patients with NBIA. ACMG Annual Clinical Genetics Meeting 2008. Abstract Number:150.

28. Malandrini A, Bonuccelli U, Parrotta E, Ceravolo R, Berti G, Guazzi GC. Myopathic involvement in two cases of Hallervorden–Spatz disease. *Brain Dev* 1995; **1**(4): 286–90.

29. Williams DJ, Ironside JW. Liver and pituitary abnormalities in Hallervorden–Spatz disease. *J Neurol Neurosurg Psychiatry* 1989; **52**(12): 1410–14.

30. Zupanc ML, Chun RW, Gilbert-Barness EF. Osmiophilic deposits in cytosomes in Hallervoden–Spatz syndrome. *Pediatr Neurol* 1990; **6**(5): 349–52.

31. Forni GL, Balocco M, Cremonesi L, Abbruzzese G, Parodi RC, Marchese R. Regression of symptoms after selective iron chelation therapy in a case of neurodegeneration with brain iron accumulation. *Mov Disord* 2008; **23**(6): 904–7.

32. Skidmore FM, Drago V, Foster P, Schmalfuss IM, Heilman KM, Streiff RR. Aceruloplasminaemia with progressive atrophy without brain iron overload: treatment with oral chelation. *J Neurol Neurosurg Psychiatry* 2008; **79**(4): 467–70.

33. Panourias IG, Themistocleous M, Sakas DE. Intrathecal baclofen in current neuromodulatory practice: established indications and emerging applications. *Acta Neurochir Suppl* 2007; **97**(1): 145–54.

34. Balas I, Kovacs N, Hollody K. Staged bilateral stereotactic pallidothalamotomy for life-threatening dystonia in a child with Hallervorden–Spatz disease. *Mov Disord* 2006; **21**(1): 82–5.

35. Castelnau P, Cif L, Valente EM *et al.* Pallidal stimulation improves pantothenate kinase-associate neurodegeneration. *Ann Neurol* 2005; **57**(5): 738–41.

36. Fung GP, Chan KY. Cervical myelopathy in an adolescent with Hallervorden–Spatz disease. *Pediatr Neurol* 2003; **29**(4): 337–40.

37. Morgan NV, Westaway SK, Morton JE *et al.* PLA2G6, encoding a phospholipase A2, is mutated in neurodegenerative disorders with high brain iron. *Nat Genet* 2006; **38**(7): 752–4.

38. Khateeb S, Flusser H, Ofir R *et al.* PLA2G6 mutation underlies infantile neuroaxonal dystrophy. *Am J Hum Genet* 2006; **79**(5): 942–8.

39. Paisan-Ruiz C, Bhatia KP, Li A *et al.* Characterization of PLA2G6 as a locus for dystonia-parkinsonism. *Ann Neurol* 2009; **65**(1): 19–023.

40. Sina F, Shojaee S, Elahi E, Paisan-Ruiz C. R632W mutation in PLA2G6 segregates with dystonia-parkinsonism in a consanguineous Iranian family. *Eur J Neurol* 2009; **16**(1): 101–4.

41. Schneider SA, Bhatia KP, Hardy J. Complicated recessive dystonia parkinsonism syndromes. *Mov Disord* 2009; **24**(4): 490–8.

42. Curtis AR, Fey C, Morris CM *et al.* Mutation in the gene encoding ferritin light polypeptide causes dominant adult-onset basal ganglia disease. *Nat Genet* 2001; **28**(4): 350–4.

43. Chinnery PF. Neuroferritinopathy. 2007 Aug 8. Available at: www.genetests.org (accessed May 8, 2009).

44. Kubota A, Hida A, Ichikawa Y *et al.* A novel ferritin light chain gene mutation in a Japanese family with neuroferritinopathy: description of clinical features and implications for genotype–phenotype correlations. *Mov Disord* 2009; **24**(3): 441–5.

45. Maciel P, Cruz VT, Constante M *et al.* Neuroferritinopathy: missense mutation in FTL causing early-onset bilateral pallidal involvement. *Neurology* 2005; **65**(4): 603–5.

46. Curtis AR, Fey C, Morris CM *et al.* Mutation in the gene encoding ferritin light polypeptide causes dominant adult-onset basal ganglia disease. *Nat Genet* 2001; **28**(4): 350–4.

47. Levi S, Cozzi A, Arosio P. Neuroferritinopathy: a neurodegenerative disorder associated with L-ferritin mutation. *Best Pract Res Clin Haematol* 2005; **18**(2): 265–76.

48. Chinnery PF, Curtis AR, Fey C *et al.* Neuroferritinopathy in a French family with late onset dominant dystonia. *J Med Genet* 2003; **40**(5): e69.

49. Caparros-Lefebvre D, Destee A, Petit H. Late onset familial dystonia: could mitochondrial deficits induce a diffuse lesioning process of the whole basal ganglia system. *J Neurol Neurosurg Psychiatry* 1997; **63**(2): 196–203.

50. Crompton DE, Chinnery PF, Bates D *et al.* Spectrum of movement disorders in neuroferritinopathy. *Mov Disord* 2005; **20**(1): 95–9.

51. McNeill A, Pandolfo M, Kuhn J, Shang H, Miyajima H. The neurological presentation of ceruloplasmin gene mutations. *Eur Neurol* 2008; **60**(4): 200–5.

52. Miyajima H, Takahashi Y, Kono S. Aceruloplasminemia, an inherited disorder of iron metabolism. *Biometals* 2003; **16**(1): 205–13.

53. Harris ZL, Takahashi Y, Miyajima H, Serizawa M, MacGillivray RT, Gitlin JD. Aceruloplasminemia: molecular characterization of this disorder of iron metabolism. *Proc Natl Acad Sci U S A* 1995; **92**(7): 2539–43.

54. Miyajima H. Aceruloplasminemia. 2008 May 15. Available at: www.genetests.org (accessed May 8, 2009).

55. Takeuchi Y, Yoshikawa M, Tsujino T *et al.* A case of aceruloplasminaemia: abnormal serum ceruloplasmin protein without ferroxidase activity. *J Neurol Neurosurg Psychiatry* 2002; **72**(4): 543–5.

56. Yamaguchi K, Takahashi S, Kawanami T, Kato T, Sasaki H. Retinal degeneration in hereditary ceruloplasmin deficiency. *Ophthalmologica* 1998; **212**(1): 11–14.

57. Kaneko K, Yoshida K, Arima K *et al.* Astrocytic deformity and globular structures are characteristic of the brains of patients with aceruloplasminemia. *J Neuropathol Exp Neurol* 2002; **61**(12): 1069–77.

58. Miyajima H, Takahashi Y, Kamata T, Shimizu H, Sakai N, Gitlin JD. Use of desferrioxamine in the treatment of aceruloplasminemia. *Ann Neurol* 1997; **41**(3): 404–7.

59. Yonekawa M, Okabe T, Asamoto Y, Ohta M. A case of hereditary ceruloplasmin deficiency with iron deposition in the brain associated with chorea, dementia, diabetes mellitus and retinal pigmentation: administration of fresh-frozen human plasma. *Eur Neurol* 1999; **42**(3): 157–62.

60. Kuhn J, Bewermeyer H, Miyajima H, Takahashi Y, Kuhn KF, Hoogenraad TU. Treatment of symptomatic heterozygous aceruloplasminemia with oral zinc sulphate. *Brain Dev* 2007; **29**(7): 450–3.

61. Chan KY, Lam CW, Lee LP, Tong SF, Yuen YP. Panthothenate kinase-associated neurodegeneration in two Chinese children: identification of a novel PANK2 gene mutation. *Hong Kong Med J* 2008; **14**(1): 70–3.

Dementia and parkinsonism

Praveen Dayalu and Kelvin L. Chou

Introduction

Dementia occurs in many disorders that cause parkinsonism. In children and young adults with both parkinsonism and dementia, the differential diagnosis includes Wilson disease (particularly because it is treatable), Huntington disease (Westphal variant), neurodegeneration with brain iron accumulation (NBIA), neuroacanthocytosis, neuroferritinopathy, spinocerebellar ataxia type 2 and HIV.

However, the vast majority of patients with both dementia and parkinsonism are middle-aged to older adults. Dementia often complicates Parkinson disease (PD) later in its course, and mild parkinsonism is not uncommon in individuals with Alzheimer disease (AD). When dementia and parkinsonism both occur early in the course of a neurological disease in an adult of middle age or older, the differential diagnosis includes dementia with Lewy bodies, corticobasal degeneration (CBD), progressive supranuclear palsy (PSP), vascular parkinsonism and prion disease. Frontal subcortical lesions can present with dementia, apathy and a parkinson-like gait disorder with freezing, shuffling or apraxia. Examples include multiple infarcts, brain tumor and hydrocephalus (including normal-pressure hydrocephalus).

Many disorders listed above are covered elsewhere in this book. The focus of this chapter will be on dementia with Lewy bodies, the most common cause of dementia with parkinsonism.

Dementia with Lewy bodies: definition

Dementia with Lewy bodies (DLB) is a progressive neurodegenerative disease affecting older adults, causing dementia, psychosis and parkinsonism. Lewy bodies, its pathological hallmark, are large intraneuronal aggregates of the synaptic protein α-synuclein, most apparent in the brain. What we now know as DLB was recognized only in the late 1980s as a distinct clinicopathological entity. Consensus clinical and pathological criteria for the disease were formalized in 1995 [1]. In 2005, these diagnostic criteria were revised to improve diagnostic sensitivity and reflect updates in our knowledge of the disorder [2]. (See "Clinical diagnostic criteria" and "Pathology.")

DLB overlaps to a large degree with Parkinson disease dementia (PDD). The term PDD is used for patients who initially develop PD that is later complicated by dementia; specifically, the parkinsonism precedes the dementia by at least one year. The term "Lewy Body dementias" encompasses both PDD and DLB, while the umbrella term "Lewy Body disease" includes the entire spectrum of PD, PDD and DLB [3].

This chapter will emphasize DLB specifically. Aside from the "one-year rule," however, there are no known definitive clinical or pathological features that truly separate DLB and PDD as distinct diseases. Therefore, most of the content of this chapter, especially the practical aspects of clinical care, are applicable to both entities.

Clinical diagnostic criteria

The following criteria are from the third report of the DLB consortium [2]. For clinical diagnosis, they allow two grades of certainty: probable DLB or possible DLB. A definitive diagnosis requires postmortem confirmation (see "Pathology").

1. Central features (essential for a diagnosis of possible or probable DLB):
   (a) Dementia, defined as progressive cognitive decline sufficient to interfere with normal social or occupational function.
   (b) Prominent or persistent memory impairment may not necessarily occur in the early stages but is usually evident with progression.
   (c) Deficits of attention, executive function and visuospatial ability may be especially prominent.

Uncommon Causes of Movement Disorders, ed. Néstor Gálvez-Jiménez and Paul J. Tuite. Published by Cambridge University Press. © Cambridge University Press 2011.

2. Core features (two core features are sufficient for a diagnosis of probable DLB, one for possible DLB):
   (a) Fluctuating cognition with pronounced variations in attention and alertness.
   (b) Recurrent visual hallucinations, typically well formed and detailed.
   (c) Spontaneous features of parkinsonism.
3. Suggestive features. (If one or more of these is present along with one or more core features, a diagnosis of probable DLB can be made. Absent any core features, one or more suggestive features are sufficient for possible DLB. Probable DLB should not be diagnosed on the basis of suggestive features alone):
   (a) REM sleep behavior disorder.
   (b) Severe neuroleptic sensitivity.
   (c) Low dopamine transporter uptake in basal ganglia demonstrated by SPECT or PET imaging.
4. Supportive features (commonly present but not proven to have diagnostic specificity):
   (a) Repeated falls and syncope.
   (b) Transient, unexplained loss of consciousness.
   (c) Severe autonomic dysfunction, e.g., orthostatic hypotension, urinary incontinence.
   (d) Nonvisual hallucinations.
   (e) Systematized delusions.
   (f) Depression.
   (g) Relative preservation of medial temporal lobe structures on CT/MRI scan.
   (h) Generalized low uptake on SPECT/PET perfusion scan with reduced occipital activity.
   (i) Abnormal (low uptake) MIBG myocardial scintigraphy.
   (j) Prominent slow wave activity on EEG with temporal lobe transient sharp waves.
5. A diagnosis of DLB is less likely:
   (a) In the presence of cerebrovascular disease evident as focal neurologic signs or on brain imaging.
   (b) In the presence of any other physical illness or brain disorder sufficient to account in part or in total for the clinical picture.
   (c) If parkinsonism only appears for the first time at a stage of severe dementia.
6. Temporal sequence of symptoms:
   (a) DLB should be diagnosed when dementia occurs before or concurrently with parkinsonism (if it is present).
   (b) The term Parkinson disease dementia (PDD) should be used to describe dementia that occurs in the context of well-established PD.

Pathology

A detailed explanation of neuropathological methodology and criteria used to diagnose DLB post mortem is beyond the scope of this text. However, neuropathological analysis is imperative in making the diagnosis definitively, so a brief review is important.

The pathological hallmarks of DLB are Lewy bodies (LB) and Lewy neurites, which are pathological aggregates of α-synuclein visible with immunohistochemical staining. The density of such pathology in the brain is systematically rated in specific regions of the brain stem (nuclei of cranial nerves IX–X, locus ceruleus, and substantia nigra); limbic and basal forebrain regions (nucleus basalis of Meynert, amygdala, transentorhinal and cingulate cortices); and neocortex (temporal, frontal, and parietal). Lewy pathology in the neocortex carries the most diagnostic "weight" for likelihood of DLB, while Lewy pathology in brain stem alone makes the diagnosis less likely. Other brain pathology is also graded, most critically Alzheimer-related pathology as measured by amyloid plaques and neurofibrillary tangles. Coexistent Alzheimer pathology is very common; so-called "pure DLB" occurs less often. Unfortunately, DLB patients with a high burden of Alzheimer pathology are less likely to be correctly diagnosed in life. They may lack core and suggestive clinical features of DLB, and present primarily with an Alzheimer-like amnestic syndrome [4,5].

Another challenge in the pathological assessment of DLB is that Lewy bodies are not specific to DLB. PD is also characterized by Lewy pathology, but beginning in the caudal brain stem and ascending rostrally over years, with neocortical structures involved late [6]. Neocortical Lewy bodies have been found in up to 30% of normal elderly brains [7], emphasizing the importance of the clinical diagnosis.

The diagnostic certainty for DLB is determined by the density and extent of Lewy pathology in proportion to any coexistent Alzheimer and vascular pathology. The more Alzheimer pathology exists, the more Lewy pathology is required for ultimate diagnosis of DLB [2,4].

α-Synuclein clearly is central in the pathogenesis of DLB. However, Lewy bodies themselves are probably not be the primary driver of neuronal dysfunction and death. Small abnormal presynaptic aggregates of α-synuclein, for example, may be a major factor in synaptic dysfunction [8]. The initial steps of the pathophysiologic cascade in DLB remain unknown.

Several key neurotransmitters are reduced in DLB, as with PD and PDD. Nigrostriatal dopaminergic deficit is a major cause of parkinsonism. Deficits in serotonin and norepinephrine occur from degeneration of their respective brain stem nuclei, resulting in psychiatric and sleep disturbances. Degeneration in the nucleus basalis of Meynert results in a marked cortical cholinergic deficit, contributing significantly to cognitive deficits and fluctuations.

Epidemiology

After AD, DLB is probably the second commonest cause of degenerative dementia in the elderly. Like the other Lewy body diseases, it has a slight male predominance. Its reported prevalence varies from 10% to 26% [9], likely due to different methodologies and populations. The incidence of DLB above age 65 is estimated at 1 per 1000 per year [10]. Onset of DLB prior to age 50 is rare.

Etiology and genetics

Like PD, the vast majority of DLB cases are sporadic and of unknown ultimate cause. The disease is thought to arise from complex interactions of genetic and environmental factors that are only beginning to be understood. Known genetic causes of DLB are heterogeneous and overlap with genetic causes of PD. Families with prominent DLB have been reported. In one, an α-synuclein mutation segregated with pure DLB (with no Alzheimer pathology), cementing the notion that this protein has a central role in DLB pathogenesis [11]. More common gene mutations are those of leucine-rich repeat kinase 2 (LRRK2) and glucocerebrosidase (GCA). LRRK2 mutations cause PD and DLB [12]. GCA mutations are associated with Lewy body disorders [13]. APOE ε4 allele may be a risk factor for DLB [14]. Mutant β-synuclein, presenilin-1, and even prion protein PRNP have all been reported in cases of DLB, but more evidence is needed before implicating these genes in the disorder.

Environmental risk factors almost certainly contribute to the genesis of DLB but are not yet known. Certain toxic exposures, such as to manganese, herbicides and insecticides, are thought to contribute to a minority of PD cases; little is known about these exposures with respect to DLB specifically. Nutritional, infectious, and behavioral factors might play a role.

Natural history and prognosis

Dementia with Lewy bodies is a progressive neurodegenerative disease. Rates of progression vary widely. With time, patients manifest increased disability and loss of independence. There is a steady decline in motor, cognitive, behavioral and autonomic function. The relative contribution by each of these factors to overall morbidity varies from patient to patient. Institutionalization is often required. Patients with advanced disease are vulnerable to complications of dementia, dysphagia, and immobility. Sepsis, aspiration, dehydration, and hip fractures are common complications. Death often occurs within 8–10 years of disease onset.

Cognitive manifestations

The pattern of neuropsychologic deficits in DLB differs from that in AD. On average, early DLB patients manifest greater impairments in attention, concentration, executive dysfunction and visuospatial function than early AD patients [15,16]. Conversely, early DLB patients show less impairment in memory than early AD patients. These observations come from aggregate data and are not reliable in individual cases. Even in pathologically proven DLB cases, extensive concurrent AD pathology can "mask" the DLB clinical phenotype and result in a clinical appearance that more strongly suggests AD [5]. Conversely, AD sometimes presents with early prominent visuospatial impairment and visual hallucinations.

Fluctuations, a core clinical diagnostic criterion in DLB, refer to noticeable alterations in arousal, attention, cognition, speech and global function. They may occur over hours or days and resemble delirium, but without any apparent cause. Unfortunately, ascertaining a history of fluctuations from caregivers is difficult. Caregivers of normal elderly and AD patients may endorse such fluctuations if the probe question is too nonspecific, such as "Does the patient have good and bad days in their performance and attention?" DLB fluctuations appear to have a more transient quality and are independent of situational demands [17]. Better discrimination is obtained by asking specifically about four features (the Mayo Fluctuations Composite Scale): (1) daytime drowsiness or lethargy; (2) daytime sleep of two or more hours; (3) staring into space for long periods; and (4) episodes of disorganized speech. Three or more features provided a positive predictive value of 83% for DLB, while two or fewer yielded a negative predictive value of 70% [18]. Another assessment option is the One Day Fluctuation Assessment scale [19].

Visual hallucinations occur in many DLB patients and satisfy a core criterion when they are recurrent and occur early in the disease. Hallucinations are often quite detailed: patients see people, animals and entire scenes in front of them. Early on, they may recognize these as hallucinations, but insight eventually is lost. Patients may be severely distressed by what they see. Typical reports include: "There is a strange woman in my bed" or "Some young men are looking into the windows; they want to rob us." Such hallucinations are a major burden for caregivers. In PD they are a strong predictor of institutionalization. Visual hallucinations correlate strongly with temporal lobe Lewy body density [20]. Auditory hallucinations may occur in some patients. Delusional thinking and paranoia are also common in DLB but lack diagnostic specificity as they are also common in other dementias such as AD.

Parkinsonism and other motor manifestations

The core parkinsonian features of rest tremor, bradykinesia, rigidity and postural instability are common in DLB, along with associated features such as masked facies, stooped posture, hypophonia and micrographia. Overall, the severity of parkinsonism as assessed with the Unified PD Rating Scale is similar between DLB, PDD and PD, but in DLB may worsen more rapidly: over two years, UPDRS scores on medications worsened by about 10 points in PDD and DLB, versus 5 points in PD subjects, though DLB subjects did receive slightly less L-dopa [21].

Rest tremor seems less common in DLB than in PD. In a study with pathological confirmation, rest tremor was present in only 55% of DLB cases versus 85% of PD cases [22]. Other case series showed a rest tremor prevalence of 47–66% in DLB versus 75% and higher in PD. Interestingly, PD patients with prominent rest tremor are less likely to develop dementia [23].

Repeated falls are a supportive feature in DLB. They occur more often in DLB patients (37%) than other demented populations (6% in AD) [24], and may also occur earlier. One explanation is greater autonomic dysfunction in DLB leading to syncope. Another is

that a postural instability-gait disorder phenotype is more common in DLB than in PD. One study reported that only 25% of DLB patients had motor asymmetry, versus 80% of PD patients [25]. Myoclonus occurs in about 19% of DLB cases, while it is virtually absent in PD [22].

DLB patients are extremely sensitive to neuroleptics [26]. Typical and atypical antipsychotics, as well as many antiemetics, may acutely exacerbate parkinsonism and impair consciousness. Serious morbidity and even death may ensue. Such neuroleptic sensitivity reactions, if they have occurred in the past, are a suggestive diagnostic feature for DLB. Neuroleptics are best avoided in this population, and should never be prescribed deliberately as a diagnostic "test."

Sleep dysfunction

Rapid eye movement (REM) sleep behavior disorder (RBD) is strongly associated with the synucleinopathies, including DLB, PD and multiple system atrophy (MSA) [27]. When dementia is present, RBD is a suggestive diagnostic feature for DLB. RBD may precede dementia by many years and is more common in males. It is characterized by the loss of muscle atonia during REM sleep with prominent motor activity; patients appear to act out their dreams. Vivid dreams may be reported. Patients can injure themselves by colliding with furniture or falling from the bed, and spouses may be hit by flailing limbs.

In these disorders, RBD is probably due to degeneration in the brain stem structures modulating REM sleep: locus ceruleus, pedunculopontine nucleus, gigantocellularis reticular nucleus and amygdala [28]. RBD occurs rarely in the tauopathies such as progressive supranuclear palsy, AD, corticobasal degeneration and Pick disease [27].

Excess daytime sleepiness is also common in DLB. This is intrinsic to the disease (as in fluctuations) but may also be caused by medications, obstructive sleep apnea and severe RBD.

Autonomic dysfunction

Autonomic dysfunction is a supportive criterion for the diagnosis of DLB, and may be more prominent than in other dementias [29]. As in PD, autonomic neural pathways are selectively involved in DLB. α-Synuclein aggregates affect the dorsal motor nucleus of vagus (DMV) [7], resulting in parasympathetic dysfunction. Cell loss and Lewy bodies are seen in the intermediolateral horn of the thoracic cord and sympathetic ganglia. Cardiac denervation is demonstrable in DLB, PD and PDD (see "Imaging and laboratory studies").

The commonest autonomic problems in the Lewy body diseases are orthostatic hypotension, urinary dysfunction, and constipation. Orthostatic hypotension is defined as a decrease in systolic blood pressure upon standing of at least 20 mmHg, or of diastolic blood pressure by at least 10 mmHg. It occurs in about 50% of DLB patients [29] and may contribute to recurrent falls as well as spells of decreased responsiveness. Orthostasis in DLB may be more prevalent and more severe than in PD, but is notably less severe than in MSA.

Orthostatic symptoms include lightheadedness and graying of vision, palpitations, tremulousness and anxiety. Syncope may occur. Symptoms are typically worst while standing or walking, often in the morning, after meals, or after a hot bath or on hot days. Contributors may include dopaminergic and antihypertensive drugs, cardiac factors and insufficient hydration; clinicians should conduct a full evaluation before simply attributing symptoms to neurodegeneration.

Urinary dysfunction is common in PD, and a few small studies suggest that it might occur even more often in DLB. Detrusor hyperactivity is the commonest pattern, causing nocturia, urgency and frequency [30].

Imaging and laboratory studies

Laboratory studies are performed in patients with suspected DLB to exclude other treatable diagnoses. Assessments for a vitamin B_{12} deficiency, thyroid disturbance and a structural brain lesion (a noncontrast CT brain is usually sufficient) are important in the evaluation of any patient with dementia. Medication lists should be reviewed for drugs that impair cognition or that cause parkinsonism (such as antipsychotics or antiemetics). Other metabolic or infectious contributors should also be considered, especially if there has been evidence of rapid decline. EEG may be necessary in some patients with dramatic fluctuations that are suspicious for seizures. Some DLB patients have prominent slow-wave activity with temporal lobe transient sharp waves, but this pattern is not diagnostically specific.

Many imaging modalities are of research interest. Given the difficulties in diagnosing DLB and separating cases from AD using clinical grounds alone, there is a broad effort to develop valid and reliable biomarkers. Nuclear imaging is especially promising. A good

imaging protocol would allow early and precise diagnosis of DLB, improving clinical care and prognostication. Improved accuracy would enhance clinical research by helping investigators select a truer population of DLB subjects, reducing "contamination" of studies with AD and other diagnoses. Ideal functional neuroimaging markers would also demonstrate change over time that correlates reliably with actual pathological degeneration, thereby potentially serving as proxy outcomes in neuroprotection trials.

For DLB specifically, dopamine transporter (DAT) imaging currently has the greatest evidence of diagnostic utility. Decreased striatal DAT binding on FP-CIT SPECT correlates well with clinically probable DLB, and discriminates clinically ascertained cases from AD [31]. Still lacking is a large study correlating DAT imaging with pathological diagnosis. Decreased DAT uptake does not separate DLB from PD or other parkinsonian disorders with striatal degeneration (such as PSP, CBD and MSA). Although decreased striatal DAT uptake is a suggestive feature in the clinical diagnosis of DLB, such imaging is not currently available for clinical use in the United States.

FDG-PET imaging is primarily used to distinguish frontotemporal dementia from AD. However, DLB patients have significant hypometabolism in the occipital lobe, especially primary visual cortex, which distinguishes them from AD patients [32]. Consistent with this, SPECT imaging shows occipital hypoperfusion in DLB relative to AD [33].

Pittsburgh Compound B (PIB), a PET ligand selective for beta amyloid, is used increasingly in Alzheimer imaging research. In one study, global cortical PIB binding was high in DLB but not in PDD, suggesting that beta amyloid may have a special role in the time course and cognitive profile of DLB [34].

Compared with AD, in DLB there is relative preservation of medial temporal lobe volume by MRI [35]. This is consistent with greater memory preservation in DLB relative to AD. Finally, cardiac *meta*-[^{123}I]iodobenzylguanidine scintigraphy is likely to show cardiac sympathetic denervation in DLB and other Lewy body diseases, but not in AD [36].

Overview of management

The main goal in DLB treatment is to maximize independence, function and quality of life while minimizing burden and stress on caregivers. The clinician must address motor, cognitive, behavioral, sleep and autonomic issues.

A major challenge is that treatments that improve certain symptoms may worsen others, requiring a "balancing act." For example, dopaminergic medications may improve motor function but may exacerbate psychosis or cognition. Whenever possible, nonpharmacological measures must be kept in mind. A mild motor decline may respond sufficiently to physical therapy. Nondistressing infrequent hallucinations may respond to reassurance only. Caregivers should be given strategies to help with psychotic symptoms such as checking around the house for signs of intrusion to validate a patient's concern, and avoiding arguments over what is or is not real.

Management of parkinsonism

In DLB, responsiveness of parkinsonism to levodopa is variable. Following acute levodopa challenge, UPDRS motor score improved by a mean 14% in DLB, versus 21% in PD [37]. In a longitudinal study of PD patients, those who were demented at 14 years had a smaller levodopa response with worse on and off disability scores than the nondemented subjects [38]. These data may reflect, in part, a higher prevalence in DLB of motor problems that are nonresponsive to levodopa, such as postural instability and dysarthria.

The pharmacologic approach to treating motor symptoms in DLB is similar to the approach in PD, with a few caveats. Amantadine, anticholinergics and dopamine agonists are generally avoided because they are more likely to worsen psychosis than levodopa. When using levodopa for DLB, it is best to "start low and go slow" [39]. Many patients are maintained at a low daily dose of 300–600 mg of levodopa, but some may tolerate higher doses.

Several nonpharmacologic measures are useful for postural instability sufficient to cause frequent falls. These include physical therapy and gait assistive devices such as walkers; stand-by supervision; and modification of the environment such as reducing clutter and adding grab bars in bathrooms. Dysphagia should be evaluated by a speech pathologist, with therapy and appropriate dietary modifications.

Management of dementia

Before initiating medications to treat cognition or psychosis, clinicians should seek correctable causes such as infection, dehydration, metabolic derangements and toxicity of medications that act on the central nervous system. Infections in the elderly may not cause fever; psychosis or delirium may be the first manifestation of a urinary tract infection or pneumonia.

The focus of pharmacologic therapy for cognitive impairment in PDD and DLB has been on the cholinesterase inhibitors. Currently there are four such drugs approved by the United States Food and Drug Administration (FDA) for use in AD: tacrine, donepezil, rivastigmine, and galantamine. The NMDA antagonist memantine is also approved for AD. Of these, only rivastigmine is FDA approved for treatment of PDD.

The rivastigmine approval for PDD was based on a large randomized, double-blind, placebo-controlled study of rivastigmine in 541 patients with PDD [40]. The mean dose of rivastigmine was 8.6 mg daily. At week 24 the rivastigmine group had a statistically significant improvement of 2.1 points on the Alzheimer's Disease Assessment Scale (ADAS-cog), versus a 0.7 point worsening in the placebo group. Scores on the Clinician's Global Impression of Change (ADCS-CGIC) significantly favored the rivastigmine group. Rivastigmine also improved scores in several secondary variables, including the Mini-mental state examination (MMSE), the Neuropsychiatric Inventory items 1–10 (NPI-10), attention, verbal fluency and the Ten Point Clock-Drawing test. Side-effects of rivastigmine were primarily gastrointestinal (nausea, vomiting, anorexia and diarrhea).

In DLB specifically, the most rigorous clinical trial of a cholinesterase inhibitor was for rivastigmine 6–12 mg versus placebo for 20 weeks, in a randomized double blind trial involving 120 subjects [41]. Almost twice as many patients on rivastigmine (63%) as on placebo (30%) showed at least a 30% improvement from baseline on the Neuropsychiatric Inventory (NPI). Performance on several secondary outcomes was significantly better with rivastigmine. Notably, measures of attention improved by 23% in the rivastigmine group and declined by 19% in the placebo group. Donepezil has smaller randomized controlled trials supporting its efficacy in PDD [42,43].

From the above studies, the American Academy of Neurology's evidence-based practice parameter concluded that rivastigmine and donepezil are probably effective in improving cognitive function and should be considered for the treatment of dementia in PD (level B recommendation) [44]. By extension, it would be reasonable to apply these therapies to DLB. There are insufficient data on tacrine, galantamine and memantine at this time.

Management of psychosis

The first step in managing psychosis is to look for correctable causes (see "Management of dementia"). If psychosis persists despite correction of the above factors, the next step is to reduce antiparkinsonian medications to their lowest tolerable levels before considering additional pharmacologic agents. There is currently no FDA-approved treatment for psychosis in these diseases. If an agent must be initiated, cholinesterase inhibitors should be tried first as they may also improve cognition, as discussed in the previous section.

Scant data support the use of cholinesterase inhibitors for psychosis in PDD or DLB. Rivastigmine has the best empirical support, with two randomized controlled trials demonstrating a reduction in hallucinations, delusions and psychosis [41,45]. Case reports exist of DLB psychosis responding to donepezil, but a large trial is still required. There are no data for the use of galantamine for psychosis in PDD or DLB.

If psychosis persists even with cholinesterase inhibition, quetiapine and clozapine can be considered as a last resort. These are currently the only atypical antipsychotics that are relatively free from extrapyramidal exacerbations, with little or no dopamine D2 receptor occupancy. Of the two, quetiapine is usually tried first because of the cumbersome weekly blood monitoring required with clozapine. However, there are other serious safety concerns, even with these drugs: the increased risk of sudden cardiac death with both atypical and typical antipsychotics [46].

Although a number of case reports or small open-label studies support the use of quetiapine or clozapine for psychosis in the PDD/DLB patient, clinical trials are lacking. A small randomized, placebo-controlled trial of quetiapine for psychosis in patients with dementia and parkinsonism (a mix of PDD and DLB) showed no benefit in the primary outcome measure (Brief Psychiatric Rating Scale) [47]. Clozapine at a mean dose of 25 mg/day was superior to placebo in reducing psychosis in PD subjects, 56% of whom had dementia, at 1 month [48].

Mild worsening of parkinsonism may occur with quetiapine treatment, but it is generally insufficient to discontinue the medication [49]. Other adverse effects include somnolence and orthostasis. Known side-effects of clozapine include sedation, sialorrhea, orthostasis and the risk of agranulocytosis.

Management of sleep dysfunction

For excess daytime somnolence, clinicians should seek out and treat medication-induced drowsiness and primary sleep disorders (e.g., obstructive sleep apnea). Wakefulness-promoting agents and stimulants have not been tested in this population; exacerbation of psychosis is a concern.

No prospective randomized trials for the treatment of RBD exist, but low-dose clonazepam at bedtime (0.25–0.5 mg) is considered the treatment of choice [2]. It is thought to work by suppressing phasic EMG activity during REM sleep [50]. The drug may impair daytime alertness or balance in some. Melatonin may be an option in these patients, with efficacy in a few open-label studies of idiopathic RBD. Nonpharmacologic safety measures include removing lamps and furniture from the bedside and placing cushions on the floor next to the bed.

Management of autonomic dysfunction

Nonpharmacologic approaches to orthostatic hypotension are vital. Increased salt and fluid intake expands blood volume. Drinking 500 ml of water can increase standing systolic blood pressure by 20 mmHg for about 2 hours [51]. Compression stockings improve venous return. Exercises such as leg crossing can help mobilize fluid centrally [52]. Elevating the head of the bed reduces supine hypertension and nocturia. Drug treatment options include midodrine and fludrocortisone. Midodrine, an α1-agonist, is the only drug FDA approved for orthostatic hypotension. Fludrocortisone, a mineralocorticoid, helps expand plasma volume. It may lower serum potassium, requiring supplementation. Both drugs can cause supine hypertension.

Urinary dysfunction can be difficult to manage. In men, prostate disease may contribute to urinary dysfunction, so a full urologic evaluation may be useful. Anticholinergic medications, such as oxybutynin and tolterodine, are the treatment of choice for detrusor hyperactivity in general, though there are no randomized control trials of these agents in PD or DLB. Moreover, their anticholinergic action in the brain may worsen cognition and psychosis. Newer agents, such as solifenacin and darifenacin, are more selective for the bladder and may prove to be safer. Trospium chloride, a nonselective anticholinergic that does not cross the blood–brain barrier, is also promising. Many patients may eventually need to be managed with intermittent or long-term catheterization.

Conclusions and future directions

There are a few common causes of parkinsonism with dementia, such as DLB and PDD, and many less common ones. DLB is a complex progressive neurodegenerative disorder affecting cognition, behavior, motor function, autonomic function and sleep. Explicit diagnostic criteria can help the clinician identify DLB, and separate it from other etiologies, especially AD. Despite this, antemortem diagnostic accuracy is limited. Available treatments are symptomatic and not neuroprotective; they are often only weakly effective and may result in significant side-effects. As with PD and PDD, α-synuclein plays a central role in the disease process; however, the initial steps that lead to neurodegeneration are still not known.

Newer developments such as molecular and metabolic nuclear imaging may eventually enter clinical practice and improve the diagnosis and care of these patients. Ultimately, what we need most are therapies that can delay the progression of the Lewy body diseases, or prevent them altogether.

References

1. McKeith IG, Galasko D, Kosaka K et al. Consensus guidelines for the clinical and pathologic diagnosis of dementia with Lewy bodies (DLB): report of the consortium on DLB international workshop. *Neurology* 1996; **47**: 1113–24.

2. McKeith IG, Dickson DW, Lowe J et al. Diagnosis and management of dementia with Lewy bodies: third report of the DLB Consortium. *Neurology* 2005; **65**: 1863–72.

3. Lippa CF, Duda JE, Grossman M et al. DLB and PDD boundary issues – diagnosis, treatment, molecular pathology, and biomarkers. *Neurology* 2007; **68**: 812–19.

4. Fujishiro H, Ferman TJ, Boeve BF et al. Validation of the neuropathologic criteria of the Third Consortium for Dementia with Lewy bodies for prospectively diagnosed cases. *J Neuropathol Exp Neurol* 2008; **67**: 649–56.

5. Merdes AR, Hansen LA, Jeste DV et al. Influence of Alzheimer pathology on clinical diagnostic accuracy in dementia with Lewy bodies. *Neurology* 2003; **60**: 1586–90.

6. Braak H, Del Tredici K, Rub U, de Vos RAI, Steur ENHJ, Braak E. Staging of brain pathology related to sporadic Parkinson's disease. *Neurobiol Aging* 2003; **24**: 197–211.

7. Jellinger KA. Lewy body-related alpha-synucleinopathy in the aged human brain. *J Neural Transm* 2004; **111**: 1219–35.

8. Kramer ML, Schulz-Schaeffer WJ. Presynaptic alpha-synuclein aggregates, not Lewy bodies, cause neurodegeneration in dementia with Lewy bodies. *J Neurosci* 2007; **27**: 1405–10.

9. Zaccai J, McCracken C, Brayne C. A systematic review of prevalence and incidence studies of dementia with Lewy bodies. *Age Ageing* 2005; **34**: 561–6.

10. Matsui Y, Tanizaki Y, Arima H et al. Incidence and survival of dementia in a general population of Japanese elderly: the Hisayama study. *J Neurol Neurosurg Psychiatry* 2009; **80**: 366–70.

11. Zarranz JJ, Alegre J, Gomez-Esteban JC et al. The new mutation, E46K, of alpha-synuclein causes Parkinson and Lewy body dementia. *Ann Neurol* 2004; **55**: 164–73.

12. Zimprich A, Biskup S, Leitner P et al. Mutations in LRRK2 cause autosomal-dominant Parkinsonism with pleomorphic pathology. *Neuron* 2004; **44**: 601–7.

13. Clark LN, Kartsaklis LA, Gilbert RW et al. Association of glucocerebrosidase mutations with dementia with Lewy bodies. *Arch Neurol* 2009; **66**: 578–83.

14. Borroni B, Grassi M, Costanzi C, Archetti S, Caimi L, Padovani A. APOE genotype and cholesterol levels in Lewy body dementia and Alzheimer disease: investigating genotype-phenotype effect on disease risk. *Am J Geriatr Psychiatry* 2006; **14**: 1022–31.

15. Kraybill ML, Larson EB, Tsuang DW et al. Cognitive differences in dementia patients with autopsy-verified AD, Lewy body pathology, or both. *Neurology* 2005; **64**: 2069–73.

16. Nelson PT, Kryscio RJ, Jicha GA et al. Relative preservation of MMSE scores in autopsy-proven dementia with Lewy bodies. *Neurology* 2009; **73**: 1127–33.

17. Bradshaw J, Saling M, Hopwood M, Anderson V, Brodtmann A. Fluctuating cognition in dementia with Lewy bodies and Alzheimer's disease is qualitatively distinct. *J Neurol Neurosurg Psychiatry* 2004; **75**: 382–7.

18. Ferman TJ, Smith GE, Boeve BF et al. DLB fluctuations – Specific features that reliably differentiate DLB from AD and normal aging. *Neurology* 2004; **62**: 181–7.

19. Walker MP, Ayre GA, Cummings JL et al. Quantifying fluctuation in dementia with Lewy bodies, Alzheimer's disease, and vascular dementia. *Neurology* 2000; **54**: 1616–24.

20. Harding AJ, Broe GA, Halliday GM. Visual hallucinations in Lewy body disease relate to Lewy bodies in the temporal lobe. *Brain* 2002; **125**: 391–403.

21. Burn DJ, Rowan EN, Allan LM, Molloy S, T O'Brien J, McKeith IG. Motor subtype and cognitive decline in Parkinson's disease, Parkinson's disease with dementia, and dementia with Lewy bodies. *Journal of Neurology Neurosurgery and Psychiatry* 2006; **77**: 585–9.

22. Louis ED, Klatka LA, Liu Y, Fahn S. Comparison of extrapyramidal features in 31 pathologically confirmed

cases of diffuse Lewy body disease and 34 pathologically confirmed cases of Parkinson's disease. *Neurology* 1997; **48**: 376–80.

23. Rajput AH, Voll A, Rajput ML, Robinson CA, Rajput A. Course in Parkinson disease subtypes: a 39-year clinicopathologic study. *Neurology* 2009; **73**: 206–12.

24. Ballard CG, Shaw F, Lowery K, McKeith I, Kenny R. The prevalence, assessment and associations of falls in dementia with Lewy bodies and Alzheimer's disease. *Dement Geriatr Cogn Disord* 1999; **10**: 97–103.

25. Gnanalingham KK, Byrne EJ, Thornton A, Sambrook MA, Bannister P. Motor and cognitive function in lewy body dementia: comparison with Alzheimer's and Parkinson's diseases. *J Neurol Neurosurg Psychiatry* 1997; **62**: 243–52.

26. Aarsland D, Perry R, Larsen JP *et al*. Neuroleptic sensitivity in Parkinson's disease and parkinsonian dementias. *J Clin Psychiatry* 2005; **66**: 633–7.

27. Boeve BF, Silber MH, Ferman TJ, Lucas JA, Parisi JE. Association of REM sleep behavior disorder and neurodegenerative disease may reflect an underlying synucleinopathy. *Mov Disord* 2001; **16**: 622–30.

28. Braak H, Rub U, Sandmann-Keil D *et al*. Parkinson's disease: affection of brain stem nuclei controlling premotor and motor neurons of the somatomotor system. *Acta Neuropathol* 2000; **99**: 489–95.

29. Allan LM, Ballard CG, Allen J *et al*. Autonomic dysfunction in dementia. *J Neurol Neurosurg Psychiatry* 2007; **78**: 671–7.

30. Ransmayr GN, Holliger S, Schletterer K *et al*. Lower urinary tract symptoms in dementia with Lewy bodies, Parkinson disease, and Alzheimer disease. *Neurology* 2008; **70**: 299–303.

31. McKeith I, O'Brien J, Walker Z *et al*. Sensitivity and specificity of dopamine transporter imaging with I-123-FP-CIT SPECT in dementia with Lewy bodies: a phase III, multicentre study. *Lancet Neurol* 2007; **6**: 305–13.

32. Minoshima S, Foster NL, Sima AAF, Frey KA, Albin RL, Kuhl DE. Alzheimer's disease versus dementia with Lewy bodies: cerebral metabolic distinction with autopsy confirmation. *Ann Neurol* 2001; **50**: 358–65.

33. Lobotesis K, Fenwick JD, Phipps A *et al*. Occipital hypoperfusion on SPECT in dementia with Lewy bodies but not AD. *Neurology* 2001; **56**: 643–9.

34. Gomperts SN, Rentz DM, Moran E *et al*. Imaging amyloid deposition in Lewy body diseases. *Neurology* 2008; **71**: 903–10.

35. Barber R, Ballard C, McKeith IG, Gholkar A, O'Brien JT. MRI volumetric study of dementia with Lewy bodies: a comparison with AD and vascular dementia. *Neurology* 2000; **54**: 1304–9.

36. Estorch M, Camacho V, Paredes P *et al*. Cardiac I-123-metaiodobenzylguanidine imaging allows early identification of dementia with Lewy bodies during life. *Eur J Nucl Med Mol Imaging* 2008; **35**: 1636–41.

37. Molloy S, McKeith IG, O'Brien JT, Burn DJ. The role of levodopa in the management of dementia with Lewy bodies. *J Neurol Neurosurg Psychiatry* 2005; **76**: 1200–3.

38. Alty JE, Clissold BG, McColl CD, Reardon KA, Shiff M, Kempster PA. Longitudinal study of the levodopa motor response in Parkinson's disease: relationship between cognitive decline and motor function. *Mov Disord* 2009; **24**: 2337–43.

39. Goldman JG, Goetz CG, Brandabur M, Sanfilippo M, Stebbins GT. Effects of dopaminergic medications on psychosis and motor function in dementia with Lewy bodies. *Mov Disord* 2008; **23**: 2248–50.

40. Emre M, Aarsland D, Albanese A *et al*. Rivastigmine for dementia associated with Parkinson's disease. *N Engl J Med* 2004; **351**: 2509–18.

41. McKeith I, Del Ser T, Spano P *et al*. Efficacy of rivastigmine in dementia with Lewy bodies: a randomised, double-blind, placebo-controlled international study. *Lancet* 2000; **356**: 2031–6.

42. Aarsland D, Laake K, Larsen JP, Janvin C. Donepezil for cognitive impairment in Parkinson's disease: a randomised controlled study. *J Neurol Neurosurg Psychiatry* 2002; **72**: 708–12.

43. Ravina B, Putt M, Siderowf A *et al*. Donepezil for dementia in Parkinson's disease: a randomised, double blind, placebo controlled, crossover study. *J Neurol Neurosurg Psychiatry* 2005; **76**: 934–9.

44. Miyasaki JM, Shannon K, Voon V *et al*. Practice Parameter: evaluation and treatment of depression, psychosis, and dementia in Parkinson disease (an evidence-based review) – Report of the Quality Standards Subcommittee of the American Academy of Neurology. *Neurology* 2006; **66**: 996–1002.

45. Burn D, Emre M, McKeith I *et al*. Effects of rivastigmine in patients with and without visual hallucinations in dementia associated with Parkinson's disease. *Mov Disord* 2006; **21**: 1899–907.

46. Ray WA, Chung CP, Murray KT, Hall K, Stein CM. Atypical Antipsychotic drugs and the risk of sudden cardiac death. *N Engl J Med* 2009; **360**: 225–35.

47. Kurlan R, Cummings J, Raman R, Thal L, Alzheimer's Disease Cooperative Study Group. Quetiapine for agitation or psychosis in patients with dementia and parkinsonism. *Neurology* 2007; **68**: 1356–63.

48. Friedman J, Lannon M, Comella C *et al*. Low-dose clozapine for the treatment of drug-induced psychosis in Parkinson's disease. *N Engl J Med* 1999; **340**: 757–63.

49. Fernandez HH, Trieschmann ME, Burke MA, Friedman JH. Quetiapine for psychosis in Parkinson's disease versus dementia with Lewy bodies. *J Clin Psychiatry* 2002; **63**: 513–5.

50. Lapierre O, Montplaisir J. Polysomnographic features of REM-sleep behavior disorder: development of a scoring method. *Neurology* 1992; **42**: 1371–4.

51. Shannon JR, Jordan J, Grogan E *et al.* The pressor response to water drinking in humans: a sympathetic reflex? *Circulation* 1998; **98**: 2484.

52. Bouvette CM, McPhee BR, OpferGehrking TL, Low PA. Role of physical countermaneuvers in the management of orthostatic hypotension: efficacy and biofeedback augmentation. *Mayo Clin Proc* 1996; **71**: 847–53.

Chapter

8

Impulsive and compulsive behaviors in Parkinson disease

Nelson Hwynn and Hubert H. Fernandez

Introduction

The traditional emphasis in Parkinson disease (PD) has been on the motor disorders of tremor, rigidity, bradykinesia and postural instability, as these were the most easily visible signs. However, in the past decade attention has expanded and also directed to non-motor manifestations that more often significantly reduce the quality of life in PD patients compared with the motor symptoms. Dopamine plays a role in the reward mechanisms. The euphoric sensations associated with drugs such as cocaine and amphetamines have been linked to dopamine transporter and D2 receptor stimulation, which also increases the attractiveness of external stimuli associated with drug intake [1]. Likewise, patients with PD can have impulse behavioral disorders such as excessive shopping, gambling and hypersexual behaviors that can be very disruptive and distressing. They can also be prone to compulsive behaviors such as repetitively acting out their urges (punding or hobbyism) owing to the dopaminergic stimulation. Dopamine dysregulation syndrome is considered another form of compulsive behavior disorder in which patients compulsively ingest dopaminergic medications [2]. Caution should be used with terminology as dopamine dysregulation syndrome can often be used in various sources of literature to refer also to all types of compulsive and impulsive behaviors as well. In this chapter, dopamine dysregulation syndrome is specifically referred to compulsively taking more dopaminergic therapy than needed for appropriate benefit of motor symptoms.

Dopamine and addiction

To understand the disorders that are presented in this chapter, it is important to consider the common underlying pathophysiology that underlies their existence; despite variabilities in how the disorders present, they share a common etiology: dopamine stimulation and hypersensitivity. Dopamine is important for voluntary movement control and the brain's reward system and modification of behavior [3]. While there are several purported mechanisms in the brain that are responsible for the development of drug addiction, there is evidence that activation of the mesocorticolimbic dopamine system plays a key role in the reinforcement effect. Mesolimbic dopamine projections to the pleasure center of the accumbens-related circuitry have been implicated in behaviors directed toward obtaining and consuming food, sex and other rewards as well as being associated with behavioral addictions [4,5]. Dopamine is a neurotransmitter thought to be associated with the euphoric sensation from using drugs. Dopaminergic cell bodies in the ventral tegmental area project to the prefrontal cortex and nucleus accumbens. The amygdala, hippocampus and hypothalamus are associated with emotional memories with drug addiction [1].

Parkinson disease results in progressive denervation of the striatum, which is often divided into two main areas. Ventral striatal degeneration leads to non-motor manifestations of loss of initiative, apathy, dysphoria, anxiety, fear and depression [3]. Overactivation of ventral striatum results in increased emotional control over behavior such as obsessive-compulsive behavior [3]. The dorsal striatum modulates voluntary movement. As this degenerates in PD, there is loss of inhibition of glutamatergic excitation of the motor cortex, leading to motor manifestations of tremor, slowness and stiffness [4]. Dorsal striatal hyperactivity leads to repetitive, stereotyped behavior in PD [3].

Current understanding postulates that pulsatile stimulation with dopaminergic medications leading to chronically intermittent stimulation of dopamine receptors leads to progressive neural adaptations and neural plasticity that change the effectiveness of transmission in neural circuits from long-term continued dopaminergic

Uncommon Causes of Movement Disorders, ed. Néstor Gálvez-Jiménez and Paul J. Tuite. Published by Cambridge University Press. © Cambridge University Press 2011.

stimulation [6,7]. Neural plasticity can be beneficial as it can help in compensation of dysfunctional activity after injury, but it can also be deleterious as in the case of impulsive and compulsive behavior disorders [7]. In normal patients, anticipation of risky behavior (involving money and sex) has been shown to result in phasic dopamine release in the nucleus accumbens, making chronic exposure to these risky behaviors addictive as well in susceptible individuals [6].

Impulse control disorders

These behaviors include pathological gambling, hypersexuality, excessive shopping and binge eating or overeating. Occasionally referred to as "behavioral addictions," impulse control disorders (ICDs) are abnormal behaviors in which patients fail to resist behaviors that result in distress or impaired social and occupational functioning and can potentially pose health risks as well [8,9]. They have been linked to the use of dopamine agonists though the selective stimulation of D3 receptors primarily confined to the limbic system that prime the reward circuits that facilitate certain behaviors [10]. In animal models, D3 receptor agonists increase motivation to obtain drugs. Bromocriptine, pramiprexole, pergolide and ropinirole all bind to D2 receptors but are also are highly potent agonists of D3 receptors [11]. Dopamine agonists were introduced in the 1980s but became widely available in the mid-1990s [12]. Many clinicians prefer to use dopamine agonists as first-line treatment, especially in younger-onset PD patients to reduce the likelihood of developing motor fluctuations and levodopa-induced dyskinesias [12,13]. Interestingly, ICD from dopamine agonist use has been associated with young age and premorbid novelty-seeking tendencies [8]. Driver-Dunckley et al. reported 1884 patients with PD, with 1281 patients on dopamine agonists (pramiprexole, ropinirole, pergolide), where 9 patients were found to experience pathological gambling [14]. Eight were on pramiprexole, one was on pergolide. None of the patients treated with levodopa alone were found to have pathological gambling. The risk of developing ICDs is 6% of Parkinson patients and about 14% of patients on dopamine agonists, although this is likely underreported for several reasons: (1) patients may be embarrassed or ashamed to disclose these aberrant behaviors to their physicians; (2) physicians do not routinely ask; and (3) even when disclosed, the behavior may not be consistently documented [10,15,16]. In a survey among PD patients, Voon et al. reported the lifetime prevalence of pathological gambling at 7.2%, of hypersexuality at 7.2%, and of compulsive shopping at 1.4% [17]. Eighty percent of ICDs can present within the first year of initiation of dopamine agonists [6]. Pathological gambling was more commonly associated with males [2,17], whereas females are thought to be more susceptible to compulsive shopping and binge eating [2]. Impulse control disorders are addictive-like behaviors that can be an extension of an individual's premorbid preference, such as excessive use of the internet or participating in sporting activities [18]. When engaged in these behaviors, individuals often feel unable to cease the activity, or forget to sleep or eat. Furthermore, they may develop withdrawal symptoms when forced to cease [18]. Reported risk factors for developing dopamine therapy-related impulse control disorders include a history of impulsivity, reward-seeking behavior, or addiction prior to initiating Parkinson disease medications [19].

In a retrospective study by Holman, out of 1356 fibromyalgia patients who were treated with dopamine agonists (mostly pramiprexole) at a mean dose of 4.5 mg at night, 21 patients developed impulse control or compulsive disorders: compulsive gambling (33%), shopping (40%), or both gambling and shopping (27%), compulsive eating (13%), cleaning (7%) and crafting (13%). These behaviors improved in 73% of patients weaned off the medication [20]. In another survey study by Driver-Dunkley et al., a small percentage of patients with restless legs syndrome treated with dopamine agonists were found to have increased urges in gambling and sexual behavior after having been started on dopaminergic medication (levodopa, ropinirole and pramiprexole) [21].

Educating patients about these potential side-effects of their medications is very important as they may not be able to make the connection themselves. Discontinuing the responsible medication may reduce or eliminate the impulse control disorder. If reduction in dopamine agonists is not possible, quetiapine or clozapine may be considered [3]. Although it is often an effective and well-tolerated medication, many clinicians are reluctant to use clozapine because of the risk of developing of agranulocytosis. In a large registry of 11 555 patients on clozapine, the cumulative incidence of agranulocytosis in the USA was 0.80% after 1 year and 0.91% after 1.5 years of use, with greatest risk occurring within the first 3 months of treatment [22]. This risk has been reduced with close monitoring of weekly white blood cell count for the first 6 months, and then every other week thereafter while the patient remains on clozapine [23].

Pathological gambling

Pathological gambling is a constantly recurring gambling disorder that is disruptive to the patient, the family, or the patient's work [24]. The International Classification of Diseases (10th edition) (ICD-10) emphasizes the continuation of gambling despite personal distress and interference with personal functioning in daily living [11,25]. Pathological gambling is more consistently seen in men than in women [26]. The risk of developing pathological gambling in all PD patients can range from 2.6% to 4.4%, which can increase to 7.2–8.0% among patients taking dopamine agonists [15]. Pathological gambling can lead to significant social, legal, and/or economic consequences that include divorce, bankruptcy, incarceration and attempted suicide [12]. This can be associated with affective disorders and substance abuse [24]. The mean latency of onset of pathological gambling from onset of dopamine agonist initiation has been estimated to be 23 months [12]. A premorbid interest in betting may be a risk factor for development of this with dopamine agonist treatment but other risk factors include male sex, young age of patients, and association with feelings of anger, anxiety and confusion [13,27]. It has been reported that pathological gamblers lost an average of $129 000 [12,28]. In a survey study by Shapiro and colleagues, most common gambling behaviors were use of slot machines (70%), scratch-off lottery tickets (50%), cards (40%), state lottery (30%), casinos (30%), and horse/dog tracks (20%) [13]. It has also been observed that compulsive gambling behavior activities increase with closer proximity to casinos [14,29,30]. Pathological gambling tends to occur during the "on-medication" states of motor fluctuations [30].

Pathological gambling has been associated with reduced activity in the ventromedial prefrontal cortex as well as the ventral striatum [15]. A recent study by Cilia et al. showed that, compared with matched healthy controls, PD patients with pathological gambling on dopamine replacement therapy exhibited overactivity in the right hemisphere of the orbitofrontal cortex, hippocampus, amygdala, insula and ventral pallidum possibly related to drug-induced overstimulation of relatively preserved reward-related neuronal systems [31].

Treatment other than educating the patient consists of reducing dopaminergic medication, if possible. Risperidone has been reported to be an effective treatment of compulsive gambling, but only in a single case study in Parkinson disease [32].

Hypersexuality

Hypersexuality can be considered a manifestation of increased libido and inappropriate frontal inhibition [18]. Hypersexuality has been estimated in PD patients to carry a lifetime prevalence rate of 2.4%. This prevalence increased to 7.2% when treated with dopamine agonists [17]. Excessive libido can lead to sexual promiscuity, constant sexual requests more than the spouse can handle, uncontrolled masturbation, or compulsive use of pornography that may lead to marital strife [19]. Patients can also display paraphilias such as voyeurism, exhibitionism, sexual masochism, zoophilia (sexual fantasies and arousals involving animals) and pedophilia [19].

In the general population, risk factors for hypersexuality are substance abuse and smoking [18,33] and hypersexuality is more commonly reported in depressed and anxious people [18,34]. In a cohort of patients with hypersexuality, Cooper et al. found them more likely to be depressed with elevated Becker Depression Inventory (BDI) scores in a majority of patients [35]. While it was traditionally thought to have been more common in males than in females, this study found hypersexuality to be equal in males and females [35].

Like other impulsive behavior disorders in PD, long-term continuous dopaminergic stimulation resulting in neuroplastic changes is thought to lead to development of hypersexuality [18]. Patients are often not forthright about disclosing hypersexual and paraphilic behaviors. Shapiro et al. described the example of a 29-year-old man with a transvestite fetishism who took 2 years to volunteer this information to his treating physicians. The patient did so only after he read an article about someone with similar issues [16]. Hypersexuality can also occur in the setting of impotence and it can accompany dopamine-replacement therapy-related penile erections [19].

If dopamine agonist and/or levodopa therapy cannot be reduced, clozapine or other atypical antipsychotics may be considered. Fernandez and Durso reported a case of a man with PD who developed paraphilias while on carbidopa/levodopa and pergolide with good response to treatment with clozapine and without significant change in pergolide and levodopa [36].

Binge eating/compulsive eating

Binge eating is defined as loss of control over eating, involving the eating large amounts of food with at least three of the following conditions: rapid eating, feeling uncomfortably full, eating large amounts of food when not hungry, eating alone because of embarrassment about the amount being eaten, feeling disgusted or guilty after overeating, and marked distress [37]. It should not occur during periods of anorexia or bulimia nervosa. Compulsive eating behavior is characterized as consumption of larger amounts of food than necessary to alleviate hunger [2]. The incidence of compulsive eating in PD may be underreported, but a small-scale study by Miwa and Kondo estimated that 8.3% of patients (out of 60 consecutive PD patients who were evaluated) exhibited alterations in food preference following the start of dopamine replacement therapy [38]. In a cohort reported by Zahodne *et al.*, out of 96 PD patients who completed questionnaires, 1 patient (1%) met all criteria for binge-eating disorder, while 8 (8.3%) had subthreshold binge eating identified by detailed questioning that the patients themselves were not aware of having [37]. Despite the general tendency of PD patients to lose weight, compulsive eating may lead to health risks such as obesity and weight gain [39]. In many cases compulsive eating and weight gain resolve with significant reduction and discontinuation of the medication [39]. Overeating has been found in higher percentages in patients with deep brain stimulation (DBS) in the subthalamic nucleus than in PD patients without DBS surgery [37]. Some other possible risk factors for patients to develop compulsive eating behaviors are younger-onset PD, premorbid histories of repetitive behaviors, or being overweight [39]. In addition, some patients develop carbohydrate craving on dopamine agonists, specifically for cookies, crackers, potato chips and pasta, as noted in a small series report by Nirenberg and Waters [39]. Carbohydrate craving by itself has been hypothesized to be "self-medication" in which consumption of sweet or starchy foods results in an increase in insulin secretion and altered tryptophan levels, resulting in increased serotonin levels that can improve dysphoria [40]. However, untreated PD patients have an intrinsic tendency to lose weight and these cases of carbohydrate craving have been linked to dopamine agonist use rather than intrinsic self-medication with carbohydrates [39].

Excessive shopping

Patients with compulsive shopping experience constant impulsive and excessive buying that can cause personal and family distress and result in financial difficulty [18]. Patients often are interested in the items that they purchase, but after the purchase interest is lost [18,41]. It has been estimated that compulsive shopping has a lifetime prevalence of 5.8% in the general adult population; it mostly involves women and has been found in people who have family history of mood disorders and substance abuse [3,42]. Estimates of prevalence in Parkinson patients are not widely available at this time. Like other forms of compulsive shopping, this usually improves significantly with reduction in dopamine agonist therapy.

Dopamine and compulsive behavioral disorders

The abnormal behaviors associated with using more dopaminergic medications than necessary for motor benefit and punding, in which patients compulsively perform meaningless, repetitive activity, are grouped under the category of compulsive behavioral disorders. The precise mechanism for compulsive behavior disorders has not been completely elucidated at this time. A hypothesis for the etiology of compulsive behaviors can be made from observations in cases where there was reduction of punding behavior and dopamine dysregulation syndrome after deep brain stimulation, where it is thought that pulsatile dopaminergic stimulation can lead to neural plasticity [43]. Neural plasticity refers to the ability to change the effectiveness of transmission in neural circuits [7]. This can be beneficial as it can help in compensation of dysfunctional activity after injury [7]. However, repeated pulsatile stimulation of dopamine may lead to "priming" of neural plastic changes that predisposes to development of compulsive behaviors. Unlike impulsive behavior disorders, which occur usually with dopamine agonists and not with levodopa, compulsive use of levodopa in dopamine dysregulation disorder occurs with high levodopa dose and not with dopamine agonists [15,44]. With repeated exposure to cocaine and amphetamines, long-lasting alterations in the nucleus accumbens and dorsal striatum lead

Table 8.1. Differences between OCD and compulsive and impulse control disorders in Parkinson disease prior to, during and after performing the act.

Event	Obsessive-compulsive behavior	Punding	Impulse control disorders
Prior to the act	Anxious / distressed / conflicted	Intense curiosity / fascination with object or activity	Strong, uncontrollable urge / impulse
During and *after* the act	Sense of relief	Sense of calmness	Pleasure / satisfaction

Reprinted with permission from Fernandez *et al.* [2].

to enhancement of the motivational impact of drug-associated stimuli and compulsive drug use [4,45].

Punding

Originally described in amphetamine addicts in Scandinavian countries [27,46], punding refers to complex behavior characterized by intense fascination with repetitive movements that traditionally has been determined to be meaningless or purposeless. Such behavior includes continual handling, collecting, examining and sorting of common objects, taking apart mechanical objects, hoarding, pointless driving, and engaging in extended monologues devoid of meaning, but can also involve some activities that may not be as meaningless, such as excessive grooming, sorting, and writing [47–49]. It does not appear to be related to depression, dementia, severity of PD, or obsessive-compulsive behaviors [48]. The frequency of punding in PD patients has been reported to be from 1.4% to 14% [50,51].

Punding in Parkinson disease is thought to be related to dopamine excess and is traditionally considered to be correlated with higher than average doses of levodopa and compulsive use of dopaminergic drugs [48,52]. There may be a "priming" effect from chronic dopaminergic stimulation that underlies the pathophysiology of punding, similar to the underlying mechanisms responsible for the development of levodopa-induced dyskinesias. Punding in fact can be seen more often in patients with tardive dyskinesias, which supports this theory [15]. Highly addictive drugs such as cocaine, amphetamines and methamphetamines all work by inhibiting dopamine transporters (DAT) and greatly increasing the concentration of dopamine in the nucleus accumbens, providing continued dopamine stimulation of this pleasure center [1].

The use of selegeline may increase the incidence of punding in patients also on dopamine agonist treatment and improve when the selegeline is removed.

This may be due to its being metabolized to amphetamine [48]. It may be difficult, yet important, to differentiate punding from obsessive-compulsive disorders (OCDs) or behaviors. Punding is driven by an intense fascination in carrying out the repetitive behavior, whereas OCD is driven by obsessive thoughts about performing certain actions, with a perceived sense of relief when those actions are carried out [53,54] (Table 8.1). After performing the task, OCD patients often perceive a relief of "sense of" tension, whereas patients who perform acts of punding find a sense of calmness rather than the relief of inner tension. Punders can be temporarily distracted from carrying out the activity but can be irritated if they are unable to resume [27]. Both OCD and punding can severely interfere with patients' normal functioning [48]. Punding activity can persist throughout the night and lead to insomnia and sleep deprivation [27]. There may be sex differences between the punding activities carried out by males and females. Males tended to take apart engines or electronic devices such as clocks, watches and radio sets, while females can have tendencies to sort through their handbags and continuously brush their hair [27].

In one of the early case reports series, Fernandez and Friedman described three women of ages ranging from 65 to 72 years, one of whom spent hours at the supermarket fascinated with cans, one would spend hours gardening and would rather wet herself rather than stop, and the third hoarded flashlights and would take them apart [48]. A case report by Nguyen *et al.* described a 54-year-old man without a history of Parkinson disease or use of dopaminergic therapy who developed a right pontine acute ischemic infarct and several days afterward developed an extreme fascination with hand-copying recipes from online recipes and websites, spending enormous amount of time in this activity. He did not feel any "relief" in his symptoms and was angered when asked to cease his activities [53].

A plausible approach to attempting to improve punding is to try to reduce the dosage of dopamine replacement therapy, if possible, but this may lead to worsening of parkinsonian symptoms. Since this not always possible without significant worsening of parkinsonism, amantadine has been considered as one approach as it helps in the treatment of levodopa-induced dyskinesias. Although there are no randomized controlled trials (RCTs) with amantadine for treatment of punding, in a case report Kashihara and Imamura described dramatic improvement of chronic punding in a PD patient without levodopa-induced dyskinesias the day after introduction of amantadine 200 mg [55]. Likewise there have been no RCTs to see whether antipsychotics would help alleviate punding, but there have been case reports documenting onset of punding associated with high doses of quetiapine use of 100–200 mg/day [56]. In the case report of punding after brain stem stroke, Nguyen and colleagues reported improvement with sertraline at 100–150 mg/day [53].

Dopamine dysregulation syndrome

Also called "hedonistic homeostatic dysregulation" [6], this is a recently described phenomenon that has been associated with impulsive personality traits and compulsive intake of medication. Patients with dopamine dysregulation syndrome (DDS) seek higher and higher doses of dopamine replacement therapy (DRT) well above doses needed to treat their motor disabilities; they complain about ineffectiveness and can increase doses against medical advice [4]. Patients can exaggerate their symptoms of stiffness and tremors or resort to bribery in an effort to get more medication [4]. The prevalence of DDS in patients in PD centers has been reported to be about 3–4% [47]. Risk factors for DDS include being male, younger-onset PD, higher novelty-seeking personality, history of heavy alcohol consumption or illegal drug use and history of affective disorder [4,57]. Impulsive behaviors can result from excessive use of dopaminergic stimulation. The sensation of need for higher doses of dopamine does not give a feeling of pleasure or satisfaction but rather is driven by the sensation of compulsive wanting and craving of more dopamine [47].

In early stages of DDS, patients can get boosts of energy and productivity without significant improvements in motor symptoms. With progression of DDS, patients note off-medication dysphoria or dopamine replacement therapy-induced euphoria [4]. Patients may develop an altered perception of "on-medication"

time and may feel "on" when markedly dyskinetic [58]. As doses continue to increase, patients may develop hypomania and mania with disorganized thinking and poor judgment. Patients may develop paranoia aimed at family and caregivers. They may also develop punding and impulse control disorders [58]. Many of these symptoms of psychosis improve with reduction of the dosage of dopaminergic stimulation.

Since the goal of treatment in patients with DDS is reduction of medication, one might expect that deep brain stimulation surgery (particularly of the subthalamic nucleus, where there is an average 50% reduction of medications) would be ideal to help treat DDS, but the evidence has been contradictory despite improvements in motor scores after surgery [57] (Table 8.2).

Treatment of DDS may be complicated and may need to involve a multidisciplinary approach with a neurologist, a psychiatrist, the patient's pharmacist and the patient's family as well. The patient needs to be gradually weaned down with close monitoring. Subcutaneous administration of apomorphine and dopamine agonists should be taken off first, then levodopa therapy weaned. Some patients develop a "high" with the rapid onset of effects [58]. There may be a worsening of depression and/or anxiety as the medications are reduced and psychiatric symptoms will need to be closely monitored, with help from a psychiatrist if needed for initiation or titration of worsening depression/anxiety [47,58]. Cognitive behavioral therapy may also be tried, but at the current time there are no random controlled trials on psychological treatments in DDS [47].

Deep brain stimulation and impulse behavior disorders

In a double-blind comparative study, no difference was seen between the motor benefits from deep brain stimulation (DBS) of the subthalamic nucleus (STN) compared with the globus pallidus interna (GPi) [59]. However, STN stimulation can lead to more medication reduction than GPi site stimulation [59]. It is therefore possible that resolution of neuropsychiatric symptoms caused by dopaminergic medications is more likely with STN stimulation owing to the greater net reduction in medication dose than with GPi stimulation [60]. Wood *et al.*, for example, reported improvement in punding behavior after unilateral STN stimulation [61]. However, reports in the literature have mixed outcomes, with some cases showing improvement or resolution of impulsive and compulsive behaviors after surgery and other reports of introduction or

Table 8.2. Review of outcomes of deep brain stimulation surgery cases for Parkinson patients who developed reported impulsive/compulsive behavioral disorders.

Author	Year	Number of patients	Target sites	Outcome
Lim *et al.* [57]	2009	21	9 b/l STN	Had pre-op ICD unchanged or worse
			5 b/l STN	Had pre-op ICD improved
			1 R STN	Had pre-op ICD unchanged or worse (unclear from paper)
			2 b/l Gpi	Had pre-op unchanged or worse
			2 b/l STN	Developed DDS after surgery
			1 b/l STN	Developed ICD after surgery
Halbig *et al.* [62]	2009	16	STN (unspecified)	Only looked at patients postoperatively 3/16 patients (19%) with STN DBS developed ICD compared with 3/37 patients (8%) with PD who were managed
Ardouin *et al.* [43]	2006	7	b/l STN	All seven had impulse control disorders preoperatively that resolved by 18 months post-STN DBS with reduction of medication dosages
Wood *et al.* [61]	2009	3	unilateral STN	Two patients had improvement in punding behaviors despite higher levodopa equivalent doses; 1 patient developed punding after surgery when pramiprexole started that resolved after pramiprexole was discontinued
Knobel *et al.* [65]	2008	1	STN	Had compulsive use of dopaminergic drugs before surgery, resolved after surgery and medication reduction
Smeding *et al.* [64]	2007	1	b/l STN	3 years after STN, admitted to health care providers that he had developed severely disruptive pathological gambling despite having had levodopa and pergolide reduced; ICD disappeared with weaning off pergolide completely
Sensi *et al* [63]	2004	1	b/l STN	Patient developed rage and kleptomania related to increased voltage that persisted at 6 months post-DBS

STN, subthalamic nucleus; b/l, bilateral; ICD, impulse control disorder; DDS, dopamine dysregulation syndrome; PD, Parkinson disease; DBS, deep brain stimulation.

worsening of such behaviors. Risk factors for development of impulse control behavior disorders in DBS include patients with a preoperative history of levodopa abuse, younger age of PD onset, shorter duration of PD, and high motivation to self-medication [60]. Impulse behavioral disorders such as hypersexuality and compulsive shopping have been attributed to high frequency STN DBS stimulation [3]. These behaviors do not always improve when dopamine agonists are reduced and discontinued. Care should be used in pre-screening these patients prior to surgery for impulsive and compulsive behavioral disorders.

References

1. Haile CN, Kosten TR, Kosten TA. Pharmacogenetic treatments for drug addiction: cocaine, amphetamine

and methamphetamine. *Am J Drug Alcohol Abuse* 2009; **35**(3): 161–77.

2. Fernandez HH, Nguyen FN, Shapiro MA, Cooper C, Wood MF, Okun MS. Compulsive behavior versus impulse control disorders: a single-center experience from the University of Florida Movement Disorders Center. *Mov Disord* 2008; **23**(9): 1335–6.

3. Wolters ECh, van der Werf YD, van den Heuvel OA. Parkinson's disease-related disorders in the impulsive-compulsive spectrum. *J Neurol* 2008; **255**(Suppl 5): 48–56.

4. Evans AH, Lees AJ. Dopamine dysregulation syndrome in Parkinson's disease. *Curr Opin Neurol* 2004; **17**(4): 393–8.

5. Moro, E. Impulse control disorders and subthalamic nucleus stimulation in Parkinson's disease: are we jumping the gun? *Eur J Neurol* 2009; **16**(4): 440–1.

6. Antonini A, Cilia R. Behavioural adverse effects of dopaminergic treatments in Parkinson's disease: incidence, neurobiological basis, management and prevention. *Drug Saf* 2009; **32**(6): 475–88.

7. Linazasoro, G. Dopamine dysregulation syndrome and levodopa-induced dyskinesia in Parkinson disease: common consequences of anomalous forms of neural plasticity. *Clin Neuropharmacol* 2009; **32**(1): 22–27.

8. Dagher A, Robbins TW. Personality, addiction, dopamine: insights from Parkinson's disease *Neuron* 2009; **61**(4): 502–10.

9. Pontone G, Williams JR, Bassett SS, Marsh L. Clinical features associated with impulse control disorders in Parkinson disease. *Neurology* 2006; **67**(7): 1118–9.

10. Bostwick JM, Kathleen AH, Stevens SR, Bower JH, Ahlskog JE. Frequency of new-onset pathologic compulsive gambling or hypersexuality after drug treatment of idiopathic parkinson disease. *Mayo Clin Proc* 2009; **84**(4): 310–6.

11. Lader, M. Antiparkinsonian medication and pathological gambling. *CNS Drugs* 2008; **22**(5): 407–16.

12. Lim SY, Evans AH, Miyasaki JM. Impulse control and related disorders in Parkinson's disease: review. *Ann N Y Acad Sci* 2008, **1142**: 85–107.

13. Shapiro MA, Chang YL, Munson SK *et al.*. The four As associated with pathological Parkinson disease gamblers: anxiety, anger, age, and agonists. *Neuropsychiatr Dis Treat* 2007; **3**(1): 161–7.

14. Driver-Dunckley E, Samanta J, Stacy M. Pathological gambling associated with dopamine agonist therapy in Parkinson's disease. *Neurology* 2003; **61**(3): 422–3.

15. Voon V, Potenza M, Thomsen T. Medication-related impulse control and repetitive behaviors in Parkinson's disease. *Curr Opin Neurol* 2007; **20**(4): 484–92.

16. Shapiro MA, Chang YL, Munson SK, Okun MS, Fernandez HH. Hypersexuality and paraphilia induced by selegeline in Parkinson's disease: Report of 2 cases. *Parkinsonism Relat Disord* 2006; **12**(6): 392–5.

17. Voon V, Hassan K, Zurowski M *et al.* Prevalence of repetitive and reward-seeking behaviors in Parkinson disease. *Neurology* 2006; **67**(7): 1254–7.

18. Merims D, Giladi N. Dopamine dysregulation syndrome, addiction and behavioral changes in Parkinson's disease. *Parkinsonism Relat Disord* 2008; **14**(4): 273–80.

19. Ferrrara JM, Stacy M. Impulse-control disorders in Parkinson's disease. *CNS Spectr* 2008; **13**(8): 690–8.

20. Holman, AJ. Impulse control disorder behaviors associated with pramipexole used to treat fibromyalgia. *J Gambl Stud* 2009; **25**(3): 425–31.

21. Driver-Dunckley ED, Noble BN, Hentz JG *et al.* Gambling and increased sexual desire with dopaminergic medications in restless legs syndrome. *Clin Neuropharmacol* 2007; **30**(5): 249–55.

22. Alvir JM, Lieberman JA, Safferman AZ, Schwimmer JL, *Schaaf JA*. Clozapine-induced agranulocytosis. Incidence and risk factors in the United States. *N Engl J Med* 1993; **329**(3): 162–7.

23. Honigfeld G, Arellano F, Sethi J, Bianchini A, Schein J. Reducing clozapine-related morbidity and mortality: 5 years of experience with the Clozaril National Registry. *J Clin Psychiatry* 1998; **59**(Suppl 3): 3–7.

24. DeCaria CM, Hollander E, Grossman R, Wong CM, Mosovich SA, Cherkasky S. Diagnosis, neurobiology, and treamtent of pathological gambling. *J Clin Psychiatry* 1996; **57**(Suppl 8): 80–83; discussion 83–4.

25. World Health Organization. *ICD-10 Classification of Mental and Behavioral Disorders*. Edinburgh: Churchill Livingstone; 1994.

26. Unwin BK, Davis MK, De Leeuw JB. Pathologic gambling. *Am Fam Physician* 2000; **61**: 741–9.

27. Evans AH, Katzenschlager R, Paviour D *et al.* Punding in Parkinson's disease: its relation to the dopamine dysregulation syndrome. *Mov Disord* 2004; **19**(4): 397–405.

28. Voon V, Hassan K, Zurowski M *et al.*. Prospective prevalence of pathologic gambling and medication association in Parkinson disease. *Neurology* 2006; **66**(11): 1750–2.

29. Jacques C, Ladouceur R. A prospective study of the impact of opening a casino on gambling behaviours: 2- and 4-year follow-ups. *Can J Psychiatry* 2006; **51**(12): 764–73.

30. Molina JA, Sáinz-Artiga MJ, Fraile A *et al.* Pathologic gambling in Parkinson's disease: a behavioral manifestation of pharmacologic treatment? *Mov Disord* 2000; **15**(5): 869–72.

31. Cilia R, Siri C, Marotta G *et al.* Functional abnormalities underlying pathological gambling in Parkinson disease. *Arch Neurol* 2008; **65**(12): 1604–11.

32. Seedat S, Kesler S, Niehaus DJ, Stein DJ. Pathological gambling behaviour: emergence secondary to treatment of Parkinson's disease with dopaminergic agents. *Depress Anxiety* 2000; **11**(4): 185–6.

33. Langstrom N, Hanson RK. High rates of sexual behavior in the general population: correlates and predictors. *Arch Sex Behav* 2006; **35**(1): 37–52.

34. Bancroft J, Vukadinovic Z. Sexual addiction, sexual compulsivity, sexual impulsivity, or what? Toward a theoretical model. *J Sex Res* 2004; **41**(3): 225–34.

35. Cooper CA, Jadidian A, Paggi M *et al.* Prevalence of hypersexual behavior in Parkinson's disease patients: not restricted to males and dopamine agonist use. *J Gen Med* 2009; **2**: 57–61.

36. Fernandez HH, Durso R. Clozapine for dopaminergic-induced paraphilias in Parkinson's disease. *Mov Disord* 1998; **13**(3): 597–8.

37. Zahodne LB, Susatia F, Bowers D, Okun MS, Fernandez HH. Binge eating in Parkinson disease: prevalence, correlates, and the contribution of deep brain stimulation. *J Neuropsychiatry Clin Neurosci* 2011; **23**(1): 56–62.

38. Miwa H, Kondo T. Alteration of eating behaviors in patients with Parkinson's disease: possibly overlooked? *Neurocase* 2008; **14**(6): 480–4.

39. Nirenberg MJ, Waters C. Compulsive eating and weight gain related to dopamine agonist use. *Mov Disord* 2006; **21**(4): 524–9.

40. Wurtman RJ, Wurtman JJ. Brain serotonin, carbohydrate-craving, obesity and depression. *Obes Res* 1995; **3**(Suppl 4): 477S–80S.

41. Lejoyeux M, Bailly F, Moula H, Loi S, Adès J. Study of compulsive buying in patients presenting obsessive-compulsive disorder. *Comp Psychiatry* 2005; **46**(2): 105–10.

42. Koran LM, Faber RJ, Aboujaoude E, Large MD, Serpe RT. Estimated prevalence of compulsive buying in the United States. *Am J Psychiatry* 2006; **163**: 1806–12.

43. Ardouin C, Voon V, Worbe Y *et al.* Pathological gambling in Parkinson's disease improves on chronic subthalamic nucleus stimulation. *Mov Disord* 2006; **21**(11): 1941–6.

44. Evans AH, Lawrence AD, Potts J, Appel S, Lees AJ. Factors influencing susceptibility to compulsive dopaminergic drug use in Parkinson disease. *Neurology* 2005; **65**(10): 1570–4.

45. Kalivas PW, McFarland K. Brain circuitry and the reinstatement of cocaine-seeking behavior. *Psychopharmacology (Berl)* 2003; **168**(1–2): 44–56.

46. Sethi, K. Levodopa unresponsive symptoms in Parkinson disease. *Mov Disord* 2008; **23** (Suppl): S521–33.

47. O'Sullivan SS, Evans AH, Lees AJ. Dopamine dysregulation syndrome: an overview of its epidemiology, mechanisms, and management. *CNS Drugs* 2009; **23**(2): 157–170.

48. Fernandez HH, Friedman JH. Punding on L-dopa. *Mov Disord* 1999; **14**(5): 836–8.

49. Nguyen FN, Chang Y, Okun MS *et al.* Prevalence and characteristics of punding and repetitive behaviors among Parkinson patients in North-Central Florida. *Int J Geriatr Psychiatry* 2009; **24**: 1–2.

50. Miyasaki MJ, Al Hassan K, Lang AE. Punding prevalence in Parkinson's disease. *Mov Disord* 2007; **22**: 1179–81.

51. Stamey W, Jankovic J. Impulse control disorders and pathological gambling in Parkinson disease. *Neurologist* 2008; **14**(2): 89–99.

52. Silveira-Moriyama L, Evans AH, Katzenschlager R, Lees AJ. Punding and dyskinesias. *Mov Disord* 2006; **21**(12): 2214–7.

53. Nguyen FH, Pauly RR, Okun MS, Fernandez HH. Punding as a complication of brain stem stroke? Report of a case. *Stroke* 2007; **38**(4): 1390–2.

54. Kluger BM, Fernandez HH. Management of non-motor manifestations of Parkinson's disease. In: Pahwa R, Simuni T, eds. *Parkinson's Disease*. New York: Oxford University Press; 2009: 83–94.

55. Kashihara K, Imamura T. Amantadine may reverse punding in Parkinson's disease: observation in a patient. *Mov Disord* 2008; **23**(1): 129–30.

56. Miwa H, Morita S, Nakanishi I, Kondo T. Stereotyped behaviors or punding after quetiapine administration in Parkinson's disease. *Parkinsonism Relat Disord* 2004; **10**(3): 177–80.

57. Lim SY, O'Sullivan SS, Kotschet K *et al.* Dopamine dysregulation syndrome, impulse control disorders and punding after deep brain stimulation surgery for Parkinson's disease. *J Clin Neurosci* 2009; **9**(16): 1148–52.

58. Giovannoni G, O'Sullivan JD, Turner K, Manson AJ, Lees AJ. Hedonistic homeostatic dysregulation in patients with Parkinson's disease on dopamine replacement therapies. *J Neurol Neurosurg Psychiatry* 2000; **68**(4): 423–8.

59. Okun MS, Fernandez HH, Wu SS *et al.* Cognition and mood in Parkinson's disease in subthalamic nucleus versus globus pallidus interna deep brain stimulation: the COMPARE trial. *Ann Neurol* 2009; **65**(5): 586–95.

60. Voon V, Kubu C, Krack P, Houeto JL, Troster AI. Deep brain stimulation: neuropsychological and neuropsychiatric issues. *Mov Disord* 2006; **21**(Suppl 14): S305–27.

61. Wood MF, Nguyen FN, Okun MS, Rodriguez RL, Foote KD, Fernandez HH. The effect of deep brain stimulation surgery on repetitive behavior in Parkinson patients: a case series. *Neurocase* 2010; **16**(1): 31–6.

62. Hälbig TD, Tse W, Frisina PG *et al.* Subthalamic deep brain stimulation and impulse control in Parkinson's disease. *Eur J Neurol* 2009; **16**(4): 493–7.

63. Sensi M, Eleopra R, Cavallo MA *et al.* Explosive-aggressive behavior related to bilateral subthalamic stimulation. *Parkinsonism Relat Disord* 2004; **10**(4): 247–51.

64. Smeding HM, Goudriaan AE, Foncke EM, Schuurman PR, Speelman JD, Schmand B. Pathological gambling after bilateral subthalamic nucleus stimulation in Parkinson disease. *J Neurol Neurosurg Psychiatry* 2007; **78**(5): 517–19.

65. Knobel D, Aybek S, Pollo C, Vingerhoets FJ, Berney A. Rapid resolution of dopamine dysregulation syndrome (DDS) after subthalamic DBS for Parkinson Disease: a case report. *Cogn Behav Neurol* 2008; **21**(3): 187–9.

Pallidal and thalamic atrophies

Kurt A. Jellinger

Introduction

Pallidal and thalamic atrophies are rare neurodegenerative diseases of both familial and sporadic occurrence, clinically featuring progressive movement disorders and morphologically by degeneration of the globus pallidus (GP) alone or in association with the subthalamic nucleus (STN), substantia nigra (SN) or other neuronal systems. An autosomal dominant basal ganglia disease with iron accumulation in the GP is neuroferritinopathy. The GP may also be involved in other neurodegenerative diseases, e.g., Huntington disease (HD).

Thalamic atrophy occurs as a rare familial or sporadic neurodegenerative syndrome of unknown etiology, is a distinctive feature of fatal familial insomnia (FFI), a prion disease, or is associated with a variety of other disorders. The essential clinical and morphologic features of both syndromes are reviewed (see also reference 1).

Pallidal atrophies
History and terminology

In 1917, Hunt described four sporadic cases of juvenile paralysis agitans with progressive rigidity, tremor and flexion dystonia [2]. One autopsy case showed neuronal loss and gliosis in GP, caudate nucleus (CN), putamen and nucleus basalis of Meynert (NBM), with degeneration of the ansa lenticularis, striopallidal and striatoluysian fibers. Hunt interpreted it as "primary atrophy of the efferent pallidal system." A female patient later developing pyramidal signs, morphologically showing pallor of the pyramidal tracts in the medulla oblongata, was considered to have "pallidopyramidal disease" [3], a term critically discussed recently [4]. Degenerative disorders of the pallidal and pallido-luysio-nigral systems, reviewed by Van Bogaert [5], are

classified into subgroups (Table 9.1). They are defined purely morphologically, and, because of much clinical and morphologic overlap among these disorders, it is not clear whether they truly represent distinct diseases. Their etiology is unknown.

Clinical findings

Depending on the pattern of morphologic lesions, salient features are choreoathetosis, torsion dystonia, akinesia with or without rigidity, and other movement disorders that gradually decrease and are often replaced by rigidity, rigido-spasticity, or abnormal postures and limb contractures. They may be associated with intellectual impairment. From the limited number of autopsy-confirmed cases, the following clinical syndromes can be distinguished.

"Pure" pallidal atrophy (PPA), a juvenile onset disorder, is characterized by isolated bilateral degeneration of the GP and of the efferent pallidal fibers. Six confirmed cases with onset at age 5–14 years [5–8] showed pes equinovarus deformity in three patients and mental retardation in two. Torsion dystonia, choreoathetosis and speech disorders due to peribuccal spasms were seen in early stages, while one patient presented with slowness in motion without rigidity [7]. Hyperflexion, hyperpronation deformity of the limbs, and abnormal proximal postures were associated with increasing involuntary movements, later by progressive akinesia, rigidity or spasticity and dystonic postures. Tendon reflexes varied; pyramidal, sensory and mental impairment could be present. Final stages showed stiffness, contractures, dystonic postures, and dysphagia with only rare torsion-dystonic movements. Death occurred between age 54 and 65 years.

Pallidoluysian atrophy (PLA), morphologically featured by symmetrical atrophy of the GP and STN, was observed in one member of a family with torticollis,

Uncommon Causes of Movement Disorders, ed. Néstor Gálvez-Jiménez and Paul J. Tuite. Published by Cambridge University Press. © Cambridge University Press 2011.

Table 9.1. Pallidal degenerations: classification and possible variants.

Pure pallidal atrophy	
Age of onset	First and second decades
Clinical features	Variable mental retardation, movement disorders (dystonia, rigidity, choreoathetosis), later akinesia
Neuropathology	Loss of neurons from globus pallidus, especially the external segment Loss of myelinated fibers from the pallidoluysian tract Mild gliosis of the subthalamic nucleus
Genetics	Autosomal-recessive or sporadic
Pallidoluysian atrophy	
Age of onset	Juvenile, adult
Clinical features	Extrapyramidal movements: dystonia, cognitive decline, ballism, rigidity, hypokinesia (juvenile onset)
Neuropathology	Neuronal loss from and gliosis of globus pallidus and subthalamic nucleus
Genetics	Autosomal-recessive or sporadic
Pallidonigral degeneration	
Age of onset	Early infantile or adulthood
Clinical features	Spasticity, opisthotonus, seizures, decerebrate state (infantile onset)
Neuropathology	Bilateral degeneration of globus pallidus and substantia nigra
Genetics	Sporadic
Pallidonigroluysian degeneration	
Age of onset	Adulthood
Clinical features	Akinesia, rigidity, pseudobulbar palsy, supranuclear gaze palsy
Neuropathology	Degeneration of external and internal segment of globus pallidus, subthalamic nucleus, ventrolateral thalamic nucleus, substantia nigra
Genetics	Sporadic
Pallidonigrospinal atrophy (debatable)	
Age of onset	17–54 years
Clinical features	Extrapyramidal movement disorder with cognitive decline leading to dementia; amyotrophy
Neuropathology	Neuronal loss from globus pallidus, substantia nigra, and spinal anterior horns Variable loss of neurons from subthalamic nucleus, pontine tegmentum Variable degeneration of corticospinal tracts (questionable)
Dentatorubropallidonigral degeneration	
Age of onset	Early adulthood, adults (wide range of onset)
Clinical features	Ataxia, chorea, dystonia, gaze palsy, dementia, spastic paraparesis, myoclonus
Neuropathology	Multiple system degeneration involving dentatorubral and pallidonigral systems, involvement of centrum medianus thalami, and other systems
Genetics	Autosomal-dominant; unstable CAG triplet repeat on chromosome 12p

presenting with dystonia, head tremor and distal abnormal movement, followed by progressive rigidity. Other patients presented with athetosis, axial torsion dystonia and complex hyperkinesias or supranuclear gaze palsy [9], tremor, dystonia and postural disorders, followed by progressive rigidity [10], ballistic movements, dystonia, ataxia, dysarthria, hypokinesia and dementia.

Pallidonigral atrophy (PNA), with symmetric degeneration of the GP and STN, was observed in two sibling Afro-American girls who, at ages 4 and 16 months, developed fever, lymphadenopathy, hepatosplenomegaly and sickle cell anemia with progressive spasticity, hyperreflexia, opisthotonus and convulsion. They died at ages 23 and 35 months [11]. A man aged 51 years developed progressive pure akinesia, freezing phenomenon and festination during 21 years, without tremor, rigidity, upward gaze palsy and dementia, not responding to L-dopa. A 54-year-old woman with negative family history developed proximal limb weakness, wasting and fasciculation, associated with rigidity, tremor and akinesia. Autopsy revealed spinal pallidonigral degeneration with neuronal loss in spinal anterior horns [12].

Pallidonigroluysian atrophy (PNLA), typified by degeneration of the GP, STN, and SN, in two unrelated adult males presented with progressive akinesia, hypomimia, parkinsonian gait, dysarthria, rigidity, upward-gaze palsy and pseudobulbar signs [13]. Similar clinical features without rigidity or tremor occurred in two unrelated men [14]. Duration of disease ranged from 5 to 8 years. Other patients presented as pure akinesia [15,16], rapid progressive hemidystonia [17], association with progressive supranuclear palsy (PSP) and adult-onset Hallervorden–Spatz disease [18] or motor neuron disease with or without dementia [19–21].

Pallidoluysian dentate atrophy (PLDA), with degeneration of the pallidoluysian and dentatorubral systems, was observed in a case of hereditary hemiballism [22], and in other sporadic and familial cases presenting with myoclonus epilepsy [23].

Pallidopyramidal disease/syndrome (PPD/S) or pallidonigrospinal degeneration (a misnomer?). The combination of recessive early-onset parkinsonism and pyramidal tract signs is known as pallidopyramidal disease. Since Davison's [3] original description of two unrelated sibling pairs from consanguineous parents and a patient reported by Hunt [2], 15 other cases have been reported, most of whom suffered from early-onset parkinsonism or L-dopa-responsive dystonia and pseudobabinski ("striatal toe"), often mistaken for pyramidal Babinski sign. However, since there is no definite postmortem proof of pyramidal lesions in any of these patients, the existence of PPD/S has recently been considered to be doubtful [4].

The autosomal-recessive Kufor–Rakeb syndrome, characterized by early-onset L-dopa-responsive parkinsonism, supranuclear upgaze palsy, spasticity and dementia caused by mutation of PARKIN 9 at chromosome 1p.36 [24], has also been designed pallidopyramidal degeneration, but reexamination was unable to confirm previous MRI findings of pyramidal degeneration [24].

Dentatorubral-pallidoluysian atrophy (DRLPA), a rare autosomal dominant spinocerebellar degeneration disorder, caused by unstable (CAG)n expression in atrophin I (ATN-1) on chromosome 12p13,31 (the normal gene includes 7–23 CAG repeats, *DRPLA* alleles contain 49–75 repeats), is clinically characterized by a variable combination of progressive dementia, ataxia, chorea, epilepsy and psychiatric disturbance [25]. The disease occurs in both Japanese and non-Asian populations [26]. Three main types of the disease were distinguished; an ataxo-choreoathetotic, a pseudo-Huntington and a myoclonic-epileptic type [27]. Early-onset patients with larger CAG repeat extension tend to have prominent myoclonic epilepsy. Patients with onset after age 20 years develop cerebellar ataxia, choreoathetosis, or dystonic movements with or without dementia, and no opsoclonus [25]. Some patients showed supranuclear palsy or nystagmus. Myelopathy with spastic paraparesis and truncal ataxia can be seen with homozygosity for intermediate-size alleles [25]. Non-Asian patients with a mean age at onset of 31 years (range 1–67 years), mainly show epilepsy, ataxia and chorea as common features. Their clinicogenetic phenomenology is similar to Asian series, with marked genetic anticipation and a clear association between repeat length, clinical phenotype and disease severity [26]. Recent studies suggest that the mutant C-terminal frequently plays a principal role in the pathologic accumulation of ATN1 in DRPLA [28]. It is now likely that DRPLA has an aspect of neuronal storage disorder and shows multiple system degeneration, the lesion distribution of which varies depending on the CAG repeat sizes in the causative gene [29].

Neuroferritinopathy is a hereditary multisystem disorder caused by mutations in the gene encoding ferritin light chain (FTL) in various pedigrees. Its clinical features include choreoathetosis, parkinsonism, focal dystonia, especially orofacial dystonia leading to dys-arthrophonia, cerebellar signs, and cognitive impairment, with great variability among affected individuals [30–31].

Natural history

The disorders of this group have an insidious onset and a slowly progressive course with onset of symptoms in familial cases between ages 5 and 40 years and in sporadic cases between 30 and 64 years. Death occurs after an illness lasting from several months to 40 years between the ages of 10 and 71 years. In DRPLA, a significant relationship between CAG repeat length, age at onset and main presenting complaints was observed [26].

Laboratory investigations and imaging

Routine laboratory data, including blood and urine analysis, ceruloplasmin, copper, endocrine screening, liver biopsy, funduscopy, slit-lamp examination and CSF levels are unremarkable, and there are no laboratory findings specific for the various forms of pallidal atrophy. EEG may be normal [6,15] or show diffuse dysrhythmia. Cranial CT is normal or shows mild atrophy of the brain stem [7]. Cranial MRI was normal [15] or showed cortical, brain stem and cerebellar atrophy, and white matter changes, particularly in adult patients with long disease duration or hypodense areas in the GP and/or in the SN [17,25,32], and later generalized brain atrophy. HMPAO-SPECT and FDG-PET revealed cortical hyperperfusion and hypermetabolism, whereas the lenticular nucleus was slightly hypometabolic [17]. EMG shows permanent activities in the flexors and extensors with variable frequency. In patients with associated motor neuron disease, both EMG and muscle biopsies revealed denervation [12]. Molecular diagnosis of DRPLA is made by analysis of the size of the CAG repeat in the *DRPLA* gene.

Genetics and epidemiology

Epidemiologic data are insufficient because of the small number of reported cases. They appear not to exhibit ethnic or racial selectivity since verified cases have been observed in Europe, Japan, East Asia, and America, including African Americans [33]. Familial occurrence with probable autosomal recessive inheritance has been observed in a kindred affecting 2 of 6 children [5] and in a family with 6 siblings [34]. PLA was seen in two North American families [11], and PLDA in three Japanese families showing dominant

inheritance [23]. DRLPA, initially reported to involve predominantly Japanese individuals with an estimated prevalence of 0.2–0.7/100 000, comparable with that of HD in the Japanese population [25], has recently been observed in many non-Asian families. Their clinicogenetic phenomenology is similar to that of Asian series [26]. Sporadic cases affecting both sexes have been reported for most subtypes [1,6].

Neuropathology

The major morphologic features of this group of disorders are bilateral neuronal loss and gliosis in the GP and/or STN and degeneration of their efferent fiber systems. These lesions vary considerably in their intensity and extent and may or may not be associated with degeneration in other neuronal systems.

"Pure" pallidal atrophy shows bilateral degeneration of the GP with accentuation of neuronal loss in the external segment and gliosis in the internal segment (Figure 9.1), degeneration of the ansa lenticularis and pallidoluysian tract, and mild gliosis in STN and substantia nigra pars reticulata (SNr) but no further CNS lesions [5,7,10,35]. The lesion pattern of PPA suggests that the GP and its efferents are selectively involved. Other cases in addition to severe neuronal loss and gliosis in the GIM and GIL with minor affection of the globus pallidus external segment (Gpe) (Figure 9.2), showed degeneration of the ansa lenticularis and fasciculus thalamicus (see [5,6]).

Pallidonigral atrophy showed bilateral cystic lesions in GP and SN with mild damage to the STN associated with an unclassified lymphoid disease [11].

Pallidoluysian atrophy shows symmetrical degeneration of the GP involving the external and less so the internal segment (Figure 9.3), with degeneration of the ansa lenticularis and STN [5,36]. Other cases revealed atrophy of the pallidonigral system or degeneration of the red nucleus and pyramidal tracts, or exhibited spreading of the lesions to the striatum and/or SN [2,10] (Figure 9.4) and slight transneuronal atrophy of the anterior thalamic nucleus and the dorsolateral STN.

Pallidonigroluysian atrophy is featured by symmetrical atrophy of the globus pallidus internal (GPi) and external (GPe) segments and STN with depigmentation and neuronal loss in SN, associated with degeneration of the ansa lenticularis, fasciculus lenticularis [37], ventrolateral thalamus and brain stem tegmentum, centrum medianum, periaqueductal gray, and superior colliculi. There are pallidonigral hyperpigmentation

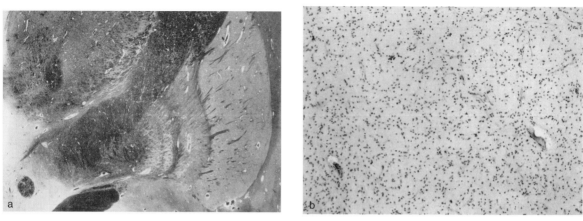

Figure 9.1. Progressive pallidal degeneration. (a) Left globus pallid us. Myelin pallor of the external and intermediary segments (GE, GIL) and of lamina medullaris incompleta pallidi. Thinning and pallor of ansa and fasciculus lenticularis. Heidenhain ×5.5. (b) Right mediolateral pallidal segment (GIM). Almost complete neuronal loss with reparative cellular gliosis. Cresyl violet ×85.

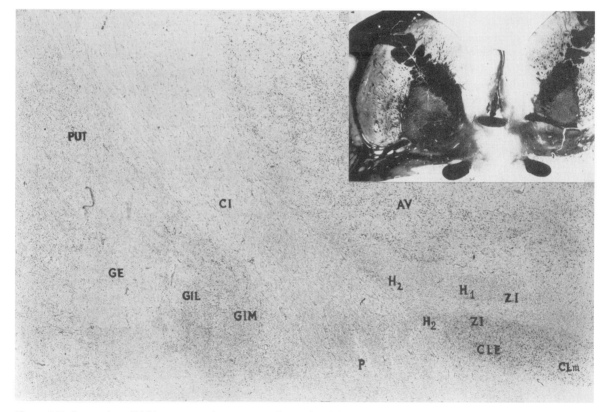

Figure 9.2. Progressive pallidal degeneration. Severe neuronal loss with cell gliosis in the inner pallidal segment (GIM, GIL) and moderate atrophy and gliosis in the external pallidum (GE). Slight gliosis in lateral parts of the corpus subthalamicum and in the nucleus of the H-field. Celloidin, Nissl ×3. Inset: slight myelin pallor in oral globus pallidus. Celloidin, Weigert. (Figure reproduced courtesy of Dr. L. van Bogaert.)

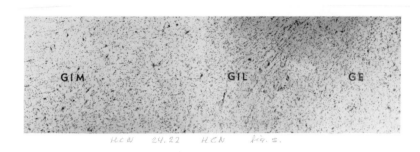

Figure 9.3. Pallidoluysian degeneration. Globus pallidus. Rarefication of neuronal cells in outer pallidal segments (GE, GIL) and lesser in the inner part (GIM) with proportional cell gliosis. Celloidin, Nissl ×50. (Figure reproduced courtesy of Dr. L. van Bogaert.)

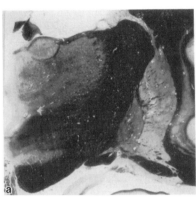 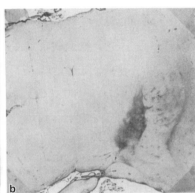

Figure 9.4. Progressive pallidal degeneration [10], (case 2). Left basal ganglia in coronal plan. (a) Slight myelin pallor in caudal pallidum, lamina medullaris externa and reduction of striopallidal bundles. Heidenhain. (b) Fibrillary gliosis of the external segment of pallidum and lesser in the inner parts, and slight gliosis in the striopallidal bundles, Kanzler-Arendt.

and axonal spheroids, ultrastructurally consisting of filaments or dense membrane-bound material, different from neuroaxonal dystrophy [14]. Pallidonigral and thalamic degeneration were recorded in an adult presenting with progressive dementia and parkinsonism; another case showed bilateral degeneration of GP, SN, and thalamus, without other pathologies [13].

Pallidoluysian dentate atrophy (PLDA) in a case of hereditary hemiballism [22] showed degeneration of GP and STN associated with degeneration of the dentatorubral system and incipient olivopontocerebellar atrophy. In two sporadic cases the prominent changes were bilateral atrophy of GP and degeneration of the dentate nuclei and their projections [38]. Four autopsy cases of three different Japanese families with myoclonus epilepsy showed degeneration of the dentate nuclei and superior cerebellar peduncles, and prominent degeneration of the pallidoluysian system, classified as "hereditary dentatocerebellar and pallidoluysian system atrophy" [23].

Combination of PNA and PNLA with motor system degeneration observed in several cases is a matter of discussion, since reexamination of the MRI findings and autopsy data did not confirm unequivocal demyelination of the pyramidal tracts (see reference 4). The same holds for Kufor–Rakeb disease [24]. In patients with FBX07 mutation, clinically presenting with equinovarus deformity, plantar extension reflexes, and spasticity of lower limbs [39], postmortem proof of pallidopyramidal degeneration is also lacking [40].

In two female patients with a combination of dystonia, hypokinesia, progressive rigidity and amyotrophy, autopsy revealed symmetrical degeneration of the GP and STN with mild involvement of SN, and degeneration of the corticospinal tracts and neuronal loss of hypoglossal nuclei and spinal anterior horns [20] (Figure 9.5).

A woman with sporadic disease (proximal limb weakness and atrophy, fasciculations, hyperreflexia, hypomimia, tremor and L-dopa-responsive parkinsonism, dying after 10 years with severe akinesia and amyotrophy) showed a combination of pallidoluysionigral atrophy, gliosis of the pontobulbar tegmentum, and degeneration of the X and XI nerve nuclei, the pyramidal tracts being intact [12].

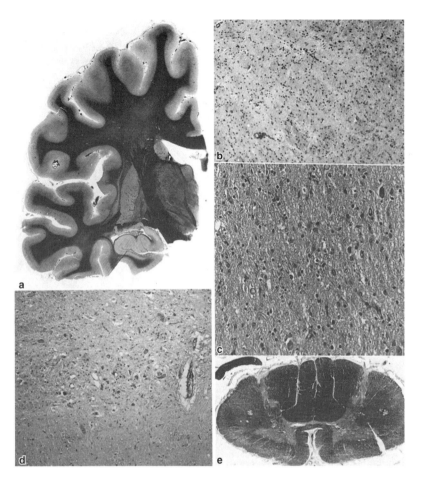

Figure 9.5. Pallidoluysionigral atrophy with amyotrophic lateral sclerosis. Coronal section of left cerebral hemispheres, atrophy and demyelination of corpus subthalamicum and pallidum, and demyelination of the ansa lenticularis (a). Neuronal loss and gliosis in inner pallidum (b) and subthalamic nucleus (c). Neuronal loss, depigmentation and gliosis in substantia nigra (d). Demyelination of the corticospinal tracts in cervical spinal cord (e). Klüver-Barrera ×1 (a), H-E ×50 (b, c, d), Loyez ×8 (e). (Reproduced from Gray *et al.* (1985) [20], by permission of the editors of *Acta Neuropathologica.*)

Dentatorubral-pallidoluysian atrophy macroscopically shows atrophy and brownish-tan discoloration of the GP, STN, dentate nucleus and pontine tegmentum; occasionally mild cortical atrophy and dilatation of the lateral ventricles. Histology reveals combined degeneration of the GPe and STN, loss of pallidosubthalamic fibers originating from the severely involved GPe and gliosis of the red nucleus. The dentate nucleus shows "grumose degeneration," myelin pallor of the dentate hilus. Pallidonigral degeneration is more marked than dentatorubral degeneration in juvenile-onset cases, and the reverse is seen in adult-onset disease [25]. Less involvement has been described in the neostriatum, thalamus, SN and inferior olives. There may be mild neuronal loss in cerebral cortex and diffuse myelin pallor in the centrum medianum, and degeneration of the spinocerebellar tracts and posterior spinal column. Eosinophilic neuronal intranuclear inclusions (NIIs) in DRPLA are immunoreactive for ubiquitin and atrophin I, the *DRPLA*

gene product [41]. Ultrastructurally, they contain a mixture of granular and filamentous structures, 10–20 nm in diameter, often surrounded by a single capsular structure, composed of granular material, immunoreactive for PML (promyelocytic leukemia protein). Ubiquitinated filamentous and polyglutamine immunoreactive inclusions involve neuronal cytoplasm in the dentate nucleus [25]. In some cases, NIIs are absent, but intracytoplasmic inclusions are seen in the pons, striatum, thalamus and STN [42]; other cases show extensive nuclear inclusions in oligodendroglia [41]. Experimental models are DRPLA transgenic mice with 129 polyglutamine stretches, which show NIIs in restricted CNS areas similar to those in the human DRPLA brain, associated with atrophy in pyramidal neurons and synaptic alterations in cerebral cortex [43]. These data suggest that neuronal atrophy and glial involvement are essential in the pathology of DRPLA closely related to polyglutamine pathogenesis.

Pallidal atrophy in other neurodegenerative diseases

Atrophy and gliosis of the GP has been observed in HD, resulting from striatopallidal fiber loss. In Hallervorden-Spatz disease (HSD) (PANK 2-related disorder), bilateral involvement of the GP with abnormal iron deposition may occur, and MRI shows low signal intensity in GP [44]; in rare nonfamilial cases, the disorder may almost be restricted to GP. Pallidal atrophy has been reported in hypoprebetalipoproteinemia, acanthocytosis, retinitis pigmentosa and pallidal degeneration (HARP syndrome), associated clinically with spasticity, dystonia and intellectual abnormality, caused by mutation in the PANK 2 gene [45,46].

Differential diagnosis

The combination of progressive rigidity and postural anomalies associated with choreoathetosis and torsion dystonia or tremor with or without pyramidal signs and mental deterioration with onset in the second decade or later, and gradually resulting in semiflexed contractures of the limbs, may suggest pallidal degeneration, particularly occurring in a family, while additional ballism may suggest PLA [5]. However, a definite diagnosis of these rare disorders is possible only by postmortem examination. Differential diagnosis has to consider: HSD, idiopathic torsion dystonia, HD, multiple system atrophy (MSA), Creutzfeldt–Jakob disease (CJD), PSP, Wilson disease, and other movement disorders [6,47]. It is vital to exclude the presence of axonal spheroids, MSA inclusions, and inclusions associated with motor neuron disease.

Management

Since the etiology of these disorders is unknown, no specific or causal treatment is available. In the presence of positive family histories, only early genetic counseling of the at risk population may be effective in reducing subsequent incidence of these diseases. Symptomatic treatment may include dopaminergic drugs in patients with prominent rigid-akinetic parkinsonian symptoms and physiotherapy, while antispastic drugs and neuroleptics may be of use in those individuals with prominent pyramidal and hyperkinetic features.

Thalamic atrophies
History and terminology

Since the description of the thalamic syndrome by Déjérine and Roussy in 1906 [48], it has not ceased to arouse the attention of neurologists. Thalamic degeneration is a rare disorder that presents clinically with variable cognitive, memory and behavioral disorders. The first case of thalamic dementia was a 40-year-old man suffering from rapidly progressive apathy, hypersomnia, memory loss, confabulation, perseveration and disorientation, accompanied by sucking and grasping reflexes and loss of pupillary response. Death occurred after 9 months. Autopsy revealed symmetric degeneration of the thalamus, lipopigmentary atrophy of neurons in cerebral cortex, atrophy of the inferior olives, and gliosis in the superior colliculi [49].

Four types of thalamic atrophy have been distinguished [1,47]: (1) thalamic degeneration in a variety of neurodegenerative diseases (Friedreich ataxia, spinocerebellar degeneration, HD, etc.), and in metabolic disorders (e.g., Wernicke syndrome, Menkes 'kinky-hair' disease or membranous lipodystrophy); (2) in epilepsy, multiple sclerosis, schizophrenia, alcoholism, Alzheimer disease and perinatal anoxia; (3) severe and preferential thalamic involvement in prion diseases (CJD) and familial fatal insomnia [50]; (4) isolated degeneration of the thalamus of unknown etiology, different from CJD and other neurodegenerative disorders, referred to as "pure" thalamic atrophy [51].

Clinical features

Symmetrical thalamic degeneration without additional CNS damage was observed in two siblings without any history of exogenous lesions, suggesting a genetically determined disorder [52]. It presents clinically with behavioral and mental disturbances, amnestic syndrome, apathy, disorientation and progressive dementia, associated with ataxia, myoclonus, hemineglect, dysarthria, optic agnosia, pyramidal signs, parkinsonism and, finally, akinetic mutism. Less than a dozen acceptable cases of pure thalamic atrophy have been described, mainly in men aged 18–60 years, with a clinical course of progressive deterioration of 6 months to 3 years and rare prolonged course up to 26 years [53–55].

Fatal familial insomnia (FFI) is characterized by alterations in the sleep–wake cycle, dysautonomia and motor signs, with variable severity and time of presentation. FFI is linked to the D178N-129M haplotype of the prion protein gene (*PRNP*). Its phenotype appears to depend on the M129V polymorphism located at codon 129 of *PRNP* [56]. Homozygotes have a disease duration of 12 ± 4 months, heterozygotes 21 ± 15 months. However, the age at disease onset does not differ between these two subgroups (mean 49 years; range 20–72 years). Studies in a large kindred revealed a wide phenotypic spectrum [57]. Early symptoms in MM patients with the frequent MM molecular subtype are insomnia, apathy, enacted dreams and vegetative symptoms. Sleep disturbances are often associated with autonomic alterations including blood pressure elevation, pyrexia, and increased heart rates [58]. Extrapyramidal signs and hallucinations occurred after around 12 weeks. Later loss of temporal and spatial orientation is followed by dysarthria and ataxia, and finally by myoclonus and pyramidal signs. In MV patients with the rare MV subtype, ataxia occurred as early as after about 4 weeks, followed by bulbar and vegetative symptoms, whereas hallucinations only occurred in late disease stages [59]. Diplopia, dysarthria, dysphagia, gait abnormalities, ataxia, pyramidal signs and seizures are generally more prominent in heterozygous patients.

Sporadic fatal insomnia, formerly known as the MM2 thalamic subtype, is rare and corresponds to the "thalamic" variant of sporadic CJD in previous classifications [56,60]. The clinical course is similar to FFI. The mean age at onset is around 50 years, with ataxia, followed by visual signs, dementia and eventually insomnia, and a range of motor abnormalities. These clinical features should be considered in patients with negative family history and negative genetic test results.

Natural history

"Pure" thalamic atrophy not related to prion diseases may involve both children and adults with progressive clinical course between 6 months and 2 years [53]. The onset of FFI is between middle and late adulthood (51 ± 7 years) with a disease duration between 8 and 72 months (mean 18.4 ± 17.3 moths), and it is ultimately fatal.

Laboratory investigations and imaging

In FFI findings of routine laboratory tests including CSF detection of tau protein and 14-3-3 protein are helpful in the diagnosis of CJD [61] and technical investigations are nonspecific [62], but polysomnography may help to support the diagnosis. In typical cases, the 24-hour EEG shows a continuous oscillation between the activity of normal wakefulness and sub-wakefulness; as the disease progresses, EEG activities typical of non-REM sleep are lost. In sporadic fatal insomnia, EEG shows nonspecific slowing [59] and MRI shows an increase of apparent diffusion coefficient of water and a metabolic pattern indicating gliosis [63]. With (^{18}F)FDG-PET, a minority of individuals had thalamic changes, whereas a majority had nonfocal cortical hypometabolism [59]. Thalamic and cingular involvement may be correlated with an early disease stage, whereas involvement of further regions depends on disease duration [62]. A targeted screening for the D178N mutation of PRNP may help establish an early FFI diagnosis.

Genetics and epidemiology

The nosological position, incidence and etiology of the rare "pure" thalamic atrophy are unknown; familial occurrence is known, but no genetic background has been detected.

For FFI and related prion diseases, genetic techniques are required to establish the presence of pathological mutations and to assist in the diagnosis of familial form, which account for 10–15% of all human prion diseases. More than 30 pathogenic mutations of the PNP have been reported to date, and cases with heterogeneous clinical phenotypes have been reported [59]. Hence, a targeted screening for mutations of *PRNP* permits an early diagnosis of FFI and related prion disorders.

Neuropathology

Isolated thalamic degeneration (pure thalamic atrophy) is characterized by bilateral symmetrical degeneration of thalamic nuclei; most severely affected are the anterior, medial and pulvinar formation and the superficial dorsal, dorsal posterior and reticular nuclei, with preservation of the magnocellular part of the medial thalamus and the small interneurons of Golgi type II [51]. The thalamic lesions are well demarcated and there are no signs of inflammation, necrosis or vacuolar lesions. The cerebral cortex usually is intact except for some neuronal loss [53], while several cases showed involvement of the inferior olives [51].

The distinctive feature of FFI is severe atrophy of the anterior ventral, dorsomedial and pulvinar thalamic nuclei, with loss of 80–90% of the neurons and severe gliosis in the absence of spongiform changes.

Other thalamic nuclei are affected less severely and more inconsistently. Atrophy of the inferior olives is the second most common change [64]. The presence and degree of cortical changes are functions of the disease duration, which is related in part to the PRNP phenotype at codon 129. MV patients developed more prominent spongiform changes in the cingulate and sylvian cortex; cases with 7–10 months' duration usually show focal spongiform degeneration in the entorhinal cortex and mild gliosis in deeper layers of the neocortex, while in cases with longer duration, progressive spongiform changes, neuronal loss and astrocytosis occur in the cerebral cortex. The cerebellar cortex, periaqueductal gray matter, raphe nucleus and reticular formation in the brain stem may also be involved. Prion protein (PrP) immunoreactivity has been reported in the cerebellum, subiculum and entorhinal cortex, particularly in cases with long clinical illness [57], rarely in the inferior olives [64].

In *sporadic fatal insomnia*, the main histological abnormalities are severe neuronal loss and gliosis in the anterior and medial thalamus but relative sparing of the posterior nuclei. Spongiform changes are usually absent in the thalamus [65] but may be identified in the cerebrum, entorhinal cortex and, occasionally, in the cerebellum. Amyloid plaques are not present, and neuronal loss and gliosis are uncommon outside the thalamus. PrP immunohistochemistry is negative in many regions, including the thalamus, but faint synaptic-like positivity can be identified in the cerebral cortex [66]. Spongiform degeneration in the thalamus and widespread abnormal prion protein (PrPSc; scrapie-associated prion protein) deposits in the brain were observed in single cases of sporadic fatal insomnia [67].

Pathophysiology

The key clinical aspects of FFI, i.e., hypovigilance and attention deficit, inability to generate EEG sleep patterns, sympathetic hyperactivity and attenuation of vegetative oscillations, are related to selective atrophy of the anteroventral and mediodorsal thalamic nuclei that constitute the limbic part of the thalamus interconnecting limbic and paralimbic regions of the cortex and subcortical structures in the limbic system including the hypothalamus. The latter, released from cortico-limbic control, is shifted to a prevalence of activating or of deactivating functions, including loss of sleep, sympathetic hyperactivity and attenuation of autonomic, circadian and endocrine oscillations. These findings

document that the limbic thalamus has a strategic position in the central autonomic network extending from the limbic cortical regions to the lower brain stem which regulates the body's homeostasis [50].

Thalamic atrophy in other neurological disorders

Thalamic atrophy has been reported in a large variety of nervous disorders, e.g., in childhood absence epilepsy [68], in medial temporal and idiopathic generalized epilepsy [69], with consistent neuronal loss in the dorsal medial thalamic nucleus in limbic epilepsy, and in both hippocampal and thalamic atrophy in temporal epilepsy [70]. Thalamic atrophy and changes in thalamic metabolism were observed in early HD [71]. Thalamic degeneration was documented in frontotemporal dementia [72], in Machado–Joseph disease [73], in Lewy body diseases and PSP [74,75], in Alzheimer disease [76], in Wernicke encephalopathy and in schizophrenia, mainly involving the mediodoral thalamic nucleus [77,78], suggesting a structural deficit in the corticothalamic systems [79]. Thalamic involvement is related to cognitive impairment in chronic multiple sclerosis [80], related to thalamocortical white matter lesions [81]. Symmetrical thalamic lesions occur after perinatal brain damage, in children after severe traumatic brain injury [82], or in persistent vegetative state [83,84].

Management

Specific/causal management of both thalamic atrophy of unknown etiology and that related to prion diseases is so far undetermined; it is restricted to symptomatic methods. For thalamic degeneration in other nervous disorders, symptomatic treatment may also be helpful.

Conclusions and future directions

The grouping together of pallidal atrophies is based on the morphologic findings of degeneration centered on the globus pallidus, either alone or in combination with damage to neuronal systems. The disorders have been grouped according to the pattern of pathological changes. Clinically, it is associated with a variety of movement disorders, with or without dementia. Some are familial and others sporadic.

It is difficult to evaluate the nosologic status of many of the cases described in the literature as their relationship to disorders that can now be better defined by molecular genetic and immunohistochemical techniques is uncertain. In particular, cases of DRPLA, spinocerebellar atrophies, MSA, and diseases characterized by inclusions seen in amyotrophic lateral sclerosis (ALS) are probably included in some of the historic series. Once these entities are excluded, a group of pallidal degenerations remains that can be classified on a purely descriptive basis, although it is not clear to what extent they represent distinct diseases.

Thalamic atrophies occur in a large variety of neurologic disorders, and can be divided into four major groups: (1) neurodegenerative and metabolic disorders in which thalamic atrophy may be prominent; (2) other CNS disorders with frequent involvement of the thalamus, such as epilepsies, multiple sclerosis, schizophrenia and Alzheimer disease; (3) preferential involvement of the thalamus in prion disorders, in particular FFI and sporadic fetal insomnia, the only ones in which the etiology is well defined and molecular biologic screening permits an early diagnosis; (4) rare cases of more or less isolated atrophy of the thalamus without relation to prions or other genetic factors, whose etiologies remain uncertain, and, as in pallidal atrophies, the elucidation of whose etiopathogeneses is a big challenge for future neurosciences.

References

1. Jellinger KA. Rare neurodegenerative disorders. In: Calne DB, ed. *Neurodegenerative Diseases.* Philadelphia: W.B.Saunders; 1994: 909–31.

2. Hunt JR. Progressive atrophy of the globus pallidus (primary atrophy of pallidal system): a system disease of paralysis agitans type. *Brain* 1917; **40**: 58–148.

3. Davison C. Pallido-pyramidal disease. *J Neuropathol Exp Neurol* 1954; **13**: 50–9.

4. Horstink M, Dekker M, Montagna P *et al.* Pallidopyramidal disease: a misnomer? *Mov Disord* 2010 ; **25**(9): 1109–15.

5. van Bogaert L. Aspects cliniques et pathologiques des atrophies pallidales et pallido-luysiennes progressives. *J Neurol Neurosurg Psychiatry* 1946; **9**: 125–57.

6. Jellinger KA. Pallidal, pallidonigral and pallidoluysionigral degenerations including associations with thalamic and dentate degenerations. In: Vinken PJ, Bruyn GW, Klawans HL, eds. *Handbook of Clinical Neurology.* Vol. 5. Amsterdam/New York: Elsevier; 1986: 445–64.

7. Aizawa H, Kwak S, Shimizu T *et al.* A case of adult onset pure pallidal degeneration. I. Clinical manifestations and neuropathological observations. *J Neurol Sci* 1991; **102**: 76–82.

8. Lange E, Poppe W, Scholtze P. Familial progressive pallidum atrophy. *Eur Neurol* 1970; **3**: 265–7.

9. Wooten GF, Lopes MB, Harris WO *et al.* Pallidoluysian atrophy: dystonia and basal ganglia functional anatomy. *Neurology* 1993; **43**: 1764–8.

10. Jellinger K. [Progressive pallidal atrophy]. *J Neurol Sci* 1962; **6**: 19–44.

11. McCormick WF, Lemmi H. Familial degeneration of the pallidonigral system. *Neurology* 1965; **15**: 141–53.

12. Serratrice GT, Toga M, Pellissier JF. Chronic spinal muscular atrophy and pallidonigral degeneration: report of a case. *Neurology* 1983; **33**: 306–10.

13. Kosaka K, Oyanagi S, Matsushita M *et al.* Multiple system degeneration and involving thalamus, reticular formation, pallido-nigral, pallido-luysian and dentatorubral systems. A case report. *Acta Neuropathol* 1977; **39**: 89–95.

14. Takahashi K, Nakashima R, Takao T *et al.* Pallido-nigro-luysial atrophy associated with degeneration of the centrum medianum. A clinicopathologic and electron microscopic study. *Acta Neuropathol* 1977; **37**: 81–5.

15. Katayama S, Watanabe C, Khoriyama T *et al.* Slowly progressive L-DOPA nonresponsive pure akinesia due to nigropallidal degeneration: a clinicopathological case study. *J Neurol Sci* 1998; **161**: 169–72.

16. Konishi Y, Shirabe T, Katayama S *et al.* Autopsy case of pure akinesia showing pallidonigro-luysian atrophy. *Neuropathology* 2005; **25**: 220–7.

17. Vercueil L, Hammouti A, Andriantseheno ML *et al.* Pallido-luysio-nigral atrophy revealed by rapidly progressive hemidystonia: a clinical, radiologic, functional, and neuropathologic study. *Mov Disord* 2000; **15**: 947–53.

18. Yamamoto T, Kawamura J, Hashimoto S *et al.* Pallido-nigro-luysian atrophy, progressive supranuclear palsy and adult onset Hallervorden–Spatz disease: a case of akinesia as a predominant feature of parkinsonism. *J Neurol Sci* 1991; **101**: 98–106.

19. Sudo S, Fukutani Y, Matsubara R *et al.* Motor neuron disease with dementia combined with degeneration of striatonigral and pallidoluysian systems. *Acta Neuropathol* 2002; **103**: 521–5.

20. Gray F, Eizenbaum JF, Gherardi R *et al.* Luyso-pallido-nigral atrophy and amyotrophic lateral sclerosis. *Acta Neuropathol* 1985; **66**: 78–82.

21. Bergmann M, Kuchelmeister K, Migheli A *et al.* Motor neuron disease with pallido-luysio-nigral atrophy. *Acta Neuropathol* 1993; **86**: 105–8.

22. Titeca J, van Bogaert L. Heredo-degenerative hemiballismus: a contribution to the question of primary atrophy of the corpus Luysii. *Brain* 1946; **69**: 251–63.

23. Oyanagi S, Naito H. [A clinico-neuropathological study on four autopsy cases of degenerative type of myoclonus epilepsy with Mendelian dominant

heredity (author's transl)]. *Seishin Shinkeigaku Zasshi* 1977; **79**: 113–29.

24. Williams DR, Hadeed A, al-Din AS *et al*. Kufor Rakeb disease: autosomal recessive, levodopa-responsive parkinsonism with pyramidal degeneration, supranuclear gaze palsy, and dementia. *Mov Disord* 2005; **20**: 1264–71.

25. Takahashi H, Yamada M, Tsuji S. Dentatorubral-pallidoluysian atrophy. In: Dickson DW, ed. *Neurodegeneration: The Molecular Pathology of Dementia and Movement Disorders*. Basel: ISN Neuropath Press; 2003: 269–74.

26. Wardle M, Morris HR, Robertson NP. Clinical and genetic characteristics of non-Asian dentatorubral-pallidoluysian atrophy: a systematic review. *Mov Disord* 2009; **24**: 1636–40.

27. Uyama E, Kondo I, Uchino M *et al*. Dentatorubral-pallidoluysian atrophy (DRPLA): clinical, genetic, and neuroradiologic studies in a family. *J Neurol Sci* 1995; **130**: 146–53.

28. Suzuki Y, Nakayama K, Hashimoto N, *et al*. Proteolytic processing regulates pathological accumulation in dentatorubral-pallidoluysian atrophy. *FEBS J* 2010; **277**: 4873–87.

29. Yamada M. Dentatorubral-pallidoluysian atrophy (DRPLA). *Neuropathology* 2010; **30**: 453–7.

30. Chinnery PF, Crompton DE, Birchall D *et al*. Clinical features and natural history of neuroferritinopathy caused by the FTL1 460InsA mutation. *Brain* 2007; **130**: 110–19.

31. Ohta E, Nagasaka T, Shindo K *et al*. [Clinical features of neuroferritinopathy]. *Rinsho Shinkeigaku* 2009; **49**: 254–61.

32. Kobayashi J, Nagao M, Kawata A *et al*. A case of late adult-onset dentatorubral-pallidoluysian atrophy mimicking central pontine myelinolysis. *J Neurol* 2009; **256**: 1369–71.

33. Becher MW, Rubinsztein DC, Leggo J *et al*. Dentatorubral and pallidoluysian atrophy (DRPLA). Clinical and neuropathological findings in genetically confirmed North American and European pedigrees. *Mov Disord* 1997; **12**: 519–30.

34. Lange E, Poppe W. [Clinical contribution to the pathological aspect of progressive atrophy of the pallidum (Van Bogaert).]. *Psychiatr Neurol (Basel)* 1963; **146**: 176–92.

35. van Bogaert L, Titeca J. Choréo-athétose dystonique (atrophie pallidale progressive pure?). *J Belge Neurol Psychiatr* 1947; **47**: 691–4.

36. Ito T, Ogasawara N. [Autopsy case of progressive atrophy of the globus pallidus]. *Rinsho Shinkeigaku* 1974; **14**: 10–16.

37. Contamin F, Escourolle R, Nick J *et al*. Atrophie pallido-nigro-luysienne: syndrome akinétique avec palilalie, rigidité oppositionnelle et catatonie. *Rev Neurol* 1971; **124**: 107–20.

38. Neumann MA. Combined degeneration of globus pallidus and dentate nucleus and their projections. *Neurology* 1959; **9**: 430–8.

39. Shojaee S, Sina F, Banihosseini SS *et al*. Genome-wide linkage analysis of a Parkinsonian-pyramidal syndrome pedigree by 500 K SNP arrays. *Am J Hum Genet* 2008; **82**: 1375–84.

40. Di Fonzo A, Dekker MC, Montagna P *et al*. FBXO7 mutations cause autosomal recessive, early-onset parkinsonian-pyramidal syndrome. *Neurology* 2009; **72**: 240–5.

41. Yamada M, Wood JD, Shimohata T *et al*. Widespread occurrence of intranuclear atrophin-1 accumulation in the central nervous system neurons of patients with dentatorubral-pallidoluysian atrophy. *Ann Neurol* 2001; **49**: 14–23.

42. Espay AJ, Bergeron C, Chen R *et al*. Rapidly progressive sporadic dentatorubral pallidoluysian atrophy with intracytoplasmic inclusions and no CAG repeat expansion. *Mov Disord* 2006; **21**: 2251–4.

43. Sakai K, Yamada M, Sato T *et al*. Neuronal atrophy and synaptic alteration in a mouse model of dentatorubral-pallidoluysian atrophy. *Brain* 2006; **129**: 2353–62.

44. Porter-Grenn L, Silbergleit R, Mehta BA. Hallervorden–Spatz disease with bilateral involvement of globus pallidus and substantia nigra: MR demonstration. *J Comput Assist Tomogr* 1993; **17**: 961–3.

45. Ching KH, Westaway SK, Gitschier J *et al*. HARP syndrome is allelic with pantothenate kinase-associated neurodegeneration. *Neurology* 2002; **58**: 1673–4.

46. Orrell RW, Amrolia PJ, Heald A *et al*. Acanthocytosis, retinitis pigmentosa, and pallidal degeneration: a report of three patients, including the second reported case with hypoprebetalipoproteinemia (HARP syndrome). *Neurology* 1995; **45**: 487–92.

47. Ince P, Wharton S, Shaw P *et al*. Diseases of movement and system degenerations. In: Ellison D, Louis D, Love S, eds. *Greenfield's Neuropathology*. 8th ed. London: Arnold Publishing; 2007: 891–1030.

48. Déjérine J, Roussy G. Le syndrome thalamique. *Rev Neurol* 1906; **14**: 521–32.

49. Stern K. Severe dementia associated with bilateral symmetrical degeneration of the thalamus. *Brain* 1939; **62**: 157–71.

50. Lugaresi E, Tobler I, Gambetti P *et al*. The pathophysiology of fatal familial insomnia. *Brain Pathol* 1998; **8**: 521–6.

51. Martin JJ, Yap M, Nei IP *et al.* Selective thalamic degeneration – report of a case with memory and mental disturbances. *Clin Neuropathol* 1983; **2**: 156–62.

52. Abuelo DN, Barsel-Bowers G, Tutschka BG *et al.* Symmetrical infantile thalamic degeneration in two sibs. *J Med Genet* 1981; **18**: 448–50.

53. Grünthal E. Über thalamische Demenz. *Monatsschr Psychiatr Neurol* 1942; **106**: 114–28.

54. Oda M. Thalamus degeneration in Japan. A review from clinical and pathological viewpoints. *Appl Neurophysiol* 1976; **39**: 178–98.

55. Siska E, Gereby G, Tariska S. [Thalamic dementia]. *Fortschr Neurol Psychiatr* 1985; **53**: 302–11.

56. Montagna P, Gambetti P, Cortelli P *et al.* Familial and sporadic fatal insomnia. *Lancet Neurol* 2003; **2**: 167–76.

57. Harder A, Jendroska K, Kreuz F *et al.* Novel twelve-generation kindred of fatal familial insomnia from Germany representing the entire spectrum of disease expression. *Am J Med Genet* 1999; **87**: 11–16.

58. Medori R, Tritschler HJ, LeBlanc A *et al.* Fatal familial insomnia, a prion disease with a mutation at codon 178 of the prion protein gene. *N Engl J Med* 1992; **326**: 444–9.

59. Krasnianski A, Bartl M, Sanchez Juan PJ *et al.* Fatal familial insomnia: clinical features and early identification. *Ann Neurol* 2008; **63**: 658–61.

60. Hirose K, Iwasaki Y, Izumi M *et al.* MM2-thalamic-type sporadic Creutzfeldt–Jakob disease with widespread neocortical pathology. *Acta Neuropathol* 2006; **112**: 503–11.

61. Krasnianski A, Schulz-Schaeffer WJ, Kallenberg K *et al.* Clinical findings and diagnostic tests in the MV2 subtype of sporadic CJD. *Brain* 2006; **129**: 2288–96.

62. Cortelli P, Perani D, Montagna P *et al.* Pre-symptomatic diagnosis in fatal familial insomnia: serial neurophysiological and [18]FDG-PET studies. *Brain* 2006; **129**: 668–75.

63. Haik S, Galanaud D, Linguraru MG *et al.* In vivo detection of thalamic gliosis: a pathoradiologic demonstration in familial fatal insomnia. *Arch Neurol* 2008; **65**: 545–9.

64. Almer G, Hainfellner JA, Brucke T *et al.* Fatal familial insomnia: a new Austrian family. *Brain* 1999; **122**(Pt 1): 5–16.

65. Janssen JC, Lantos PL, Al-Sarraj S *et al.* Thalamic degeneration with negative prion protein immunostaining. *J Neurol* 2000; **247**: 48–51.

66. Ironside JW, Ghetti B, Head MW *et al.* Prion diseases. In: Ellison D, Louis D, Love S, eds. *Greenfield's Neuropathology*. 8th ed. London: Arnold Publishing; 2007: 1197–273.

67. Piao YS, Kakita A, Watanabe H *et al.* Sporadic fatal insomnia with spongiform degeneration in the thalamus and widespread PrPSc deposits in the brain. *Neuropathology* 2005; **25**: 144–9.

68. Chan CH, Briellmann RS, Pell GS *et al.* Thalamic atrophy in childhood absence epilepsy. *Epilepsia* 2006; **47**: 399–405.

69. Gong G, Concha L, Beaulieu C *et al.* Thalamic diffusion and volumetry in temporal lobe epilepsy with and without mesial temporal sclerosis. *Epilepsy Res* 2008; **80**: 184–93.

70. Stewart CC, Griffith HR, Okonkwo OC *et al.* Contributions of volumetrics of the hippocampus and thalamus to verbal memory in temporal lobe epilepsy patients. *Brain Cogn* 2009; **69**: 65–72.

71. Feigin A, Tang C, Ma Y *et al.* Thalamic metabolism and symptom onset in preclinical Huntington's disease. *Brain* 2007; **130**: 2858–67.

72. Radanovic M, Rosemberg S, Adas R *et al.* Frontotemporal dementia with severe thalamic involvement: a clinical and neuropathological study. *Arq Neuropsiquiatr* 2003; **61**: 930–5.

73. Tokumaru AM, Kamakura K, Maki T *et al.* Magnetic resonance imaging findings of Machado–Joseph disease: histopathologic correlation. *J Comput Assist Tomogr* 2003; **27**: 241–8.

74. Brooks D, Halliday GM. Intralaminar nuclei of the thalamus in Lewy body diseases. *Brain Res Bull* 2009; **78**: 97–104.

75. Halliday GM, Macdonald V, Henderson JM. A comparison of degeneration in motor thalamus and cortex between progressive supranuclear palsy and Parkinson's disease. *Brain* 2005; **128**: 2272–80.

76. de Jong LW, van der Hiele K, Veer IM *et al.* Strongly reduced volumes of putamen and thalamus in Alzheimer's disease: an MRI study. *Brain* 2008; **131**: 3277–285.

77. Danos P, Schmidt A, Baumann B *et al.* Volume and neuron number of the mediodorsal thalamic nucleus in schizophrenia: a replication study. *Psychiatry Res* 2005; **140**: 281–9.

78. Cullen TJ, Walker MA, Parkinson N *et al.* A postmortem study of the mediodorsal nucleus of the thalamus in schizophrenia. *Schizophr Res* 2003; **60**: 157–66.

79. Kim JJ, Kim DJ, Kim TG *et al.* Volumetric abnormalities in connectivity-based subregions of the thalamus in patients with chronic schizophrenia. *Schizophr Res* 2007; **97**: 226–35.

80. Houtchens MK, Benedict RH, Killiany R *et al.* Thalamic atrophy and cognition in multiple sclerosis. *Neurology* 2007; **69**: 1213–23.

81. Henry RG, Shieh M, Amirbekian B *et al.* Connecting white matter injury and thalamic atrophy in clinically isolated syndromes. *J Neurol Sci* 2009; **282**: 61–6.

82. Fearing MA, Bigler ED, Wilde EA *et al.* Morphometric MRI findings in the thalamus and brainstem in children

after moderate to severe traumatic brain injury. *J Child Neurol* 2008; **23**: 729–37.

83. Kinney HC, Korein J, Panigrahy A *et al.* Neuro-pathological findings in the brain of Karen Ann Quinlan. The role of the thalamus in the persistent vegetative state. *N Engl J Med* 1994; **330**: 1469–75.

84. Uzan M, Albayram S, Dashti SG *et al.* Thalamic proton magnetic resonance spectroscopy in vegetative state induced by traumatic brain injury. *J Neurol Neurosurg Psychiatry* 2003; **74**: 33–8.

Restless legs syndrome and sleep-related disorders

Giacomo Della Marca and Alberto Albanese

History

"Wherefore to some, when being at bed they betake themselves to sleep, presently in the arms and legs leapings and contractions to the tendons, and so great restlessness and tossing of their members ensue, that the diseased are no more able to sleep than if they were in a place of the greatest torture" [1]. Thomas Willis provided in 1672 what is thought to be the first clinical description of restless legs syndrome (RLS), which would be considered as a distinct clinical entity only centuries later, when Ekbom commented: "The syndrome is so common and causes such suffering, that it should be known to every physician" [2]. Following this seminal paper, RLS has also been known as Ekbom syndrome. This peculiar symptomatology has since attracted the interest of physicians but it has remained an elusive entity because of diagnostic uncertainties. The link between iron and RLS was formally made in 1953 when Nordlander put forward the theory that iron insufficiency caused RLS, and used large doses of intravenous iron to treat it [3]. More recently, evidence of the involvement of the dopaminergic system (in particular the deficiency of dopamine D2 receptors) suggested the use of dopaminergic agonists in the treatment of RLS, which proved to be highly effective [4]. In 2006, the US Food and Drug Administration (FDA) approved the use of pramipexole for the treatment of moderate to severe RLS. In 1995, the International Restless Legs Syndrome Study Group (IRLSSG) established consensus diagnostic criteria [5], which were further revised in 2003 [6]. Notably, in the latest formulation of diagnostic criteria, the presence of sleep disorders is considered no longer essential for the diagnosis of RLS, but rather an associated feature. Nevertheless, since insomnia and disruption of sleep quality are common in RLS patients, the International Classification of Sleep Disorders (ICSD, 2nd edition) [7] retains RLS among sleep-related movement disorders, a group of sleep disorders defined as "relatively simple, usually stereotyped, movements that disturb sleep." In the previous edition of the ICSD, RLS was included among parasomnias. RLS is frequently encountered by clinical neurologists, both in the field of movement disorders and in sleep medicine. It has been estimated that up to 15% of patients who refer for insomnia to sleep disorders centers in Italy suffer from RLS [8].

Clinical findings

Restless legs syndrome is a complex disorder, with sensory and motor manifestations. The most prominent features are sensory symptoms, which consist of very unpleasant sensations felt mostly deep inside the limbs, unilaterally or bilaterally, affecting the calf, the ankle, the knee, or the entire lower limb. Unpleasant sensation can be variously described: pin pricks, internal itch, or creeping or crawling sensations are usually reported. In some patients, pain is the most prominent symptom and this can lead to the syndrome being misdiagnosed as a chronic pain problem. RLS is often a progressive condition, and symptoms may gradually worsen with age; with progression, an involvement of the upper limbs occurs in about half of the patients [9]. Dysesthesia is worsened by immobility, and patients start to complain after sitting or lying down for a while [10]. Voluntary movements reduce the discomfort. Typically, after sitting or lying for a while, the patient feels an urge to move – walking, stretching, or bending the legs – and the movement brings partial and temporary relief of the sensory discomfort. Since both immobility and sleepiness facilitate the occurrence of RLS, most patients report difficulty in falling asleep or are forced to wake up in the middle of the night, rise from the bed and walk around to relieve the discomfort. The severity of RLS fluctuates according to a circadian

Uncommon Causes of Movement Disorders, ed. Néstor Gálvez-Jiménez and Paul J. Tuite. Published by Cambridge University Press. © Cambridge University Press 2011.

pattern with a maximum occurring in the late evening or during the night (between midnight and 01:00) and a minimum in the morning between 09:00 and 11:00 [11]. Many patients therefore report insomnia, which involves either difficulty in falling asleep or, less frequently, nocturnal awakenings due to leg discomfort.

The prevalence of restless legs syndrome has long been underestimated for [12] and the disorder is considered to be underdiagnosed. Some years ago, a slogan used by the RLS Foundation in the USA said: "Restless legs syndrome: the most common medical condition you have never heard of." The main reason for underdiagnosis is the variability and elusiveness of clinical features. In the last decade, a variety of epidemiological studies have been performed in various countries [13–17]. It has been observed that RLS is a relatively common disorder, especially if mild forms with minimal or inconstant symptoms are considered. Its prevalence ranges between 2.5% and 10% of the general population [18]. RLS has a female preponderance of almost 2:1, which is related to the number of pregnancies: nulliparous women have the same incidence risk as age-matched men, whereas the risk for RLS increases progressively for women with one, two, three or more pregnancies [19]. However, if only severe forms are taken in account (those with symptoms occurring more than twice per week and resulting in a significant impairment of the quality of life), RLS prevalence ranges between 1.5% and 4.2% [20]. The age of onset seems to have a bimodal distribution with a peak occurring at age 20 years and a smaller peak in the fifth decade [21]. Familial cases are frequent and have a younger age of onset [22].

Onset of RLS may occur from childhood to >80 years of age [6]. The natural course varies widely but RLS is generally regarded as a chronic condition with a progressive increase of symptoms. The severity of RLS can vary greatly from one patient to another, and also in the same patient through lifetime. Periods of remission, followed by sudden relapses, are common, especially in young adults [6, 9]. Nevertheless, in most cases the syndrome has a progressive course, and its severity increases with advancing age. RLS may cause daytime sleepiness, fatigue, emotional disturbances, anxiety and depression [23], and it represents a major cause of impairment of quality of life [24–26].

Restless legs syndrome may be a primary disorder or a syndrome secondary to a variety of causes, including renal failure, a number of neuropathies [27–31], deficiencies of iron or magnesium [32–34], and Crohn disease [35,36]. RLS has also been reported in 25% of patients diagnosed with rheumatoid arthritis and Sjögren syndrome [37]. Uremia is the most frequent cause of secondary RLS. Uremic RLS appears to deteriorate faster and to become more severe than idiopathic RLS. Moreover, uremic RLS patients appear to have a decreased response to dopamine agonists [38]. RLS is significantly associated with multiple sclerosis (MS) [39]. In particular, severe motor and sensory disability and cervical cord damage represent a significant risk factor for RLS in MS patients [40]. RLS seems to be associated with diabetes mellitus, impaired glucose tolerance, and impaired fasting glucose; in particular, the occurrence of RLS in association with thermal dysesthesias may reflect the involvement of small sensory fibers in the form of hyperexcitable C fibers or A-delta fiber deafferentation [41]. A study of small sensory fibers hypothesized that two forms of RLS exist: one is triggered by painful dysesthesias associated with small sensory fiber loss, has later onset, and no family history; the other is without involvement of small sensory fiber loss, and has earlier onset age, positive family history for RLS, and no pain. The authors of this study hypothesize that patients with the small sensory fiber loss subtype of RLS will preferentially respond to neuropathic pain medications [42]. In a study by Iannaccone *et al.* [30], all patients exhibited two or more electrical, psychophysiological, and/or morphological features of peripheral axonal neuropathy. Morphometric analysis of the sural nerve showed a significant reduction in myelinated fiber density and *g* ratio (axon diameter/fiber diameter) in the RLS group compared with eight control biopsy specimens. These results suggest that axonal neuropathy is often present in patients with RLS.

The clinical features of RLS are not easy to distinguish and may be confused with other neurological conditions, such as akathisia, nocturnal leg cramps, symptoms of peripheral neuropathy, lumbosacral radiculopathy, and painful legs and moving toes. The severity of RLS symptoms and their impact on the patients' daily life can be measured with the 10-item IRLSSG scale [43]. This is a validated subjective scale that has been shown to have internal consistency once the diagnosis is established [44]. Unfortunately, there are no objective rating instruments. The PLM (periodic limb movements) indexes, during wake or sleep, have been proposed as tools for objective rating of RLS severity; nevertheless, these indices have low specificity, and cannot be considered reliable. Measurement of quality of life is considered a useful tool for trial-based assessments of treatments for RLS [45, 46]. Nevertheless, at present, the IRLSSG scale is the most widely adopted rating tool in therapeutic trials.

Diagnostic issues

Diagnostic criteria for RLS have been standardized by the IRLSSG (see Table 10.1) [5, 6]. The diagnosis is clinical, based on four criteria considered essential to the diagnosis: (1) an urge to move the legs accompanied or caused by uncomfortable and unpleasant sensations in the legs; (2) the symptoms worsen during periods of rest or inactivity; (3) symptoms are partially or totally relieved by movement; (4) the urge to move or unpleasant sensations are worse in the evening or at night than during the day or only occur in the evening or at night. The four diagnostic criteria can easily be evaluated by history, and a single screening questionnaire based on these essential criteria has been reported to have high sensitivity and specificity [47]. In cases in which diagnostic uncertainty exists, other features may be helpful: in particular, the occurrence of family history of RLS, improvement with dopaminergic treatment, and presence of periodic limb movements during sleep (PLMS). The response to treatment is particularly relevant and a diagnostic levodopa test has been proposed. This consists of the administration of a single dose of 100/25 mg levodopa/peripheral decarboxylase inhibitor and subsequent observation for 2 hours. Before

drug intake, and in the ensuing 15-minute interval, the patients rate the severity of their "symptoms in the legs" and their "urge to move the legs" using a 100 mm visual analogue scale. It has been reported that this test yields 88% sensitivity for "symptoms in the legs" and 80% sensitivity for "urge to move the legs," with specificity of 100% for both items [48].

Periodic limb movements (PLM) are often encountered in patients with RLS. Previously defined as "nocturnal myoclonus" [49, 50], PLM occur during sleep in the majority of patients with RLS, although they may either occur during wake (PLMW) or during sleep (PLMS). PLM are repetitive, stereotyped movements of the lower limbs, which consist of a slow, tonic dorsiflexion of the big toe, the ankle, the knee and even the hip. They appear after sleep onset, during light sleep, and are organized in sequences, consisting of several movements (at least four), each lasting 0.5 to 5 seconds, with a frequency of 1.5 to 3 per minute. In some individuals with RLS, involuntary twitching movements of the legs may appear during wakefulness, typically when they are sitting or lying. These movements may be periodic (PLMW) or aperiodic [9]. In polysomnographic recordings, PLMS may be recorded with surface EMG, especially from quadriceps and anterior tibialis muscles. They may occur in association with EEG arousals, or not [51–53]; however, a more sophisticated analysis of sleep microstructure based on the detection of cyclic alternating pattern (CAP) reveals

Table 10.1. Diagnostic criteria for RLS.

Essential criteria	An urge to move the legs, usually accompanied by uncomfortable or unpleasant sensations in the legs
	Unpleasant sensations or the urge to move begin or worsen during periods of rest or inactivity such as lying or sitting
	Unpleasant sensations or the urge to move are partly or totally relieved by movement such as walking, bending, stretching, at least for as long as the activity continues
	Unpleasant sensations or the urge to move are worse in the evening or at night than during the day, or only occur in the evening or night
Supportive criteria	Positive response to dopaminergic treatment
	Periodic limb movements (during wakefulness or sleep)
	Positive family history of the restless legs syndrome suggestive of an autosomal dominant mode of inheritance.
Associated features	Natural clinical course of the disorder (progressive in most cases))
	Sleep disturbance (insomnia)
	Medical and neurological examination (in particular, low serum ferritin <50 μg/l makes the diagnosis of RLS more likely)

Reproduced with permission from reference 9.

that PLMS are closely related to fluctuation of the levels of arousal during non-REM (NREM) sleep [53]. When PLMS are associated with arousals, they may lead to significant sleep disruption and daytime somnolence. With the progression of the disease, as happens for sensory symptoms, which spread to upper limbs, periodic limb movements can also affect the upper limbs [54]. Although they occur in more than 80% of the cases of RLS [9], periodic movements are not specific for the diagnosis since they have been observed in many other sleep disorders (narcolepsy [55], obstructive sleep apnea [56], REM behavior disorder [55]), and even as an isolated phenomenon.

The differential diagnosis should primarily include peripheral neuropathies, radiculopathies, neuroleptic-induced akathisia and arthritis [9]. Akathisia, particularly, may mimic some motor manifestations of RLS. It is characterized by unpleasant sensations of restlessness leading to inability to sit still or remain motionless. In most cases, akathisia is secondary to medications, mainly neuroleptics and antidepressants [57], but it can also occur in Parkinson disease (PD) and related syndromes [57]. On the other hand, several polyneuropathies may cause symptoms, such as paresthesias or dysesthesias, which overlap with the sensory symptoms of RLS. In most cases, the relief of symptoms with voluntary movement and the presence of a clear circadian rhythm of symptoms, and the association with PLM may help in the diagnosis. Nocturnal cramps, are sudden, intense and involuntary contractions of single muscles or muscle groups, usually in the calf or the foot, that may arise during wakefulness or sleep; they cause severe pain, with tenderness or discomfort persisting for hours after cramps [7]. The syndrome of "painful legs and moving toes" is characterized by spontaneous causalgic pain in the lower extremities associated with peculiar involuntary movements of the lower extremities, especially the toes and feet; the pain is diffuse, intractable, aching and deep [58]. The movement disorder consists of persistent writhing movements in the digits that cannot be limited voluntarily. Electromyography may reveal complex patterns of rhythmic activity with normal recruitment of motor units involving several myotomes. Response to drug treatment may be helpful in the differential diagnosis when GABAergic agents are efficacious on pain and movements. It should be recalled that overt pain is a relatively uncommon symptom of RLS and it also missing in the so-called "painless legs and moving toes" variant. In the case of peripheral neuropathies and radiculopathies, the distribution of sensory impairment, tendon reflexes abnormalities, and the neurophysiological findings help orient the diagnosis.

RLS and PD

The main reason why RLS and PD have been often considered to be interrelated is that both diseases can be treated with dopaminergic medications. However, RLS patients present specific complications of dopaminergic therapy, specifically augmentation, whereas PD patients develop different side-effects, namely, dyskinesias. Some studies indicate that the prevalence of RLS is increased in PD patients. These data are difficult to interpret because current diagnostic criteria for RLS have not been validated in PD. Moreover, many PD patients suffer from motor restlessness due to parkinsonism, a condition that may be mistaken for RLS. It has been hypothesized that the medical treatment of PD patients unmasks subclinical RLS in some cases due to augmentation [59]. However, a number of biological data separate RLS from motor restlessness associated with PD. Imaging techniques show that RLS have normal presynaptic dopamine transporter density, whereas receptor density is reduced in PD patients [60,61]. Ultrasound studies show that PD patients present a hyperechogenic substantia nigra (speaking in favor of increased iron concentration), whereas RLS patients show hypoechogenicity compared with control subjects [62]. Moreover, reduced iron and H-ferritin staining has been observed in the substantia nigra of RLS patients, [63] in contrast to increased iron content in the substantia nigra of PD patients [63].

Several data indicate that RLS may be at least partially caused by spinal mechanisms and that the gate control system for pain may be disrupted. In genetic studies, no reports have identified disease loci associated with RLS or motor restlessness associated with PD [64]. In summary, clinical, neuroimaging and neurophysiologic investigations do not support a pathological relationship between RLS and PD. All findings suggest that similar neuronal populations are involved in the pathophysiology of both diseases, albeit in a different manner [64]. According to Ondo et al., "there is no evidence that RLS symptoms early in life predispose to the subsequent development of PD" [65]. Interestingly, in a report by Kedia et al. [66], the emergence of RLS was observed in 11 of 195 PD patients after deep brain stimulation of the subthalamic nucleus. This suggests that the emergence of RLS could be related to a reduction of antiparkinsonian medication following deep brain stimulation.

111

Classically, idiopathic and secondary forms of RLS are distinguished. Symptomatic RLS is commonly associated with iron deficiency (in particular with serum ferritin levels below 50 µg/L), pregnancy [67], end-stage renal disease [68], or spinal cord lesions [69]. Pregnant women have at least two or three times higher risk of experiencing RLS than the general population [70]. During pregnancy, RLS disease frequently appears in the third trimester, and tends to disappear after delivery [71]. RLS is also frequent in end-stage renal disease; dialysis treatment is associated with increased odds for RLS, whereas RLS may ameliorate after kidney transplantation [72,73]. Although nerve [42] or muscle [74] abnormalities have occasionally been reported, no clear peripheral morphological abnormality can be associated with RLS. RLS responsive to dopamine agonist treatment was observed in a patient who received bilateral above-knee amputation of the lower limbs [75].

Natural history

Primary RLS is a disorder in itself and should be differentiated from secondary RLS. The natural history of primary RLS is only partially known. Several studies suggest that RLS has a chronic course and tends to worsen with age until the seventh decade [76]. On the other hand, there may be complete remissions of symptoms, even if for few months only, in up to 15% of cases, regardless of the therapy. The long-term evolution of RLS is still poorly known, mainly in the mild-to-moderate forms. With disease progression, sensory and motor symptoms spread from lower to upper limbs. Moreover, the progression of RLS leads to a progressive loss of circadian rhythm, and onset of symptoms extends from night-time to day-time. Disruption of sleep may become more and more severe, resulting in sleepiness, fatigue, anxiety and depression. A variety of studies demonstrate that severe, long-lasting, RLS affects not only quality of sleep but also many aspects of quality of life, including social functioning, daily functioning, and emotional well-being [24,77,78].

Laboratory investigations

Neurophysiologic evaluations may help reaching the diagnosis and assist in monitoring the progression of RLS.

A provocation test called the "suggested immobilization test" (SIT) has been introduced as an assessment tool [79,80]. The SIT stems from the clinical observation that symptoms occur at rest: the patient remains in bed or sits in a comfortable chair, at a 45° angle, with legs outstretched, for 60–90 minutes. Limb movements are recorded using surface EMG from bilateral anterior tibialis muscles. This allows testers to detect the appearance of PLM. Leg discomfort is subjectively estimated by the patient every 5 minutes, on a 100-mm horizontal visual analogue scale. The test is considered positive if leg discomfort or PLM occur. The time of administration of the SIT could significantly influence leg motor activity; therefore, it is mandatory to administer the SIT late in the evening, when RLS symptoms are more severe and sensitive to immobility. Although it cannot be considered a "gold standard" test for assessing RLS, the SIT is a clinical and research tool allowing the measurement of RLS symptoms [79]. A "forced immobilization test" has been also proposed, in which the legs are immobilized in a stretcher [81].

Polysomnography (PSG) is a common neurophysiologic test aimed at measuring a variety of sleep variables. Rather than allowing the diagnosis, which is based essentially on the clinical evaluation, PSG measures the impact of RLS and PLMS on the sleep pattern (Figure 10.1). Although PSG is not a mandatory tool for the diagnosis or the clinical assessment of RLS [82], it helps assessing the patients with associated sleep-related comorbidities. When performed, diagnostic PSG must include the recording of EEG, electro-oculography (EOG), EMG of submental muscles and bilateral EMG of anterior tibialis (Figure 10.2). PSG allows the evaluation of the impact of RLS on the sleep pattern, by measuring sleep latency, sleep duration, nocturnal awakenings, arousals and PLMS indexes [52]. Patients with RLS have prolonged sleep onset latencies, shorter total sleep time, lower sleep efficiency, higher arousal index, higher number of stage shifts, and longer REM sleep latency [83]. These measures can be useful in monitoring the progression of RLS symptoms as well as the response to medication.

Actigraphy is a method of inferring sleep from the presence or absence of movement, recorded by a sensor placed at the wrist or, less frequently, at the ankle. It has been validated against polysomnography in trials with people without insomnia [84]. Actigraphy may be helpful in the assessment and follow-up of RLS, because it may enhance accuracy of diagnosis and may allow monitoring of response to treatments [85].

A complete evaluation of the iron status is mandatory for the clinical assessment of patients with RLS. This includes dosing iron, ferritin and transferrin.

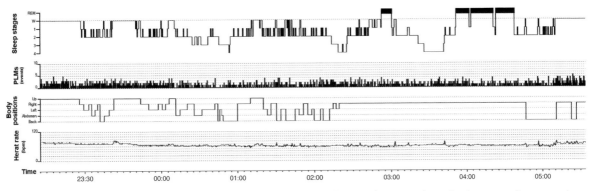

Figure 10.1 Polysomnographic study of a patient with severe RLS and PLMS. The upper histogram shows the sleep stages (hypnogram). PLMs: time course of PLM, expressed as number of events. The body position recording shows the continuous motor activity in the first part of the night. The lower trace shows the heart rate. (Data from the Catholic University sleep laboratory.)

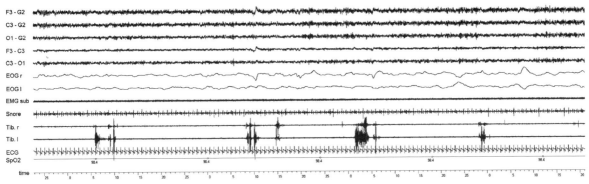

Figure 10.2 Polysomnographic recording showing PLMS. Montage includes (from top to bottom) EEG (F3, C3 and O1), right and left EOG, surface EMG of submental and tibialis anterior muscles (right and left), snoring sound, peripheral hemoglobin saturation and time. A sequence of bilateral, synchronous periodic limb movements is visible in the recording from tibialis anterior bilaterally (arrows). (Data from the Catholic University sleep laboratory.)

In order to identify, or rule out, secondary causes of RLS, the laboratory assessment should include dosage of serum glucose (for detecting underlying diabetes), creatinine (to assess renal function), and serum creatine kinases (to detect myopathies and cramps). Electromyography and nerve conduction studies may help to assess concurrent peripheral neuropathies or radiculopathies.

Genetics

Up to 60% of patients with primary RLS report a positive family history [86]. Compared with nonfamilial cases, these usually have a younger age at onset and a more slowly progressive course [87]. Twin studies showed a high concordance rate for RLS (>80%) in identical twins [88,89]. This suggests that there is a substantial genetic contribution in the etiology of RLS. To date, no gene has been identified, although linkage studies in RLS families have identified eight loci associated with familial RLS [19].

Genome-wide association studies are increasingly used to determine regions of the genome that may contain loci influencing the risk of neurological disorders [90]. Currently, six loci for RLS have been mapped in RLS families, on chromosomes 12q, 14q, 9p, 2q, 20p, and 6p (RLS1-RLS6), with recessive or autosomal dominant transmission. Recent genome-wide association studies have identified allelic variants within intronic or intergenic regions of MEIS1 (myeloid ecotropic viral integration site homeobox 1), BTBD9, (BTB/POZ domain containing protein 9) MAP2K5 (mitogen-activated protein kinase kinase 5)/LBXCOR1 (ladybird homeobox co-repressor 1) and PTPRD (receptor-type tyrosine-protein phosphatase delta) [19]. Many of these genes are developmental factors: MEIS1 is part of a transcriptional regulatory network that specifies

113

spinal motor neuron pool identity and connectivity and therefore may have a function in the motor part of RLS or PLM. The MAP2K5 gene, a member of the mitogen-activated protein kinase family, and the adjacent LBXCOR1 gene is annotated downstream of MAP2K5 acting as a transcriptional co-repressor of LBX1 [19]. This gene plays a critical role in the development of sensory pathways in the dorsal horn of the spinal cord that relay pain and touch [19].

A genome-wide linkage analysis performed in a large RLS family of Italian origin, with 12 affected members in three generations, provided evidence for linkage on chromosome 19p [91], but when this study was replicated in a set of 159 trios of European origin, it suggested evidence for a further RLS locus [91]. These findings support the picture of RLS as a genetically heterogeneous complex trait, which reflects the known clinical heterogeneity of this syndrome.

Pathology

There are no known pathological abnormalities in idiopathic RLS patients [92]. Conversely, several studies have identified neuropathological abnormalities in secondary RLS, in particular in the morphology of peripheral nerves, concerning both sensory and small, dolorific thermofibers [41,42].

Only a single postmortem study is available in idiopathic RLS, and it investigated only four patients [92]. In this postmortem study of brain and spinal cord, Lewy bodies were not identified and alpha-synuclein immunohistochemistry was negative. Neurofibrillary tangle pathology was variable and nonspecific [92]. These findings suggest that tau- or alpha-synuclein brain pathology is not a component of primary RLS. The lack of diagnostic microscopic pathology suggests that the pathological substrate of primary RLS is neurochemical or receptor based [92].

The striking clinical response to dopaminergic agents suggests an involvement of dopaminergic pathways in RLS. Several neuroimaging studies have supported the hypothesis of impaired dopaminergic neurotransmission [93–95]. No animal model of RLS is available; however, a rat study analyzed the effects of bilateral lesions of the A11 dopaminergic cell group, which is located in the midbrain close to the hypothalamus and projects into the cortex, the limbic system and the spinal cord. A11 lesions induced behavioral modifications similar symptoms of human primary RLS [96]. These behavioral modifications were at least partially reversed by administration of pramipexole.

A11 cells are the only neurons providing dopaminergic innervation to the spinal cord. Since they are in close proximity to the hypothalamic circadian pacemaker [9], their dysfunction could explain the peculiar circadian fluctuations of symptoms in RLS.

Iron metabolism also plays a role in the pathogenesis of RLS. Patients with RLS have reduced iron depletion, assessed by demonstrating low ferritin levels both in serum [97] and in the cerebrospinal fluid (CSF) [98]. Furthermore, RLS is commonly observed in conditions known to be associated with iron abnormalities, such as pregnancy, dialysis following renal failure, and iron deficiency anemia [99]. Serum ferritin levels may be low in RLS despite normal measures of serum iron. Moreover, some patients have abnormally reduced CSF ferritin levels despite normal serum ferritin levels [100]. A magnetic resonance imaging (MRI) study found decreased iron levels in the substantia nigra and, to a lesser degree, in the putamen of patients with primary RLS [101]. Haba-Rubio *et al.* demonstrated decreased regional iron levels in the substantia nigra, red nucleus, and pallidum of two patients with hemochromatosis and severe RLS [102]. Moreover, a neuropathological study showed a defect in the regulation of the transferrin receptors in RLS, resulting in impaired iron acquisition by the brain [63]. Taken together, these studies support the hypothesis that RLS is associated with a primary abnormality of CNS iron metabolism, but the relationship between dopaminergic dysfunction and CNS iron metabolism remains to be determined [99]. It is thought that iron deficiency reduces dopamine-transporter function by yet unknown mechanisms [103]. Dopaminergic pathways are sensitive to regional brain iron deficiency, and iron deficiency reduces the density of dopamine transporters in the striatum and nucleus accumbens and reduces dopamine uptake into striatal synaptosomes.

Management

A general principle is that not all patients with symptoms of RLS or PLMS need medical treatment: most patients with sporadic or only mild symptoms, and who do not experience significant impairment, do not to require pharmacological treatment, as this may cause augmentation and worsening of the symptoms [19]. In the general population, the prevalence of patients with severe RLS that require treatment is estimated as 2–3% [20,75]. In a population-based German survey, a majority of patients with RLS refused treatment [104]. Before considering drug prescription, sleep hygiene

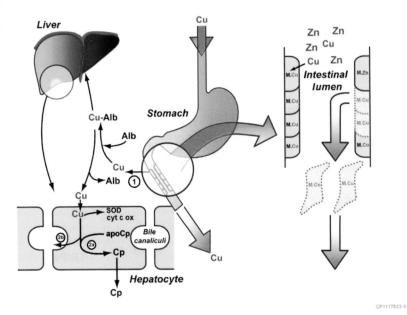

CP1117823-9

Figure 5.2. **Mechanism of action of zinc in reducing copper absorption and sites of defect in copper deficiency.** Excretion of copper into the gastrointestinal tract is the major pathway that regulates copper homeostasis and prevents deficiency or toxicity. The zinc-induced inhibition of copper absorption could be the result of competition for a common transporter or a consequence of induction of metallothionein in enterocytes. Metallothionein has a higher binding affinity for copper than for zinc. Copper is retained within the enterocytes and lost as the intestinal cells are sloughed off. Failure to mobilize absorbed copper from intestinal cells forms the basis of Menkes disease (1). In Wilson disease there is decreased incorporation of copper into ceruloplasmin (2a) and impaired biliary excretion of copper (2b). *Abbreviations:* Cu, copper; Zn, zinc; Cp, ceruloplasmin; M, metallothionein; alb, albumin; SOD, superoxide dismutase; cyt c ox, cytochrome *c* oxidase. (Reproduced from reference 82.)

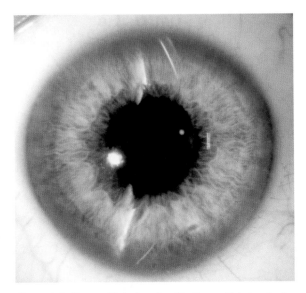

Figure 5.4. **Kayser–Fleischer ring.** The Kayser–Fleischer ring is due to copper accumulation in the Descemet's membrane in the limbic area of the cornea. It is frequently seen in patients with WD, particularly so in those who have neurologic manifestations. The ring is frequently not seen in those with only hepatic involvement.

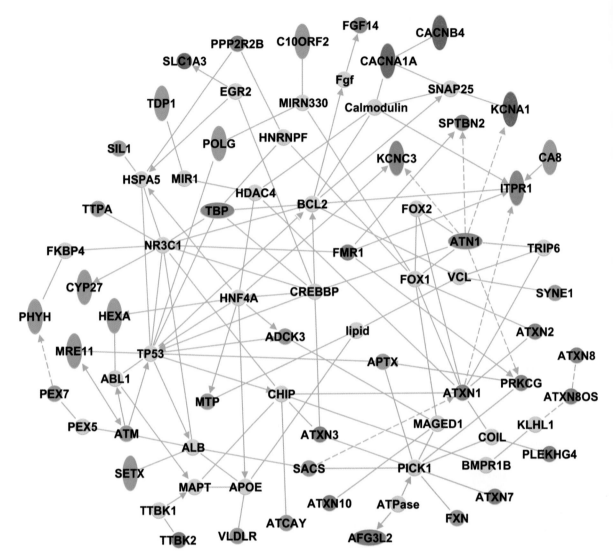

Figure 19.5. Hereditary ataxia gene products form a social network. The 19 autosomal dominant cerebellar ataxia genes (blue), the 21 auto-somal recessive cerebellar ataxia genes (green), the 1 X-linked cerebellar ataxia gene (pink), and the 4 episodic ataxia genes (red) discussed in this chapter were analyzed using Ingenuity pathway analysis software (http://www.ingenuity.com) and representative relationships are shown. CACNA1A causes both an autosomal dominant and an episodic ataxia and is therefore depicted in purple. Additional gene products that bridge the various ataxia gene products are shown in orange. The relationships between genes are shown as direct (solid lines) or indir-ect (dashed lines). Not all known interactions are shown and proteins may be further connected by interactions not depicted here. All interac-tions are from the Ingenuity database or from additional references [40,68,69].

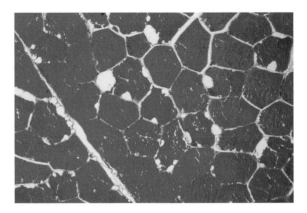

Figure 22.1. McArdle disease (myophosphorylase deficiency). (Courtesy of Dr. Richard Prayson.)

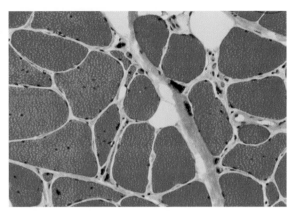

Figure 22.2. Myotonic dystrophy. (Courtesy of Dr. Richard Prayson.)

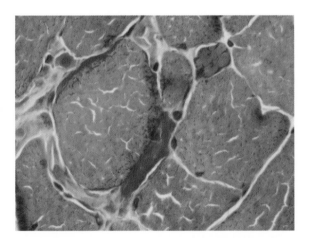

Figure 24.2. A typical ragged red fiber in mitochondrial disease demonstrated by modified Gomori trichrome staining of a skeletal muscle biopsy. (Courtesy of Dr. Ehud Lavi, Weill Cornell Medical College, New York NY.)

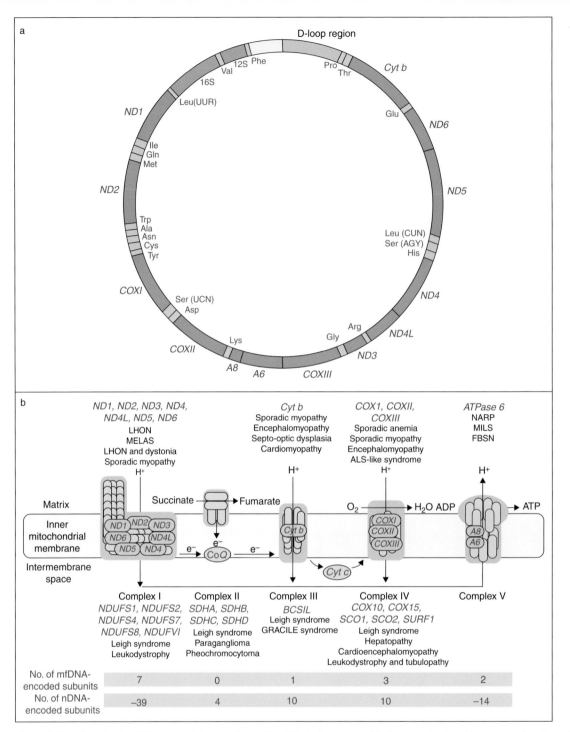

Figure 24.3. The mitochondrial genome in human disease. Panel (a) depicts a map of the human mitochondrial genome. Protein-coding genes (red): complex I (*ND*); cytochrome *c* oxidase (*COX*); cytochrome *b* subunit of complex III (*Cyt b*); adenosine triphosphate (ATP) synthase (*A6, A8*). Protein-synthesis genes (blue): 12S and 16S ribosomal RNAs, 22 transfer RNAs; D-loop region. Panel (b) depicts subunits of the respiratory chain: nuclear DNA encoded (blue); mtDNA encoded (red). Protons (H⁺) are pumped by Complexes I, III and IV from matrix to the intermembrane space, and return via Complex V activity, resulting in ATP synthesis. Coenzyme Q (CoQ) and cytochrome *c* (Cyt *c*) function in electron transfer. Mitochondrial disorders are denoted beneath. Genes responsible for a subset of specific respiratory-chain disorders are also shown beneath corresponding protein complexes, as follows: *ATPase 6*, ATP synthase 6; *BCS1L*, cytochrome *b–c* complex assembly protein (Complex III); *NDUF*, NADH dehydrogenase–ubiquinone oxidoreductase; *SCO*, synthesis of cytochrome oxidase; *SDHA, SDHB, SDHC, SDHD*: succinate dehydrogenase subunits; *SURF1*: surfeit gene 1. Disorders included are as follows: ALS, amyotrophic lateral sclerosis; FBSN, familial bilateral striatal necrosis; LHON, Leber hereditary optic neuropathy; MELAS: mitochondrial encephalomyopathy, lactic acidosis, and strokelike episodes; MILS, maternally inherited Leigh syndrome; NARP, neuropathy, ataxia, and retinitis pigmentosa; GRACILE, growth retardation, aminoaciduria, lactic acidosis, and early death. (Reproduced from reference [12] with permission. Copyright © 2003 Massachusetts Medical Society. All rights reserved.)

measures should be recommended and the causes of secondary RLS should be sought, particularly iron deficiency. Caffeine, nicotine and alcohol, especially if consumed in the evening, can worsen RLS symptoms and patients should be alerted to the possible effects of these common stimulants and sedatives [105]. A moderate level of daily physical exercise is of benefit. Some drugs may aggravate symptoms, such as neuroleptics, antiemetics, antinausea medications, gastrointestinal medications (such as metoclopramide), some sedatives and antihistamines [105].

Iron supplementation must be considered in all patients with serum ferritin <50 μg/l. Ferrous sulfate (325 mg t.i.d.) should be administered together with vitamin C (250–500 mg t.i.d.). Iron supplementation is often poorly tolerated, and gastrointestinal discomfort, especially constipation, is a relevant drawback. Nevertheless, in many RLS patients symptoms are refractory to iron supplementation. It is conceivable that oral iron supplements commonly recommended for RLS are ineffective because of poor absorption and poor tolerability at efficacious doses. Intravenous iron dextran has been shown to increase brain iron content, and it can occasionally cause a dramatic improvement of refractory RLS; nevertheless, these results are cannot be predicted by any clinical feature observed in the patients.

Dopaminergic drugs are the first-choice therapy for patients who need treatment. Levodopa was first tried, but its use is currently limited by the high incidence of augmentation [106]. Still, levodopa is highly effective, particularly in patients with mild symptomatology or in those who only have PLMS. In particular, levodopa is indicated in patient who have intermittent symptoms, and in those who need occasional or low-dose treatment (maximum 200 mg daily) [105]. The advantage of using levodopa in such patients is that a number of side-effects of dopaminergic treatment (nausea, lightheadedness, headache, sleepiness) are less frequent with low doses of levodopa than with dopamine agonists.

Dopamine agonists, in particular non-ergoline derivatives, are the first choice drugs for RLS with daily symptoms [107–112]. They ameliorate motor symptoms, as well as sleep structure, and reduce PLMS [113]. The use of ergolinic dopamine agonists, such as pergolide and cabergoline, which have longer half-life and lower risk of augmentation, is limited by the occurrence of fibrotic ergolinic side-effects [114]. Treatment should start with very low dosage in single

administration, and should be progressively up-titrated [105,115]. Adverse effects, such as dyskinesias, hallucinations, sleep attacks and psychosis, may occur in RLS patients, and have lower incidence compared to those observed in PD, probably because patients with RLS have a normal dopamine system and require much lower doses [105].

Augmentation is the main complication of long-term dopaminergic treatment for RLS. It was described for the first time in 1996 [106], and consists of an overall worsening of symptoms, which includes earlier occurrence during the day, faster appearance when at rest, diffusion to the upper limbs and trunk, and shorter duration of benefit from treatment [116]. Diagnostic criteria for augmentation have been standardized in order to differentiate this condition from insufficient response to treatment. Augmentation usually requires modification of the therapeutic strategy, and in particular decrease of dopaminergic stimulation. Augmentation occurs if onset of symptoms is anticipated by at least 2 hours during the day compared to before start of treatment. This leads to a paradoxical overall increase of symptom intensity, inducing a vicious cycle of medication dosage increase; the latency to symptoms at rest becomes shorter than before treatment and symptoms extend to other body parts; severity of symptoms requires change of treatment [103]. All of these modifications must occur for a diagnosis of augmentation. For assessment and quantification of the severity of augmentation, the European RLS Study Group has developed and validated an Augmentation Severity Rating Scale (ASRS) [117]. Augmentation is reported in up to 60% of patients treated with levodopa and to a lesser extent in patients treated with dopamine agonists [103].

The mechanisms of augmentation are only partially clarified. According to a model, augmentation is triggered by prolonged and intense dopaminergic stimulation, due to dopaminergic therapy [103]. This results in an overstimulation of the D1 receptor compared with the D2 and D3 receptors, mainly at the spinal cord level. The risk of augmentation is enhanced by iron deficiency causing a dysfunction of dopamine-transport, increased extracellular dopamine concentration and further dopamine overstimulation. Sleep deprivation also contributes to the development of augmentation. To reduce the risk of augmentation it is required to use low dosages of dopaminergic drugs, to correct iron levels and to switch to alternative drugs as soon as augmentation starts [103]. Once augmentation occurs, it should be avoided to increase dopaminergic drugs to high dosages, as this induces a vicious cycle capable of worsening the symptomatology. This condition is similar to medication overuse headache, when prolonged exposure to analgesic drugs favors nociception.

A variety of anticonvulsants have also been used in RLS, including carbamazepine [118], valproate [119], lamotrigine [120] and levetiracetam [121]. Carbamazepine has long been the first choice drug before the introduction of dopamine agonists. Gabapentin, an antiepileptic drug structurally related to gamma-aminobutyric acid, is generally effective and well tolerated [122]; it reduces PLMS and improves sleep architecture [123]. At present, anticonvulsants can be considered a second-line class of drugs, which can be used when dopaminergic agents are ineffective or contraindicated.

There is no evidence for the efficacy of hypnotics in the treatment of RLS. A common presentation of RLS is with severe insomnia refractory to treatment with sedative-hypnotic drugs. Clonazepam, the most commonly used drug in this class, was reported to be no more effective than placebo in a controlled trial [124].

Several opioids have been tested in the treatment of RLS: oxycodone [125], methadone [126], morphine [127], tramadol [128]. Most of them are effective, with a low risk of addiction. Potential side-effects include sedation, urinary retention and constipation. Long-term treatment requires a careful monitoring of dependence and respiratory function. Opioids are the treatment of choice once the cascade of augmentation with dopaminergic drugs has been activated.

Conclusions

Restless legs syndrome is a complex sensory-motor disorder, characterized by a peculiar circadian prevalence yielding to a close relation of symptoms with sleep. Consistent advances have been achieved in the last few decades concerning the pathophysiology and treatment of RLS. The introduction of dopaminergic agents has provided an effective symptomatic treatment for a condition that was considered poorly responsive to therapies. On the other hand, dopaminergic drugs have deeply modified the disease course, causing great amelioration in most patients, but also a peculiar worsening, defined as augmentation, in a minority of them.

A number of points need to be further clarified. In first place, the genetics of RLS is still poorly understood. Furthermore, the roles of iron and dopaminergic transmission have been highlighted but not fully clarified.

The mechanism of augmentation, which has become the most relevant clinical issue in the treatment of RLS, also needs further clarification. It seems conceivable that the development of neuroimaging techniques, and the development of animal models will help to address these issues.

References

1. Willis T. *De anima brutorum*. London: Wells & Scott; 1672.

2. Ekbom KA. Restless legs syndrome. *Acta Med Scand* 1945; **158**(Suppl.): 4–124.

3. Nordlander NB. Therapy in restless legs. *Acta Med Scand* 1953; **145**(6): 453–57.

4. Lin SC, Kaplan J, Burger CD, Fredrickson PA. Effect of pramipexole in treatment of resistant restless legs syndrome. *Mayo Clin Proc* 1998; **73**(6): 497–500.

5. Walters AS. Toward a better definition of the restless legs syndrome. The International Restless Legs Syndrome Study Group. *Mov Disord* 1995; **10**(5): 634–42.

6. Allen RP, Picchietti D, Hening WA, Trenkwalder C, Walters AS, Montplaisi J. Restless legs syndrome: diagnostic criteria, special considerations, and epidemiology. A report from the restless legs syndrome diagnosis and epidemiology workshop at the National Institutes of Health. *Sleep Med* 2003; **4**(2): 101–19.

7. International Classification of Sleep Disorders. *American Academy of Sleep Medicine. Diagnostic and Coding Manual.* 2nd ed. Westchester, IL: American Academy of Sleep Medicine; 2005: 1–208.

8. Terzano MG, Parrino L, Cirignotta F *et al.* Studio Morfeo: insomnia in primary care, a survey conducted on the Italian population. *Sleep Med* 2004; **5**(1): 67–75.

9. Trenkwalder C, Paulus W, Walters AS. The restless legs syndrome. *Lancet Neurol* 2005; **4**(8): 465–75.

10. Michaud M, Lavigne G, Desautels A, Poirier G, Montplaisir J. Effects of immobility on sensory and motor symptoms of restless legs syndrome. *Mov Disord* 2002; **17**(1): 112–15.

11. Trenkwalder C, Hening WA, Walters AS, Campbell SS, Rahman K, Chokroverty S. Circadian rhythm of periodic limb movements and sensory symptoms of restless legs syndrome. *Mov Disord* 1999; **14**(1): 102–10.

12. Trenkwalder C. Restless legs syndrome: overdiagnosed or underdiagnosed? *Nat Clin Pract Neurol* 2007; **3**(9): 474–5.

13. Cho YW, Shin WC, Yun CH *et al.* Epidemiology of restless legs syndrome in Korean adults. *Sleep* 2008; **31**(2): 219–23.

14. Rijsman R, Neven AK, Graffelman W, Kemp B, de Weerd A. Epidemiology of restless legs in The Netherlands. *Eur J Neurol* 2004; **11**(9): 607–11.

15. Tison F, Crochard A, Leger D, Bouee S, Lainey E, El Hasnaoui A. Epidemiology of restless legs syndrome in French adults: a nationwide survey: the INSTANT Study. *Neurology* 2005; **65**(2): 239–46.

16. Van De Vijver DA, Walley T, Petri H. Epidemiology of restless legs syndrome as diagnosed in UK primary care. *Sleep Med* 2004; **5**(5): 435–40.

17. Ziaei J, Saadatnia M. Epidemiology of familial and sporadic restless legs syndrome in Iran. *Arch Iran Med* 2006; **9**(1): 65–7.

18. Garcia-Borreguero D, Egatz R, Winkelmann J, Berger K. Epidemiology of restless legs syndrome: the current status. *Sleep Med Rev* 2006; **10**(3): 153–67.

19. Trenkwalder C, Hogl B, Winkelmann J. Recent advances in the diagnosis, genetics and treatment of restless legs syndrome. *J Neurol* 2009; **256**(4): 539–53.

20. Allen RP, Walters AS, Montplaisir J *et al*. Restless legs syndrome prevalence and impact: REST general population study. *Arch Intern Med* 2005; **165**(11): 1286–92.

21. Whittom S, Dauvilliers Y, Pennestri MH *et al*. Age-at-onset in restless legs syndrome: a clinical and polysomnographic study. *Sleep Med* 2007; **9**(1): 54–9.

22. Hanson M, Honour M, Singleton A, Crawley A, Hardy J, Gwinn-Hardy K. Analysis of familial and sporadic restless legs syndrome in age of onset, gender, and severity features. *J Neurol* 2004; **251**(11): 1398–401.

23. Hornyak M. Depressive disorders in restless legs syndrome: epidemiology, pathophysiology and management. *CNS Drugs* 2010; **24**(2): 89–98.

24. Cuellar NG, Strumpf NE, Ratcliffe SJ. Symptoms of restless legs syndrome in older adults: outcomes on sleep quality, sleepiness, fatigue, depression, and quality of life. *J Am Geriatr Soc* 2007; **55**(9): 1387–92.

25. Mallon L, Broman JE, Hetta J. Restless legs symptoms with sleepiness in relation to mortality: 20-year follow-up study of a middle-aged Swedish population. *Psychiatry Clin Neurosci* 2008; **62**(4): 457–63.

26. Kallweit U, Siccoli MM, Poryazova R, Werth E, Bassetti CL. Excessive Daytime sleepiness in idiopathic restless legs syndrome: characteristics and evolution under dopaminergic treatment. *Eur Neurol* 2009; **62**(3): 176–9.

27. Ramchandren S, Chervin RD. The relationship between restless legs syndrome and neuropathy. *Mov Disord* 2007; **22**(4): 588; author reply 9.

28. Gemignani F, Marbini A. Restless legs syndrome and peripheral neuropathy. *J Neurol Neurosurg Psychiatry* 2002; **72**(4): 555.

29. Gemignani F, Marbini A, Di Giovanni G *et al*. Cryoglobulinaemic neuropathy manifesting with restless legs syndrome. *J Neurol Sci* 1997; **152**(2): 218–23.

30. Iannaccone S, Zucconi M, Marchettini P *et al*. Evidence of peripheral axonal neuropathy in primary restless legs syndrome. *Mov Disord* 1995; **10**(1): 2–9.

31. Callaghan N. Restless legs syndrome in uremic neuropathy. *Neurology* 1966; **16**(4): 359–61.

32. Rijsman RM, de Weerd AW. Secondary periodic limb movement disorder and restless legs syndrome. *Sleep Med Rev* 1999; **3**(2): 147–58.

33. Bartell S, Zallek S. Intravenous magnesium sulfate may relieve restless legs syndrome in pregnancy. *J Clin Sleep Med* 2006; **2**(2): 187–8.

34. Hornyak M, Voderholzer U, Hohagen F, Berger M, Riemann D. Magnesium therapy for periodic leg movements-related insomnia and restless legs syndrome: an open pilot study. *Sleep* 1998; **21**(5): 501–5.

35. Gemignani F. A further cause of secondary restless legs syndrome: Crohn's disease. *Inflamm Bowel Dis* 2010; **16**(2): 280–1.

36. Weinstock LB, Bosworth BP, Scherl EJ *et al*. Crohn's disease is associated with restless legs syndrome. *Inflamm Bowel Dis* 2010; **16**(2): 275–9.

37. Ondo W, Tan EK, Mansoor J. Rheumatologic serologies in secondary restless legs syndrome. *Mov Disord* 2000; **15**(2): 321–3.

38. Enomoto M, Inoue Y, Namba K, Munezawa T, Matsuura M. Clinical characteristics of restless legs syndrome in end-stage renal failure and idiopathic RLS patients. *Mov Disord* 2008; **23**(6): 811–6; quiz 926.

39. Manconi M, Ferini-Strambi L, Filippi M *et al*. Multicenter case-control study on restless legs syndrome in multiple sclerosis: the REMS study. *Sleep* 2008; **31**(7): 944–52.

40. Manconi M, Rocca MA, Ferini-Strambi L *et al*. Restless legs syndrome is a common finding in multiple sclerosis and correlates with cervical cord damage. *Mult Scler* 2008; **14**(1): 6–93.

41. Gemignani F, Brindani F, Vitetta F, Marbini A, Calzetti S. Restless legs syndrome in diabetic neuropathy: a frequent manifestation of small fiber neuropathy. *J Peripher Nerv Syst* 2007; **12**(1): 50–3.

42. Polydefkis M, Allen RP, Hauer P, Earley CJ, Griffin JW, McArthur JC. Subclinical sensory neuropathy in late-onset restless legs syndrome. *Neurology* 2000; **55**(8): 1115–21.

43. Walters AS, LeBrocq C, Dhar A *et al*. Validation of the International Restless Legs Syndrome Study Group rating scale for restless legs syndrome. *Sleep Med* 2003; **4**(2): 121–32.

44. Wunderlich GR, Evans KR, Sills T *et al*. An item response analysis of the international restless legs syndrome study group rating scale for restless legs syndrome. *Sleep Med* 2005; **6**(2): 131–9.

45. Abetz L, Vallow SM, Kirsch J, Allen RP, Washburn T, Earley CJ. Validation of the Restless Legs Syndrome

Quality of Life questionnaire. *Value Health* 2005; **8**(2): 157–67.

46. Atkinson MJ, Allen RP, DuChane J, Murray C, Kushida C, Roth T. Validation of the Restless Legs Syndrome Quality of Life Instrument (RLS-QLI): findings of a consortium of national experts and the RLS Foundation. *Qual Life Res* 2004; **13**(3): 679–93.

47. Ferri R, Lanuzza B, Cosentino FI *et al.* A single question for the rapid screening of restless legs syndrome in the neurological clinical practice. *Eur J Neurol* 2007; **14**(9): 1016–21.

48. Stiasny-Kolster K, Kohnen R, Moller JC, Trenkwalder C, Oertel WH. Validation of the "L-DOPA test" for diagnosis of restless legs syndrome. *Mov Disord* 2006; **21**(9): 1333–9.

49. Coccagna G, Lugaresi E. Restless legs syndrome and nocturnal myoclonus. *Int J Neurol* 1981; **15**(1–2): 77–87.

50. Lugaresi E, Cirignotta F, Coccagna G, Montagna P. Nocturnal myoclonus and restless legs syndrome. *Adv Neurol* 1986; **43**: 295–307.

51. EEG arousals: scoring rules and examples: a preliminary report from the Sleep Disorders Atlas Task Force of the American Sleep Disorders Association. *Sleep* 1992; **15**(2): 173–84.

52. Zucconi M, Ferri R, Allen R *et al.* The official World Association of Sleep Medicine (WASM) standards for recording and scoring periodic leg movements in sleep (PLMS) and wakefulness (PLMW) developed in collaboration with a task force from the International Restless Legs Syndrome Study Group (IRLSSG). *Sleep Med* 2006; **7**(2): 175–83.

53. Parrino L, Boselli M, Buccino GP, Spaggiari MC, Di Giovanni G, Terzano MG. The cyclic alternating pattern plays a gate-control on periodic limb movements during non-rapid eye movement sleep. *J Clin Neurophysiol* 1996; **13**(4): 314–23.

54. Chabli A, Michaud M, Montplaisir J. Periodic arm movements in patients with the restless legs syndrome. *Eur Neurol* 2000; **44**(3): 133–8.

55. Hornyak M, Feige B, Riemann D, Voderholzer U. Periodic leg movements in sleep and periodic limb movement disorder: prevalence, clinical significance and treatment. *Sleep Med Rev* 2006; **10**(3): 169–77.

56. Drigo R, Fontana M, Coin A, Ferraresso A, Enzo E, Zambotto FM. APAP titration in patients with mild to moderate OSAS and periodic limb movement syndrome. *Monaldi Arch Chest Dis* 2006; **65**(4): 196–203.

57. Poewe W, Hogl B. Akathisia, restless legs and periodic limb movements in sleep in Parkinson's disease. *Neurology* 2004; **63**(8 Suppl 3): S12–6.

58. Spillane JD, Nathan PW, Kelly RE, Marsden CD. Painful legs and moving toes. *Brain* 1971; **94**(3): 541–56.

59. Lee JE, Shin HW, Kim KS, Sohn YH. Factors contributing to the development of restless legs syndrome in patients with Parkinson disease. *Mov Disord* 2009; **24**(4): 579–82.

60. Tribl GG, Asenbaum S, Klosch G *et al.* Normal IPT and IBZM SPECT in drug naive and levodopa-treated idiopathic restless legs syndrome. *Neurology* 2002; **59**(4): 649–50.

61. Eisensehr I, Wetter TC, Linke R *et al.* Normal IPT and IBZM SPECT in drug-naive and levodopa-treated idiopathic restless legs syndrome. *Neurology* 2001; **57**(7): 1307–9.

62. Schmidauer C, Sojer M, Seppi K *et al.* Transcranial ultrasound shows nigral hypoechogenicity in restless legs syndrome. *Ann Neurol* 2005; **58**(4): 630–4.

63. Connor JR, Boyer PJ, Menzies SL *et al.* Neuropathological examination suggests impaired brain iron acquisition in restless legs syndrome. *Neurology* 2003; **61**(3): 304–9.

64. Moller JC, Unger M, Stiasny-Kolster K, Oertel WH. Restless Legs Syndrome (RLS) and Parkinson's disease (PD)-related disorders or different entities? *J Neurol Sci* **289**(1–2): 135–7.

65. Ondo WG, Vuong KD, Jankovic J. Exploring the relationship between Parkinson disease and restless legs syndrome. *Arch Neurol* 2002; **59**(3): 421–4.

66. Kedia S, Moro E, Tagliati M, Lang AE, Kumar R. Emergence of restless legs syndrome during subthalamic stimulation for Parkinson disease. *Neurology*. 2004; **63**(12): 2410–2.

67. Goodman JD, Brodie C, Ayida GA. Restless leg syndrome in pregnancy. *BMJ* 1988; **297**(6656): 1101–2.

68. Winkelman JW, Chertow GM, Lazarus JM. Restless legs syndrome in end-stage renal disease. *Am J Kidney Dis* 1996; **28**(3): 372–8.

69. de Mello MT, Lauro FA, Silva AC, Tufik S. Incidence of periodic leg movements and of the restless legs syndrome during sleep following acute physical activity in spinal cord injury subjects. *Spinal Cord* 1996; **34**(5): 294–6.

70. Manconi M, Govoni V, De Vito A *et al.* Pregnancy as a risk factor for restless legs syndrome. *Sleep Med* 2004; **5**(3): 305–8.

71. Manconi M, Govoni V, De Vito A *et al.* Restless legs syndrome and pregnancy. *Neurology* 2004; **63**(6): 1065–9.

72. Molnar MZ, Novak M, Ambrus C *et al.* Restless Legs Syndrome in patients after renal transplantation. *Am J Kidney Dis* 2005; **45**(2): 388–96.

73. Winkelmann J, Stautner A, Samtleben W, Trenkwalder C. Long-term course of restless legs syndrome in dialysis patients after kidney transplantation. *Mov Disord* 2002; **17**(5): 1072–6.

74. Larsson BW, Kadi F, Ulfberg J, Aulin KP. Skeletal muscle morphology in patients with restless legs syndrome. *Eur Neurol* 2007; **58**(3): 133–7.

75. Hanna PA, Kumar S, Walters AS. Restless legs symptoms in a patient with above knee amputations: a case of phantom restless legs. *Clin Neuropharmacol* 2004; **27**(2): 87–9.

76. Hening W, Walters AS, Allen RP, Montplaisir J, Myers A, Ferini-Strambi L. Impact, diagnosis and treatment of restless legs syndrome (RLS) in a primary care population: the REST (RLS epidemiology, symptoms, and treatment) primary care study. *Sleep Med* 2004; **5**(3): 237–46.

77. Kushida C, Martin M, Nikam P *et al.* Burden of restless legs syndrome on health-related quality of life. *Qual Life Res* 2007; **16**(4): 617–24.

78. Abetz L, Allen R, Follet A *et al.* Evaluating the quality of life of patients with restless legs syndrome. *Clin Ther* 2004; **26**(6): 925–35.

79. Michaud M. Is the suggested immobilization test the "gold standard" to assess restless legs syndrome? *Sleep Med* 2006; **7**(7): 541–3.

80. Michaud M, Poirier G, Lavigne G, Montplaisir J. Restless legs syndrome: scoring criteria for leg movements recorded during the suggested immobilization test. *Sleep Med* 2001; **2**(4): 317–21.

81. Montplaisir J, Boucher S, Nicolas A *et al.* Immobilization tests and periodic leg movements in sleep for the diagnosis of restless leg syndrome. *Mov Disord* 1998; **13**(2): 324–9.

82. Hornyak M, Kotterba S, Trendwalder C. Consensus statement from the German Sleep Society: indications for performing polysomnography in the diagnosis and treatment of restless leg syndrome. *Sleep Med* 2002; **3**(5): 457–8.

83. Hornyak M, Feige B, Voderholzer U, Philipsen A, Riemann D. Polysomnography findings in patients with restless legs syndrome and in healthy controls: a comparative observational study. *Sleep* 2007; **30**(7): 861–5.

84. Lichstein KL, Stone KC, Donaldson J *et al.* Actigraphy validation with insomnia. *Sleep* 2006; **29**(2): 232–9.

85. Allen RP. Improving RLS diagnosis and severity assessment: polysomnography, actigraphy and RLS-sleep log. *Sleep Med* 2007; **8**(Suppl 2): S13–8.

86. Ferini-Strambi L, Bonati MT, Oldani A, Aridon P, Zucconi M, Casari G. Genetics in restless legs syndrome. *Sleep Med* 2004; **5**(3): 301–4.

87. Allen RP, Earley CJ. Defining the phenotype of the restless legs syndrome (RLS) using age-of-symptom-onset. *Sleep Med* 2000; **1**(1): 11–9.

88. Allen RP. Article reviewed: Restless legs syndrome in monozygotic twins: clinical correlates. *Sleep Med* 2001; **2**(2): 169–71.

89. Ondo WG, Vuong KD, Wang Q. Restless legs syndrome in monozygotic twins: clinical correlates. *Neurology* 2000; **55**(9): 1404–6.

90. Gubitz AK, Gwinn K. Mining the genome for susceptibility to complex neurological disorders. *Curr Mol Med* 2009; **9**(7): 801–13.

91. Caylak E. The genetics of sleep disorders in humans: narcolepsy, restless legs syndrome, and obstructive sleep apnea syndrome. *Am J Med Genet* A 2009; **149A**(11): 2612–26.

92. Pittock SJ, Parrett T, Adler CH, Parisi JE, Dickson DW, Ahlskog JE. Neuropathology of primary restless leg syndrome: absence of specific tau- and alpha-synuclein pathology. *Mov Disord* 2004; **19**(6): 695–9.

93. Cervenka S, Palhagen SE, Comley RA *et al.* Support for dopaminergic hypoactivity in restless legs syndrome: a PET study on D2-receptor binding. *Brain* 2006; **129**(Pt 8): 2017–28.

94. Ruottinen HM, Partinen M, Hublin C *et al.* An FDOPA PET study in patients with periodic limb movement disorder and restless legs syndrome. *Neurology* 2000; **54**(2): 502–4.

95. Turjanski N, Lees AJ, Brooks DJ. Striatal dopaminergic function in restless legs syndrome: ^{18}F-dopa and ^{11}C-raclopride PET studies. *Neurology* 1999; **52**(5): 932–7.

96. Ondo WG, He Y, Rajasekaran S, Le WD. Clinical correlates of 6-hydroxydopamine injections into A11 dopaminergic neurons in rats: a possible model for restless legs syndrome. *Mov Disord* 2000; **15**(1): 154–8.

97. Matthews WB. Letter: Iron deficiency and restless legs. *Br Med J* 1976; **1**(6014): 898.

98. Mizuno S, Mihara T, Miyaoka T, Inagaki T, Horiguchi J. CSF iron, ferritin and transferrin levels in restless legs syndrome. *J Sleep Res* 2005; **14**(1): 43–7.

99. Mahowald MW. Restless legs syndrome: the CNS/iron connection. *J Lab Clin Med* 2006; **147**(2): 56–7.

100. Earley CJ, Connor JR, Beard JL, Malecki EA, Epstein DK, Allen RP. Abnormalities in CSF concentrations of ferritin and transferrin in restless legs syndrome. *Neurology* 2000; **54**(8): 1698–700.

101. Allen RP, Barker PB, Wehrl F, Song HK, Earley CJ. MRI measurement of brain iron in patients with restless legs syndrome. *Neurology* 2001; **56**(2): 263–5.

102. Haba-Rubio J, Staner L, Petiau C, Erb G, Schunck T, Macher JP. Restless legs syndrome and low brain iron levels in patients with haemochromatosis. *J Neurol Neurosurg Psychiatry* 2005; **76**(7): 1009–10.

103. Paulus W, Trenkwalder C. Less is more: pathophysiology of dopaminergic-therapy-related augmentation in restless legs syndrome. *Lancet Neurol* 2006; **5**(10): 878–86.

104. Happe S, Vennemann M, Evers S, Berger K. Treatment of individuals with known and unknown restless legs syndrome in the community. *J Neurol* 2008; **255**(9): 1365–71.

105. Hening WA. Current guidelines and standards of practice for restless legs syndrome. *Am J Med* 2007; **120**(1 Suppl 1): S22–7.

106. Allen RP, Earley CJ. Augmentation of the restless legs syndrome with carbidopa/levodopa. *Sleep* 1996; **19**(3): 205–13.

107. McLean AJ. The use of the dopamine-receptor partial agonist aripiprazole in the treatment of restless legs syndrome. *Sleep* 2004; **27**(5): 1022.

108. Stiasny-Kolster K, Kohnen R, Schollmayer E, Moller JC, Oertel WH. Patch application of the dopamine agonist rotigotine to patients with moderate to advanced stages of restless legs syndrome: a double-blind, placebo-controlled pilot study. *Mov Disord* 2004; **19**(12): 1432–8.

109. Porter MC, Appiah-Kubf LS, Chaudhuri KR. Treatment of Parkinson's disease and restless legs syndrome with cabergoline, a long-acting dopamine agonist. *Int J Clin Pract* 2002; **56**(6): 468–74.

110. Tergau F, Wischer S, Wolf C, Paulus W. Treatment of restless legs syndrome with the dopamine agonist alpha-dihydroergocryptine. *Mov Disord* 2001; **16**(4): 731–5.

111. Kruszewski SP, Shane J. Efficacy and safety of pramipexole in restless legs syndrome. *Neurology* 2007; **68**(19): 1641; author reply 2.

112. McCormack PL, Siddiqui MA. Pramipexole: in restless legs syndrome. *CNS Drugs* 2007; **21**(5): 429–37; discussion 38–40.

113. Partinen M, Hirvonen K, *JAMA* L *et al.* Efficacy and safety of pramipexole in idiopathic restless legs syndrome: a polysomnographic dose-finding study – the PRELUDE study. *Sleep Med* 2006; **7**(5): 407–17.

114. Horvath J, Fross RD, Kleiner-Fisman G *et al.* Severe multivalvular heart disease: a new complication of the ergot derivative dopamine agonists. *Mov Disord* 2004; **19**(6): 656–62.

115. Vignatelli L, Billiard M, Clarenbach P *et al.* EFNS guidelines on management of restless legs syndrome and periodic limb movement disorder in sleep. *Eur J Neurol* 2006; **13**(10): 1049–65.

116. Garcia-Borreguero D, Allen RP, Benes H *et al.* Augmentation as a treatment complication of restless legs syndrome: concept and management. *Mov Disord* 2007; **22**(Suppl 18): S476–84.

117. Garcia-Borreguero D, Kohnen R, Hogl B *et al.* Validation of the Augmentation Severity Rating Scale (ASRS): a multicentric, prospective study with levodopa on restless legs syndrome. *Sleep Med* 2007; **8**(5): 455–63.

118. Larsen S, Telstad W, Sorensen O, Thom E, Stensrud P, Nyberg-Hansen R. Carbamazepine therapy in restless legs. Discrimination between responders and non-responders. *Acta Med Scand* 1985; **218**(2): 223–7.

119. Eisensehr I, Ehrenberg BL, Rogge Solti S, Noachtar S. Treatment of idiopathic restless legs syndrome (RLS) with slow-release valproic acid compared with slow-release levodopa/benserazid. *J Neurol* 2004; **251**(5): 579–83.

120. Youssef EA, Wagner ML, Martinez JO, Hening W. Pilot trial of lamotrigine in the restless legs syndrome. *Sleep Med* 2005; **6**(1): 89.

121. Della Marca G, Vollono C, Mariotti P *et al.* Levetiracetam can be effective in the treatment of restless legs syndrome with periodic limb movements in sleep: report of two cases. *J Neurol Neurosurg Psychiatry* 2006; **77**(4): 566–7.

122. Albanese A, Filippini G. Gabapentin improved sensory and motor symptoms in the restless legs syndrome. *ACP J Club* 2003; **139**(1): 17.

123. Garcia-Borreguero D, Larrosa O, de la Llave Y, Verger K, Masramon X, Hernandez G. Treatment of restless legs syndrome with gabapentin: a double-blind, cross-over study. *Neurology* 2002; **59**(10): 1573–9.

124. Boghen D, Lamothe L, Elie R, Godbout R, Montplaisir J. The treatment of the restless legs syndrome with clonazepam: a prospective controlled study. *Can J Neurol Sci* 1986; **13**(3): 245–7.

125. Walters AS, Wagner ML, Hening WA *et al.* Successful treatment of the idiopathic restless legs syndrome in a randomized double-blind trial of oxycodone versus placebo. *Sleep* 1993; **16**(4): 327–32.

126. Ondo WG. Methadone for refractory restless legs syndrome. *Mov Disord* 2005; **20**(3): 345–8.

127. Lindvall P, Ruuth K, Jakobsson B, Nilsson S. Intrathecal morphine as a treatment for refractory restless legs syndrome. *Neurosurgery* 2008; **63**(6): E1209; author reply E1209.

128. Lauerma H, Markkula J. Treatment of restless legs syndrome with tramadol: an open study. *J Clin Psychiatry* 1999; **60**(4): 241–4.

Dystonic syndromes

Susanne A. Schneider and Christine Klein

History

Dystonia is defined as involuntary twisting and repetitive movement resulting in abnormal postures [1] due to sustained muscle co-contractions of agonist and antagonist muscles. The term "dystonia" embraces three different meanings: first, dystonia can be a physical sign; second, dystonia can be a syndrome of sustained muscle contractions; and third, dystonia may refer to a disease such as "idiopathic (or primary) dystonia" [2].

Historically, one of the first descriptions of the condition may be that from 1901 by Destarac of a teenage girl with generalized dystonia affecting the neck, arm, pelvis muscles and feet. In 1908 Schwalbe described several patients and noted hereditability of dystonia. However, he also attributed a number of the physical features to being psychologically driven. Oppenheim coined the term "dystonia." In 1919 Mendel described findings of a series of 33 cases and noted that many of the patients had a Jewish background. Much was written following this, documenting the details of the clinical manifestations, and the debate about its inheritance continued. It took until the 1990s for the first gene responsible for some cases of generalized torsion dystonia, then termed *DYT1*, to be successfully localized to chromosome 9 [3,4] and it could later be calculated that the mutation within the Ashkenazi Jewish population, where this *DYT1*-associated form of dystonia is 5- to 10-fold more common compared to non-Jewish populations, may have taken its origin some 350 years ago according to Risch *et al.*(see reference 27). It is clear that this discovery has opened a new era in the understanding of this disorder and since then numerous genetic causes and mechanisms have been identified, some of which will be discussed in the following.

Clinical findings

Dystonias can be classified in various ways, including according to clinical features or by etiological cause.

The clinical categorization is based on age at onset, site of onset, and distribution of symptoms (focal, segmental, multifocal, generalized). Early-onset dystonia typically starts in the lower limbs, tends to generalize and commonly has a genetic origin. In contrast, adult-onset dystonia usually spares the lower extremities, frequently involves neck or cranial muscles and has a tendency to remain focal. This late-onset variant affects more women than men and appears to be sporadic in most cases (for review see reference 5), although some 15–30% of patients do have a positive family history.

By etiology, dystonias can be classified into primary and secondary forms. In the primary forms, dystonia is the only sign of the disease (with the exception of tremor [dystonic tremor/ tremor associated with dystonia] which may or may not be additionally present). The cause of primary dystonia is by definition either unknown or genetic. In the secondary forms, dystonia is usually only one of several disease manifestations and the cause may be genetic or due to other insults (e.g., lesions, trauma, drugs/toxins, metabolic disorders). Inconsistencies remain about how to categorize the heterodegenerative disorders and dystonia-plus syndromes.

In recent years, a growing number of genetic causes associated with dystonia have been recognized. The monogenic forms have been "classified" according to the gene loci. However, loci are being assigned chronologically according to appearance in the literature and thus, this list of "DYTs" cannot be considered a classification in the true sense of the word. Rather, it represents an assortment of clinically and genetically heterogeneous disorders associated with monogenic dystonia.

Uncommon Causes of Movement Disorders, ed. Néstor Gálvez-Jiménez and Paul J. Tuite. Published by Cambridge University Press. © Cambridge University Press 2011.

The prevalence of dystonia in Europeans, as diagnosed by adult neurologists with specialist movement disorders (and botulinum toxin) clinics, for primary dystonia was 152 per million in a European prevalence study [6]. Focal dystonia was most frequent with 117 per million, followed by cervical dystonia, blepharospasm and writer's cramp (57, 36 and 14 per million). As mentioned above, more women than men tend to have segmental and focal dystonias with the exception of writer's cramp. Data for secondary dystonia suggest prevalence rates of 10 700 per million in the general community aged 50–89 years [7]. Of the various cases, in a Brazilian sample of 46 patients with secondary dystonia, tardive dystonia (35%) and perinatal brain injury (30%) were most common, followed by stroke (13%), encephalitis (7%) and Wilson disease (4%) [8].

Onset is usually gradual, and with some exceptions, a sudden onset usually hints at a secondary cause such as a lesion following a vascular event and should give rise to further investigations. There are, however, genetic forms in which onset may be rather rapid, including rapid-onset dystonia-parkinsonism (DYT12) [9] and DYT6 dystonia [10].

Additional terminology is commonly used for some forms of dystonia. Torticollis, for example, refers to focal dystonia affecting the neck muscles and may present as torticollis per se (meaning turning of the neck), antecollis (involuntary turning of the head forwards), retrocollis (involuntary turning of the head backwards) or laterocollis (head bent sideways). Blepharospasm refers to dystonia of the orbicularis oculi muscle. Meige syndrome is a combination of oromandibular dystonia plus blepharospasm. There are also a number of focal dystonias that are induced by a specific task, such as writing (writing dystonia/writer's cramp), and are sometimes referred to as occupational cramps. Finally, there are some forms of dystonias, the group of paroxysmal dyskinesias, that occur episodically and are of only brief duration [11,12]. Here, specific triggers may bring on attacks, for instance, alcohol, caffeine, sudden or prolonged movements and exercise. All these manifestations of dystonia can be primary or secondary.

Natural history

Before making the diagnosis of a primary form, secondary causes must be excluded, and the natural history depends on the underlying etiology. For example, in secondary dystonia due to exposure to neuroleptic drugs, once developed, tardive dystonia is usually persistent [13]. There is a chance of remission, and discontinuation of neuroleptics seems the most important factor related to this. However, other factors such as duration of exposure also influence the prognosis. For example, in one study patients with up to 10 years on neuroleptics had a five times greater chance of remission than those with more than 10 years' exposure [13].

The natural course of primary dystonias has also been studied, with particular attention on the DYT1 variant. The clinical course is highly variable (phenotypic heterogeneity): the clinical status of carriers of the *DYT1* gene mutation ranges from severe generalized dystonia to mild focal dystonia (like writer's dystonia) [14]. Notably, however, 70–80% of mutation carriers remain unaffected in that they do not exhibit any dystonia at all. The natural course among the 30–40% of symptomatic cases is influenced by clinical factors such as age of onset, site of onset, and distribution of symptoms that have prognostic significance [15–17]. The most extensive investigation was done on 267 patients DYT1 dystonia (168 Ashkenazi Jews and 99 non-Jews) [16]. Unfortunately, the paper does not provide information about correlation of the clinical course with different therapeutic modalities. This was studied in more recent reports [18,19]. There is a tendency for stabilization of the clinical course after the age of 25 years and there seems to be no direct relationship to therapeutic modalities [20]. Others [21] have suggested that earlier treatment could slow down the disease progression.

Laboratory investigations

The diagnosis of dystonia is made on the clinical impression. The possible presence or absence of other neurological features including other movement disorders, eye movement abnormalities, pyramidal signs, cerebellar signs, involvement of the peripheral nervous system, etc. should be carefully established. The clinician should also look for (or exclude) the presence of other clinical signs such as ophthalmological abnormalities (like the Kayser–Fleischer ring), a hepatomegaly, skeletal abnormalities, etc. In the presence of clinical findings that are not compatible with a primary form of dystonia, laboratory investigations can help to diagnose a secondary form. Investigations include blood tests, urine studies, neuroimaging, a slit-lamp examination, neurophysiologic studies, muscle biopsy, lumbar puncture, and genetic testing (see Table 11.1). Investigations are expected to be normal in primary dystonia.

Table 11.1. Recommended investigations in a patient with dystonia.

Investigation	Primary dystonia		In patients with features suggestive of secondary dystonia	Diagnosis to be excluded (incomplete list)
	Early onset	Late onset	Independent of age of onset	
CCT, MRT	+	+	+	Vascular disease, malformations, neoplasms, calcifications
EEG	+		+	
Slit-lamp examination	+	+	+	Wilson disease
CSF	+		+	
Muscle biopsy			+	Mitochondrial disease (Leigh disease)
Gene test (*DYT1*)	+	(+)		*DYT1* dystonia
Blood test				
Full blood count, liver/kidney function test, coagulation parameters	+	+	+	
Ceruloplasmin, copper	+	+	+	Wilson disease
Serology: lues, etc.	+	+	+	Infections (lues, Tbc, AIDS, SSPE)
Anti-nuclear/thyroid antibodies	+		+	Immune disease (SLE)
Immunoelectrophoresis			+	Ataxia telangiectasia
Amino acids			+	Metabolic disease affecting the amino acid metabolism (e.g., homocystinuria)
Lysosomal enzymes, long-chain fatty acids			+	Metabolic disease affecting fat metabolism (e.g., gangliosidosis, metachromatic leukodystrophy)
Acanthocytes in peripheral blood smear			+	Neuroacanthocytosis, McLeod syndrome
Alpha-fetoprotein			+	Ataxia telangiectasia
Urine				
Copper	+	+	+	Wilson disease
Amino acids	+		+	Metabolic disease affecting the amino acid metabolism
Oligosaccharides/ mucopolysaccharides			+	

Overall, in patients with a late-onset and a non-progressive focal form of dystonia, a primary course is most likely, whereas young-onset cases should be investigated further for genetic causes or treatable metabolic diseases.

Genetics

Certain features may be suggestive of a genetic cause. These include an early age of onset, a specific clinical picture (for example, diurnal variation of the dystonia with worsening throughout the day suggesting dopa-responsive dystonia), certain ethnic backgrounds (for example, DYT1 dystonia is more common among Ashkenazi Jews; DYT3 is typically seen in Filipinos [22]) and a positive family history. We emphasize, however, that a genetic etiology should also be considered in those with a negative family history. Here, too small a family size, reduced penetrance, variable expressivity, and *de novo* mutations, but also nonpaternity and adoption, may appear as "pseudo"-negative family history.

Currently at least twenty different types of dystonia can be distinguished genetically, which are referred to as DYT1–20 (Table 11.2). In addition to this growing list of DYT loci, in recent years advances have been made in the genetics underlying conditions presenting with a mixed phenotype of dystonia *and* parkinsonism with or without additional features such as pyramidal involvement (for review see reference 23).

With the exception of five rare forms (DYT2, 3, 5b, 16 and 17), the different types follow an autosomal dominant pattern of transmission with reduced penetrance. In at least one form (DYT11) maternal imprinting also plays a role [24]. Genes have been identified for seven of these monogenic dystonias (DYT1, 3, 5, 6, 8, 9, 11, 12 and 18), and the chromosomal location is known for all but two forms (DYT2 and DYT4).

Genetic testing has become commercially available for several of the monogenic dystonias: DYT1 (due to mutations in the *TOR1A* gene), DYT5a (dopa-responsive dystonia due to dominantly inherited mutations in the *GCHI* gene) and DYT5b (dopa-responsive dystonia due to recessively inherited mutations in the *tyrosine hydroxylase* gene; *TH*), DYT6 (associated with mutations in the *THAP1* gene), DYT8 (due to mutations in the *myofibrillogenesis regulator 1* gene, *MR-1*); DYT11 (myoclonus-dystonia with mutations or deletions of the *SGCE* gene), DYT12 (due to mutations in the *Na/K ATPase alpha 3*; *ATP1A3*) and DYT9/DYT18 (due to mutations in the *SLC2A1* gene encoding the GLUT1 transporter).

Some of the other genes including DYT3, are currently being analyzed in selected research laboratories only. The website http://www.geneclinics.org can help to find a laboratory that offers testing.

It is important to realize that a negative gene test result does not fully exclude a mutation in that gene; firstly, because the sensitivity and specificity of many methods is less than 100%; secondly, because introns and promoter regions are usually not sequenced and variations in these areas remain difficult to interpret; and thirdly, in addition to mutations in the gene per se, entire or parts of genes may be deleted (whole gene deletion; exon deletion) or multiplied, also referred to as gene dosage alterations. Examples are the *GTP cyclohydrolase I* gene (*GCHI*) [25] and the *SGCE* gene [26]. However, routine methods that are used for mutational analysis fail to pick these up and alterations are detected only if gene dosage analysis is explicitly performed.

In addition to confirmation of the diagnosis in a patient, genetic testing can be used to identify at-risk individuals on the basis of their mutational status. For both symptomatic and nonsymptomatic gene mutation carriers, knowledge of the genetic status has implications regarding prognosis and therapeutic management decisions and with respect to family planning. Prenatal testing also plays a special role. Dystonia testing guidelines have been proposed for DYT1 [16]. Genetic testing guidelines are still being formulated for the other forms.

Some of the genetic forms of dystonia, DYT1, DYT5, DYT6 and DYT11, will be discussed in more detail in the following.

DYT1 dystonia (dystonia musculorum deformans, Oppenheim dystonia, early-onset generalized dystonia)

DYT1 dystonia typically presents as early-onset, generalized dystonia. It is caused by a mutation (typically a 3-base-pair (bp) deletion [GAG]) in the *TOR1A* gene located on chromosome 9. The frequency in the Ashkenazi Jewish population is estimated to be at least 1/9000 and 5- to 10-fold higher than in non-Jewish populations [27]. Inheritance of DYT1 dystonia is autosomal dominant. Penetrance is reduced to about 30%, which is partly due to other genetic factors. One example is the D216H polymorphism, which plays a protective role if present within the nonaffected "trans" allele, thus the gene copy that was inherited from the mutation-negative parent [28]. Although

Table 11.2. Monogenic forms of dystonia (DYT1–20)

Designation	Dystonia type	Mode of inheritance	Gene locus	Gene product	Genetic testing[a]
DYT1	Early-onset generalized torsion dystonia (TD)	Autosomal dominant	9q	Deletion in torsin A	Commercially available
DYT2	Autosomal recessive TD	Autosomal recessive	Unknown	Unknown	Unavailable
DYT3	X-linked dystonia parkinsonism; "lubag"	X-chromosomal recessive	Xq	Disease-specific changes 3 in DYT3 region	Available in selected research laboratories
DYT4	"Non-DYT1" TD; whispering dysphonia	Autosomal dominant	Unknown	Unknown	Unavailable
DYT5	Dopa-responsive dystonia; Segawa syndrome	Autosomal dominant / Autosomal recessive	14q / 11p	GTP-cyclohydrolase I / Tyrosine hydroxylase	Commercially available / Available in selected research laboratories
DYT6	Adolescent-onset TD of mixed type	Autosomal dominant	8p	THAP1	Commercially available
DYT7	Adult onset focal TD	Autosomal dominant	18p	Unknown	Unavailable
DYT8	Paroxysmal nonkinesigenic dyskinesia	Autosomal dominant	2q	Myofibrillogenesis regulator 1	Commercially available
DYT9[c]	Paroxysmal choreoathetosis with episodic ataxia and spasticity	Autosomal dominant	1p35	Glucose transporter 1 (same as DYT18)	Commercially available
DYT10	Paroxysmal kinesigenic choreoathetosis	Autosomal dominant	16p-q	Unknown	Unavailable
DYT11	Myoclonus-dystonia	Autosomal dominant	7q	Epsilon-sarcoglycan	Commercially available
DYT12	Rapid-onset dystonia-parkinsonism	Autosomal dominant	19q	Na$^+$/K$^+$ ATPase alpha 3	Commercially available
DYT13	Multifocal/segmental dystonia	Autosomal dominant	1p	Unknown	Unavailable
DYT15[b]	Myoclonus-dystonia	Autosomal dominant	18p	Unknown	Unavailable
DYT16	Generalized dystonia parkinsonism	Autosomal recessive	2q	Protein kinase interferon-inducible double-stranded RNA-dependent activator	Commercially available
DYT17	Young-onset generalized dystonia	Autosomal recessive	20p	Unknown	Unavailable
DYT18[c]	Paroxysmal exercise-induced dyskinesia	Autosomal dominant	1p35	Glucose transporter 1	Commercially available

Table 11.2. (*cont.*)

Designation	Dystonia type	Mode of inheritance	Gene locus	Gene product	Genetic testing[a]
DYT19	Paroxysmal kinesigenic dyskinesia 2 (episodic kinesigenic dyskinesia 2)	Autosomal dominant	16q	Unknown	Unavailable
DYT20	Paroxysmal nonkinesigenic dyskinesia 2	Autosomal dominant	2q31	Unknown	Unavailable

[a] Note that some gene tests may (only) be available on a research basis (see www.geneclinics.org for laboratories offering molecular testing on diagnostic and/or research grounds). To choose the appropriate gene test, it is helpful clinically and genetically to think of autosomal recessive syndromes, autosomal dominant syndromes and X-linked syndromes. Furthermore, genetic testing in general has implications not only for the diagnosis and therapy but also, of course, for family planning and counseling of family members.
[b] DYT14 was recently omitted and reclassified as DYT5.
[c] DYT9 was found to be due to mutations in the same gene as DYT18.

unusual phenotypes in genetically proven cases have been described [29,30], clinical experience shows that if symptoms do not occur prior to 28 years of age in mutation carriers, they will usually remain unaffected for the rest of their life.

The encoded protein, torsin A, is a member of the superfamily of ATPases and associated with a number of different functions including protein processing and degradation, organelle biogenesis, intracellular trafficking and vesicle recycling [31]. Torsin A is expressed throughout the body, with high levels in specific neuronal populations in the adult human brain, including in the substantia nigra, thalamus and cerebellum [32].

DYT6

Other loci associated with early-onset or adolescent-onset generalized dystonia include DYT6 dystonia [10] and advances have been made recently regarding this form [10,33,34]. DYT6 dystonia was originally described in three Mennonite families [35]. It is inherited in an autosomal dominant manner with reduced penetrance [10]. It presents as focal or generalized dystonia. However, in contrast to DYT1 dystonia, there seems to be a rostrocaudal gradient, and prominent bulbar findings. Overall, the data on DYT6 dystonia are still very limited. In addition to the original paper when the gene was identified [34], so far there are only few published studies, including one familial-based and one genetic screening study [10,33], overall suggesting that, among patients with early-onset nonfocal dystonia, mutations in *THAP1* may not be an uncommon cause.

[11C]Raclopride and PET imaging of regional glucose metabolism showed significant reductions in caudate and putamen D2 receptor availability and these changes were greater in DYT6 relative to DYT1 mutation carriers. There was, however, no significant difference between manifesting and nonmanifesting carriers [36].

The *THAP1*-encoded THAP1 protein belongs to the family of sequence-specific DNA-binding factors. THAP1 was shown to function as a nuclear proapoptotic protein, it regulates endothelial cell proliferation, and is considered to function as a transcription factor [37–39].

DYT5 dystonia (dopa-responsive dystonia; Segawa syndrome)

Dopa-responsive dystonia (DRD) is characterized by the triad of childhood-onset dystonia with or without parkinsonism, diurnal fluctuation of symptoms, and a dramatic and sustained response to levodopa. Cerebrospinal fluid analysis may demonstrate decreased catecholamine metabolites. The most common form of DRD (DYT5a) is dominantly inherited and associated with mutations in the *GTP cyclohydrolase I* (*GCHI*) gene, which encodes the enzyme GTPCH that catalyzes the first step in the dopamine synthesis. Mutations in *GCHI* can be identified in 40–60% of clinically typical DRD patients [40]. In addition, exon deletions have been demonstrated [25] that are not detectable by conventional screening methods (see above) and may account for at least another 10% of the "mutation-negative" cases.

Recessive forms of DRD also occur and may be due to mutations in the tyrosine hydroxylase (*TH*) gene (DYT5b). Other autosomal recessively inherited genes associated with dopa-responsive dystonia-plus syndromes include those encoding 6-pyruvoyl-tetrahydropterin synthase (6-PTPS), sepiapterin reductase (SPR), dihydropterine reductase (DHPR) and aromatic L-amino acid decarboxylase (AADC) (for review see reference 41) and the encoded pathways may be involved in the same metabolic pathways of biopterin and dopamine synthesis.

DYT11 – myoclonus-dystonia

As the name suggests myoclonus-dystonia (M-D) is characterized by the combination of myoclonic jerks –rapid, brief muscle contractions – plus dystonia, which leads to abnormal postures. Symptom onset is usually in childhood or early adolescence [42,43].

The myoclonic jerks here are typically brief lightning-like movements most often affecting the neck, trunk and upper limbs. Legs are less prominently affected. There is often a dramatic beneficial response of the myoclonic jerks to alcohol, but with rebound effect. Approximately half of affected individuals have focal or segmental cervical or arm dystonia [42]. Thus, in contrast to DYT1 dystonia, onset of dystonia in the lower limbs is rare. There may also be non-motor features of psychiatric involvement (depression, anxiety, panic attacks, obsessive-compulsive disorder [OCD], personality disorders and addiction) [44].

Mutations in the *epsilon-sarcoglycan* gene (*SGCE*) [44] on chromosome 7 have been identified that are inherited in an autosomal dominant manner with reduced penetrance due to maternal genomic imprinting [45] of the *SGCE* gene. The gene has 12 exons and the function remains unknown. All types of mutations have been reported in the *SGCE* gene, including nonsense, missense, deletions, insertions leading to frame shifts and splicing errors, and also larger deletions of entire exons and *de novo* mutations [26,42,44,46].

A recent comprehensive study reviewed 22 articles on *SGCE* screening covering 558 index patients [26]; 83% of patients with genetically confirmed *SGCE* mutations had a positive family history. Patients in whom *SGCE* mutations were excluded had a positive family history in 25% of cases. Some mutations appeared more commonly (c.304C>T). There were no obvious genotype–phenotype correlations among *SGCE* mutation carriers and no clear genotype:phenotype differences between *SGCE* mutation-positive and mutation-negative cases. However, in addition to genetic variations affecting the *SGCE* gene only, there are also reports of larger deletions affecting neighboring genes as well ("genomic deletions") with consequences for the clinical phenotype. For example, if the *COL1A2* gene is also affected, patients may be affected by additional osteoarthritis, osteoporosis or delayed skeletal development [26,47]. Other clinical manifestations associated with the neighboring genes include a split-hand/split-foot malformation, sensorineural hearing loss and cavernous cerebral malformations [47]. Such findings emphasize the importance of a careful clinical examination, which also includes other (non-motor) features [26].

Finally, there is evidence of genetic heterogeneity after mutations in the *SGCE* gene were excluded in a large Canadian family with a clinical presentation compatible with typical M-D. This family was linked to chromosome 18p, and this was designated the DYT15 locus, but the gene is as yet unknown [48].

Further genetic forms of dystonia

Other clinically distinct forms of hereditary dystonia have been described that are rarer (see Table 11.2), including some for which gene lesions have not yet been identified. This includes the group of paroxysmal dyskinesias (DYT8, DYT10 as well as DYT19 and DYT20) that are defined as abnormal involuntary movements that are intermittent or episodic in nature. The episodes are sudden in onset and without change in consciousness. Subgroups can be distinguished according to triggering factors and include the nonkinesigenic variant (PNKD), the kinesigenic variant (PKD), and the exercise-induced variant (PED) (for review see reference 49).

Pathology

Pathological findings correlate with the etiology, for example with vascular or strategic lesions in the corresponding secondary form. With respect to the primary dystonias, only few pathological descriptions have been described in the literature [50–55]. Here routine postmortem studies are typically normal [50–55]. Using more sophisticated techniques, in *DYT1*-related dystonia presence of brain stem perinuclear inclusion bodies in cholinergic and other neurons in the periaqueductal gray matter, pedunculopontine nucleus, cuneiform nucleus and reticular formation was demonstrated that were immunoreactive for ubiquitin, ubiquitin–protein conjugates, lamin A/C, and torsin A [56]. Such findings were not present in a cohort of non-DYT1 adult-onset primary dystonia patients with focal forms [57].

In the X-linked recessive form of Lubag dystonia–parkinsonism (XDP; DYT3), there is loss of calcineurin-expressing neurons with accompanying gliosis in the striosome compartment of the striatum [58]. This is in line with the results of in-vivo neuroimaging studies that illustrate a moderate decrease of putaminal dopamine transporter activity using FP-CIT SPECT and decreased dopamine D2 receptor expression using IBZM SPECT [59].

In dopa-responsive dystonia (DYT5), severely hypomelanized dopaminergic neurons in the substantia nigra and locus ceruleus in the absence of Lewy bodies have been observed [60].

Management

Management in dystonia syndromes [61] is symptom-based, but options are overall quite effective. On the other hand, pathogenesis-targeted treatment is still elusive (with the exception of dopa-responsive dystonia and Wilson disease). In general, there are three types of therapeutic pillars that can by themselves or in combination be beneficial for dystonia patients. These are medication (given orally or via injections), surgical interventions and supportive methods. General goals are relieving the involuntary movements, correcting the abnormal posture, preventing contractures, reducing pain, and improving function and quality of life [62].

Oral medications mainly include levodopa (in fact, all young-onset cases should have a trial of levodopa to investigate for dopa-responsive dystonia), anticholinergics and benzodiazepines. This is the first choice in patients with generalized forms. Botulinum toxin can be injected into affected muscles every three to four months, where it blocks release of acetylcholine into the synapse and thereby reduces the muscle tone. It is particularly useful for focal forms of dystonia. Surgical interventions include peripheral and central procedures such as selective peripheral denervation [63] and deep brain stimulation of the globus pallidus [64]. Supportive therapy provides an important adjunct to medical and surgical treatments and among others includes physiotherapy, ergotherapy and speech therapy.

Conclusions and future directions

Grand advances have been made in the field of dystonia in the last century. While dystonia was (at least partly) considered to have a psychological basis at the beginning of the twentieth century, the discovery of the genetic basis has opened a new era in the understanding of this disorder. It is likely that the number of known genetic causes will continue to grow, which may shed light on underlying mechanisms. This in turn will hopefully help to design target-oriented therapeutics in a "from bench to bedside" manner.

References

1. Fahn S. Concept and classification of dystonia. *Adv Neurol* 1988; **50**: 1–8.

2. Quinn N. Parkinsonism and dystonia, pseudo-parkinsonism and pseudodystonia. *Adv Neurol* 1993; **60**: 540–3.

3. Ozelius LJ, Kramer PL, De Leon D *et al.* Strong allelic association between the torsion dystonia gene (DYT1) and loci on chromosome 9q34 in Ashkenazi Jews. *Am J Hum Genet* 1992; **50**: 619–28.

4. Ozelius LJ, Hewett JW, Page CE *et al.* The early-onset torsion dystonia gene (DYT1) encodes an ATP-binding protein. *Nat Genet* 1997; **17**: 40–48.

5. Klein C, Breakefield XO, Ozelius LJ. Genetics of primary dystonia. *Semin Neurol* 1999; **19**: 271–80.

6. Epidemiological Study of Dystonia in Europe (ESDE) Collaborative Group. A prevalence study of primary dystonia in eight European countries. *J Neurol* 2000; **247**: 787–92.

7. Wenning GK, Kiechl S, Seppi K *et al.* Prevalence of movement disorders in men and women aged 50–89 years (Bruneck Study cohort): a population-based study. *Lancet Neurol* 2005; **4**: 815–20.

8. Ferraz HB, Andrade LA. Symptomatic dystonia: clinical profile of 46 Brazilian patients. *Can J Neurol Sci* 1992; **19**: 504–507.

9. Brashear A, Dobyns WB, de Carvalho AP *et al.* The phenotypic spectrum of rapid-onset dystonia-parkinsonism (RDP) and mutations in the ATP1A3 gene. *Brain* 2007; **130**: 828–35.

10. Djarmati A, Schneider SA, Lohmann K *et al.* Mutations in THAP1 (DYT6) are associated with generalised dystonia with prominent spasmodic dysphonia – a genetic screening study. *Lancet Neurol* 2009; **8**: 447–52.

11. Demirkiran M, Jankovic J. Paroxysmal dyskinesias: clinical features and classification. *Ann Neurol* 1995; **38**: 571–9.

12. Fahn S. The paroxysmal dyskinesias. In: Marsden CD, Fahn S, eds. *Movement Disorders*. Oxford: Butterworth Heinmann; 1994: 310–45.

13. Kiriakakis V, Bhatia KP, Quinn NP *et al.* The natural history of tardive dystonia. A long-term follow-up study of 107 cases. *Brain* 1998; **121**(Pt 11): 2053–66.

14. Kabakci K, Hedrich K, Leung JC *et al.* Mutations in DYT1: extension of the phenotypic and mutational spectrum. *Neurology* 2004; **62**: 395–400.

15. Almasy L, Bressman S, De Leon D. Ethnic variation in the clinical expression of idiopathic torsion dystonia. *Mov Disord* 1997; **12**: 715–21.

16. Bressman SB, Sabatti C, Raymond D *et al.* The DYT1 phenotype and guidelines for diagnostic testing. *Neurology* 2000; **54**: 1746–52.

17. Green P, Kang UJ, Fahn S. Spread of symptoms in idiopathic torsion dystonia. *Mov Disord* 1995; **10**: 143–52.

18. Scott BL. Evaluation and treatment of dystonia. *South Med J* 2000; **93**: 746–51.

19. Adler CH. Strategies for controlling dystonia. *Postgrad Med* 2000; **108**: 151–60.

20. Anca MH, Zaccai TF, Badarna S *et al.* Natural history of Oppenheim's dystonia (DYT1) in Israel. *J Child Neurol* 2003; **18**: 325–30.

21. Greene P. Baclofen in the treatment of dystonia. *Clin Neuropharmacol* 1992; **15**: 276–88.

22. Lee LV, Pascasio FM, Fuentes FD *et al.* Torsion dystonia in Panay, Philippines. *Adv Neurol* 1976; **14**: 137–51.

23. Schneider SA, Bhatia K, Hardy J. Complicated recessive dystonia parkinsonism syndromes. *Mov Disord* 2009; **24**: 490–9.

24. Grabowski M, Zimprich A, Lorenz-Depiereux B *et al.* The epsilon-sarcoglycan gene (SGCE), mutated in myoclonus-dystonia syndrome, is maternally imprinted. *Eur J Hum Genet* 2003; **11**: 138–44.

25. Furukawa Y, Guttman M, Sparagana SP *et al.* Dopa-responsive dystonia due to a large deletion in the GTP cyclohydrolase I gene. *Ann Neurol* 2000; **47**: 517–20.

26. Grunewald A, Djarmati A, Lohmann-Hedrich K *et al.* Myoclonus-dystonia: significance of large SGCE deletions. *Hum Mutat* 2008; **29**: 331–2.

27. Risch N, de LD, Ozelius L *et al.* Genetic analysis of idiopathic torsion dystonia in Ashkenazi Jews and their recent descent from a small founder population. *Nat Genet* 1995; **9**: 152–9.

28. Risch NJ, Bressman SB, Senthil G *et al.* Intragenic cis and trans modification of genetic susceptibility in DYT1 torsion dystonia. *Am J Hum Genet* 2007; **80**: 1188–93.

29. Gasser T, Windgassen K, Bereznai B *et al.* Phenotypic expression of the DYT1 mutation: a family with writer's cramp of juvenile onset. *Ann Neurol* 1998; **44**: 126–28.

30. Edwards M, Wood N, Bhatia K. Unusual phenotypes in DYT1 dystonia: a report of five cases and a review of the literature. *Mov Disord* 2003; **18**: 706–11.

31. Vale RD. AAA proteins. Lords of the ring. *J Cell Biol* 2000; **150**: F13–F19.

32. Augood SJ, Keller-McGandy CE, Siriani A *et al.* Distribution and ultrastructural localization of torsinA immunoreactivity in the human brain. *Brain Res* 2003; **986**: 12–21.

33. Bressman SB, Raymond D, Fuchs T *et al.* Mutations in THAP1 (DYT6) in early-onset dystonia: a genetic screening study. *Lancet Neurol* 2009; **8**: 441–6.

34. Fuchs T, Gavarini S, Saunders-Pullman R *et al.* Mutations in the THAP1 gene are responsible for DYT6 primary torsion dystonia. *Nat Genet* 2009; **41**: 286–8.

35. Almasy L, Bressman SB, Raymond D *et al.* Idiopathic torsion dystonia linked to chromosome 8 in two Mennonite families. *Ann Neurol* 1997; **42**: 670–3.

36. Carbon M, Niethammer M, Peng S *et al.* Abnormal striatal and thalamic dopamine neurotransmission: Genotype-related features of dystonia. *Neurology* 2009; **72**: 2097–103.

37. Cayrol C, Lacroix C, Mathe C *et al.* The THAP-zinc finger protein THAP1 regulates endothelial cell proliferation through modulation of pRB/E2F cell-cycle target genes. *Blood* 2007; 109.

38. Roussigne M, Cayrol C, Clouaire T *et al.* THAP1 is a nuclear proapoptotic factor that links prostate-apoptosis-response-4 (Par-4) to PML nuclear bodies. *Oncogene* 2003; **22**: 2432–42.

39. Bessiere D, Lacroix C, Campagne S *et al.* Structure-function analysis of the THAP zinc finger of THAP1, a large C2CH DNA-binding module linked to Rb/E2F pathways. *J Biol Chem* 2008; **283**: 4352–63.

40. Nygaard TG, Wooten GF. Dopa-responsive dystonia: some pieces of the puzzle are still missing. *Neurology* 1998; **50**: 853–5.

41. Friedman J, Standaert DG. Neurogenetics of dystonia and paroxysmal dyskinesias. *Neurogenetics: Scientific and Clinical Advances*. New York: Marcel Dekker; 2005: 403–26.

42. Asmus F, Zimprich A, Tezenas Du MS *et al.* Myoclonus-dystonia syndrome: epsilon-sarcoglycan mutations and phenotype. *Ann Neurol* 2002; **52**: 489–92.

43. Quinn NP, Rothwell JC, Thompson PD *et al.* Hereditary myoclonic dystonia, hereditary torsion dystonia and hereditary essential myoclonus: an area of confusion. *Adv Neurol* 1988; **50**: 391–401.

44. Zimprich A, Grabowski M, Asmus F *et al.* Mutations in the gene encoding epsilon-sarcoglycan cause myoclonus-dystonia syndrome. *Nat Genet.* 2001; **29**: 66–9.

45. Muller B, Hedrich K, Kock N *et al.* Evidence that paternal expression of the epsilon-sarcoglycan gene accounts for reduced penetrance in myoclonus-dystonia. *Am J Hum Genet* 2002; **71**: 1303–11.

46. Hedrich K, Meyer EM, Schule B *et al.* Myoclonus-dystonia: detection of novel, recurrent, and de novo SGCE mutations. *Neurology* 2004; **62**: 1229–31.

47. Asmus F, Hjermind LE, Dupont E *et al.* Genomic deletion size at the epsilon-sarcoglycan locus determines the clinical phenotype. *Brain* 2007; **130**: 2736–45.

48. Grimes DA, Han F, Lang AE *et al.* A novel locus for inherited myoclonus-dystonia on 18p11. *Neurology* 2002; **59**: 1183–6.

49. Schneider SA, Bhatia K. Paroxysmal dyskinesias – an overview. In: Jankovic J, Tolosa E, eds. *Parkinson's Disease and Movement Disorders*. 5th ed. Philadelphia: Lippincott Williams & Wilkins; 2006: 459–67.

50. Altrocchi PH, Forno LS. Spontaneous oral-facial dyskinesia: neuropathology of a case. *Neurology* 1983; **33**: 802–5.

51. Bhatia K, Daniel SE, Marsden CD. Orofacial dystonia and rest tremor in a patient with normal brain pathology. *Mov Disord* 1993; **8**: 361–2.

52. Gibb WR, Lees AJ, Marsden CD. Pathological report of four patients presenting with cranial dystonias. *Mov Disord* 1988; **3**: 211–21.

53. Kulisevsky J, Marti MJ, Ferrer I *et al.* Meige syndrome: neuropathology of a case. *Mov Disord* 1988; **3**: 170–5.

54. Zweig RM, Hedreen JC, Jankel WR *et al.* Pathology in brainstem regions of individuals with primary dystonia. *Neurology* 1988; **38**: 702–6.

55. Zweig RM, Hedreen JC. Brain stem pathology in cranial dystonia. *Adv Neurol* 1988; **49**: 395–407.

56. McNaught KS, Kapustin A, Jackson T *et al.* Brainstem pathology in DYT1 primary torsion dystonia. *Ann Neurol* 2004; **56**: 540–7.

57. Holton JL, Schneider SA, Ganesharajah T *et al.* Neuropathology of primary adult-onset dystonia. *Neurology* 2008; **70**: 695–9.

58. Kaji R, Goto S, Tamiya G *et al.* Molecular dissection and anatomical basis of dystonia: X-linked recessive dystonia-parkinsonism (DYT3). *J Med Invest* 2005; **52**(Suppl): 280–3.

59. Tackenberg B, Metz A, Unger M *et al.* Nigrostriatal dysfunction in X-linked dystonia-parkinsonism (DYT3). *Mov Disord* 2007; **22**: 900–2.

60. Grotzsch H, Pizzolato GP, Ghika J *et al.* Neuropathology of a case of dopa-responsive dystonia associated with a new genetic locus, DYT14. *Neurology* 2002; **58**: 1839–42.

61. Albanese A, Barnes MP, Bhatia KP *et al.* A systematic review on the diagnosis and treatment of primary (idiopathic) dystonia and dystonia plus syndromes: report of an EFNS/MDS-ES Task Force. *Eur J Neurol* 2006; **13**: 433–44.

62. Jankovic J. Treatment of dystonia. *Lancet Neurol* 2006; **5**: 864–72.

63. Munchau A, Palmer JD, Dressler D *et al.* Prospective study of selective peripheral denervation for botulinum-toxin resistant patients with cervical dystonia. *Brain* 2001; **124**: 769–83.

64. Kupsch A, Benecke R, Muller J *et al.* Pallidal deep-brain stimulation in primary generalized or segmental dystonia. *N Engl J Med* 2006; **355**: 1978–90.

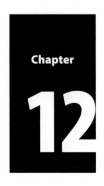

Chapter

12

Hemifacial spasm
Unusual causes and differential diagnosis

Danita Jones and Néstor Gálvez-Jiménez

Hemifacial spasm

Hemifacial spasm (HFS) is a brief, clonic jerking movement of the facial muscles that has been classically associated with vascular compression of the root exit zone of the seventh (facial) cranial nerve. The compression presumably is associated with demyelination and resultant ephaptic "aberrant" transmission. The spasm itself begins as a unilateral involuntary, intermittent clonic or tonic contraction of the orbicularis oculi muscle, usually spreading in a downward manner involving the other facial muscles. Causes of HFS other than vascular compression are exceedingly rare (Table 12.1).

Facial nerve anatomy

The facial nerve is a mixed nerve consisting of a motor and sensory root. The motor branch has its origin at the pontine motor nucleus of the facial nerve located anterior and laterally to cranial nerve (CN) VI nucleus (abducens nucleus), medial to the trigeminal sensory nucleus (CN V) and posterior to the superior border of the olive. Its motor fibers travel dorsal and medial and surround CN VI nucleus before proceeding anterior and lateral to the pyramidal tract, and then exiting at the pontomedullary junction (called by some anatomists the apparent origin of the nerve). Its sensory component originates at the geniculate ganglia nerve cells traversing the brain stem into the sensory trigeminal nucleus and nucleus of the tractus solitarius. This branch provides sensory innervations to the tragus, antitragus, external auditory meatus, tongue, soft palate and submandibular and sublingual salivary glands. CN VII also has sympathetic elements from the internal carotid artery that together with the superior and deep petrosal nerves form the vidian nerve. Another branch of the eighth nerve, the chorda tympani, carries sensory innervations to the anterior

two-third of the tongue via the lingual nerve, a branch of the trigeminal nerve. The terminal branches of the facial nerve may be divided into those to the muscles above the zygomaticus area and those below the zygomaticus region. The main purpose of the facial nerve is to provide facial expression. The posterior belly of the digastric is also innervated by branches of the facial nerve. There appears to be a somatotopic distribution of the facial nerve fibers within the main trunk of the facial nerve. The neurons innervating the lower facial muscles are primarily found in the lateral portion of the facial motor nucleus, whereas neurons innervating the upper facial muscles are located in the dorsal nuclei region. The medial propriobulbar fiber system, which tends to distribute its fibers bilaterally, chiefly comes from neurons in the medial part of the lateral tegmental field. These findings help to explain the pathophysiological changes and facial reflexes seen in patients with intracranial or extracranial facial nerve damage [1]. In Figure 12.1 the topographic anatomy of the facial nerve is precisely presented, which helps explain the peripheral distribution of symptoms due to extrinsic compression.

History

Perhaps the first description of what we now call hemifacial spasm was made by Schultze in 1875 and first cited in the English language by Gowers in his *Manual of Diseases of the Nervous System* in 1888 [2]. According to Gowers, Schultze's patient was a 56-year-old man with right facial spasm, increased by movement of the jaw or face. At autopsy, a left vertebral artery aneurysm was found to compress the facial nerve. It is interesting that it was an aneurysmal compressive lesion and not the typical overriding anterior inferior cerebellar artery (AICA) that caused the HFS. Gowers used the term facial spasm to describe these movements and divided

Uncommon Causes of Movement Disorders, ed. Néstor Gálvez-Jiménez and Paul J. Tuite. Published by Cambridge University Press. © Cambridge University Press 2011.

Table 12.1. Unusual causes of hemifacial spasm.

Vascular with resultant compression
Overriding anterior inferior cerebellar artery (most common cause)
Basilar artery ectasia
Vertebrobasilar artery complex ectasia
Vertebral artery aneurysm
Arteriovenous malformation
Venous compressions
Medullary venous malformations
Tumors
Epidermoid
Lipoma
Meningioma
Neurinoma/schwannoma
Cholesteoma
Arachnoid cyst (posterior fossa)
Paget disease
Occipital falcine meningioma
Pontine glioma
Pontine infarction
Fourth ventricle ganglioma
Syringobulbia
Multiple sclerosis
Central or peripheral facial nerve trauma
Hypothyroidism
Idiopathic intracranial hypertension (pseudotumor cerebri)
Craniovertebral anomalies
Trigeminal neuralgia (tic convulsive/tic douloureux)
Parotid gland tumors
Focal motor seizures
Arterial hypertension
Psychogenic HFS

the causes of such facial spasms into those generated by either an abnormal cortical discharge, nuclear (pontine) alterations, or nerve-trunk pathology. He stated that pressure on the nerve may "excite the nerve fibers directly, as electrical stimulation does, and may … maintain or intensify the muscle contractions" [2]. He also noted that usually facial spasm commences during adult life and typically affects women. He emphasized the onset of the spasm at the orbicularis oculi with

further unilateral spread to the zygomatic and other facial muscles. From his own observations, Gardner concluded that HFS should be considered a reversible state due to chronic pressure of the seventh nerve resulting in local demyelination and ephaptic electrical transmission correctable with surgical decompression [1].

The term hemifacial spasm is credited to Ehni and Woltman of the Mayo Clinic, who described 106 individuals with hemifacial movements; all of which had no gross brain pathology [3]. They emphasized the predominance of this condition in women, with a sex ratio of 3:2, an average age at onset of 45 years (range 17–70), and involvement beginning most often in the eyelids in 65% of patients [3,4]. The spasms were bilateral in 5%. They also first reported that HFS was often aggravated by anxiety and fatigue. In some of their cases, vertigo, facial weakness and hearing difficulties were found. Since their report pre-dated modern neuroimaging and neurophysiological techniques, small posterior fossa tumors, e.g., seventh nerve acoustic neuromas, may have been missed in those individuals who had accompanying features. Thus despite Ehni and Woltman associating HFS with no obvious "gross disease in the posterior fossa" they did not necessarily exclude causes in their cryptogenic cases. Thus one approach is to consider HFS a clinically defined condition and to search for underlying etiologies.

Even though HFS is due to vascular pathology compressing the exiting nerve root of nerve VII, one should be aware of other causes. There are few reports where cerebellopontine angle tumors can present with features of HFS. In Gardner and Sava's original series of 19 patients at the Cleveland Clinic Foundation in 1961, not a single case was caused by a posterior fossa tumor [1]. Kay and Adams found no masses in 16 patients treated with posterior fossa surgery [5]. In eight cases of symptomatic HFS reported by Nagata et al., a cerebellopontine angle mass was found in only two [6]. Another individual had an extension of a glossopharyngeal neurinoma through the jugular foramen with upward compression of the facial nerve. A fourth person had a tentorial meningioma with downward compression of the structures in the cerebellopontine angle. The remaining four patients had vascular malformations or an aneurysm. Loeser and Chen found in 450 operated cases of HFS that cerebellopontine angle tumors were responsible for HFS in 0.9% of cases [7]. Most cases were due to arterial compression (89%), venous compression (4%), aneurysm (0.4%) and arteriovenous malformations (0.2%). In a review of

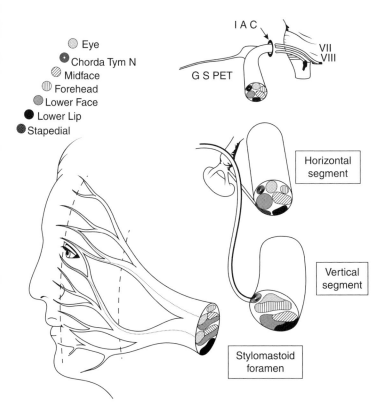

- Eye
- Chorda Tym N
- Midface
- Forehead
- Lower Face
- Lower Lip
- Stapedial

IAC

GS PET

VII
VIII

Horizontal segment

Vertical segment

Stylomastoid foramen

Figure 12.1. Topographic anatomy of the facial nerve. IAC = internal auditory canal; GS PET = greater petrosal nerve. (Reproduced with permission from May M and Schaitkin BM. *The Facial Nerve*. 2nd ed. New York: Thieme; 2000.)

the subject in 1988, of 1688 reported cases only 1% of such cases were due to cerebellopontine angle tumors [4]. Singh *et al.* reported a 46-year-old man with right HFS caused by a cerebellopontine angle epidermoid tumor that was believed to have caused displacement of the AICA against the root exit zone of the seventh nerve [8]. This case is unusual in that the onset and clinical presentation of HFS did not follow the normal progression of symptoms. Here the patient began with symptoms in the lower face (orbicularis oris) rather than the normal onset of the orbicularis oculi. Along with the onset of the lower face hemifacial spasm, there was associated tinnitus. Both the hemifacial spasm and the tinnitus disappeared after surgery. Altinos *et al.* reported two patients with typical onset and progression of the HFS from the orbicularis oculi to the rest of the facial muscles caused by a cerebellar arachnoid cyst in the posterior fossa with anterior displacement of the cerebellar hemisphere that displaced the facial nerve into close proximity with the AICA [9]. After separating the facial nerve from the AICA, the symptoms disappeared in 3 weeks. Inoue *et al.* reported a 66-year-old man with intermittent twitching of the right inferior orbicularis oculi spreading to other areas of the right hemiface [10]. His examination showed the presence

of mild facial weakness along with the right hemifacial spasm and mild hearing loss. MRI of the brain demonstrated the presence of a hyperintense mass in the right cerebellopontine angle area. Surgery showed that a lipoma had displaced the seventh and eighth nerves along with downward compression of the ninth, tenth, and eleventh cranial nerves. A similar case was reported by Levin and Lee in a medical student [11]. Nagata *et al.* reported four patients with posterior fossa tumors in whom the tumor compressed the seventh nerve without having an associated vascular loop [12]. In three such cases the hemifacial spasm improved after surgery. Two of these cases were due to a meningioma, one a neurinoma, and one an epidermoid. In a series of 18 patients with a cerebellopontine angle epidermoid tumor, three had hemifacial spasm [13].

The majority of the reported cases caused by a posterior fossa tumor have other symptoms; most notably tinnitus, hearing loss and unsteady gait. Ohashi *et al.*, in a series of 27 patients with HFS, found 20 with abnormalities in a neuro-otological examination, such as abnormal brain stem auditory evoked response (50%) and electronystagmography (50%), with alterations in saccadic eye movements, optokinetic nystagmus, pursuit eye movements and positional or rotational nystagmus [14].

Other rare causes include schwannomas, meningiomas (e.g., occipital falcine), pontine glioma, pontine infarction, fourth ventricle ganglioglioma, multiple sclerosis, craniovertebral anomalies (e.g., Paget disease), cerebellopontine angle venous malformation, vertebrobasilar ectasia, syringobulbia, sarcomas, cholesteatomas, trauma, entrapment by a parotid gland tumor and psychogenic. Reported associations with hypothyroidism and idiopathic intracranial hypertension have also been made [15–26]. A few cases of HFS alone or in combination with trigeminal neuralgia have been reported as a false localizing sign in patients who had a contralateral posterior fossa mass or acoustic neuroma [27,28].

There are three reports of HFS secondary to parotid gland tumor [29–31]. The direct compression resulting in local ischemic changes has been demonstrated intraoperatively in all three reported cases. Unfortunately, our third patient refused surgical exploration and was lost to follow-up, and the mechanism in our case is uncertain. In this case, HFS was present only in the lower face, suggesting involvement of the buccomandibular facial nerve branches as they exit the parotid gland. This atypical onset of HFS should suggest to the clinician a cause other than a vascular loop and, as this case demonstrated, a peripheral compressive facial nerve lesion may cause repetitive facial contraction.

Oliveira *et al.* reported the association of arterial hypertension and HFS [32]. In their study they found that 66.7% of patients with HFS had arterial hypertension compared with 38.2% of patients with blepharospasm, which served as a control. They hypothesized that arterial hypertension increased the tortuosity of the posterior circulation arteries, resulting in secondary brain stem or facial nerve root compression. These findings have been disputed by some [33].

In addition to the various cases above, there have been few reports of HFS as a result of facial nerve lesions following trauma [33]. HFS, in these reports, is the consequence of lesions distal to the stylomastoid foramen due to facial trauma or laceration. In our experience, the normal "expected" downward progression of facial muscle involvement is not observed. Rather, the spread of muscle involvement seems to spread upward toward the upper facial muscles, or remain localized to the most affected peripheral facial nerve branches. Kindling, according to the above authors, may account for increased firing at the facial nucleus, resulting in an increase in the rate of neuronal firing producing HFS. Posttraumatic HFS may have a central, a peripheral,

or perhaps a combination of the pathophysiologic mechanisms. The pathological changes associated with traumatic peripheral nerve injuries consists of demyelination, as well as axon swelling or loss. Seddon's peripheral nerve injury classification, one of the most commonly used, separates injuries into either neurotmesis or complete nerve transaction, axonotmesis or axonal loss but with stromal continuity and neuroapraxia indicating demyelination. We had two cases of crushing injuries to the peripheral nerve resulting in HFS, which spread upward to the remaining muscles innervated by the facial nerve (unpublished observations). Observations of facial nerve trauma, either stretching or crushing, have resulted in different pathological changes to the nerve. Stretching injuries result in demyelination with minimal axonal loss, whereas the crushing group results in predominantly axonal loss with wallerian degeneration and demyelination leading to incomplete recovery. After investigation for the more common etiologies of HFS, the diagnosis of HFS was made. Both patients responded well to botulinum toxin therapy. Of note, it was also found that trauma-induced HFS may also present after a period of facial weakness.

Pathophysiology

Although most cases of HFS are due to vascular compression at the exit root zone, causes other than vascular loops may result in HFS. It is not clear why most cases of vascular compression result in HFS as compared with space-occupying lesions in the cerebellopontine angle area or peripheral nerve. Various hypotheses regarding the genesis of HFS have been proposed. The most widely accepted theory was proposed by Gardner and Sava in 1962 [1]. This hypothesis has been supported by electrophysiological recordings by Nielsen, Moller and Auger, which indicate that the focal compression of the facial nerve causes ectopic excitation and ephaptic transmission (crosstalk) of electrical impulses in adjacent nerve fibers with new synapse formation at the site of the compression [34–38]. Nielsen has demonstrated focal conduction slowing at the same site [34,35]. We hypothesized that the constant "hammering" of each cardiac pulse affects the myelin sheath over time, acting perhaps as a new injury effect, while slow growth results in distortion of the facial nerve with less likelihood of inducing local demyelination and ephaptic/transaxonal communication with new synapse formation. It is believed that this peripheral injury may antidromically alter the facial motor nucleus, resulting in uninhibited firing. Moller has presented evidence to suggest that the symptoms of HFS are caused by hyperactivity in the facial motor nuclei and the trigeminal facial system [36,37]. Martinelli *et al.* reported three cases of HFS evolving from peripheral traumatic facial nerve lesions to support the role of antidromically mediated intrinsic changes in the facial motor nucleus [38]. Furthermore, Ishikawa *et al.* have demonstrated hyperexcitability of the facial motor neurons by showing prolongation of facial nerve F waves in those with HFS at the site of the symptoms [39]. Some have questioned the validity of this hypothesis, and the pathophysiology of HFS remains controversial. As indicated by Kotterba *et al.*, electromyography shows short bursts of high-frequency normal motor unit discharges as well as blink reflexes, resulting in increased R2-recovery curves [40]. Facial muscles do not act on joints, have no proprioceptors, and receive neither reciprocal nor recurrent inhibition on their motor neurons. The lack of axon collaterals and muscle proprioceptors reduces postexcitatory and reflex mechanisms to a minimum, allowing central inhibition to operate in isolation. Kotterba *et al.* used transcranial magnetic stimulation as a diagnostic tool to differentiate between HFS and somatoform disorder [40]. The authors explained how, within the hemifacial spasm group, TMS revealed unchanged H-reflexes as an indicator of spinal motor neuron excitability. After electrical stimulation of the facial nerve, EMG suppression was short lasting. They found blinklike responses and M-waves could be elicited during the silent period after TMS, thus indicating that facial motor neurons were not refractory to reflex activation. It was then concluded that facial motor neurons respond easily to trigeminal stimulation, receiving only mild to short-lasting excitation of the corticobulbar inhibitory descending projections. The results of this study suggested a central mechanism in the genesis of HFS.

Differential diagnosis

When evaluating someone with presumed HFS, one should consider other forms of facial dystonia such as benign essential blepharospasm (BEB), facial myokymia, and Meige syndrome (see Table 12.2). BEB, a form of focal dystonia, is easily differentiated from HFS. Patients with BEB by definition have the abnormal contraction of the orbicularis oculi bilaterally, which is usually symmetric and synchronous. As discussed in Kowal *et al.*, the eyelids are frequently and involuntarily forced shut [41]. This can result in functional blindness.

Table 12.2. Differential diagnosis of hemifacial spasm.

Blepharospasm
Tardive dyskinesias and Meige syndrome
Chorea
Facial myoclonus
Tics and Tourette syndrome
Hemimasticatory spasm
Facial myokymia
Focal motor seizures
Palatal myoclonus with facial muscle involvement
Whipple disease
Facial myorrhythmia in patients with dystonia (especially segmental or generalized dystonia)
Facial stereotypes and mannerisms
Psychogenic hemifacial spasm as part of other psychogenic movement disorders syndromes in the same patient
Bruxism
Trigeminal neuralgia (tic convulsive/tic douloureux) and other atypical facial pain

BEB is usually idiopathic and begins in adulthood. The condition itself is usually progressive, beginning with early irritation and discomfort in the eyelids; often described as a sandlike sensation in the eyes. There is some data to suggest that dryness in the eyes or other ocular pathology may increase the chance of developing BEB due to the accompanying increased sensory afferent signaling from changes in the eyes. This leads to a increased eye blinking and frequent, forceful involuntary closure of the eyes. Both eyes are usually affected symmetrically and the condition rarely resolves spontaneously. In the study performed by Kowal *et al.*, the average age of onset for BEB was 61 years whereas the average age of onset for HFS was 59 years [41]. Patients differ in their presenting symptoms in that those with blepharospasm complain of blinking, lid closure, sore or dry eyes, blurred vision, squinting, grittiness and lid twitching. BEB is exacerbated by stress and sunlight; driving may be one of the times of greatest disability due to the changes in light–dark contrast that lead to more pronounced symptoms. Over time, there is gradual progression of BEB, with the frequency of blinking attacks increasing and the duration of attacks being more prolonged, eventually leading to lid closure. Patients with HFS complain of lid and facial twitching, blinking and closure or ptosis. HFS gradually worsens, with lid twitching becoming more frequent and leading to lid closure and involvement of the muscles in the cheek and face. A second condition, entitled facial myokimia, is characterized by slow undulating vermian ("bag of worms") movements classically affecting the orbicularis oculi musculature – most often of the lower lid but they may involve the upper lid [42,43]. These movements may be brought on by caffeine or fatigue. Typically they are benign without an underlying cause; however, rarely pontine tumors, multiple sclerosis, inflammatory neuropathies, e.g., acute inflammatory demyelinating polyneuropathy (also known as Guillan–Barré syndrome), basilar artery ectasia, syringobulbia or prior radiation are associated (33,43–46). A secondary cause is to be suspected when the facial myokimia affects the lower face; nonetheless clinical judgment is needed when individuals present with facial movements as to whether imaging is appropriate to evaluate for a posterior fossa pathology [44,45]. A third condition that needs to be distinguished from HFS is a craniofacial dystonia called Meige syndrome, which is a combination of blepharospasm and oromandibular dystonia, with a mean age of onset of 65 years. The typical bilateral nature of this condition allows it to be distinguished from HFS. Also, unlike in HFS, the movements in Meige syndrome may be present with action; for example, speaking may generate tongue and lower facial involvement whereas with HFS the spasms are at rest and can be brought on with facial movements but are not manifest at the time of the movement.

Hemimasticatory spasm is another condition to consider in someone with abnormal facial movements. In these cases there are involuntary movements of the masticatory and other jaw-closing muscles such as the masseter, temporalis and medial pterygoids on one side of the face. Usually, this abnormal hyperkinetic movement disorder is associated with hemifacial atrophy, but this is not always the rule. This has been our experience and that of others [47–49].

Another challenge is to determine whether the facial movements are due to nonneurological factors. Since a considerable portion of patients initially diagnosed with psychogenic disorders are later proven to have an organic neurological disease, one needs to be cautious. Specifically with HFS, the intermittent clonic and tonic contractions of the facial nerve-innervated muscles are often induced by stress and fatigue, as well as voluntary movements of the eyes, so it may be considered to be psychogenic or a conversion reaction. However, reports of psychogenic hemifacial spasm are extremely rare. In a study by Lesser and Fahn, only one of 85 patients with psychiatric illness presented as dystonia [50]. However, patients with dystonia are frequently referred for psychiatric treatment at the time of initial symptom onset. This raises the importance of recognizing the correct diagnosis in order to ensure correct and efficient treatment. In addition, a psychogenic disorder frequently coexists with an organic neurological disease similar to patients with epilepsy who also may be diagnosed with nonepileptic "psychogenic" seizures. No exact figures are available on the true prevalence of psychogenic HFS in the literature on psychogenic movement disorders. In a review of the topic, we found that psychogenic facial movements lumped together with psychogenic blepharospasm accounted for 1.5% of 259 cases of psychogenic movement disorders seen at two large movement disorders [51]. In all cases, the following clues suggested that the HFS and accompanying movement disorders were of psychogenic origin: abrupt onset, static course, multiple somatizations and secondary gain. Clinically, the character of the movements was variable with exacerbations and reduction with attention or distraction, response to placebo and abrupt discontinuation of the abnormal movements after psychiatric intervention. In all instances the psychogenic HFS was accompanied by other psychogenic movements including tremor, myoclonus and dystonic spasms. The presence of other movements, which is also a hallmark of psychogenic disorders, still makes it challenging for a clinician who is cautious to prematurely conclude that the movements are not organic (51–53).

Tonic contraction of the face, as a manifestation of a focal motor seizure affecting the motor cortex, may mimic HFS. The nature of the movements may be quite similar but the duration of the twitching tends to be longer with a seizure, though in some cases they are very brief. If there is accompanying cortical epileptic spread there may be movements in the ipsilateral arm and possibly a generalized tonic-clonic seizure. Unilateral facial weakness may be seen. Brain imaging with electroencephalographic studies are useful in diagnosing and characterizing the underlying process in this seizure disorder. Lastly, one may wish to consider facial tics in the differential. Typically these present during childhood, adolescence or young adulthood in contrast to later age of onset for HFS. The movements may be unilateral or bilateral eye blinking, grimacing, etc. Often other tics that have waxed or waned may provide a clue. Associated features such as attention deficit hyperactivity disorder, learning disabilities, or obsessive compulsive traits may be seen in the individual or in their family history.

The introduction of botulinum toxin injections for the treatment of organic dystonic disorders opens a new nonsurgical therapy. In general, botulinum toxin is a useful treatment. The neurotoxin is injected directly into the affected muscle, causing chemical denervation.

Conclusion

When HFS is the initial clinical presentation followed by other cranial nerve involvement, the chance of finding a lesion other than an acoustic neuroma is greatly increased and a meningioma or cholesteatoma becomes important differential diagnostic considerations. Careful documentation of impaired corneal reflexes, deafness, papilledema, sensory loss in a trigeminal distribution, and facial paralysis suggests an acoustic neuroma. Furthermore, the onset of HFS in the lower facial musculature should alert the physician to search for secondary causes of HFS. We therefore recommend that contrast-enhanced brain MRI be performed in patients with HFS, especially in those with an atypical presentation, to search for possible treatable causes of HFS other than a vascular loop.

Acknowledgment

Portions of this chapter were updated from an earlier publication entitled "Unusual causes of HFS" published in *Seminars in Neurology* 2001.

References

1. Gardner WT, Sava GA. Hemifacial spasm: a reversible pathophysiologic state. *J Neurosurg* 962; **19**: 240–7.

2. Gowers WR. *A Manual of Disease of the Nervous System.* Vol 2. Darien, CT: Hafner; 1970: 248–59.

3. Ehni G, Woltman HW. Hemifacial spasm. *Arch Neurol Psychiatry* 1945; **53**: 205–11.

4. Digree K, Corbett JA. Hemifacial spasm: differential diagnosis, mechanism and treatment. *Adv Neurol* 1988: **49**: 151–76.

5. Kay AH, Adams CBT. Hemifacial spasm: a long term followup of patients treated by posterior fossa surgery and facial nerve wrapping. *J Neurol Neurosurg Psychiatry* 1981; **4**: 1101–3.

6. Nagata S, Matsushima T, Fujii K et al. Hemifacial spasm due to tumor, aneurysm, or arteriovenous malformation. *Surg Neurol* 1992; **38**: 204–9.

7. Loeser JD, Chen J. Hemifacial spasm: treatment by microsurgical facial nerve decompression. *Neurosurgery* 1983; **13**: 141–6.

8. Singh Ak, Jain VK, Chhabra DK et al. Hemifacial Spasm and Cerebellopontine angle epidermoid: case report and review. *Neurol Res* 1994; **16**: 321–3.

9. Altinos N, Kars Z, Cepoglu C. Rare causes of hemifacial spasm: report of two cases. *Clin Neurol Neurosurg* 1991; **93**: 155–8.

10. Inoue T, Maeyama R, Ogawa H. Hemifacial spasm resulting from cerebellopontine angle lipoma: case report. *Neurosurgery* 1995; **36**: 846–50.

11. Levin JM, Lee JE. Hemifacial spasm due to cerebellopontine angle lipoma: case report. *Neurology* 1987; **37**: 337–9

12. Nagata S, Matsuchima T, Fujji M et al. Hemifacial spasm due to tumor, aneurysm or arteriovenous malformation. *Surg Neurol* 1992; **38**: 204–9.

13. Auger RG, Piepgras DG. Hemifacial spasm associated with epidermoid tumors of the cerebellopontine angle. *Neurology* 1989; **39**: 577–80.

14. Ohashi N, Yasumara S, Mizukoshi K et al. Involvement of the 8th cranial nerve and the brainstem in patients with hemifacial spasm. *Acta Otolaryngol* 1991; **111**: 1060–4.

15. Kim Y, Tanaka A, Kimura M et al. Arteriovenous malformation in the cerebellopontine angle presenting as hemifacial spasm. *Neurol Med Chir (Tokyo)* 1991; **31**: 109–12.

16. Ing Eb, Savino PJ, Bosley TM et al. Hemifacial spasm and osteitis deformans. *Am J Ophthalmol* 1995; **119**: 376–7.

17. Linazasoro F, Marti Masso JF. Paget's disease and hemifacial spasm. *Neurology* 1992; **42**: 1643–4.

18. Bhayani R, Goel A. Occipital falcine meningioma presenting with ipsilateral hemifacial spasm: a case report. *Br J Neurosurg* 1996; **10**: 603–5.

19. Westra I, Dummond GT. Occult pontine glioma in a patient with hemifacial spasm. *Can J Ophthalmol* 1991; **26**: 148–51.

20. Bill DC, Hanieh A. Hemifacial spasm in an infant due to 4th ventricular ganglioglioma. *J Neurosurg* 1991; **75**: 134–7.

21. Vermersch P, Petit H, Marion MH et al. Hemifacial spasm due to pontine infarction. *J Neurol Neurosurg Psychiatry* 1991; **54**: 1018.

22. Barraquer-Bordas L, Zamora S, Abello-Villa P. Espasmo hemifacial y sordera central bilateral en el cuadro clinic de una siringobulbia. *Rev Esp Oto Oftalmol* 1955; **17**: 17–22.

23. Genes D, Rechart W, Fernandez-Real JM et al. Hemifacial spasm and hypothyroidism. *Lancet* 1993; **342**: 1112.

24. Selky AK, Purvin VA. Hemifacial spasm. An unusual manifestation of idiopathic intracranial hypertension. *J Neuroophthalmol* 1994; **14**: 196–8.

25. Kerbert CW, Margolis MT, Newton TH. Tortuous vertebrobasilar system: a cause of cranial nerve signs. *Neuroradiology* 1972; **4**: 74–7.

26. Maroun FB, Jacob JC, Weir BKA *et al.* Hemifacial spasm and craniovertebral anomaly. Can *J Neurol Sci* 1990; **17**: 424–6.

27. Matsuura N, Kondo A. Trigeminal neuralgia and hemifacial spasm as false localizing sign in patients with contralateral mass of the posterior cranial fossa: report of three cases. *J Neurosurg* 1996; **84**: 1067–71.

28. Nishi T, Matsukado Y, Nagahiro S *et al.* Hemifacial spasm due to contralateral acoustic neuroma: a case report. *Neurology* 1987; **37**: 339–42.

29. Destee A, Bouchez P, Pellegrini P *et al.* Hemifacial spasm associated with a mixed benign parotid gland tumor. *J Neurol Neurosurg Psychiatry* 1985; **48**: 189–90.

30. Nussbaum M. Hemifacial spasm associated with a benign parotid tumor. *Ann Otol* 1977; **86**: 73–4.

31. Gandon J, Trotoux J, Peghegre R *et al.* Bilan de 158 parotidectomies et problèmes histologiques poses par le tumeurs mixtes des glandes salivaires. *Ann Otolaryngol (Paris)* 1979; **96**: 261–80.

32. Oliveira LD, Cardoso F, Vargas AP. Hemifacial spasm and arterial hypertension. *Mov Disord* 1999; **14**: 832–5.

33. Tan EK, Jankovic J. Hemifacial spasm and hypertension: how strong is the association? *Mov Disord* 2000; **15**: 363–5.

34. Nielsen VK. Pathophysiology of hemifacial spasm: I. Ephaptic transmission and ectopic excitation. *Neurology* 1984; **34**: 418–26.

35. Nielsen VK. Electrophysiology of the facial nerve in hemifacial spasm: II. Ectopic/ephaptic excitation. *Muscle Nerve* 1985; **8**: 545–55.

36. Moller AR. Hemifacial spasm: ephaptic transmission or hyperexcitability of the facial motor nucleus? *Exp Neurol* 1987; **98**: 110–19.

37. Moller AR. The cranial nerve vascular compression syndrome: II. A review of pathophysiology. *Acta Neurochir (Wien)* 1991; **113**: 24–30.

38. Auger RG. Hemifacial spasm: clinical and electrophysiologic observations. *Neurology* 1979; **29**: 1261–72.

39. Ishikawa J, Takase M, Ohira T *et al.* Effect of repetitive stimulation on lateral spreads and F-waves in hemifacial spasm. *J Neurol Sci* 1996; **142**: 99–106.

40. Kotterba, S., Tegenthoff, M., Malin, J.-P. Hemifacial spasm or somatoform disorder: postexcitatory inhibition after transcranial magnetic cortical stimulation as a diagnostic tool. *Acta Neurol Scand* 2000; **101**: 305–10.

41. Kowal L, Davies R, Kiely P. Facial muscle spasms: an Australian study. Australian and *N Z J Ophthalmol* 1998. **26**: 123–8.

42. Chalk CH, Litchy WJ, Ebersold MH *et al.* Facial myokymia and unilateral basilar invagination. *Neurology* 1988; **38**: 1811–12.

43. Galvez-Jimenez, Nestor, M.D, Hanson, Maurice, M.D., Desai, Mehul, M.D. Unusual causes of hemifacial spasm. *Seminars in Neurology* 2001. **21**: 75–83.

44. Riaz G, Campbel WW, Carr J *et al.* Facial myokymia and syringobulbia. *Arch Neurol* 1990; **47**: 472–4.

45. Tenser RB, Corbett J. Myokymia and facial contraction in brainstem glioma. *Arch Neurol* 1974; **30**: 425–7.

46. Paty DW, Ebers GC. *Multiple Sclerosis: Contemporary Neurology Series*. Philadelphia: FA Davis; 1998.

47. Thompson PD, Carroll WM. Hemimasticatory and hemifacial spamsl: a common pathophysiology? *Clin Exp Neurol Proc Aust Assoc Neurol* 1982; **19**: 274–76.

48. Thompson PD, Carroll WM. Hemimasticatory spasm: a peripheral paroxysmal cranial neuropathy? *J Neurol Neurosurg Psychiatry* 1983; **46**: 274–6.

49. Auger RG, Litchy Wj, Cascino TL *et al.* Hemimasticatory spasm: clinical and electrophysiological observations. *Neurology* 1992; **42**: 2263–6.

50. Lesser, Ronald, M.D., Fahn, Stanley, M.D. Dystonia: a disorder often misdiagnosed as a conversion reaction. *Am J Psychiatry* 1978; **135**(3): 349–52.

51. Galvez-Jimenez N, Lang AE. Psychogenic movement disorders. In: Watt RL, Koller WC, eds. *Movement Disorders: Neurologic Principles and Practice*. New York: McGraw-Hill; 1997: 715–32.

52. Williams DT, Ford B, Fahn S. Phenomenology and psychopathology related to psychogenic movement disorders. In: Weiner WJ, Lang AE, eds. *Behavioral Neurology in Movement Disorders*. New York: Raven Press; 1994: 231–57.

53. Fahn S, Williams DT. Psychogenic dystonia. In: Fahn S, Marsden CD, Calne DB, eds. *Dystonia 2*. New York: Raven Press; 1988: 431–55.

Chapter 13

Tardive dyskinesias and other drug-induced movement disorders

Santiago Perez-Lloret and Marcelo Merello

Spontaneous and drug-induced movement disorders in psychiatric patients

A variety of movement disorders can accompany neuropsychiatric conditions and need to be differentiated from those induced by drugs [1,2]. Chorea or dystonia in Huntington disease for example, may be difficult to distinguish from tardive dyskinesia (TD) caused by antipsychotics drugs (APDs) often prescribed for psychiatric symptoms of the disease. Myoclonus, tics, tremor and even parkinsonism can be seen as part of conversion disorders, of malingering or even of Munchausen syndrome. There are also a variety of complex repetitive hyperkinetic disorders presenting as mannerisms, stereotypy and compulsions that may appear identical to certain movement disorders such as tics or dystonia, further complicating differential diagnosis. Lastly, hypokinetic conditions including bradyphrenia, catatonia, rigidity, catalepsy, negativism and mutism are generally difficult to distinguish from various forms of drug-induced parkinsonism.

Drug-induced movement disorders (DMIDs) were identified soon after marketing of APDs began in the 1950s. Initially, use of these drugs was linked to acute adverse extrapyramidal syndromes including acute dystonia, akathisia and parkinsonism [3]. Later, TD was also recognized as an adverse drug reaction to APDs.

Initially, some clinicians were reluctant to accept the possibility that TD was a direct result of APD treatment, considering it more likely to be a manifestation of chronic psychotic disorders [4]. This skepticism was due to several factors, including: (1) abnormal outcome after discontinuation of APDs; (2) the presence of spontaneous movement disorders in untreated schizophrenics; and (3) clinicians' reluctance to attribute

serious and persistent iatrogenic adverse effects to a class of drugs that had revolutionized the treatment of psychosis [5,6].

Clinical syndromes

Abnormal involuntary movements or extrapyramidal reactions are common adverse events; though initially described after APD use, they have also been linked to other psychiatric or nonpsychiatric drugs such as serotonin-specific reuptake inhibitors, metoclopramide or some calcium-channel blockers, among others [7–11].

Accompanying symptoms and time to onset of DIMDs vary significantly and include parkinsonism as well as motor restlessness (akathisia), dystonia and the entire spectrum of hyperkinesias (namely, chorea, stereotypies, myoclonus, dystonia and tics) [12]. They can be categorized as acute (immediate), continuous (insidious) or persistent (tardive) (Table 13.1) [13]. Dystonia represents the most important acute drug reaction, often intensifying so rapidly and to such a degree of severity that patients present directly to the emergency room and may require hospitalization. Continuous DIMDs persist only while the offending drug is being administered and remit after its discontinuation, either immediately or a variable of time after discontinuation. They include akathisia, tremor, parkinsonism, chorea and myoclonus. Finally, tardive syndromes consist of a variety of DIMDs appearing long after the beginning of drug use. Typically, discontinuation of the offending drug will not relieve persistent DIMD [13].

Acute and continuous syndromes

Acute dystonia

Ninety-five percent of acute dystonic movements develop within 96 hours of starting treatment, characterized by jerks or prolonged muscle spasms often

---

Uncommon Causes of Movement Disorders, ed. Néstor Gálvez-Jiménez and Paul J. Tuite. Published by Cambridge University Press. © Cambridge University Press 2011.

Table 13.1. Classification of drug-induced movement disorders.

Category	Abnormal movement	Principal characteristics
Acute (immediate)	Dystonia	Sustained involuntary muscular contractions or spasms resulting in abnormal postures or twisting and repetitive movements. Symptoms are associated with distress, with or without pain.
Continuous (insidious)	Akathisia	Subjective feeling of restlessness and need to move. Objective symptoms: walking in place, foot tapping, rocking while seated.
	Parkinsonism	Tremor, rigidity and slowness of movements affecting bilateral upper and lower extremities. Gait imbalance, masked facies, micrographia and stooped posture may be present.
	Tremor	They can be postural, intentional or action tremors. Their frequency can vary between 4 and 12 Hz.
	Chorea	Irregular, sudden-onset, explosive, purposeless movements.
	Myoclonus	Brief, involuntary, muscular jerks.
Persistent (tardive)	Dyskinesia Dystonia Akathisia Myoclonus Tics Tremor	Tardive dyskinesia: choreoathetoid involuntary movements affecting the orofacial region and tongue. Lip smacking, chewing movements and tongue protrusion are common. Symptoms are not painful but are highly distressing.

involving the craniocervical region (eyes, mouth, throat, neck) or even oculogyric crises [11,14].

Involvement of the trunk and limbs as observed in idiopathic dystonia is less common in TD [11,14]. Acute dystonic reactions can be dramatic, and at times severe enough to warrant life-saving measures, for example, involvement of laryngeal muscles causing acute respiratory distress.

Risk factors are listed in Table 13.2 and differential diagnoses in Table 13.3 [11,14]. Psychogenic dystonia may be suspected in cases in which dystonia disappears whenever patients believe they are unobserved, or when other psychogenic movement disorders or nonorganic neurological features are present, or when symptoms of somatization disorder are present, or in the static form of dystonia. When patients clearly obtain secondary (for example, financial) gain from the disorder, a malingering state may be considered. Catatonia is often accompanied by symptoms such as rigidity, akinesis, cerea flexibilitas and mutism, which are not seen in acute dystonia and are not related to drug treatment. The main difference between acute and tardive dystonia is that the latter occurs only after months or years of treatment with APDs and does not improve rapidly after administration of anticholinergics.

Acute akathisia

Akathisia (Greek meaning "not to sit") consists in difficulty remaining still and a subjective sense of restlessness [7,15]. It is a recognized adverse drug reaction of APDs, antiemetics and antidepressants among others medications[15]. Difficult to detect reliably, it may present unexpectedly in a variety of clinical settings and be accompanied by unpleasant oral or genital paresthesias and burning or lancinating pain not responding to conventional treatments.

Risk factors for akathisia are shown in Table 13.2 and differential diagnoses in Table 13.3 [7]. Restless legs syndrome (RLS) is characterized by muscle discomfort, pain and restlessness, or crawling sensations relieved by walking. Unlike akathisia, which ceases during sleep, RLS occurs mostly at night. Hyperactivity associated with anxiety states is often indistinguishable from akathisia, especially in psychotic patients on neuroleptics. However, sympathetic overactivity, e.g., excessive sweating, palpitations, hyperventilation, tremulousness and dilated pupils, characteristic of anxiety and panic attacks, is not seen in patients with akathisia. In bipolar affective disorders, akathisia can be confused with spontaneous mania, although usually milder and short-lived. In addition, spontaneous

Table 13.2. Risk factors for drug-induced movement disorders.

Acute dystonia	Akathisia	Drug-induced parkinsonism	Tremors	Tardive dyskinesia
Male sex	Advanced age	Older age	Older age	Age
Age under 30 years	Presence of an	Female sex	Liver failure	Presence of affective
Previous episode of	affective disorder	AIDS	CNS lesions	disorders
acute dystonia	Cognitive	Dementia	Anxiety	Drug dose
Recent cocaine use	impairment	Genetic		Alcoholism
Hypocalcemia	Female sex	predisposition		Diabetes mellitus
Dehydration	History of akathisia			Electroconvulsive treatment
Hypoparathyroidism	Iron deficiency			Iron deficiency
	Mental retardation			Mental retardation
				Organic brain disorder
				Female sex
				Genetic factors

Table 13.3. Differential diagnoses for each drug-induced movement disorders.

Acute dystonia	Akathisia	Drug-induced parkinsonism	Tremor	Tardive dyskinesia
Psychogenic dystonia	Restless legs syndrome	Other causes of parkinsonian syndromes (such as Parkinson disease, the parkinsonian form of multiple system atrophy, vascular parkinsonism, etc.)	Parkinsonisms	Tardive akathisia
Catatonia	Anxiety states		Hyperthyroidism	Spontaneous buccolingual dyskinesias of the elderly
Tardive dystonia	Dyskinesias (in Parkinson disease patients)		Hypoglycemia	Edentulous dyskinesias
Others			Other	Stereotyped movements in schizophrenia
				Drug-induced chorea or dyskinesias
				Other choreic syndromes

mania is usually accompanied by delusions, hallucinations and bizarre behavior.

Dyskinesia, in contrast to akathisia is often unilateral, or if bilateral tends to be more pronounced in the more severely affected arm and leg. As a rule, it increases in severity approximately 1–2 hours after each levodopa and/or dopamine agonist dose, although not always.

Parkinsonism

Drug-induced parkinsonism (DIP) is the second most common cause of parkinsonian syndrome [9]. The diversity of drugs involved in the production of DIP and the wide range of clinical disorders in which they are used poses a tough diagnostic challenge [16].

DIP is characterized by its symmetrical presentation with bradykinesia dominating the overall clinical picture [9,17]. Typical resting tremor is not frequently observed, but when present is postural and of higher frequency than in idiopathic disease. It develops insidiously after the offending drug is introduced; taking weeks or months to manifest fully.

Risk factors are listed in Table 13.2 and differential diagnoses in Table 13.3 [9]. DIP should be suspected in older patients, more prone to be taking different medications for underlying chronic conditions, including whenever symmetrical symptoms are present, disease onset is not compatible with idiopathic Parkinson disease or akinesia, and postural tremor predominate over rigidity and rest tremor [16,17]. Other drug-induced symptoms like akathisia or tardive dyskinesia can provide clues to the origin of parkinsonian syndrome.

Drug-induced parkinsonism may persist long after the offending drug has been withdrawn, sometimes for as long as a year or more [9]. In the majority of cases, however, it subsides gradually over a period of weeks or months. Patients show global improvement soon after drug withdrawal; cognitive and mood disturbances subside more slowly, while tremor may persist for 18 months after discontinuation of the drug in a significant number of patients. In those in whom parkinsonism becomes persistent and irreversible even after drug-withdrawal, diagnosis of latent idiopathic parkinsonism should be considered.

Tremors, chorea and myoclonus

Tremor is classified according to the behavior it is associated with [18]. Resting tremor is usually 4–6 Hz, occurs with the limb supported against gravity, and decreases with movement. Action or postural tremor varies widely in amplitude and frequency and occurs with maintained posture or movement. Finally, intentional tremor is terminal kinetic tremor (typically <5 Hz), with larger amplitude during final stages of target-directed movements. Drugs may induce tremor in any of these categories. D2-blockers (such as classical APDs or metoclopramide, among others) can cause resting tremor, often in the context of a parkinsonian syndrome. Antidepressants can induce rapid, low-amplitude postural tremors. Tremor induced by antiepileptics may be postural, but rest tremor can also occur. Intention tremors can be induced by beta-stimulants such as salbutamol.

Drug-induced tremors are generally dose-responsive (i.e., increasing the drug dose worsens the tremor, or decreasing the dose ameliorates the tremor) and display lack of progression, unlike tremors in Parkinson disease and essential tremor [18]. Risk factors and differential diagnoses are shown in Tables 13.2 and 13.3.

Choreas are irregular, sudden-onset, explosive, purposeless movements [19]. They usually include facial, shoulder or finger movements. They are facilitated by emotion and attention and inhibited by rest, calm and sleep. They are infrequently caused by drugs, except for the well-known levodopa-induced dyskinesias in parkinsonian patients. That said, contraceptives can cause choreas, especially in the case of patients with antecedents of rheumatic fever. Antiepileptics such as phenytoin can also be related to choreas.

Myoclonus consists of brief, involuntary muscular jerks that can generate movement or not [19]. Penicillins are frequent causes of myoclonus. It can also occur with antiepileptic or antidepressants overdose, in the context of an encephalopathy.

Tardive dyskinesia and other syndromes

Tardive syndromes (TD, tardive myoclonus, tardive tics, tardive dystonia, tardive akathisia and tardive tourettism) occur most frequently after prolonged APD exposure [10]. They often run a persistent course despite cessation of the triggering drug therapy. In some instances they may become permanent and irreversible. They should be considered in patients presenting abnormal involuntary movements after at least 3 months' total cumulative neuroleptic exposure, although they are more common after longer periods of exposure (1–2 years) [8,12]. They can develop even after APD dose reduction (unmasked TD), or even after the causative drug has been withdrawn (covert or withdrawal TD).

Tardive dyskinesia

Tardive dyskinesia consists of involuntary movements usually involving muscles of the tongue, lips, mouth or face (i.e., the so-called "buccolinguomasticatory syndrome") [1,4,8,12]. Upper facial muscles are less frequently affected by involuntary movements, but it is possible to see increased blinking, blepharospasm, arching of the eyebrows, ocular torsion and deviation.

Other parts of the body can be affected, though less frequently, and a wide range of movements can be observed including myoclonic jerks, tics, chorea and dystonia. Gait can be abnormal, with a broad base, leg jerking and repetitive irregular flexion and extension of the knees [1,3,8]. While standing in place, affected individuals tend to shift their weight from one leg to the other or exhibit pacing or marching in place. The diaphragm and accessory respiratory muscles are often involved, causing a fast and irregular breathing pattern (respiratory dyskinesia). The movements are more pronounced when the patient is alert or excited and disappear during sleep. Patients can sometimes suppress the movements through intense voluntary effort.

Table 13.2 shows risk factors for TD, and differential diagnoses are shown in Table 13.3 [1]. Movements in TD are somewhat different from typical chorea, tending to be more patterned, repetitive and stereotypic. Although patients frequently show apparent restlessness, indistinguishable from tardive akathisia, the subjective component is rarely present and, surprisingly, a large number of patients are unaware of the presence of abnormal involuntary movements; associated parkinsonian syndrome is quite frequent in these patients and should immediately suggest DIMD.

Other tardive syndromes

Dystonic phenomena account in up to 20% of tardive syndromes found in psychiatric inpatients and is similar to acute dystonia [10,20]. The differential diagnosis of tardive dystonia should include other disorders presenting dystonic phenomena such as idiopathic torsion dystonia, Wilson disease, and other symptomatic dystonias [1]. The primary difference between tardive dystonia and acute dystonia is that the former is characterized by persistent muscle contraction whereas muscle contraction is transient in the latter.

Motor and vocal tics following chronic neuroleptic treatment can occasionally be seen as part of the tardive syndrome. This type of clinical presentation has been described and referred to as tardive tourettism [21]. In a small number of cases, myoclonus can be the predominant feature of TD. Tardive tremor has also been added to the clinical spectrum of TD [21]. Painful sensations localized in the mouth or genital regions, alone or in association with dyskinesias, are also believed to be another clinical manifestation of TD. Pain may on occasion be so distressing as to overshadow all other concurrent psychiatric and motor manifestations.

Causal agents and pathophysiology

A nonexhaustive list of the drugs implicated in DIMDs is provided in Table 13.4. There follows a description of the main drug classes commonly associated with DMIDs.

Movement disorders caused by typical and atypical antipsychotics

Centrally acting dopamine receptor blockers, such as haloperidol and phenothiazine APDs, are the agents most commonly associated with DIMD [1,10]. The proposed mechanism for these adverse drug reactions is dopamine receptor blockage at the level of the striatum. DIMD are less frequently associated with the atypical APDs, but dose-related movement disorders occur with olanzapine, risperidone and quetiapine at higher doses as well [22]. Mechanisms underlying DIMDs are complex and not fully understood, but are probably related to alterations within subcortical brain regions (e.g., basal ganglia and thalamus) and do not involve the corticospinal pyramidal motor system.

Incidence of *acute dystonia* in treated patients varies from 2% to 64% according to different series and pathogenesis remains unclear. All APDs bind to D2 receptors, it has therefore been suggested that blockage of these receptors in the caudate, putamen and globus pallidus is partly responsible for causing acute dystonia [23].

Drug-induced parkinsonism is observed on average in about 4% of patients taking neuroleptics [24,25]. The risk of DIP in patients treated with low doses of atypical neuroleptics (≤1 mg of risperidone daily, or equivalent doses of related compounds) is lower than that of the classical neuroleptics, but is similar when typical and atypical neuroleptics are used at high doses.

DIP is caused by several mechanisms interfering with the normal nigrostriatal dopamine neuron function. Generally, compounds responsible for DIP block striatal dopamine D2 receptors, requiring blockade to exceed 75% in order to trigger DIP [26]. The lower DIP risk observed for atypical APDs than for the classic ones probably derives from the fact that in addition to a less potent dopaminergic blocking action, they bind preferentially to other subtypes of receptors. Several recent reports suggest that certain neuroleptics produce DIP not only in relation to excessive blockade of dopamine receptors but also mediated through direct and persistent toxic effects on nigrostriatal dopamine neurons [27].

The commonest drugs causing *akathisia* are classic APDs, and less frequently the atypical ones [28]. The underlying pathophysiological mechanism of akathisia is thought to be an imbalance between cortical and nigrostriatal dopaminergic innervation, favoring increased functional activity of the mesolimbic and nigrostriatal systems, in particular the nucleus accumbens [7].

The annual incidence of *APD-induced TD* is about 5% overall, including transient (3%) and persistent (2%) TD [6]. Risk of TD has been shown to be lower with atypical APDs than with classic ones. A recent review of clinical trials on several modern antipsychotics versus haloperidol in schizophrenia showed that risperidone, olanzapine, quetiapine, amisulpride or ziprasidone induced TD in 2.1% of cases, which is lower than the aforementioned annual TD rate for classic APDs. Indeed; among patients under 50 years old, risk of new-onset TD with haloperidol (5.4%) was 6.8 times greater than with atypical APDs [29]. Conversely, TD incidence with modern drugs among patients over 50 years old was similar to rates in younger individuals exposed to haloperidol, suggesting an important agent–age interaction [29]. The incidence of TD varied remarkably little among modern agents except for increased risk with higher doses of risperidone.

The pathophysiologic basis of TD remains speculative, but various neurochemical hypotheses have been proposed, including striatal dopaminergic

143

Table 13.4. Drugs inducing movement disorders.

Principal indication/s	Drug	Acute dystonia	Akathisia	Drug-induced parkinsonism	Tardive dyskinesias	Tremors	Myoclonus	Other choreas	Tic
Anesthetics/SNC depressors	Propofol	x [62]	x [62]					x [43]	
	Procaine			x [63]					
	Ethanol (toxic or withdrawal)			x [63]		xx [18]			
Antibiotics	Amphotericin B			[64]		x [18]			
	Penicillin						xx [19]		
	Cephalosporins						xx [19]		
	Chloroquine	x [11]							
	Aciclovir					x [18]		x [43]	
	Vidarabine					xx [18]			
	Cotrimoxazol					x [18]			
	Foscarnet	x [65]							
Anticephaleic	Sumatriptan	x [66]							
	Methysergide		x [43]						
Anticholinergic	Trihexphenidyl				x [37]			x [13]	
Anti-dementia, urinary retention	Donepezil			x [9]					
	Rivastigmine			x [9]					
	Pyridostigmine			x [67]					
	Bethanocol			x [63]					
Anticonvulsants	Valproic acid		x [43]	x [9,67]		xx [18]	x [19]	x [43]	
	Carbamazepine	x [11]			x [11,37]			x [43]	
	Topiramate								
	Phenytoin	x [11]	x [43]	x [9,67]	x [68]		xx [19]	x [13]	
	Phenobarbital				x [68]	x [18]	x [19]	x [43]	
	Gabapentin	x [69]				x [18]	xx [70]	x [43]	
	Lamotrigine		xx [13]			x [18]			
	Tiagabine					x [18]			

Category	Drug						
	Oxcarbazepine							x[18]
	Levetirazepam							
	Ethosuximide		x[63]	x[9]				x[43]
	Pregabaline		x[45]	x[45]				
Antidepressants	Tricyclics	x[19]	xx[11]	x[7]	x[10,37]	xx[18]	x[19]	x[13]
	SSRIs	xx[11]	xx[7]	x[9,33,67,71]	xx[33,37]	xx[18,33]	x[19,33]	x[13]
	Trazodone			x[63]			x[19]	
	Buproprion			x[63]			x[19]	
	Venlafaxine						x[19]	
	Nefazodone						x[19]	
	Mirtazapine						x[19]	
Antiemetics	Metochlopramide	xx[11]	xx[71]	xx[9,71]	xx[10,37,71]	xx[18]	xx[19]	
	Domperidone	x[72]						
	Clebopride		x[73]					
Anti-mania	Lithium	xx[11]	xx[7]	xx[9,67,71]	x[10,37,71]	xx[18]	x[19]	x[43]
Antipsychotics	Typical	xx[11]	xx[7,71]	xx[7,71]		xx[37]	xx[19]	x[19,37]
	Atypical	x[7,22]	x[7,22]	x[7,22]	x[7,22]		x[7,19,22]	
Anti-vertigo	Prochlorperazine/tiethylperazine		xx[9]	xx[9]				
	Cinnarizine/flunarizine	x[11]	x[10,71]	x[10,71]	x[10,71]			
Anxiolytics	Buspirone	x[74]	x[74]	x[74]	x[74]	x[43]	x[19,74]	
	Diazepam	x[68]	x[43]	x[43]	x[43]	x[19]	x[19]	
	Clonazepam					x[19]		
	Lorazepam		x[71]	x[71]	x[10]		x[19]	
Asthma/allergies	Chlorpheniramine	x[63]	xx[67]	xx[67]	x[68]	x[43]		
	Theophylline			x[43]	x[43]	x[43]		
	B2-adrenergic agonists	xx[13]				xx[18]		
Cancer	Cytosine arabinoside		x[67]	x[67]		x[18]		
	Vincristine		x[67]	x[67]				

Table 13.4. (*cont.*)

Principal indication/s	Drug	Acute dystonia	Akathisia	Drug-induced parkinsonism	Tardive dyskinesias	Tremors	Myoclonus	Other choreas	Tic
	Methotrexate			x [67]					
	5-Fluoruracil			x [67]					
	Doxyrubicin			x [75]					
	Thalidomide					x [18]			
	Ifosfamide					x [18]			
	Vincristine					x [18]			
	Interferon alfa					xx [18]		x [43]	
Cardiovascular disorders	Amiodarone			xx [9,67]	x [76]	xx [18,19]	x [76]		
	Procainamide					xx [18]			
	Pindolol					x [18]			
	Diltiazem/verapamil	x [77]		x [9,67,71,77]					
Endocrine disorders/ conditions	Levothyroxine		xx [13]			xx [18,43]			
	Calcitonin					x [18]			
	Oral contraceptives			x [43]	x [78]			x [13]	
	Corticosteroids		xx [13]						
	Velaripride (menopause)	x [67]		x [79]	x [79]	x [79]		x [79]	
	Hypoglycemics			x [40]		x [43]			
	Anabolic steroids				x [78]			x [43]	
Hyperkinetic movement disorders	Tetrabenezine/ reserpine /Metil-Tyr		x [80]	xx [9]	xx [37,43]				
Immunosuppression	Ciclosporin/ tacrolimus			x [67]		xx [18,19]			
NSAIDs	Naproxen sodium			x [63]					
Opiates	Meperidine		x [43]	x [67]			x [11,22]		
	Morphine						xx [19]		
	Oxycodone						x [68]		

	Methadone			x [81]		x [68]	x [43]	
	Fentanyl			x [37]	x [82]			
	Tramadol				x [19]			
Reflux/gastric ulcers	Cimetidine		x [68]		x [18]		x [13]	
	Ranitidine		x [68]		x [18]		x [13]	
	Misoprostol		x [83]		x [18]			
	Lansoprazole							
	Bismuth					xx [13]		
Stimulants	Methamphetamine/amphetamines		x [18]		x [18]		x [13]	x [19,37]
	Cocaine	x [11]	x [38]	x [39]	x [18]		xx [43]	x [19,37]
	Methylphenidate	x [38]					xx [13]	x [19,37]

x = uncommon/single report; xx= common (frequency >10%).

hypersensitivity, basal ganglia cholinergic deficiency, dysfunctions of striatonigral gamma-aminobutyric acid (GABA)-mediated neurons, glutamate-induced excitotoxicity, and oxidative stress [30–32]. It has been proposed that the APD use results in increased dopamine turnover, followed by excess free radical production and subsequent damage to striatal GABAergic fibers, with reduced inhibitory activity on motor circuits [30–32]. Concurrently, chronic blockade of dopamine receptors results in excessive glutamate activity and resultant excitotoxicity. Likewise, chronic dopamine receptor blockade results in receptor hypersensitivity and persistent changes within basal ganglia motor circuits.

Movement disorders caused by antidepressants

Movement disorders often complicate pharmacologic treatment of psychiatric disorders. Frequently, these drugs are antidepressants. On one hand, the traditional, tricyclic antidepressants, such as amitriptyline and imipramine, rarely produce movement disorders except for high-frequency, postural tremors that have been linked to their serotonergic properties [18]. On the other hand, selective serotonin reuptake inhibitors (SSRIs) produce a variety of hypokinetic and hyperkinetic movement disorders, including tremor, dystonia, bruxism, myoclonus and other hyperkinesias with higher frequency [33]. Recent reports showed that akathisia is the most frequent SSRI-related movement disorder, followed by dystonia, parkinsonism and dyskinesia [33].

The most plausible hypotheses for the induction of movement disorders by SSRIs are related to the interaction between the serotonergic and dopaminergic systems [34–36]. SSRIs would induce a 5HT2 receptor-mediated inhibition of nigral dopaminergic release in the striatum, thus causing the movement disorders.

Movement disorders induced by stimulants

Stimulants have been known to produce a variety of movement disorders such as tremors, myoclonus, DIP, dystonia or stereotypic behavior among stimulant users and abusers at very low rate [18,19,37–39].

Cocaine inhibits dopamine reuptake thus incrementing dopamine at first, but chronic use is associated with depletion of striatal dopamine level [39]. Thus it can cause both parkinsonism and dyskinesias, for instance. Methylphenidate and amphetamines increase presynaptic dopamine release and block its reuptake [40], causing choreas and tics but not parkinsonism. Amphetamines also increase norepinephrine brain levels, probably responsible for associated parkinsonian syndrome and tremor [40].

Movement disorders by other drugs

Movement disorders are also associated with other medications, including antiemetics, which may block central dopamine receptors (droperidol, metoclopramide or prochlorperazine), lithium, or calcium-channel blockers (cinnarizine, flunarizine) among others. Many of these drugs are widely prescribed and can be leading causes of DMID. Metoclopromide for example has emerged as the most common cause of tardive dyskinesia in some movement disorder clinics [41,42].

Tremor commonly occurs with lithium treatment and occasionally chorea [19,43]. The antiepileptic drug valproate is commonly associated with tremor [44]. Pregabalin has been shown to cause parkinsonism [45]. Interference with substance P neurotransmission in the basal ganglia is the proposed mechanism. For many years, chorea has been recognized as a complication of estrogen- and progesterone-containing products [46]. Psychotherapeutic combination products containing an APD, such as perphenazine/amitriptyline, should not be overlooked as causative agents.

Parkinsonism induced by cinnarizine or flunarizine is still a serious medical problem in some countries owing to the wide use of these products in the elderly, of whom up to one-third may suffer an irreversible deficit [47]. The pathophysiologic mechanisms underlying calcium-channel blocker-induced movement disorders remains uncertain, but is most likely due to D2-receptor block [48].

Diagnosis and laboratory investigations

During the course of any drug treatment, movement disorders not necessarily related to intake may occur. Nonetheless, prescription drugs should always be considered a differential diagnosis for any movement disorder, especially if the patient is on an agent known to induce them. It should be kept in mind that subjects may not readily recall all the medications they receive.

Causality assessment is indispensable but many times difficult. The following aspects of the event should be considered [49–51]:

- Timing in relation to drug intake. When symptoms begin soon after treatment starts, diagnosis may be easy; however, connecting symptoms to long-term drug use may be difficult.
- Plausibility of the event. If the event result from a known pharmacodynamic property of the drug (i.e., D2-blockage properties of neuroleptics), it may be easier to connect to the drug. Nonetheless, in some cases DMID pathophysiology may not be known.
- Exclusion of other causes. DMID may be diagnosed only after exclusion of every other possible cause for the event observed.
- Dechallenge may be of aid when feasible. Disappearance of DMID after drug discontinuation is indicative of a link to the drug. Nonetheless, some DMIDs such as TD do not disappear after drug discontinuation.

Clinical observation is crucial for DMID differential diagnosis. For DIP and TD however, some diagnostic tools are available. Firstly, since response to chronic levodopa therapy is an important factor in distinguishing PD from a parkinsonian syndrome, it follows that acute dopaminergic challenge with either levodopa or apomorphine may have similar predictive value. Indeed, it has been shown that acute levodopa challenge has 70.9% sensitivity and 81.4% specificity for predicting eventual PD diagnosis [52]. Schizophrenic patients with DIP show a noteworthy absence of response to levodopa or apomorphine during a levodopa acute challenge [53].

Assessment of dopaminergic nigrostriatal pathway integrity can also be useful in distinguishing DMID, in which they are intact, from Parkinson disease, in which they are not. This can be accomplished by imaging with positron emission tomography or single-photon emission computed tomography using ligands binding to dopaminergic nigrostriatal system markers [54].

Homovanillic acid (HVA) assay in cerebrospinal fluid (CSF) may be useful to differentiate DIP from idiopathic PD [55]. HVA levels in patients with idiopathic PD are slightly reduced compared to normal controls. Most patients treated with neuroleptics have a short-term HVA level increase in CSF, probably related to compensatory increased firing of nigrostriatal dopamine neurons in response to dopamine receptor blockade.

Neuroimaging studies may helpful for TD diagnosis as anomalies in basal ganglia and other brain regions in schizophrenic patients with TD have been identified [56]. These anomalies include caudate nuclei, left lentiform nuclei, and temporal sulcus volume differences as well as reduction in T2 relaxation time in the left caudate nuclei.

Management and natural history

Sometimes careful patient evaluation in combination with clinical perspicacity and diagnostic tools when available will result in DMID diagnosis. If possible, the offending drug should be discontinued. This sole measure will probably suffice for most patients, but in some instances extra measures will need to be taken.

In most instances, *acute dystonia* presents spontaneous resolution shortly after drug withdrawal. Nonetheless, if treatment is needed, such as in the case of stridor, anticholinergics, antihistamines and/or benzodiazepines can be of help [11,57]. Intramuscular or intravenous administration of anticholinergic drugs (biperiden 5 mg or procyclidine 5 mg) or antihistamines (promethazine 50 mg) is usually effective within 20 minutes. Occasionally, second or third injections are necessary. After resolution, treatment with anticholinergics should be continued for at least 24 to 48 hours to prevent recurrence.

Anticholinergics have been commonly prescribed as a preventive treatment of *DIP* in patients treated with APDs without strong evidence to support this use. Preliminary unconfirmed evidence supporting the use of vitamin E as a neuroprotective has been published [9].

Once DIP is diagnosed, the best possible treatment is discontinuation of the causative drug [9]. Complete recovery is uncertain and 10–30% of patients will continue to have symptoms several months after the discontinuation. At least 10% of patients will develop a persistent and progressive parkinsonian syndrome, difficult to differentiate from idiopathic PD. When these particular patients are treated with levodopa or dopamine agonists they respond well, but after–5 years they develop fluctuations and dyskinesias confirming idiopathic PD.

Propranolol has been reported to be effective in the treatment of *akathisia* [7]. Akathisia associated with use of serotonin reuptake inhibitors may be prevented or reduced by concomitant treatment with alprazolam [58]. Antiserotoninergic drugs may also be useful in the treatment of akathisia [7]. Lithium-induced akathisia was claimed to be particularly responsive to mianserin.

Although low serum iron is commonly associated with neuroleptic-induced tardive akathisia, the value of iron supplements is doubtful and may even be harmful.

The best treatment for *tardive dyskinesia* is prevention. To accomplish this, the lowest effective dose of antipsychotics should be identified for each patient and regularly rechecked. After TD develops, drug withdrawal is followed by improvement in from 0% to 92% of patients, depending on the study [8]. This wide range is due to multiple factors including patient variables (for example, age), treatment variables (drug dose and cumulative exposure), and temporal aspects (early diagnosis, duration of treatment, and duration of TD follow-up). Age is consistently correlated with TD improvement, with younger patients more likely to improve. It may take up to 5 years for complete remission to occur. Shorter neuroleptic exposure and age under 60 years after onset of TD are correlated with greater likelihood of remission. Dyskinesias may reappear, however, when APDs are reinstituted. In a significant number of patients, they may become irreversible despite APD cessation.

Treatment of TD is a clinical challenge. Unfortunately, no drugs are uniformly safe and effective over extended treatment periods. Reducing dopaminergic function is the most effective way of suppressing (masking) TD [59]. This strategy is justified only in those rare cases when TD is severe, debilitating, or life-threatening. Functional reduction of dopamine can be achieved with presynaptic depletion (reserpine) or by false transmission (methyldopa). Anticholinergics and other drugs have not produced consistent results, and thus cannot be recommended [60]. Tetrabenzine has been successfully used for tardive dyskinesia, tardive tremor and tardive tourettism treatment [61]. Botulinum toxin can be used to treat tardive dystonia [61].

Conclusion

Movement disorders are common adverse drug reactions. They should be considered when treatment with possible offending drugs is initiated. Off-label use of movement disorder-inducing drugs or use beyond recommended doses should be discouraged. If a patient must receive a movement disorder-inducing drug, minimal doses should be prescribed and careful follow up is recommended.

In this chapter we have provided an extensive albeit not exhaustive list of potential offending agents. In this light, clinicians should remain alert, as DMID may be encountered with either innovative, insufficiently studied drugs or with old well-known drugs used in new or wider populations or under new therapeutic regimens. Future research should also focus on identifying new treatments for DMID, which at present are sorely lacking.

Acknowledgments
We thank Professor Jean-Louis Montastruc for his bibliographical contributions.

References
1. Haddad PM, Dursun SM. Neurological complications of psychiatric drugs: clinical features and management. *Hum Psychopharmacol* 2008; **23**(Suppl 1): 15–26.

2. Casey DE. Spontaneous and tardive dyskinesias: clinical and laboratory studies. *J Clin Psychiatry* 1985; **46**: 42–7.

3. Tarsy D. History and definition of tardive dyskinesia. *Clin Neuropharmacol* 1983; **6**: 91–9.

4. Paulson, GW. Historical comments on tardive dyskinesia: a neurologist's perspective. *J Clin Psychiatry* 2005; **66**(2): 260–4.

5. Brown P, Funk SC. Tardive dyskinesia: barriers to the professional recognition of an iatrogenic disease. *J Health Soc Behav* 1986; **27**: 116–32.

6. Tarsy D, Baldessarini RJ. Epidemiology of tardive dyskinesia: is risk declining with modern antipsychotics? *Mov Disord* 2006; **21**: 589–98.

7. Bakheit A. The syndrome of motor restlessness – a treatable but under-recognised disorder. *Postgrad Med J* 1997; **73**: 529–30.

8. Casey DE. Tardive dyskinesia. *West J Med* 1990; **153**: 535–41.

9. Mena MA, de Yebenes JG. Drug-induced parkinsonism. *Expert Opin Drug Saf* 2006; **5**: 759–71.

10. Orti-Pareja M, Jimenez-Jimenez FJ, Vazquez A *et al.* Drug-induced tardive syndromes. *Parkinsonism Relat Disord* 1999; **5**: 59–65.

11. van Harten PN, Hoek HW, Kahn RS. Acute dystonia induced by drug treatment. *BMJ* 1999; **319**: 623–6.

12. Caligiuri MR, Jeste DV, Lacro JP. Antipsychotic-Induced movement disorders in the elderly: epidemiology and treatment recommendations. *Drugs Aging* 2000; **17**: 363–84.

13. Rodnitzky RL. Drug-induced movement disorders. *Clin Neuropharmacol* 2002; **25**: 142–52.

14. Casey DE. Neuroleptic-induced acute dystonia. In: Lang AE, Weiner WJ, eds. *Drug-induced Movement Disorders.* Mount Kisko, NY, Futura; 1992: 21–40.

15. Akagi H, Kumar TM. Lesson of the week: akathisia: overlooked at a cost. *BMJ* 2002; **324**: 1506–7.

16. Esper CD, Factor SA. Failure of recognition of drug-induced parkinsonism in the elderly. *Mov Disord* 2008; **23**: 401–4.

17. Gershanik OS. Drug-induced parkinsonism in the aged. Recognition and prevention. *Drugs Aging* 1994; **5**: 127–32.

18. Morgan JC, Sethi KD. Drug-induced tremors. *Lancet Neurol* 2005; **4**: 866–76.

19. Montastruc JL, Durrieu G. Drug-induced tremor and acute movement disorders. *Therapie* 2004; **59**: 97–103.

20. Burke RE, Fahn S, Jankovic J et al. Tardive dystonia: late-onset and persistent dystonia caused by antipsychotic drugs. *Neurology* 1982; **32**: 1335–46.

21. Jankovic J. Tardive syndromes and other drug-induced movement disorders. *Clin Neuropharmacol* 1995; **18**: 197–214.

22. Gareri P, De FP, De FS et al. Adverse effects of atypical antipsychotics in the elderly: a review. *Drugs Aging* 2006; **23**: 937–56.

23. Rupniak NM, Jenner P, Marsden CD. Acute dystonia induced by neuroleptic drugs. *Psychopharmacology (Berl)* 1986; **88**: 403–19.

24. Noyes K, Liu H, Holloway RG. What is the risk of developing parkinsonism following neuroleptic use? *Neurology* 2006; **66**: 941–3.

25. Rochon PA, Stukel TA, Sykora K et al. Atypical antipsychotics and parkinsonism. *Arch Intern Med* 2005; **165**: 1882–8.

26. Remington G, Mamo D, Labelle A et al. A PET study evaluating dopamine D2 receptor occupancy for long-acting injectable risperidone. *Am J Psychiatry* 2006; **163**: 396–401.

27. Ulrich S, Sandmann U, Genz A. Serum concentrations of haloperidol pyridinium metabolites and the relationship with tardive dyskinesia and parkinsonism: a cross-section study in psychiatric patients. *Pharmacopsychiatry* 2005; **38**: 171–7.

28. Owens DG. Extrapyramidal side-effects and tolerability of risperidone: a review. *J Clin Psychiatry* 1994; **55**(Suppl): 29–35.

29. Correll CU, Leucht S, Kane JM. Lower risk for tardive dyskinesia associated with second-generation antipsychotics: a systematic review of 1-year studies. *Am J Psychiatry* 2004; **161**: 414–25.

30. Casey DE. Pathophysiology of antipsychotic drug-induced movement disorders. *J Clin Psychiatry* 2004; **65**(Suppl 9): 25–8.

31. Galili R, Mosberg, Gil-Ad I et al. Haloperidol-induced neurotoxicity – possible implications for tardive dyskinesia. *J Neural Transm* 2000; **107**: 479–90.

32. Silvestri S, Seeman MV, Negrete JC et al. Increased dopamine D2 receptor binding after long-term treatment with antipsychotics in humans: a clinical PET study. *Psychopharmacology (Berl)* 2000; **152**: 174–80.

33. Jimenez-Jimenez FJ, Molina JA. Extrapyramidal symptoms associated with selective serotonin reuptake inhibitors. *CNS Drugs* 2000; **14**: 367–79.

34. Davies J, Tongroach P. Neuropharmacological studies on the nigro-striatal and raphe-striatal system in the rat. *Eur J Pharmacol* 1978; **51**: 91–100.

35. Dray A, Davies J, Oakley NR et al. The dorsal and medial raphe projections to the substantia nigra in the rat: electrophysiological, biochemical and behavioural observations. *Brain Res* 1978; **151**: 431–42.

36. Di Mascio M, Di Giovanni G, Di Matteo V, Prisco S, Esposito E. Selective serotonin reuptake inhibitors reduce the spontaneous activity of dopaminergic neurons in the ventral tegmental area. *Brain Res Bull* 1998; **46**: 547–54.

37. Blayac JP, Pinzani V, Peyriere H et al. Drug-induced movement disorders: tardive syndromes. *Therapie* 2004; **59**: 113–19.

38. Chung WS, Chiu HP. Drug-induced akathisia revisited. *Br J Clin Pract* 1996; **50**: 270–8.

39. Weiner WJ, Rabinstein A, Levin B et al. Cocaine-induced persistent dyskinesias. *Neurology* 2001; **56**: 964–5.

40. Ross RT. Drug-induced parkinsonism and other movement disorders. *Can J Neurol Sci* 1990; **17**: 155–62.

41. Kenney C, Hunter C, Davidson A et al. Metoclopramide, an increasingly recognized cause of tardive dyskinesia. *J Clin Pharmacol* 2008; **48**: 379–84.

42. Pasricha PJ, Pehlivanov N, Sugumar A et al. Drug Insight: from disturbed motility to disordered movement – a review of the clinical benefits and medicolegal risks of metoclopramide. *Nat Clin Pract Gastroenterol Hepatol* 2006; **3**: 138–48.

43. Jimenez-Jimenez FJ, Garcia-Ruiz PJ, Molina JA. Drug-induced movement disorders. *Drug Saf* 1997; **16**: 180–204.

44. Nouzeilles M, Garcia M, Rabinowicz A et al. Prospective evaluation of parkinsonism and tremor in patients treated with valproate. *Parkinsonism Relat Disord* 1999; **5**: 67–8.

45. Perez-Lloret S, Amaya M, Merello M. Pregabalin-induced parkinsonism: a case report. *Clin Neuropharmacol* 2009; **32**(6): 353–4.

46. Vela L, Sfakianakis GN, Heros D et al. Chorea and contraceptives: case report with pet study and review of the literature. *Mov Disord* 2004; **19**: 349–52.

47. Garcia-Ruiz PJ, Garcia de YJ, Jimenez-Jimenez FJ et al. Parkinsonism associated with calcium channel blockers: a prospective follow-up study. *Clin Neuropharmacol* 1992; **15**: 19–26.

48. Chouza C, Scaramelli A, Caamano JL et al. Parkinsonism, tardive dyskinesia, akathisia, and depression induced by flunarizine. *Lancet* 1986; **1**: 1303–4.

49. Rehan HS, Chopra D, Kakkar AK. Physician's guide to pharmacovigilance: terminology and causality assessment. *Eur J Intern Med* 2009; **20**: 3–8.

50. Edwards IR, Aronson JK. Adverse drug reactions: definitions, diagnosis, and management. *Lancet* 2000; **356**: 1255–9.

51. Montastruc JL, Sommet A, Lacroix I *et al*. Pharmacovigilance for evaluating adverse drug reactions: value, organization, and methods. *J Bone Spine* 2006; **73**: 629–32.

52. Merello M, Nouzeilles MI, Arce GP *et al*. Accuracy of acute levodopa challenge for clinical prediction of sustained long-term levodopa response as a major criterion for idiopathic Parkinson's disease diagnosis. *Mov Disord* 2002; **17**: 795–8.

53. Merello M, Starkstein S, Petracca G *et al*. Drug-induced parkinsonism in schizophrenic patients: motor response and psychiatric changes after acute challenge with L-dopa and apomorphine. *Clin Neuropharmacol* 1996; **19**: 439–43.

54. Tolosa E, Coelho M, Gallardo M. DAT imaging in drug-induced and psychogenic parkinsonism. *Mov Disord* 2003; **18**(Suppl 7): S28–S33.

55. Bowers MB, Jr., Heninger GR. Cerebrospinal fluid homovanillic acid patterns during neuroleptic treatment. *Psychiatry Res* 1981; **4**: 285–90.

56. Khiat A, Kuznetsov Y, Blanchet PJ *et al*. Diffusion-weighted imaging and magnetization transfer imaging of tardive and edentulous orodyskinesia. *Mov Disord* 2008; **23**: 1281–5.

57. Povlsen UJ, Pakkenberg H. Effect of intravenous injection of biperiden and clonazepam in dystonia. *Mov Disord* 1990; **5**: 27–31.

58. Amsterdam JD, Hornig-Rohan M, Maislin G. Efficacy of alprazolam in reducing fluoxetine-induced jitteriness in patients with major depression. *J Clin Psychiatry* 1994; **55**: 394–400.

59. Jeste DV, Wyatt RJ. Therapeutic strategies against tardive dyskinesia. Two decades of experience. *Arch Gen Psychiatry* 1982; **39**: 803–16.

60. Jeste DV, Wyatt RJ. In search of treatment for tardive dyskinesia: review of the literature. *Schizophr Bull* 1979; **5**: 251–93.

61. Jankovic J. Treatment of hyperkinetic movement disorders. *Lancet Neurol* 2009; **8**: 844–56.

62. Brooks DE. Propofol-induced movement disorders. *Ann Emerg Med* 2008; **51**: 111–12.

63. Montastruc JL, Llau ME, Rascol O *et al*. Drug-induced parkinsonism: a review. *Fundam Clin Pharmacol* 1994; **8**: 293–306.

64. Mott SH, Packer RJ, Vezina LG *et al*. Encephalopathy with parkinsonian features in children following bone marrow transplantations and high-dose amphotericin B. *Ann Neurol* 1995; **37**: 810–14.

65. Dubow JS, Panush SR, Rezak M *et al*. Acute dystonic reaction associated with foscarnet administration. *Am J Ther* 2008; **15**: 184–6.

66. Oterino A, Pascual J. Sumatriptan-induced axial dystonia in a patient with cluster headache. *Cephalalgia* 1998; **18**: 360–1.

67. Nguyen N, Pradel V, Micallef J *et al*. Drug-induced parkinson syndromes. *Therapie* 2004; **59**: 105–12.

68. Lang AE. Miscellaneus drug-induced movement disorders. In: Lang AE, Weiner WJ, eds. *Drug-induced Movement Disorders*. Mount Kikco: Futura; 1992: 339–81.

69. Reeves AL, So EL, Sharbrough FW *et al*. Movement disorders associated with the use of gabapentin. *Epilepsia* 1996; **37**: 988–90.

70. Asconape J, Diedrich A, DellaBadia J. Myoclonus associated with the use of gabapentin. Epilepsia 2000; **41**: 479–81.

71. Jimenez-Jimenez FJ, Orti-Pareja M, Yuso-Peralta L *et al*. Drug-induced parkinsonism in a movement disorders unit: A four-year survey. *Parkinsonism Relat Disord* 1996; **2**: 145–9.

72. Bonuccelli U, Nocchiero A, Napolitano A *et al*. Domperidone-induced acute dystonia and polycystic ovary syndrome. *Mov Disord* 1991; **6**: 79–81.

73. Montagna P, Gabellini AS, Monari L *et al*. Parkinsonian syndrome after long-term treatment with clebopride. *Mov Disord* 1992; **7**: 89–90.

74. LeWitt PA, Walters A, Hening W *et al*. Persistent movement disorders induced by buspirone. *Mov Disord* 1993; **8**: 331–4.

75. Bower JH, Muenter MD. Temporary worsening of parkinsonism in a patient with Parkinson's disease after treatment with paclitaxel for a metastatic grade IV adenocarcinoma. *Mov Disord* 1995; **10**: 681–2.

76. Werner EG, Olanow CW. Parkinsonism and amiodarone therapy. *Ann Neurol* 1989; **25**: 630–2.

77. Dick RS, Barold SS. Diltiazem-induced parkinsonism. *Am J Med* 1989; **87**: 95–96.

78. Shale H, Tanner C. Pharmacological options for the management of dyskinesias. *Drugs* 1996; **52**: 849–60.

79. De L, V, Morgante G, Musacchio MC *et al*. The safety of veralipride. *Expert Opin Drug Saf* 2006; **5**: 695–701.

80. Sachdev P. The epidemiology of drug-induced akathisia: Part I. Acute akathisia. *Schizophr Bull* 1995; **21**: 431–9.

81. Clark JD, Elliott J. A case of a methadone-induced movement disorder. *Clin J Pain* 2001; **17**: 375–7.

82. Petzinger G, Mayer SA, Przedborski S. Fentanyl-induced dyskinesias. *Mov Disord* 1995; **10**: 679–80.

83. Angles A, Bagheri H, Saivin S *et al*. Interaction between lansoprazole and bromocriptine in a patient with Parkinson's disease. *Therapie* 2002; **57**: 408–10.

Unusual causes of tremor

Julia Johnson and Mark Stacy

Introduction

Classification of tremor

Tremor is defined as a rhythmical, involuntary oscillatory movement of a body part and remains the most common of all movement disorders [1]. Tremor is most commonly seen in the upper extremities but can also occur in the lower extremities, head, trunk, lips, chin and vocal cords. The diagnosis of a particular tremor and its phenomenological classification depend on a definition of the activation conditions during which the tremor occurs and which body parts are affected. Presently, the following definitions and related criteria are based on the consensus statement of the Movement Disorder Society on tremor [1].

Rest tremor is present in a body part that is not voluntarily activated and is completely supported against gravity. Tremor seen in parkinsonism is typically a rest tremor. This tremor disappears with onset of movement but, once partial stability is attained in a new position, the tremor returns [1,2]. Action tremor is any tremor occurring on voluntary activation of the muscle. This includes postural, kinetic, intention, task specific and isometric tremor. Postural tremor is present while voluntarily maintaining a position against gravity. This common form of tremor can be seen in physiological tremor, cerebellar tremor, essential tremor and other forms. Kinetic tremor occurs during any voluntary movement, including goal-directed and non-goal-directed movements. Examples of kinetic tremors are primary writing tremor, vocal tremor and orthostatic tremor. Simple kinetic tremor occurs during voluntary movements that are non-goal-directed. Intention tremor is present when the amplitude increases during visually guided target directed movements. Typically the tremor amplitude fluctuates significantly as the target is approached. This type of tremor can be seen

in disorders of the cerebellum. Task-specific kinetic tremor may appear or become exacerbated during specific activities such as writing in primary writing tremor. Isometric tremor occurs as a result of muscle contraction against a rigid stationary object (Table 14.1).

Common tremors

Common tremors include physiologic tremor, essential tremor and parkinsonian tremor.

Physiologic tremor can occur in any normal subject during action and posture. It is a fine action tremor with a frequency between 6 and 12 Hz. When exacerbated by anxiety or certain medical conditions such as hyperthyroidism, it is termed enhanced physiologic tremor. The most common pathological tremor is essential tremor (ET), a predominantly postural and action tremor that may be sporadic but usually runs in families. It is usually slowly progressive over time. ET typically involves the hands and forearms but may spread to affect the head, face, voice, tongue and legs. About 50% of the patients improve with ingestion of alcohol [3]. There is class A evidence to support the use of propranolol, primidone and topiramate for the treatment of essential tremor and the combination of propranolol and primidone is more effective at suppressing the tremor than either drug alone [3,4]. Other treatment options include gabapentin, botulinum toxin injections and deep brain stimulation (DBS). Resting tremor is one of the cardinal signs of Parkinson disease. It is the commonest initial symptom of the disease, found in more than 50% of patients at the time of diagnosis, and is highly correlated with the specific diagnosis [4]. The frequency of a classical parkinsonian resting "pill rolling" tremor is 4–6 Hz but it can be higher in the early stages of the disease. In addition to resting tremor, rest and postural tremor combinations and different forms of postural and

---

Uncommon Causes of Movement Disorders, ed. Néstor Gálvez-Jiménez and Paul J. Tuite. Published by Cambridge University Press. © Cambridge University Press 2011.

Table 14.1. Tremor classification.

Tremor type	Definition	Example
Rest tremor	Disappears with onset of movement but, once partial stability is attained in a new position, the tremor returns	Parkinsonism
Action tremor	Produced by voluntary contraction of muscle including postural, kinetic and isometric tremor	See below
Postural tremor	Tremor is present while voluntarily maintaining a position against gravity	Tremor with outstretched arms
Intention tremor	Tremor is present when the amplitude increases during visually guided target directed movements	Cerebellar tremor
Kinetic tremor	Tremor occurring during any voluntary movement	Tremor during finger-to-nose test
Task specific tremor	Kinetic tremor that appears or becomes more exacerbated during specific activities	Primary writing tremor, musician's tremor, sport tremor
Isometric tremor	Tremor occurring as result of muscle contraction against a rigid stationary object	Tremor while making a fist or squeezing the examiner's finger

action tremor occurs in up to 40% of patients [3,5,6]. Besides levodopa, anticholinergics, clozapine and dopamine agonists can be effective for the treatment of parkinsonian resting tremor, but the use of some of these medications may be limited by side-effects. A kinetic tremor with an intention component is considered to be characteristic of cerebellar pathology, although various clinical forms of tremor have been described in cerebellar disorders. The frequency and amplitude of cerebellar tremor is usually irregular with a frequency between 3 and 5 Hz [2]. Head titubation or slow oscillations of the arms about the shoulders, or legs about the hip can also be seen in cerebellar disorders.

There are numerous reviews about different types of tremors available. This manuscript focuses on uncommon forms of tremors.

Uncommon forms of tremors

Holmes tremor

Holmes tremor is also known as rubral tremor, midbrain tremor, myorhythmia and Benedikt syndrome. This type tremor is usually associated with an underlying structural lesion in the central nervous system, including stroke, vascular malformations and tumors. While most often attributed to midbrain pathology, lesions in the thalamus have also been described. The criteria for Holmes tremor include the presence of both resting and intention tremor with a slow frequency of mostly less than 4.5 Hz [1]. It often involves proximal

and distal muscles, is irregular and can also have a postural component [3,7]. The tremor usually affects the upper extremities but there are reported cases of Holmes tremor involving the lower extremities [8]. There is a typical variable delay of mostly 2 weeks to 2 years between the occurrence of the lesion and the first appearance of the tremor. Functional neuroimaging may demonstrate reduced tracer uptake using both SPECT (DaTSCAN) and ^{18}F-dopa PET in the ipsilateral putamen and caudate. It is generally accepted that the pathophysiologic basis of Holmes tremor is a combined lesion of the cerebellothalamic and nigrostriatal systems [1,3].

No proven treatment is available. Some patients respond to levodopa, anticholinergics or clonazepam. Levetiracetam has also been used successfully in one case report [9]. Several patients have undergone DBS with the thalamus as a target [10].

Primary orthostatic tremor

Primary orthostatic tremor is a rare condition, characterized by a subjective feeling of unsteadiness during stance that improves during walking and sitting. Only in severe cases does it occur during gait. Patients report feeling unsteady when standing with eyes closed, even though there is little change in postural sway [11,12]. Falls are uncommon but have been observed mostly in elderly patients with orthostatic tremor. The age of onset may vary from the third through the seventh decade of life and men and women seem to be affected equally [2]. Standing may induce a visible or palpable fine-amplitude tremor of 13–18 Hz and the diagnosis can be confirmed by a surface EMG recording [1]. The pathophysiology of this condition is unknown but it has been described as a variant of essential tremor [13]. The tremor is considered to originate centrally, because the 13–14 Hz tremor frequency is too high to originate in lower-extremity reflex loops. In addition, a central source of oscillation is needed to produce the synchronicity of EMG pattern with all affected muscles [7,11]. Like other tremors, orthostatic tremor is associated with increased cerebellar blood flow on positron emission imaging (PET) [14].

Orthostatic tremor has been documented to be responsive to clonazepam and primidone. Gabapentin has been shown to be effective in small double-blinded trials [15]. Case reports of treatment with valproic acid, levodopa and propranolol showed variable success [7,16]. Chronic spinal cord stimulation found to be beneficial in two patients with medically intractable orthostatic tremor [17]. In contrast to essential tremor, orthostatic tremor usually does not respond to ethanol [18].

Palatal tremor

Palatal tremor (palatal myoclonus) is divided into two distinct clinical entities: symptomatic and essential. Symptomatic palatal tremor is caused by a lesion in the brain stem and cerebellum, usually in the triangle of Guillain and Mollaret, and is associated with subsequent olivary hypertrophy, demonstrated on magnetic resonance imaging (MRI). Clinically, it is characterized by rhythmic movements of the soft palate and often other brain stem-innervated or extremity muscles [1].

Essential palatal tremor is not associated with brain pathology. Besides rhythmic movements of the soft palate involving the tensor veli palatini, the patient often reports a clicking sound, perhaps linked to the eustachian tube opening and compression. Extremity or eye muscles are not involved [1,19].

Treatment may not be necessary if the tremor does not cause discomfort or disability. Patients with essential palatal tremor with a complaint of an ear click may request treatment. The disability in patients with symptomatic palatal tremor is often due to other clinical symptoms of the underlying brain stem or cerebellar lesion. Clonazepam, trihexyphenidyl and valproic acid have been tried and described in case reports [20]. Botulinum toxin A injections into the soft palate have reported to be safe and effective [21].

Peripheral neuropathy-associated tremor

Several acquired and hereditary peripheral neuropathies are associated with the development of tremor. Demyelinating neuropathies, especially dysgammoglobulinemic neuropathies, are frequent causes of such tremors. Other peripheral neuropathies that are associated with tremor include Guillain–Barré syndrome, diabetic neuropathy, uremic neuropathy, hereditary motor and sensory neuropathy type 1 (HMSN type 1), neuropathy associated with alcoholism, and chronic inflammatory demyelinating polyneuropathy (CIDP). Amiodarone can cause both tremor and neuropathy [2].

The tremor is mostly a postural and kinetic tremor. The frequency in hand muscles can be lower than in proximal muscles in patient with gammopathies. Patients usually present with sensory disturbances, although tremor can be a presenting symptom [1,3]. It is important to note that abnormal position sense is not a required condition for the diagnosis. The sensory loss and velocity of nerve conduction studies usually have little or no relation to the frequency and amplitude of neuropathic tremor [11].

The pathophysiology of this tremor is thought to be due to an interaction of peripheral and central factors. PET activation studies have indicated overactivity in both cerebellar hemispheres, similar to essential tremor [3].

There is no proven treatment for this type of tremor. Successful treatment of the underlying neuropathy only rarely improves the tremor. Occasionally, patients respond to treatment with propranolol and primidone, medications effective for essential tremor. One patient with peripheral neuropathy underwent successful thalamic ventralis intermedius nucleus (VIM) deep brain stimulation [22].

Drug-induced and toxin-induced tremor

Numerous drugs are known to produce tremor. Tremor secondary to drugs or toxins can take many forms including enhanced physiological tremor, precipitated essential tremor, rest tremor secondary to parkinsonism and tremor due to cerebellar pathology, or can be associated with peripheral neuropathy [2]. Identification of drug-induced tremor requires a careful and thorough history. A temporal relation with the start of the medication, lack of progression and exclusion of other medical causes support the diagnosis [23]. On examination, the patient may exhibit a mix of atypical features with symptoms occurring at rest or with postural holding or action. Interestingly, the tremor may also be asymmetric in amplitude but not in frequency.

Tricyclic antidepressants are known to produce a high-frequency, low-amplitude postural tremor consistent with an enhanced physiological tremor. The tremor may respond to reductions of the dose. Lithium is also associated with enhancement of physiological tremor and increases with increasing serum lithium levels. Monoamine oxide inhibitors and other antidepressants can induce or exacerbate action tremors. An estimated 20% of patients started on a selective serotonin reuptake inhibitor (SSRI) without prior history of tremor may develop this symptom [23].

The anticonvulsant valproic acid is the most common tremorogenic drug among antiepileptic therapies [23]. It appears particularly prone to induce an action and postural tremor, usually 3–14 months after initiation. The tremor occurs when the medication is administered in sufficiently high doses for prolonged periods but may also occur even when the dose is within the therapeutic range. It usually abates with dose reduction within several weeks [23]. Other anticonvulsants including primidone, gabapentin and topiramate can be helpful in the treatment of essential tremor and other tremors [23].

Amiodarone, a cardiac antiarrhythmic drug, can cause postural and action tremor along with ataxia. Immunosuppressants such as ciclosporin and tacrolimus are known to produce a tremor of low-amplitude and frequency [2,23]. A few chemotherapeutic drugs including tamoxifen, thalidomide and cytarabine are associated with tremor [23].

Tremor is one of the neurological manifestations that can occur as a complication of dopamine-blocking agents. It can present in the form of resting tremor in drug induced parkinsonism, rabbit syndrome in which the tremor is involving mainly the lips, and tremor in association with dopamine blocking drugs, such as traditional antipsychotic agents (e.g., haloperidol or thioridizine) and antiemetics (e.g., metoclopramide, prochlorperazine) [2,24]. Catecholamine-depleting drugs (reserpine, tetrabenzine) may also cause a resting tremor as part of a parkinsonian syndrome.

Chronic exposure to manganese can lead to parkinsonism with resting tremor. Manganese intoxication usually occurs in the setting of occupational exposure but it has also been described in association with total parenteral nutrition and chronic liver disease. Manganese intoxication is associated with signal changes in the basal ganglia that can be detected on MRI imaging [25]. Chronic inorganic exposure to mercury can have neurotoxic effects including a fine rapid tremor. There is a relatively consistent association between exposure to pesticides and Parkinson disease [26]. Exposure to chlordecone, an organochlorine pesticide, has been described to result in occurrence of tremor. Exposure to dioxin (referred to as agent orange) resulted in tremor in 35 of 47 railroad workers during a chemical spillage [2].

The treatment for drug-induced tremors and toxin-induced tremors is usually to stop the medication or exposure to the toxin. Tardive tremor may respond to tetrabenazine, clozapine and trihexyphenidyl.

Food-, alcohol- and nicotine-induced tremor

A tremor is considered to be food- or beverage-induced if it occurs in a reasonable timeframe following ingestion of that particular food or beverage. Tremor secondary to ingestion of certain food or beverages can enhance physiological tremor [2].

Alcohol can suppress essential tremor and the history of tremor response to alcohol can be of diagnostic value. Tremor is a symptom of alcohol withdrawal and may occur after a period of relative or absolute abstinence. Alcohol withdrawal tremor is a postural tremor that may persist for more than a year in the abstinence of alcohol use. Chronic alcoholism can result in cerebellar degeneration and can be associated with an intention tremor [27].

Coffee, tea and other caffeinated drinks can induce a new tremor or may exacerbate a previously existing tremor. Tremor is among the acute effects of nicotine exposure [28].

In a recent study, smokers were found to have more kinetic hand tremor than nonsmokers, more apparent in women than in men [29]. A previous study failed to elicit any significant influence of nicotine on tremor [30].

Psychogenic tremor

Psychogenic tremor is the most common form of psychogenic movement disorders and has a higher incidence in females than in males. The diagnosis is largely based on the clinical history and careful examination and observation of the tremor.

The following criteria suggest psychogenic tremor [1]:

1. Sudden onset of the condition and/or remission.
2. Unusual clinical combinations of rest, postural and/or intention tremors.
3. Decrease of tremor amplitude during distraction.
4. Variation of tremor frequency during distraction or during voluntary movements of the contralateral hand.
5. Coactivation sign of psychogenic tremor. Voluntary, variable force can be felt in both directions of the movement when tested at the wrist.
6. History of somatization.
7. Appearance of additional and unrelated neurologic signs.

Often, there is a history of symptoms for a year or longer before the patients seeks medical attention. EMG recordings are of limited diagnostic utility. The diagnosis of psychogenic tremor is, however, usually not a diagnosis of exclusion. The presence of characteristic features on history and clinical examination can usually permit an accurate diagnosis [2]. Treatment of psychogenic tremor is challenging. Some patients may respond to propranolol to desensitize the muscle spindles, which is necessary to maintain the clonus mechanism in patients with psychogenic tremor [7,31]. Physiotherapy aiming at relaxation of muscles during voluntary movements can be beneficial. Treatment of the underlying psychiatric condition may result in an improvement of the tremor; psychotherapy or biofeedback therapy is helpful in only a minority of patients. Early diagnosis and therapeutic intervention improve the outcome [32].

Dystonic tremor

A clear definition of dystonic tremor remains elusive. The Consensus Statement of the Movement Disorder Society in 1998 [1] defined dystonic tremor as "a tremor in a body part that is affected by dystonia." The tremor is mainly postural and kinetic [1]. It is usually absent during muscle relaxation, is exacerbated by muscle contraction, and can be associated with myoclonus [2]. Dystonic tremor can manifest as a jerky irregular action tremor with variable frequency due to sustained muscle spasms that can last several seconds. It can be distinguished from essential tremor as it is irregular

and remains localized. Occasionally, a dystonic tremor can occur prior to the manifestation of dystonia. An example of dystonic tremor is tremulous spasmodic torticollis or dystonic head tremor [3]. Tremulous cervical dystonia is frequently suppressed by sensory tricks (geste antgoniste), whereas essential tremor is not [33]. In a review of 42 patients with idiopathic torsion dystonia, tremor was found in 14% [34]. In a series of 271 patients with cervical dystonia, 71% were found to have associated tremor [35]. In another series of 308 patients, 10% with varieties of dystonia had a tremor [2]. The occurrence of a dystonic head tremor with a parietal lesion has also been reported [36].

Dystonic tremor can be distinguished from tremor associated with dystonia. This type is defined as a tremor that occurs in a body part not affected by dystonia while the patient has dystonia elsewhere [1]. An example would be a patient with cervical dystonia with an upper extremity postural tremor.

Many specialists believe that most isolated focal and task-specific tremors such as writer's cramp and other occupational cramps are a form of dystonia, although it remains unclear whether some cases represent variants of essential tremor. Primary writer's cramp, embouchure dystonia and the "yips" are described under task-specific tremor.

The treatment of the underlying dystonia with botulinum toxin can result in significant improvement of the dystonic tremor. Deep brain stimulation of the subthalamic area has also been reported to be beneficial in a patient with tremor and dystonia [2]. There are no controlled therapeutic trials for task-specific dystonia. Medications for essential tremor are usually tried and are beneficial to some patients [11].

Task-specific tremor

Task-specific tremors are a rare form of tremor that involves skilled, highly learned motor behaviors. Examples include writing, playing a musical instrument, swinging a golf club or the use of tools. Often, the patients develop tremor in their professional activity (e.g., playing golf or playing the piano) but other skilled movements remain unaffected. In most cases it remains unclear whether these task-specific tremors represent a type of essential tremor or a variant of dystonia or are due to a distinct pathophysiologic entity [1].

Primary writing tremor (PWT) is the most frequent type of task-specific tremor and occurs almost exclusively during this activity. It was first described in 1979 by Rothwell and has been extensively studied since [37,38]. It is sometimes difficult to differentiate PWT from a tremor that occurs in patients with writer's cramp, as some patients with PWT also have dystonic posturing. The exact etiology of PWT is still uncertain and it remains unclear whether it represents a form of an essential tremor or a dystonic tremor variant. PET studies of patients with PWT displayed bilateral cerebellar activation only, whereas those with essential tremor displayed bilateral cerebellar activation and activation in the red nucleus and thalamus [39]. No significant changes, in particular no development of dystonia or parkinsonism, were seen in 21 patients with PWT who were followed for a minimum of 1 year [38].

The "yips" was first defined as a motor phenomenon affecting golfers during the performance of shots requiring fine motor control, such as chipping and putting and was thought to represent a form of focal dystonia [40]. The psychological characteristics of a small group of cricket bowlers who experience the yips have also been reported [41]. Other sports-related task-specific dystonias affect billiard players, dart throwers, tennis and baseball players [42]. A recent study suggested two types of the yips: type I is related to impaired movement initiation and execution, whereas type II is related to performance anxiety [43].

Medications used for ET such as primidone or propranolol may be helpful in one-third of patients with PWT [38]. Overall, oral pharmacologic treatment for task-specific tremor is disappointing, however. Botulinum toxin injections have been used with some success [38]. DBS with the electrode implanted in the VIM has been tried successfully [44].

Posttraumatic tremor

Tremor in association with a physical trauma can occur in the setting of central or peripheral injury. Usually, there is an interval of days to years before the onset of the tremor [2]. Additionally, there are often other associated neurological symptoms such as rigidity or hemiparesis in patients with a central (upper motor neuron) injury. Most cases tremor resulting from severe head injuries result from damage to the midbrain [45]. Posttraumatic palatal tremor has been described in a patient with diffuse axonal injury involving the left superior cerebellar peduncle [46].

Tremor resulting from peripheral nerve injury can often be associated with neurological abnormalities such as dystonia or reflex sympathetic dystrophy.

In one study from Deuschl et al., 12 out of 21 patients with reflex sympathetic dystrophy were found to have a distal tremor with a mean frequency of 7.2 Hz, consistent with an enhanced physiologic tremor [47]. The tremor disappeared after treatment of the underlying reflex sympathetic dystrophy. Besides injury to the limb, whiplash-type neck injury has been associated with tremors [42,48,49].

Treatment of the underlying condition can be beneficial, but success is dependent on the nature of the injury and lesion. If the cause or lesion cannot be identified, therapies are less satisfactory. Peripherally induced tremors are generally resistant to conventional medical therapy, although botulinum toxin injections may transiently relieve the tremor [50]. Stereotactic thalamotomy and thalamic deep brain stimulation have been tried with success [51,52]. Several medications have been studied in the treatment of posttraumatic tremor with variable results including clonazepam, propranolol and valproic acid [2,53].

Isolated voice tremor

Isolated voice tremor occurs in two variants. The first resembles spasmodic dysphonia and is a form of focal dystonia. The second presents with a pure voice tremor and is considered a variant of essential tremor [1].

Dystonic tremor presents with a dysphonic and trembling voice and is more likely to occur if the tremor is not present during emotional speech production or singing. In abductor spasmodic dysphonia, which is caused by intermittent abduction of the vocal folds, patients exhibit a breathy, effortful voice quality with abrupt termination of voicing, resulting in aphonic, whispered segments of speech. Conversely, adductor spasmodic dysphonia is caused by irregular hyperabduction of the vocal folds. Patients with this type of dysphonia exhibit a choked, strained vocal quality with abrupt initiation and termination of voicing, resulting in short breaks in phonation [2].

Voice tremor also occurs in other conditions, such as cerebellar diseases and Parkinson disease, but usually in association with other clinical manifestations. Isolated voice tremor in contrast is usually limited to the two previously mentioned conditions.

Spasmodic dysphonia responds to botulinum toxin injections. One patient with Holmes tremor and vocal tremor was found to have improvement of vocal tremor after bilateral thalamic VIM stimulation [54].

Tremor in systemic diseases

HIV

Clinically relevant movement disorders are identified in 3% of patients with HIV infection seen at tertiary referral centers. Tremor and hemiballism-hemichorea are the most common hyperkinesias seen in patients who are HIV positive, but other movement disorders diagnosed in these patients include dystonia, chorea, myoclonus, tics, paroxysmal dyskinesias and parkinsonism [55]. Unilateral postural tremor and action tremor resulting from thalamic toxoplasmosis in a patient with AIDS has been reported [56]. There is a higher incidence of tremor in HIV positive patients that are treated with trimethoprim-sulfamethoxazole [57]. Symptomatic treatment of the tremor is often disappointing.

Hypoxia

Although rare, several movement disorders may arise as a consequence of hypoxic injury, including tremor, myoclonus, dystonia, akinetic-rigid syndromes and chorea. Anoxic injury to the basal ganglia can result in postural tremor along with bradykinesia and gait disturbance [2]. There are two main hypotheses attempting to explain the selective vulnerability of basal ganglia to hypoxic insults. The "vascular hypothesis" states that selective hypoperfusion results from the vascular supply of the basal ganglia. The second theory is the "metabolic hypothesis," which postulates that factors intrinsic to the striatum, such as intrinsically high oxidative metabolism or high density of excitatory amino acid receptors, results in hypoxic damage [58].

Liver disease

Hyperintense globus pallidus on T1-weighted MRI is present in most patients with advanced liver disease. Pujol et al. evaluated the relationship between the signal intensity of the globus pallidus and clinical or laboratory data of 77 patients eligible for liver transplantation. There was a significant correlation between the intensity of the signal, the presence of postural tremor, and the Child–Pugh score (as indication of severity of liver disease) among other laboratory markers. MRI repeated in 21 patients 10–20 months after transplantation showed a disappearance of the lesion in all cases [59]. Acquired hepatocerebral degeneration is a neurological disorder characterized by parkinsonism, ataxia and other movement disorders. It can be associated with various forms of advanced liver disease [60]. Tremor in Wilson disease is described below.

Wilson disease

Tremor has been reported as the most frequent neurological manifestation of Wilson disease in some series [61]. This symptom usually starts in one limb and may eventually spread to the whole body. It may vary from mild resting tremor in fingers to coarse tremor in all extremities, trunk, and head. Machado et al. reviewed the neurological manifestations of 119 patients with Wilson disease and found that 5% had a resting tremor and 55% had a postural tremor among other neurological symptoms [62]. Dramatic improvement of tremor has been reported with chelation therapy [63].

Thyroid disorders

A persistent fine tremor is the most common movement abnormality that presents in thyrotoxicosis and occurs in the majority of patients of all ages. It occurs both at rest and with movement and is a rhythmic, involuntary muscular contraction characterized by oscillations (to-and-fro movements) of a part of the body. Tremor is most commonly seen in the hands but can affect various body parts such as the head, facial structures, vocal cords, trunk and legs. Successful treatment of thyrotoxicosis results in improvement of the tremor [64]. Tan et al. described a patient with Graves disease who presented with orthostatic tremor without other systemic manifestations [65].

Anti-phospholipid syndrome

Movement disorders have only rarely been reported in association with anti-phospholipid syndrome (APS). Martino et al. reported three cases of APS who presented with movement disorders, including tremor, tics, myoclonus, and a corticobasal syndrome. Mild executive dysfunction was observed in all three patients. Two of these patients were successfully treated with mild oral anticoagulation [66].

Stroke

Isolated tremor as a result from stroke is rare. Lesions in the thalamus have been found to be associated with the development of tremors. Moroo et al. described three patients with postural and kinetic tremor whose MRI scans showed ischemic lesions in the midthalamus [67]. Dethy et al, reported a patient with a hemibody tremor following an ischemic lacunar stroke in the left centrum semiovale and left caudate [68]. Besides Holmes tremor (midbrain; described above), bilateral cerebellar strokes have also been reported to cause a "yes-yes" head tremor [69].

Tremor in children

Tremor in childhood is not commonly described but may be underappreciated [70]. Children with tremor comprise 10–20% of those with pediatric movement disorders. Tremor may occur in isolation or in association with other neurologic symptoms or systemic disorders. About 5–30% of adults with ET report symptom onset during childhood. Childhood-onset ET is usually hereditary, begins at a mean age of 6 years, and affects boys three times as often as girls [71].

Spasmus nutans is a disorder of infancy, typically described as the triad of head tremor, head tilt and nystagmus. The head tremor is usually a "no-no" tremor and of variable frequency. Isolated chin tremor is a rare autosomal dominant hereditary tremor syndrome characterized by high-frequency tremor of the mentalis muscles or of the chin, typically starting in early childhood [72]. Some patients may respond to botulinum toxin injections [73]. Metabolic disorders may represent with a variety of neurologic symptoms, including tremors. In one study, 10–30% of patients with phenylketonuria developed kinetic or postural tremors [74]. Pyruvate carboxylase deficiency and homocysteinuria have also been associated with tremors [70,75]. Other hereditary disorders that can present with tremors include juvenile Huntington disease, mitochondrial disorders, Wilson disease, fragile X and dystonia. Additional tremors in childhood are similar to those that can occur later in life and include drug induced tremors, psychogenic tremors and tremors secondary to underlying metabolic abnormalities.

Differential diagnosis

Tremors can present in many different forms and phenotypes. Some tremors are easy to diagnose but other movement disorders can be misinterpreted as tremors. Rhythmic myoclonus is a syndrome that has been proposed by several authors as intermittent brief muscle jerks that can be irregular or rhythmic and arise from the CNS [1]. Cortical tremor is a specific form of rhythmic myoclonus and is not considered a tremor. It presents with high-frequency, irregular, tremorlike postural and kinetic myoclonus almost indistinguishable from high-frequency postural tremor. Electrophysiological tests including electroencephalography (EEG), electromyography (EMG) and somatosensory evoked potentials (SSEP) are helpful for the differential diagnosis [1]. Cortical tremor can be acquired or hereditary and generally responds to the same drugs as used for cortical myoclonus such as clonazepam and levetiracetam [11]. Asterixis is a negative myoclonus with sudden periodic decreases of EMG activity. When the EMG pauses are long (>200 ms), typical flapping tremor during tonic contraction can result. Asterixis is usually bilateral and commonly results from metabolic or endocrine dysfunction or intoxication. Unilateral asterixis can be caused by focal lesions of the contralateral hemisphere. Epilepsia partialis continua (EPC) is a focal status epilepticus that can produce rhythmic jerks of an extremity and may therefore be misinterpreted as tremor. Physical exercise, sensitive stimulation or psychic exertion may increase the amplitude and frequency of the jerks. Lack of tremor history, epileptiform discharges on EEG, short EMG bursts, and jerk-locked averaging are supportive of the diagnosis [1].

Conclusions

Besides common tremors such as action and postural type symptoms associated with essential tremor and resting tremor seen in Parkinson disease, there are a variety of less commons forms of tremors. The pathophysiology of many tremors remains unclear despite significant research advances during the past decades. Advances in the treatment of tremors include the use of deep brain stimulation, which can be effective for many forms of disabling tremor. Pharmacological treatment is widely available but not always successful.

References

1. Deutschl G, Bain PG, Brin M and Ad Hoc Scientific Committee. Consensus statement of the Movement Disorder Society on tremor. *Mov Disord* 1998; **13**: 2–23.

2. Manyam B. Uncommon forms of tremor. In: Watts RL, Koller WC, eds. *Movement Disorders, Neurologic Principles and Practice*. 2nd ed. New York: McGraw-Hill; 2004.

3. Bain PG. Tremor. *Parkinsonism Relat Disord* 2007; **13**(Suppl 3): S369–74.

4. Bain PG. The effectiveness of treatments for essential tremor. *Neurologist* 1997; 305–21.

5. Fishman PS. Paradoxical aspects of parkinsonian tremor. *Mov Disord* 2008; 168–73.

6. De Jong H. Action tremor in Parkinson's disease. *J Nerv Ment Dis* 1926; **64**: 1.

7. Deutschl G, Volkmann J, Raethjen J. Differential diagnosis, pathophysiology and therapy. In: Jankovic J, Tolosa E, eds. *Parkinson's Disease and Movement Disorders*. 5th ed. Philadelphia: Lippincott Williams & Wilkins; 2007.

8. Baysal L, Acarer A, Celebisoy N. Post-ischemic Holmes' tremor of the lower extremities. *J Neurol* 2009; **256**(12): 2079–81.

9. Ferlazzo E, Morgante F, Rizzo V *et al*. Successful treatment of Holmes tremor by levetiracetam. *Mov Disord* 2008: **23**(14): 2101–3.

10. Nikkhah G, Propkop T, Hellwig B, Lucking CH, Ostertag CB. Deep brain stimulation of the nucleus ventralis intermedius for Holmes (rubral) tremor and associated dystonia caused by upper brainstem lesions: report of two cases. *J Neurosurg* 2004; **100**: 1079–83.

11. Elble RJ. Tremor: clinical features, pathophysiology, and treatment. *Neurol Clin* 2009; **27**(3): 679–95.

12. Bacsi AM, Fung VS, Colebatch JG. Sway patterns in orthostatic tremor: impairment of postural control mechanisms. *Mov Disord* 2005; **20**(11): 1469–75.

13. FitzGerald PM, Jankovic J. Orthostatic tremor: An association with essential tremor. *Mov Disord* 1991; **6**: 60.

14. Wills AJ, Thompson PD, Findley LJ, Brooks DJ. A positron emission tomography study of primary orthostatic tremor. *Neurology* 1996; **46**(3): 747–52.

15. Rodriguez JP, Edwards DJ, Walters SE *et al*. Gabapentin can improve stability and quality of life in primary orthostatic tremor. *Mov Disord* 2005; **20**: 865–70.

16. Willis AJ, Brusa L, Wang HC, Brown P, Marsden CD. Levodopa may improve orthostatic tremor: case report and trial of treatment. *J Neurosurg Psychiatry* 1999; **66**(5): 681–4.

17. Krauss JK, Weigel R, Blahak C *et al*. Chronic spinal cord stimulation in medically intractable orthostatic tremor. *J Neurol Neurosurg Psychiatry* 2006; **77**(9): 1013–16.

18. Gerschlager W, Münchau A, Katzenschlager R *et al*. Natural history and syndromic associations of orthostatic tremor: a review of 41 patients. *Mov Disord* 2004; **19**(7): 788–95.

19. Pearce JMS. Palatal myoclonus (syn. palatal tremor). *Eur Neurol* 2008; **60**: 312–15.

20. Fabiani G, Teive HA, Sá D *et al*. Palatal myoclonus: report of two cases. *Arq Neuropsiquiatr* 2000; **58**(3B): 901–4.

21. Penney SE, Bruce IA, Saeed SR. Botulinum toxin is effective and safe for palatal tremor: a report of five cases and a review of the literature. *J Neurol* 2006; **253**(7): 857–60.

22. Růzicka E, Jech R, Zárubová K, Roth J, Urgosík D. VIM thalamic stimulation for tremor in a patient with IgM paraproteinaemic demyelinating neuropathy. *Mov Disord* 2003; **18**(10): 1192–5.

23. Morgan JC, Sethi KD. Drug-induced tremors. *Lancet Neurol* 2005; **4**(12): 866–76.

24. Stacy M, Jankovic J. Tardive tremor. *Mov Disord* 1992; **7**: 53–7.

25. Aschner M, Erikson KM, Hernández EH, Tjalkens R. Manganese and its role in Parkinson's disease: from transport to neuropathology. *Neuromol Med* 2009; **11**(4): 252–66.

26. Brown TP, Rumsby PC, Capleton AC, Rushton L, Levy LS Pesticides and Parkinson's disease – is there a link? *Environ Health Perspect* 2006; **114**(2): 156–64.

27. Koller W, O'Hara R, Durus W, Bauer J. Tremor in chronic alcoholism. *Neurology* 1985; **35**: 1660.

28. Ellingsen DG, Bast-Pettersen R, Efskind J *et al*. Hand tremor related to smoking habits and the consumption of caffeine in male industrial workers. *Neurotoxicology* 2006; **27**(4): 525–33.

29. Louis ED. Kinetic tremor: differences between smokers and non-smokers. *Neurotoxicology* 2007; **28**(3): 569–75.

30. Zdonczyk D, Royse V, Koller WC: Nicotine and tremor. *Clin Neuropharmacol* 1988; **11**: 282.

31. Abila B, Wilson JF, Marshall RW, Richens A. The tremorolytic action of beta-adrenoceptor blockers in essential, physiological and isoprenaline-induced tremor is mediated by beta-adrenoceptors located in a deep peripheral compartment. *Br J Clin Pharmacol* 1985; **20**(4): 369–76.

32. McKeon A, Ahlskog JE, Bower JH *et al*. Psychogenic tremor: long term prognosis in patients with electrophysiologically-confirmed disease. *Mov Disord* 2009; **24**: 72–6.

33. Masuhr F, Wissel J, Müller J, Scholz U, Poewe W. Quantification of sensory trick impact on tremor amplitude and frequency in 60 patients with head tremor. *Mov Disord* 2000; **15**(5): 960–4.

34. Marsden CE, Harrison MJG. Idiopathic torsion dystonia (dystonia musculorum, deformans): a review of forty-two patients. *Brain* 1974; **97**: 793.

35. Jankovic J, Leder S, Warner D, Schwatz K. Cervical dystonia: clinical findings and associated movement disorders. *Neurology* 1991; **41**: 1088.

36. Kim JW, Lee PH. Dystonic head tremor associated with a parietal lesion. *Eur J Neurol* 2007; **14**: e32–3.

37. Rothwell JC, Traub MM, Marsden CD. Primary writing tremor. *J Neurol Neurosurg Psychiatry* 1979; **42**: 1106.

38. Bain PG, Findley LJ, Britton TC, Rothwell JC *et al*. Primary writing tremor. *Brain* 1995; **118**: 1461–72.

39. Wills AJ, Jenkins IH, Thompson PD *et al*. A positron emission study of cerebral activation associated with essential and writing tremor. *Arch Neurol* 1995; **52**: 299.

40. McDaniel KD, Cummings JL, Shain S. The "yips": a focal dystonia of golfers. *Neurology* 1989; **39**: 192–5.

41. Bawden M, Maynard I. Towards an understanding of the personal experience of the "yips" in cricketers. *J Sports Sci* 2001; **19**(12): 937–53.

42. Adler CH. Sports-related task-specific dystonia: the yips. In: Stacy M, ed. *Handbook of Dystonia*. New York: Informa Healthcare; 2007.

43. Stinear CM, Coxon JP, Fleming MK, Lim VK, Prapavessis H, Byblow WD. The yips in golf: multimodal evidence for two subtypes. *Med Sci Sports Exerc* 2006; **38**(11): 1980–9.

44. Racette BA, Dowling J, Randle J *et al.* Thalamic stimulation for primary writing tremor. *J Neurol* 2001; **248**: 380.

45. Pascual-Castroviejo I, Pascual Pascual SI, Viaño J, Martínez V. Posttraumatic intention tremor: report of a case with a lesion in the mesencephalic area. *Neurologia* 2000; **15**(3): 128–31.

46. Sharma P, Eesa M, Poppe AY, Goyal M. Teaching NeuroImage: posttraumatic palatal tremor. *Neurology* 2008; **71**(13): e30.

47. Deuschl G, Blumberg H, Lücking CH. Tremor in reflex sympathetic dystrophy. *Arch Neurol* 1991; **48**(12): 1247–52.

48. Ellis RJ. Tremor and movement disorders after whiplash type injuries. *J Neurol Neurosurg Psychiatry* 1997; **87**: 1884–6.

49. Ellis SJ. Tremor and other movement disorders after whiplash type injuries. *J Neurol Neurosurg Psychiatry* 1997; **63**(1): 110–12.

50. Jankovic J. Peripherally induced movement disorders. *Neurol Clin* 2009; **27**(3): 821–32.

51. Andrew J, Fowler CJ, Harrison MJG, Kendall BE. Posttraumatic tremor due to vascular injury and its treatment by stereotactic thalamotomy. *J Neurol Neurosurg Psychiatry* 1982; **45**: 560.

52. Umemura A, Samadani U, Jaggi JL, Hurtig HI, Baltuch GH. Thalamic deep brain stimulation for posttraumatic action tremor. *Clin Neurol Neurosurg* 2004; **106**(4): 280–3.

53. Jacob PC, Pratap Chand R. Posttraumatic rubral tremor responsive to clonazepam. *Mov Disord* 1998; **13**(6): 977–8.

54. Moringlane JR, Pützer M, Barry WJ. Bilateral high-frequency electrical impulses to the thalamus reduce voice tremor: acoustic and electroglottographic analysis – a case report. *Eur Arch Otorhinolaryngol* 2004; **261**(6): 334–6.

55. Cardoso F. HIV-related movement disorders: epidemiology, pathogenesis and management. *CNS Drugs* 2002; **16**(10): 663–8.

56. Micheli F, Grañana N, Scorticati MC, Giannaula RJ, Reboredo G. Unilateral postural and action tremor

resulting from thalamic toxoplasmosis in a patient with acquired immunodeficiency syndrome. *Mov Disord* 1997; **12**(6): 1096–8.

57. Floris-Moore MA, Amodio-Groton MI, Catalano MT. Adverse reactions to trimethoprim/sulfamethoxazole in AIDS. *Ann Pharmacother* 2003; **37**(12): 1810–3.

58. Venkatesan A, Frucht S. Movement disorders after resuscitation from cardiac arrest. *Neurol Clin* 2006; **24**(1): 123–32.

59. Pujol A, Pujol J, Graus F *et al.* Hyperintense globus pallidus on T1-weighted MRI in cirrhotic patients is associated with severity of liver failure. *Neurology* 1993; **43**(1): 65–9.

60. Ferrara J, Jankovic J. Acquired hepatocerebral degeneration. *J Neurol* 2009; **256**(3): 320–2.

61. Stremmel W, Meyerrose KW, Niederau C, Hefter H, Kreuzpaintner G, Strohmeyer G. Wilson disease: clinical presentation, treatment, and survival. *Ann Intern Med* 1991; **115**: 720–6.

62. Machado A, Chien HF, Deguti MM *et al.* Neurological manifestations in Wilson's disease: report of 119 cases. *Mov Disord* 2006; **21**(12): 2192–6.

63. Frucht S, Sun D, Schiff N, Eidelberg D, Gilliam TC. Arm tremor secondary to Wilson's disease. *Mov Disord* 1998; **13**(2): 351–3.

64. Kung AW. Neuromuscular complications of thyrotoxicosis. *Clin Endocrinol (Oxf)* 2007; **67**(5): 645–50.

65. Tan EK, Lo YL, Chan LL. Graves disease and isolated orthostatic tremor. *Neurology* 2008; **70**(16 Pt 2): 1497–8.

66. Martino D, Chew NK, Mir P, Edwards MJ, Quinn NP, Bhatia KP. Atypical movement disorders in antiphospholipid syndrome. *Mov Disord* 2006; **21**(7): 944–9.

67. Moroo I, Hirayama K, Kojima S. Involuntary movements caused by thalamic lesion. *Rinsho Shinkeigaku* 1994; **34**(8): 805–11.

68. Dethy S, Luxen A, Bidaut LM, Goldman S. Hemibody tremor related to stroke. *Stroke* 199; **24**(12): 2094–6.

69. Finsterer J, Muellbacher W, Mamoli B. Yes/yes head tremor without appendicular tremor after bilateral cerebellar infarction. *J Neurol Sci* 1996; **139**(2): 242–5.

70. Keller S, Dure LS. Tremor in childhood. *Semin Pediatr Neurol* 2009; **16**: 60–70.

71. Ferrara J, Jankovic J. Epidemiology and management of essential tremor in children. *Paediatr Drugs* 2009; **11**(5): 293–307.

72. Jarman PR, Wood NW, Davis MT *et al.* Hereditary geniospasm: linkage to chromosome 9q13-q21 and evidence for genetic heterogeneity. *Am J Hum Genet.* 1997; **61**(4): 928–33.

73. Mahant P, Stacy M, Sivakumar K. Treatment of hereditary geniospasm with botulinum toxin. *6th International*

Congress of Parkinson's Disease and Movement Disorders, 2000.

74. Perez-Duenas B, Valls-Sole J, Fernandez-Alverez E *et al.* Characterization of tremor in pheylketonuric patients. *J Neurol* 2005; **252**: 1328–34.

75. Garcia-Cazorla A, Rabier D, Touati G *et al.* Pyruvate carboxylase deficiency: metabolic characteristics and new neurological aspects. *Ann Neurol* 2006; **59**: 121–7.

Chapter 5

Psychogenic movement disorders

Alberto J. Espay

History and terminology

As bizarre clinical features may be components of "organic" movement disorders, clinicians have been understandably cautious about diagnosing psychogenic movement disorders (PMDs), for which examples of misdiagnoses abound in the literature [1,2]. To this date, PMDs are overwhelmingly diagnosed in an exclusionary manner despite the availability of diagnostic criteria that should facilitate a positive or inclusionary diagnosis. It is not surprising that advances in a disorder that has resided on the fringes of neurology have been hindered by poor diagnostic accuracy, variability in estimates of prevalence, and insufficient understanding of the pathophysiology. Dystonia, in particular, has undergone historical cycles wherein it has alternated between being considered strictly a psychiatric disturbance and a neurological disorder. An additional layer of complexity is illustrated by the insufficient consensus among experts about the origin and nomenclature of the focal posturing suggestive of dystonia. For example, posttraumatic cervical dystonia [3] has also been termed posttraumatic painful torticollis [4] to emphasize the psychogenic etiology in many of these patients. Similarly, in the legs and feet, the entity of complex regional pain syndrome type 1 (formerly, "reflex sympathetic dystrophy"), which consists of spasms, fixed dystonic posturing, tremor and various other jerks, has been revisited as mostly representing a psychogenic disorder, largely falling within the constructs of fixed dystonia [5] and tremor [6]. As a result of the variability in the diagnostic certainty of PMDs, therapeutic options potentially considered only among those with organic disorders have been proposed for patients with PMD [7].

This chapter will focus on the historic elements and phenomenology that should raise suspicion for a psychogenic origin of various movement disorders, the emerging body of literature regarding their pathophysiology, and the management strategies that will assist the clinician in improving the outcome of patients affected by this disabling disorder.

Clinical findings

The essential feature of PMD is that the clinical course and examination findings do not follow known neurological patterns. The specific historical and examination features that should raise the clinical suspicion for PMD are listed in Table 15.1. Particularly suggestive is the sudden onset of an inconsistent and variable abnormal movement [8]. Mixed phenomenologies are common. A single patient may exhibit distractible tremor, inconsistent gait abnormalities, incongruous posturing and paroxysmal limb movements. Similarly, other neurological complaints and abnormalities are often present, such as give-way weakness, nonanatomical sensory loss, speech impediment, and variable visual field defects. Occasionally, patients exhibit a combination of psychogenic and organic movement disorders [9], which can be a very difficult diagnostic challenge.

Concurrent legal action in the form of lawsuits is common, particularly when a precipitating event is a motor vehicle accident. Associated pain is a common associated complaint. While it cannot help in distinguishing psychogenic from organic cervical dystonia, it raises suspicion for a psychogenic etiology in other PMD phenotypes.

The range of phenomenological presentations for PMD is discussed next.

Psychogenic dystonia

In general, a focal posturing or twisting that does not follow any of the "rules" of dystonia should be suspected to be psychogenic in nature. These movements

---

Uncommon Causes of Movement Disorders, ed. Néstor Gálvez-Jiménez and Paul J. Tuite. Published by Cambridge University Press. © Cambridge University Press 2011.

Table 15.1. Historical and examination features that help raise suspicion for a psychogenic movement disorder.[a]

History	Observation	Neurological examination
Abrupt onset	**Distractibility**	**False weakness**
Paroxysmal, spontaneous	Fixed posturing	**Nonanatomical sensory loss**
remissions Incongruous movements	Variability in severity	**Entrainment of tremor**
Inconsistent over time	Variability in body distribution	**Co-contraction sign in tremor**
Multiple somatizations	Speech impediment	**Astasia-abasia**
False sensory complaints		Variable resistance to passive
Self-inflicted injuries		movements
Obvious emotional		Excessive pain to passive
disturbances[b]		Movements
		Variable visual field defects

[a] Features listed in bold type fall under the heading "inconsistent with organic disease," one of the "primary criteria" by Shill and Gerber [19].
[b] Only element required for "possible" psychogenic dystonia (this diagnostic category is least helpful for diagnosis and management).

tend to be fixed rather than position-specific; they are present at rest and may not be affected or induced by action; they exhibit equal severity at rest and during action; they often generalize or involve the legs; and they are unresponsive to, or paradoxically worsened with, sensory tricks (an unusual exception has been reported [10]) [5,11]. Trauma can be the precipitating event in the majority of individuals [5]. The overall phenotype varies according to the topographical distribution. In the cervical region (posttraumatic psychogenic torticollis), patients have pronounced laterocollis (tilted head) with ipsilateral shoulder elevation and contralateral shoulder depression [4]. In the hands, patients often demonstrate fixed flexion of the wrist and fingers with preservation of the pincer function, which preserves handwriting (Figure 15.1a). In psychogenic dystonia affecting the foot, the typical posture is fixed plantar ankle flexion and toe flexion at rest, often with secondary autonomic capillary dysfunction (Figure 15.1b). In any distribution, there often is active resistance to passive movements. Manipulations themselves may trigger or exacerbate pain.

Psychogenic gait

Any gait that is disproportionately effortful ("huffing and puffing" shortly after initiation), inefficient (using more force or balancing than truly needed; swaying often without falling), and variable in stride, cadence and base of support is likely psychogenic. The phenomenology of psychogenic gait can be varied. In a large group of PMD patients, Baik and Lang identified buckling of the knee as the most common pattern (followed by *astasia-abasia*) of *isolated* gait impairment

(Figure 15.2). Excessive slowness was more common when gait impairment was part of a constellation of other psychogenic movements [12]. The historic term *astasia-abasia* has been retained to imply the discrepancy between the normalcy of primary motor and sensory leg functions, when supine or sitting, and the inability to use the legs during stance (*abasia*) and straight walking (*astasia*) [13]. Psychogenic gait can also be a product of psychogenic or give-way leg weakness. In these cases, the motor function discrepancy can be brought to the fore by having these patients perform complex tasks, such as jumping on one foot or squatting. A variation of the theme, the "chair test," inspired by the Paul Blocq's observations, was proposed by Okun and colleagues as useful in supporting the diagnosis [14]. All but one of nine patients with psychogenic gait sitting in a swivel chair with wheels propelled themselves forward and backward much better than when walking in the upright position, whereas patients with organic gait disorders performed similarly in both conditions [14].

Psychogenic tremor

As the most common PMD phenotype, psychogenic tremor can be diagnosed with a clinically definite degree of certainty when the oscillating and rhythmic activity of a patient's limb can be shown to be variable in amplitude and distribution, distractible (suppressed by performance of complex tasks), entrainable (its frequency changes to match the induced tapping rate of an unaffected limb), and capable of being modulated (altered in amplitude with nonphysiologic interventions, such as a vibrating tuning fork on the forehead) [15, 16].

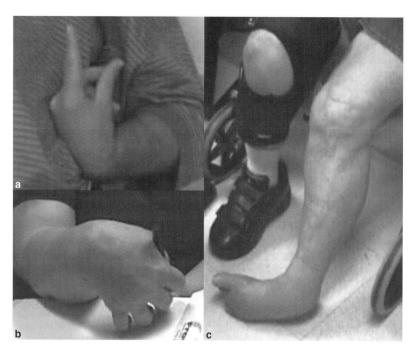

Figure 15.1. Typical posture of patients with clinically definite posttraumatic psychogenic dystonia affecting the hand. (a, b) Patients have a fixed flexion of the wrist and fingers except the thumb and index finger (a) preserving the pincer function, thus allowing handwriting. (c) Typical fixed-dystonia phenotype affecting the foot. There is plantar ankle flexion and toe flexion, often with skin discoloration suggesting secondary autonomic capillary dysfunction.

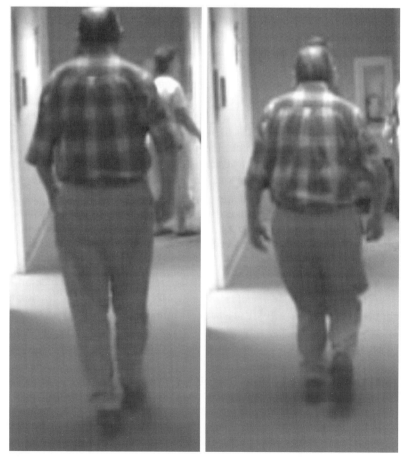

Figure 15.2. Paroxysmal knee buckling during walking is shown by a patient with clinically definite psychogenic gait.

Psychogenic myoclonus

Rapid jerks of variable frequency and amplitude, typically, but not always, involving more than one body region, that disappear with distraction or suggestion indicate a psychogenic etiology. This phenotype can reach a diagnostic category of "documented" by demonstrating a triphasic pattern of agonist and antagonist muscles and the presence of a premovement *Bereitschaftspotential* (see Laboratory investigations below).

Psychogenic parkinsonism

This phenotype, among the rare presentations of PMD, can be recognized by the presence of deliberate slowing of movements without decrement in amplitude of rapid alternating movements. Tremor, when present, is of equal magnitude at rest, on posture, and during action. Variable passive resistance substitutes true muscle rigidity. There may be an associated disproportionally poor response to the pull test (without history of falls) and knee buckling during gait. Dopamine transporter (DAT) imaging, when available, can help support a diagnosis of PMD by excluding underlying nigrostriatal dysfunction [17].

Diagnostic criteria

PMDs are not diagnoses of exclusion: clinically definite PMD relies on clinical findings and requires no additional neurological investigations other than electrophysiologic testing in the setting of challenging tremor or myoclonus presentations. Fahn and Williams proposed a number of historical and examination features suggestive for PMD and defined four categories of certainty: documented, clinically established, probable, and possible [2,18]. Two additional diagnostic criteria have been proposed since then (Table 15.2). The Fahn and Williams criteria remained the only diagnostic tool to positively define PMD until recently. The diagnosis requires the presence of at least one of the elements of the history and examination shown in bold type in the columns of Table 15.1 or the presence of incongruous or inconsistent movements to meet clinically probable degree of certainty. "Incongruous" movements include rapid onset with fixed posture at rest, active resistance to passive manipulation, etc.; "inconsistent" movements include disappearance or marked worsening with suggestion and absence of posturing on surreptitious observation. Persistent, sudden and dramatic relief occurring spontaneously or in response to suggestion or placebo distinguishes "documented" from "clinically established" PMD. Either clinically established or documented PMDs were later classified as "clinically definite" PMD [18]. A "probable" PMD category can be reached by the presence of psychogenic or "false" neurological signs or multiple somatizations, in the absence of incongruous or inconsistent movements, or nonphysiologic findings on examination.

Pitfalls in diagnostic criteria

Because "obvious emotional disturbance" is the only criterion required to establish "possible" PMD, and this can accompany organic movement disorders, it does not reliably distinguish any PMDs from their organic counterparts. Furthermore, overt psychopathology is often not evident at presentation even when patients exhibit a personality disorder or subclinical depression. It is common for the initial general psychiatric interview to fail to uncover an obvious causative psychopathology (which may prompt the psychiatrist to doubt the psychogenic nature of the disorder and question the diagnosis). Due to these issues, the "possible" and even "probable" categories of diagnostic certainty have been dropped from the Gupta and Lang proposed criteria.

The Shill and Gerber criteria were proposed as an attempt to enhance the value of the Fahn and Williams criteria, particularly by introducing disease modeling to the list of items and generating measures of specificity and sensitivity [19]. However, the disease-model criterion is nonspecific and presumes an unproven etiology, and a PMD diagnosis could be made without consideration of the neurological symptoms, limiting their use [20]. Other problems may arise when applying these criteria: (1) all the diagnostic categories of certainty (including "possible") require at least one secondary criterion, which many clearly psychogenic patients do not fulfill; (2) a patient who just misses the "clinically definite" category of diagnostic certainty may not be any more likely to meet the "clinically probable" category because it requires the presence of the two secondary criteria, which, again, may be absent; (3) accordingly, there is no diagnostic certainty grade corresponding to a patient who fulfills primary criteria but no secondary criteria; (4) finally, it is not specified how many "factors suggesting a movement disorder inconsistent with organic disease" are necessary to meet the primary criterion of "inconsistent with organic disease."

Table 15.2. Diagnostic criteria for PMDs.

	Fahn and Williams [3, 18]	Shill and Gerber [19]	Gupta and Lang [41]
1. Documented PMD	Movements relieved by psychotherapy, suggestion, or placebo, or spontaneous symptom resolution when the patient feels unobserved	*Clinically definite* (replacing Documented and Clinically established) PMD[a]: 3 of the following "primary criteria": inconsistent with organic disease (items in bold in Table 15.1),	Movements relieved by psychotherapy, suggestion, or placebo, or spontaneous symptom resolution when the patient feels unobserved
2. Clinically established PMD	Movements incongruent with organic disease or inconsistent symptoms plus other false neurological signs, multiple somatizations, or a documented psychiatric illness **(Documented or Established defines** *Clinically definite*) [18]	excessive pain or fatigue, previous exposure to a disease model, and potential for secondary gain; and at least one "secondary criterion": multiple somatizations (other than pain and fatigue) involving at least three different organ systems, and obvious psychiatric disturbance	A. Clinically established plus other features – as Fahn and Williams B. Clinically established minus other features – unequivocal clinical features incompatible with organic disease C. Laboratory-supported definite – electrophysiological evidence of PMD (for tremor and myoclonus)
3. Probable PMD	Movements are incongruent or inconsistent with no other features, or consistent/congruent but with 'false' neurological signs or multiple somatizations	Two primary criteria and two secondary criteria	Not applicable
4. Possible PMD	Suspicion for disorder based on the patient's obvious emotional disturbance alone	One primary criterion and two secondary, or two primary criteria and one secondary	Not applicable

[a] "Clinically proven" PMD was defined as remitting with psychotherapy, witnessed to remit when the patient feels unobserved, or when premovement *Bereitschaftspotential* was documented on EEG (for myoclonus only) [19].

Laboratory investigations

The diagnosis of PMD is largely clinical, following the established criteria discussed above. A major pitfall is the attainment of the diagnosis in an exclusionary manner, that is, by ruling out a large a list of organic disorders without considering the relevant findings on presentation and examination. The diagnosis of clinically probable or clinically definite PMD should be made following one of the diagnostic set of criteria discussed above.

Supportive laboratory investigations are available for tremor and myoclonus. Psychogenic tremor can be "laboratory supported" when surface EMG electromyography documents the key elements of entrainability and co-contraction sign [21] (Figure 15.3). Variability in tremor frequency as measured by accelerometry can also be used to support this diagnosis [22]. Psychogenic myoclonus will always have a burst duration greater than 100 ms and a triphasic rather than

co-contraction pattern of activation of agonist and antagonist muscles [8]. Suppression with nonphysiologic interventions is common. The most important laboratory investigation for psychogenic myoclonus is the documentation by electroencephalography of a premovement potential or *Bereitschaftspotential* preceding the movements using the technique of EMG back-averaging [23]. The presence of a premovement potential beginning around 1 second prior to the onset of abnormal movements indicates that the myoclonic jerks are generated by voluntary effort and are therefore psychogenic (Figure 15.4).

Psychopathology

Although the majority of patients do not carry psychiatric diagnoses prior to the onset of PMD, formal neuropsychiatric assessment has shown that some patients meet the *Diagnosis and Statistical Manual of Mental Disorders* criteria for somatoform disorder, motor conversion disorder subtype [24]. Psychological conflict,

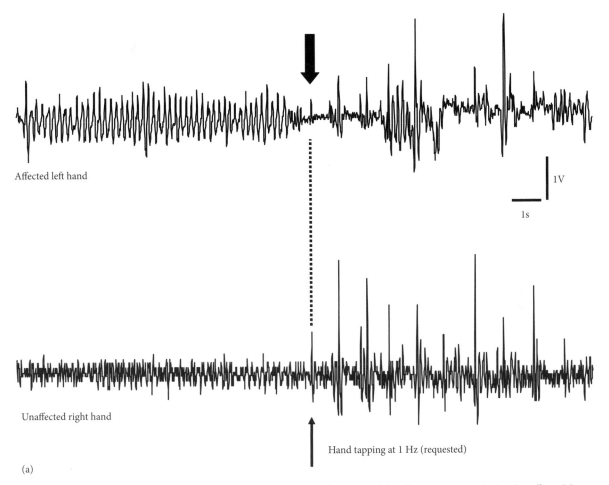

Affected left hand

1V

1s

Unaffected right hand

Hand tapping at 1 Hz (requested)

(a)

Figure 15.3. Electrophysiologic findings in psychogenic tremor. (a) Accelerometry of the affected (upper tracing) and unaffected (lower tracing) hands. Note that the pathological tremor rate is entrained (thick arrow) at the 1-Hz rate; the patient is asked to tap with the unaffected hand (thin arrow). (b) EMG of antagonistic flexor–extensor muscle pairs (two upper tracings) and accelerometry (lowest tracing) of the affected hand. The co-contraction sign is demonstrated by the increased EMG amplitude on both of these muscles (*), immediately preceding the spontaneous reemergence of the tremor, as recorded by accelerometry.

stress, or both are converted into physical symptoms as a result of a primary gain (symptoms keep intrapsychic conflicts from conscious awareness and restore psychological equilibrium at a price) or secondary gain (symptoms relieve social or occupational obligations and may result in legal or financial gain) [25]. In either case, patients are unaware of the underlying psychological conflict and firmly believe their symptoms to be organic. Depression and anxiety disorder are the most common psychiatric Axis I diagnoses in somatoform disorders of motor conversion disorder subtype [18]. The combination of depression, a personality disorder and poor schooling has been found to be highly correlated with the development of any motor conversion disorder [26].

The most intractable and disabling form of somatoform disorder is somatization disorder, overwhelmingly more common among young women, often themselves members of the extended health care fabric in developed countries [25]. In such disorder, patients may develop symptoms attributable to several different organ systems that are not due to physical illness. To meet criteria for somatization disorder, it is required that the spectrum of symptoms involve, in addition to the nervous system, the gastrointestinal and genitourinary tracts. A rare psychopathology behind PMD is factitious disorder, where illness is feigned for the purpose of obtaining medical care. These patients most often have a personality disorder. By far, the rarest form of PMD is malingering, a deliberate and

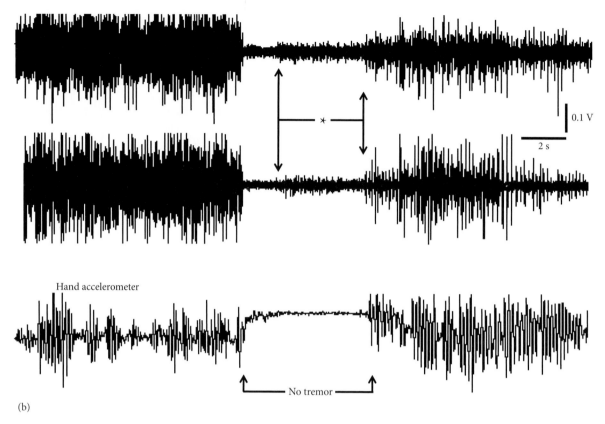

0.1 V

2 s

Hand accelerometer

— No tremor —

(b)

Figure 15.3. (*cont.*)

consciously deceiving enactment of illness in order to evade responsibilities or obtain benefits [27]. Although the popular press may portray malingering as a common driving force behind psychogenic disorders, its rarity can be emphasized by the fact that, over the last five years, no such patients have been identified in our practice, where PMD reaches nearly 4% of all patients evaluated. Malingering and factitious disorders need to be distinguished from conversion and somatization, as the management strategies outlined below do not apply to the former.

Pathophysiology

Preliminary evidence suggests that in individuals experiencing a conversion, primary perception is intact but modulation of sensory and motor planning is impaired by disruption of the anterior cingulate cortex and limbic brain regions [28]. Reduced activation of the somatosensory cortices has been reported during conversion anesthesia [29, 30].

Positron emission tomography (PET) functional imaging was used to evaluate a patient with motor conversion disorder manifested as psychogenic left-sided paralysis. PET revealed loss of activation of the right (contralateral) primary motor cortex but activation in the right orbitofrontal and anterior cingulate cortex when the patient attempted to move the affected leg [31]. Therefore, these two areas may have an inhibitory effect on motor cortex activation in the setting of psychogenic disorders. It has also been reported that hypnotic paralysis caused an identical activation and deactivation pattern [32]. An additional method of assessing brain activity that quantifies cerebral blood flow changes – single-photon emission computerized tomography (SPECT) with ^{99m}Tc-ECD – was applied to seven patients with psychogenic unilateral sensorimotor loss. There was decreased perfusion to the thalamus and basal ganglia on the side contralateral to the perceived deficit, suggesting that striato-thalamo-cortical motor circuits may also have a role in the pathogenesis of psychogenic disorders [33]. The

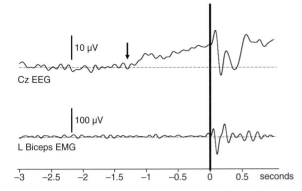

Figure 15.4. *Bereitschaftspotential.* Electroencephalographic activity demonstrates a slow positive potential beginning (arrow) around 1 second prior to the onset of movement (noted by the vertical bar at time 0), which is maximal over the vertex (CZ electrode). (Figure courtesy of Dr. Guillermo Paradiso.)

perfusion asymmetries disappeared in the four recovered patients. More recently, functional magnetic resonance imaging (fMRI) was applied to four patients with psychogenic ankle weakness. These patients activated a network of areas beyond those of healthy subjects, including the inferior frontal gyrus, putamen and left insula, and deactivated right middle frontal and orbitofrontal cortices [34]. Interestingly, this pattern of activation overlapped with but was different from the activation pattern associated with simulated weakness in healthy subjects.

Electrophysiologic studies in a cohort of 10 patients with psychogenic dystonia showed abnormal reduction of cortical inhibition, increased cutaneous silent period, and diminished reciprocal inhibition of the H reflex at intermediate (around 20 ms) and long latencies (around 100 ms), abnormalities comparable to those in patients with organic dystonia [35]. These findings suggest that the production or maintenance of abnormal posture is sufficient to alter cortical and spinal excitability or, alternatively, that the neuronal excitability itself might represent an underlying trait or endophenotype predisposing to different clinical forms of dystonia. The latter possibility was strengthened by a similar study carried out on patients with unilateral fixed dystonia in whom the cortical abnormalities were bilateral [36].

A promising electrophysiologic assessment in patients with dystonic postures of the neck of uncertain origin is frequency analysis of electromyographic (EMG) activity. This shows coherence between sternocleidomastoid and splenius muscles in the 4–7 Hz band in cervical dystonia, while normal subjects have a significant peak in the autospectrum of the splenius

EMG at 10–12 Hz [37]. It remains to be determined whether this assessment can be translated as a tool to distinguish psychogenic torticollis from organic cervical dystonia.

Finally, there has been much debate about the potential role of peripheral injury in the generation of segmental dystonia, but a cause-effect relationship has not been established. The most studied form of posttraumatic dystonia is associated with complex regional pain syndrome type I (CRPS I; also known as reflex sympathetic dystrophy). The validity of type I limb CRPS as an organic sensory, autonomic, and motor disturbance has been questioned as most of these patients have a mixture of incongruous abnormal movements associated with a variety of pseudoneurological signs [6,38]. Traumatic injury was documented to be the common precipitating event in almost 70% of the 103 patients with "fixed dystonia" reported be Schrag and colleagues, many of whom fulfilled criteria for a somatoform disorder [5].

Management

When a clinically definite (documented or clinically established) diagnosis of PMD has been reached, the delivery of diagnosis should be made with certainty, leaving no margin of doubt to patients that may open the option of additional neurological investigations. This satisfies the following goals: (1) it avoids the misperception by the patient that his or her condition remains undiagnosed ("nobody tells me what's wrong"); (2) it prevents unnecessary, costly and potentially dangerous neurological investigations and treatments; and (3) it paves the way for the institution of a multidisciplinary team to work on a committed patient to the same agenda.

The method of delivering the diagnosis is critical to ensuring follow-up. Validation of distress and disability are important to ensure continued reliance in the patient–physician relationship and compliance with the proposed ongoing care [39]. This can be best achieved by specifically stating to the patient that his or her symptoms are common in specialized clinics and very much real (translation to patient: "not in your mind"), that they do not imply a psychiatric abnormality ("you are not crazy") but do represent subconscious expressions of stress not under direct conscious or voluntary control ("you are not making this up"), and that they are clearly substantial enough to interfere with daily activities and force continued deterioration ("you are disabled and can get worse if nothing is done"). One may then "quiz" patients with such statements as "let's see if we are on the same page: first, are you crazy?" Hesitations should be immediately corrected with reassurance: "no, you are not crazy." Confirmation of patients' understanding facilitates acceptance of the diagnosis, which is the strongest predictor of favorable outcome after psychotherapy [40].

The main role of the neurologist is in continuing to provide follow-up (reexamination, reassurance, and simplification of pharmacotherapy, among others) and coordinating the care with a clinical psychologist, physical therapist and psychiatrist, if warranted, all of whom should be instructed as to the nature of PMD and goals of therapy. Patients are informed that success of treatment hinges on the strict adherence to the three-pronged approach of (1) completely accepting the diagnosis without seeking other opinions, (2) establishing a long-term, trusting relationship with a psychologist and committedly complying with the therapy sessions, and (3) ongoing neurological follow-up to document incremental gains or highlight any slippage. The last also sends the message that an "overnight cure" is not expected: only dedication and hard work can be relied upon to attain slow but steady progress. Psychiatrists experienced in dealing with these patients can be an asset mostly when depression and anxiety are major underlying psychopathologies. However, the psychiatrist's input should not be used to confirm or rule out the diagnosis because the presence or (apparent) absence of psychopathology does not prove or refute the psychogenic origin of these disorders [41].

The response to antidepressants depends on the identification of the underlying psychopathology. Voon and Lang have shown that response to antidepressants, as measured by the Montgomery Asberg Depression Rating Scale, is favorable when conversion disorder is the primary diagnosis [42]. Patients with somatization disorder, primary hypochondriasis, and factitious disorder or malingering do not benefit from antidepressants [42]. Cognitive behavioral therapy is a promising approach to the management of PMD and efforts are ongoing to delve into its efficacy in a systematic fashion [43].

Prognosis

The largest systematic study of PMD comprised a cohort of prospectively assessed individuals with the "syndrome of fixed dystonia," who overwhelmingly met criteria for clinically definite psychogenic dystonia [5]. While the prognosis was poor overall, remissions did occur among the minority of patients who underwent

multidisciplinary treatments, particularly including psychotherapy and physiotherapy [5]. Probably the most reliable demographic predictor of resolution in PMD is a short duration of psychogenic neurologic deficits [44–46]. When medical attention is given within one year of the onset of "medically unexplained motor symptoms," there is a highly significant chance for major or full recovery (odds ratio [95% confidence interval], 0.11 [0.02–0.67]) [44]. The presence of an Axis I diagnosis of depression or anxiety may also increase the chance of eventual resolution [44,46], probably because these patients have a specific target of additional therapy. Outcome is poorer in somatization disorder than conversion disorder [47]. For motor conversion disorder, poor predictive factors are the presence of a personality disorder, especially of histrionic type, a concomitant somatic disease (Axis III diagnosis), and a low DSM-IV Axis V score (patient-reported assessment of global functioning) [46].

Among patients with conversion disorder in general, between 50% and 60% will have a complete remission of their neurologic symptoms, 20%–30% will show some improvement, and 10–50% will be unchanged or worse [44,46,48]. Caution is advised when interpreting these numbers as the diagnostic certainty for conversion disorder may be questioned in certain retrospective chart reviews. In one study, 11 of 73 conversion disorder patients received a neurological diagnosis at some point during a 10-year follow-up period [48], although this is probably much less common in more recent experience [44].

Conclusions

Psychogenic movement disorder is not a diagnosis of exclusion: the clinically definite category of diagnostic certainty relies on specific history and neurological examination findings and requires no additional investigations, except to document cases of psychogenic tremor and myoclonus. Absence of overt psychopathology is never a solid argument against the diagnosis of PMD when clinical features support its classification as clinically definite. The category of "clinically possible" is neither helpful to the patient nor sufficient for the neurologist, since an organic disease must be ruled out first. Given the complexity of the presentations, only a neurologist with substantial expertise on organic movement disorders should make the diagnosis of PMD and provide follow-up to these patients. A multidisciplinary team of clinical psychologists, physiotherapists, a psychiatrist, and other allied health personnel with expertise in PMD is critical to helping address the underlying psychopathology and facilitate rehabilitation. Unfortunately, neither management guidelines nor proven therapies currently exist for PMD patients.

Since prognosis in PMD worsens with increasing duration of symptoms, early diagnosis and initiation of psychological, physical therapy and psychiatric assessments are expected to improve the likelihood of recovery. Clearly, further research on pathogenesis and disease-specific therapies is required given the pronounced disability that these patients accrue over time. PMD remain a significant, costly and neglected public health problem.

References

1. Lesser RP, Fahn S. Dystonia: a disorder often misdiagnosed as a conversion reaction. *Am J Psychiatry* 1978; **135**: 349–52.

2. Fahn S, Williams DT. Psychogenic dystonia. *Adv Neurol* 1988; **50**: 431–55.

3. Goldman S, Ahlskog JE. Posttraumatic cervical dystonia. *Mayo Clin Proc* 1993; **68**: 443–8.

4. Sa DS, Mailis-Gagnon A, Nicholson K, Lang AE. Posttraumatic painful torticollis. *Mov Disord* 2003; **18**: 1482–91.

5. Schrag A, Trimble M, Quinn N, Bhatia K. The syndrome of fixed dystonia: an evaluation of 103 patients. *Brain* 2004; **127**: 2360–72.

6. Verdugo RJ, Ochoa JL. Abnormal movements in complex regional pain syndrome: assessment of their nature. *Muscle Nerve* 2000; **23**: 198–205.

7. Romito LM, Franzini A, Perani D *et al*. Fixed dystonia unresponsive to pallidal stimulation improved by motor cortex stimulation. *Neurology* 2007; **68**: 875–6.

8. Brown P, Thompson PD. Electrophysiological aids to the diagnosis of psychogenic jerks, spasms, and tremor. *Mov Disord* 2001; **16**: 595–9.

9. Ranawaya R, Riley D, Lang A. Psychogenic dyskinesias in patients with organic movement disorders. *Mov Disord* 1990; **5**: 127–33.

10. Munhoz RP, Lang AE. Gestes antagonistes in psychogenic dystonia. *Mov Disord* 2004; **19**: 331–2.

11. Lang AE. Psychogenic dystonia: a review of 18 cases. *Can J Neurol Sci* 1995; **22**: 136–43.

12. Baik JS, Lang AE. Gait abnormalities in psychogenic movement disorders. *Mov Disord* 2007; **22**: 395–9.

13. Okun MS, Koehler PJ. Paul Blocq and (psychogenic) astasia abasia. *Mov Disord* 2007; **22**: 1373–8.

14. Okun MS, Rodriguez RL, Foote KD, Fernandez HH. The "chair test" to aid in the diagnosis of psychogenic gait disorders. *Neurologist* 2007; **13**: 87–91.

15. Deuschl G, Bain P, Brin M. Consensus statement of the Movement Disorder Society on Tremor. Ad Hoc Scientific Committee. *Mov Disord* 1998; **13**(Suppl 3): 2–23.

16. Koller W, Lang A, Vetere-Overfield B *et al*. Psychogenic tremors. *Neurology* 1989; **39**: 1094–9.

17. Kagi G, Bhatia KP, Tolosa E. The role of DAT-SPECT in movement disorders. *J Neurol Neurosurg Psychiatry* 2010; **81**: 5–12.

18. Williams DT, Ford B, Fahn S. Phenomenology and psychopathology related to psychogenic movement disorders. In: Weiner WJ, Lang AE, eds. *Behavioral Neurology of Movement Disorders*. New York: Raven Press; 1995: 231–57.

19. Shill H, Gerber P. Evaluation of clinical diagnostic criteria for psychogenic movement disorders. *Mov Disord* 2006; **21**: 1163–8.

20. Voon V, Lang AE, Hallett M. Diagnosing psychogenic movement disorders-which criteria should be used in clinical practice? *Nat Clin Pract Neurol* 2007; **3**: 134–5.

21. McAuley JH, Rothwell JC, Marsden CD, Findley LJ Electrophysiological aids in distinguishing organic from psychogenic tremor. *Neurology* 1998; **50**: 1882–4.

22. Zeuner KE, Shoge RO, Goldstein SR, Dambrosia JM, Hallett M. Accelerometry to distinguish psychogenic from essential or parkinsonian tremor. *Neurology* 2003; **61**: 548–50.

23. Papa SM, Artieda J, Obeso JA. Cortical activity preceding self-initiated and externally triggered voluntary movement. *Mov Disord* 1991; **6**: 217–24.

24. Pringsheim T, Lang AE. Psychogenic dystonia. *Rev Neurol (Paris)* 2003; **159**: 885–91.

25. Hurwitz TA. Somatization and conversion disorder. *Can J Psychiatry* 2004; **49**: 172–8.

26. Binzer M, Eisemann M. Childhood experiences and personality traits in patients with motor conversion symptoms. *Acta Psychiatr Scand* 1998; **98**: 288–95.

27. LoPiccolo CJ, Goodkin K, Baldewicz TT. Current issues in the diagnosis and management of malingering. *Ann Med* 1999; **31**: 166–74.

28. Black DN, Seritan AL, Taber KH, Hurley RA. Conversion hysteria: lessons from functional imaging. *J Neuropsychiatry Clin Neurosci* 2004; **16**: 245–51.

29. Mailis-Gagnon A, Giannoylis I, Downar J *et al*. Altered central somatosensory processing in chronic pain patients with "hysterical" anesthesia. *Neurology* 2003; **60**: 1501–7.

30. Ghaffar O, Staines WR, Feinstein A. Unexplained neurologic symptoms: an fMRI study of sensory conversion disorder. *Neurology* 2006; **67**: 2036–8.

31. Marshall JC, Halligan PW, Fink GR, Wade DT, Frackowiak RS. The functional anatomy of a hysterical paralysis. *Cognition* 1997; **64**: B1–B8.

32. Halligan PW, Athwal BS, Oakley DA, Frackowiak RS. Imaging hypnotic paralysis: implications for conversion hysteria. *Lancet* 2000; **355**: 986–7.

33. Vuilleumier P, Chicherio C, Assal F, Schwartz S, Slosman D, Landis T. Functional neuroanatomical correlates of hysterical sensorimotor loss. *Brain* 2001; **124**: 1077–90.

34. Stone J, Zeman A, Simonotto E *et al.* FMRI in patients with motor conversion symptoms and controls with simulated weakness. *Psychosom Med* 2007; **69**: 961–9.

35. Espay AJ, Morgante F, Purzner J, Gunraj CA, Lang AE, Chen R. Cortical and spinal abnormalities in psychogenic dystonia. *Ann Neurol* 2006; **59**: 825–34.

36. Avanzino L, Martino D, van de Warrenburg BP *et al.* Cortical excitability is abnormal in patients with the "fixed dystonia" syndrome. *Mov Disord* 2008; **23**: 646–52.

37. Tijssen MA, Marsden JF, Brown P. Frequency analysis of EMG activity in patients with idiopathic torticollis. *Brain* 2000; **123**(Pt 4): 677–86.

38. Kurlan R, Brin MF, Fahn S. Movement disorder in reflex sympathetic dystrophy: a case proven to be psychogenic by surveillance video monitoring. *Mov Disord* 1997; **12**: 243–5.

39. Clark MR Psychogenic disorders: a pragmatic approach for formulation and treatment. *Semin Neurol* 2006; **26**: 357–65.

40. Espay AJ, Goldenhar LM, Voon V, Schrag A, Burton N, Lang AE. Opinions and clinical practices related to diagnosing and managing patients with psychogenic movement disorders: an international survey of movement disorder society members. *Mov Disord* 2009; **24**: 1366–74.

41. Gupta A, Lang AE. Psychogenic movement disorders. *Curr Opin Neurol* 2009; **22**: 430–6.

42. Voon V, Lang AE. Antidepressant treatment outcomes of patients with psychogenic movement disorder. *J Clin Psychiatry* 2005; **66**(12): 1529–34.

43. LaFrance WC, Jr., Friedman JH. Cognitive behavioral therapy for psychogenic movement disorder. *Mov Disord* 2009; **24**: 1856–57.

44. Crimlisk HL, Bhatia K, Cope H, David A, Marsden CD, Ron MA. Slater revisited: 6 year follow up study of patients with medically unexplained motor symptoms. *BMJ* 1998; **316**: 582–6.

45. Couprie W, Wijdicks EF, Rooijmans HG, van Gijn J. Outcome in conversion disorder: a follow up study. *J Neurol Neurosurg Psychiatry* 1995; **58**: 750–2.

46. Binzer M, Kullgren G. Motor conversion disorder. A prospective 2- to 5-year follow-up study. *Psychosomatics* 1998; **39**: 519–27.

47. Kent DA, Tomasson K, Coryell W. Course and outcome of conversion and somatization disorders. A four-year follow-up. *Psychosomatics* 1995; **36**: 138–44.

48. Mace CJ, Trimble MR. Ten-year prognosis of conversion disorder. *Br J Psychiatry* 1996; **169**: 282–8.

Myoclonus

Era Hanspal and Steven Frucht

Definition

Myoclonus is defined as brief, involuntary shocklike movements. These brief jerks may be due to the contraction of one or more muscles, or occur by quick lapses of muscle contraction in active postural muscles (negative myoclonus, asterixis) [1].

Using a medical records linkage system, Caviness and colleagues studied the incidence and prevalence of myoclonus in Olmstead County, Minnesota, from 1976 to 1990. They reported an average annual incidence rate of 1.3 cases per 100 000 person-years. The prevalence in 1990 was 8.6 cases per 100 000. The prevalence of myoclonus is smaller than that of other hyperkinetic movement disorders such as essential tremor, which has an estimated prevalence as high as 50.5 cases per 1000 [2].

Marsden and colleagues proposed a classification system in 1982, which has been revised by several authors since. Myoclonus can be classified on the basis of clinical presentation (phenomenology), anatomy or pathophysiology, or etiology. It is useful to approach myoclonus from a combination of these classifications as it helps in deciding on treatment options.

Classification
Phenomenology

Clinically, there is a wide expression of myoclonus. Jerks can be focal or segmental, affecting one part or region of the body; they can be multifocal, affecting different parts at different times; or generalized. If they occur repetitively in rhythmic fashion, they can appear like a tremor. Myoclonus may be present with action, or be stimulus-provoked.

Pathophysiology

Anatomic or pathophysiologic classification divides myoclonus into the following groups: cortical, subcortical (brain stem), spinal cord, and peripheral.

Cortical myoclonus, as the name suggests, is initiated by a cortical discharge. This discharge, often focal, is generated in the sensorimotor cortex as a result of insufficient inhibition of neuronal networks. The time of subsequent transmission via corticospinal pathways to muscle is fixed and can be measured by electrophysiologic studies (typically 50 ms).

Cortical myoclonus is usually focal and reflex-induced [3], although it can also be multifocal or generalized, depending on how the discharge is spread through the cortical pathways [4]. It may also be repetitive as in epilepsia partialis continua. Its stimulus sensitivity is commonly elicited by a tendon tap, or a pin prick, but can also be produced by emotional excitation (see Table 16.1).

Epilepsia partialis continua, cortical reflex myoclonus, progressive myoclonic epilepsies and neurodegenerative diseases with cortical involvement (Alzheimer disease, Creutzfeldt–Jakob disease, Huntington disease, and Parkinson disease and other Lewy body disorders) are other conditions in which the myoclonus seen is of cortical origin.

Myoclonus originating from the brain stem can be generalized, as in reticular myoclonus, and the startle syndromes (hyperekplexia), or segmental, as in palatal myoclonus. Brainstem reticular myoclonus may follow cerebral anoxia and is likely responsible for the generalized muscle jerks that are seen in many toxic myoclonic syndromes. It is characterized by a generalized axial myoclonic jerk that starts in muscles innervated by the lower brain stem, and then spreads rostrally up the brain stem and caudally down the spinal cord [5].

Uncommon Causes of Movement Disorders, ed. Néstor Gálvez-Jiménez and Paul J. Tuite. Published by Cambridge University Press. © Cambridge University Press 2011.

Table 16.1. Causes of cortical myoclonus.

Focal

- Epilepsia partialis continua
  - Rasmussen encephalitis
  - Cerebrovascular disease
  - Tumor
  - Granuloma
  - Focal encephalitis
  - Trauma
  - Subarachnoid hemorrhage
  - Subdural hemorrhage

Generalized/multifocal

- Progressive myoclonic epilepsy
  - Lafora body disease
  - Neuronal ceroid lipofuscinosis (Batten disease)
  - Unverricht–Lundborg disease
  - MERRF
  - Sialidosis
- Progressive myoclonic ataxia
- Post-anoxic disease
- Viral encephalitis (SSPE, CJD)
- Toxic
  - Drugs such as anesthetics, anticonvulsants, withdrawal of benzodiazepines, lithium, monoamine oxidase inhibitors, and levodopa
- Metabolic encephalitis
  - Heavy metals, bismuth
  - Action myoclonus renal failure syndrome
- Neurodegenerative disorders
  - Parkinson disease
  - Huntington disease
  - Multiple system atrophy
  - Corticobasal ganglionic degeneration
  - Alzheimer disease
  - Creutzfeldt–Jakob disease

Palatal myoclonus may occur after a lesion in the brain stem or cerebellum within the Guillain–Mollaret triangle. This anatomic triangle consists of the dentate nucleus, the red nucleus and the inferior olive; denervation of the inferior olive leads to olivary hypertophy, which can be seen on magnetic resonance imaging. The resulting movements are rhythmic (1.5–3 Hz) and may synchronously involve the eyes, face, tongue, larynx and even diaphragm [6]. The movements are usually bilateral and symmetric and may persist in sleep. When no lesion is found in neuroimaging studies, there is an associated "ear click" that is audible and often bothersome to the patient.

Exaggerated startle syndromes consist of an excessive motor response to an unexpected stimulus. The stimulus may be auditory, somatic, or visual. The "jump" is usually caused by a flexion of the neck and trunk and abduction and flexion of the arm [1]. Falls are common, often causing injuries; however, there is no loss of consciousness associated with the falls. At times local brain stem pathology such as anoxic injury, inflammatory lesions, or hemorrhage can be identified. Exaggerated startle syndromes also exist as a hereditary disorder with autosomal dominant inheritance [1]. Hereditary hyperekplexia has been found to be linked to a point mutation in the alpha-1 subunit of the glycine-receptor [7]. Other mutations have been found in the presynaptic glycine transporter as well [8]. Glycine acts as an inhibitory neurotransmitter in spinal neurons; physiologic studies suggest that there is abnormal inhibition in hyperekplexia.

Myoclonus originating from the spinal cord can be of two clinical types. Spinal segmental myoclonus is rhythmic and persists during sleep. It is thought to be due to a loss of inhibitory interneurons in the posterior horns of the spinal cord. This inhibition can be demonstrated physiologically [1]. The second type, propriospinal myoclonus, produces truncal flexion and is often triggered by a stimulus (such as testing of the muscle stretch reflex), although it may occur spontaneously. The thoracic cord is usually involved first, followed by slow caudal and rostral spread through the long propriospinal fibers. The causes for such cases of propriospinal myoclonus are not always clear. At times there is evidence of spinal cord injury from trauma, infection, or tumor [1,3].

Peripheral myoclonus is rare and can be caused by lesions directly to the peripheral nerve that produce a hyperactive discharge [9]. Lesions can include trauma, tumor, or radiation. Hemifacial spasm is listed in this category. An interesting phenomenon was first described by Weir Mitchell in 1872, in which he recorded jerks and spasms of the remaining stump after amputation. When reported by Marion and colleagues, they found that the jerking movement was often preceded by lancinating pain, and appeared weeks to months after surgery; they were often stimulus sensitive as well. This movement could last as long as 40 years post procedure. This movement has since been considered to be a form of peripheral myoclonus and is called "jumpy stumps"[10].

Etiology

Classification by etiology divides myoclonus into the following categories: physiologic, essential, epileptic, and symptomatic. Physiologic myoclonus occurs in healthy individuals [11]. There is minimal to no disability and symptoms generally do not progress. As such, physiologic myoclonus rarely requires treatment. The physical examination can be expected to be normal. Examples of physiologic myoclonus include hiccups and jerks seen in sleep, or in sleep transitions. Partial jerks are usually multifocal and occur in distal muscle groups. Larger jerks are created when axial and proximal muscles are involved. Periodic movements of sleep also fall under this classification and usually involve flexion of the toes, foot, and sometimes knee and hip [12].

Essential myoclonus, better known as myoclonus-dystonia, has no associated neurologic deficit. The most prominent finding on examination is myoclonus. There is often very slow or absent progression and disability is mild [13]. Essential myoclonus can be sporadic, but hereditary forms also exist. The characteristic features of the inherited forms include onset before age 10 years, inheritance in an autosomal dominant fashion, and a benign clinical course that does not affect lifespan. There is an absence of cerebellar ataxia, spasticity, dementia, or seizures [14].

Dystonia is a common feature of hereditary essential myoclonus. The dystonia is of variable severity, although often mild, and presents as cervical or limb dystonia. The disease course is usually benign without functional disability; it is compatible with a normal lifespan [15,16]. Mutations in the epsilon-sarcoglycan gene (*SGCE* or DYT11) on chromosome 7q21 are found in 30–40% of patients. Less commonly, myoclonus dystonia is associated with mutation of the DYT15 locus on chromosome 18p11. The myoclonus can be exacerbated by muscle activation and often improves greatly with alcohol ingestion [11]. Neuropsychiatric features such as depression, addiction, and obsessive-compulsive disorder have also been reported in mutation carriers [17].

When no cause is evident, palatal myoclonus is classified as essential. In this form there is often an audible "ear click" due to contraction of the tensor veli palatini.

This ear click may be bothersome and many times is difficult to treat. There are often no other muscle groups involved as with symptomatic palatal myoclonus [1]. These patients tend to be younger at presentation.

In epileptic myoclonus, the clinical picture is dominated by seizures. This category includes the myoclonic epileptic syndromes: infantile spasms (West syndrome), severe myoclonic epilepsy of infancy, benign myoclonic epilepsy of infancy, Lennox–Gastaut syndrome, myoclonic astatic syndrome, cryptogenic myoclonus, juvenile myoclonic epilepsy and the progressive myoclonic epilepsies.

Symptomatic myoclonus is produced by another neurologic or nonneurologic disorder. The list is long and includes storage diseases, spinocerebellar degeneration, basal ganglia degenerations, dementias, encephalopathies, metabolic and toxic encephalopathies, posthypoxic injury, or focal injury by trauma, tumor, or stroke.

Evaluation

The evaluation of myoclonus begins with careful observation and examination. Consideration should be made of the area of involvement, stimulus sensitivity and rhythmicity. Myoclonus due to toxic/metabolic causes is often treatable and careful scrutiny of laboratory work and medications should be undertaken. Electophysiologic studies further aid in diagnosis and localization, and help distinguish myoclonus from other involuntary movements, such as dystonia or chorea. There are several studies that may be used, including electromyography (EMG), electroencephalography (EEG), EEG-EMG polymyography, evoked potentials, and jerk-locked back-averaging technique [1,3].

Electromyography demonstrates the sudden and brief motor contraction of myoclonus, often in bursts of 10–50 ms duration. In cases of negative myoclonus, as seen in asterixis, the silent period can be seen with examination of muscles in isometric contraction [5]. EMG bursts of 100 ms duration can be seen in essential myoclonus, whereas jerks longer than 100 ms are likely to be dystonic in origin [18].

Simultaneous EEG-EMG polygraphy reveals the relationship between EEG activity and the muscle jerk. The duration, distribution and stimulus sensitivity of EMG activity in affected muscles suggests the origin of the jerks as peripheral nerve, spinal cord, or cortex [1,18].

Jerk-locked back-averaging is a technique in which the simultaneously recorded EEG can be back-averaged with respect to the myoclonus. In this way small EEG potentials that might otherwise by unrecognizable can be related temporally to the myoclonus [18].

The evaluation of cortical myoclonus has certain characteristic findings. On EEG there are often multifocal or generalized spike-and-wave discharges. EMG correlates reveal burst duration typically less than 75 ms [4]. In cortical reflex myoclonus, there is an exaggerated cortical response to somatosensory stimuli that produces the jerk. Following the presentation of the stimuli, the somatosensory cortex generates a giant somatosensory evoked potential (SEP). This relationship is seen as the time correlation in the jerk-locked EMG to back-averaged EEG; a focal sharp wave is seen 10–40 ms before the myoclonic jerk.

Subcortical myoclonus has EMG bursts of <100 ms, and time-locked correlation is present on jerk-locked back-averaged studies. Subcortical myoclonus is also suggested when reflex myoclonus triggered by peripheral stimuli occurs after a latency that is too short to involve cortical pathways. However, it should be noted that brain stem myoclonus does not have a preceding cortical discharge as muscles are activated from the XI nucleus. As such, palatal myoclonus does not show any EEG abnormality, unless accompanied by other cerebral diseases. Psychogenic myoclonus is suggested if stimulus-evoked jerks are of very variable latency and longer than voluntary reaction time.

Treatment

There are few randomized controlled trials of medications for myoclonus and no FDA-approved treatments. All medications, therefore, are used off-label [19]. Myoclonus is often difficult to abolish completely and patients tend to be very susceptible to medication side-effects. As such, the goal of therapy should be functional improvement. The most successful medications for the treatment of myoclonus are the anticonvulsants. As a class, these medications usually enhance the inhibitory activity of gamma-aminobutyric acid (GABA). Unlike the therapeutic approach to epilepsy, in which management with a single agent is preferred, polypharmacy is often required for myoclonus [1].

Epileptic and cortical myoclonus respond best to drugs such as sodium valproate and clonazepam. Sodium valproate is the drug of choice in treatment of juvenile myoclonic epilepsy. Conventionally therapy is initiated with valproate, and clonazepam added if monotherapy is not achieved. In several small, open-label and clinical observational studies, levetiracetam

has been demonstrated to be effective in cortical myoclonus and progressive myoclonic epilepsy [20]. Piracetam is not available in the United States, but is the only agent that has been studied in a controlled, randomized, double–blind study [21,22].

Posthypoxic myoclonus may also respond to the above-mentioned therapies, but it may also respond to GABA [23].

There is less evidence available for the treatment of subcortical, spinal and peripheral myoclonus. There are reports of success with topiramate, tetrabenazine, valproic acid and clonazepam [24].

Finally, some types of myoclonus are refractory to treatment. Palatal myoclonus and negative myoclonus (asterixis) are often in this category. Botulinum toxin injection of the levator or tensor veli palatine muscles may be helpful [25] in reducing the bothersome ear click of essential palatal myoclonus.

References

1. Fahn S, Jankovic J. *Principles and Practices of Movement Disorders*. Philadelphia: Elsiever; 2007: 519–40.

2. Louis ED, Ottman R, Hauser WA. How common is the most common adult movement disorder? Estimates of the prevalence of essential tremor throughout the world. *Mov Disord* 1998; **13**(1): 5–10.

3. Rowland LP, ed. *Merritt's Textbook of Neurology*. 11th ed. Baltimore: Williams & Wilkins; 1995.

4. Brown P, Day BL, Rothwell JC *et al*. Intrahemispheric and interhemispheric spread of cerebral cortical myoclonic activity and its relevance to epilepsy. *Brain* 1991; **114**: 2333.

5. Hallet M, Chadwich D, Adam J, Marsden CD. Reticular reflex myoclonus: a physiological type of human posthypoxic myoclonus. *J Neurol Neurosurg Psychiatry* 1977a; **40**: 253–64.

6. Deuschl G, Mischke G, Schenk E *et al*. Symptomatic and essential rhythmic palatal myoclonus. *Brain* 1990; **113**: 1645–72.

7. Shiang R, Ryan SG, Shu YZ *et al*. Mutations in the alpha 1 subunit of the inhibitory glycine receptor cause the dominant neuralgic disorder, hyperekplexia. *Nat Genet* 1993; **5**: 351–8.

8. Rees, MI, Harvey K, Pearce BR *et al*. Mutations in the gene encoding GlyT2 (SLC6A5) define a presynaptic component of human startle disease. *Nat Genet* 2006; **38**: 801–6.

9. Chang VC, Frucht, SJ. Myoclonus. *Curr Treat Options Neurol* 2008; **10**: 222–9.

10. Steiner JC, DeJesus PV, Mancall EL. Painful jump in amputation stumps: pathophysiology of a "sore circuit." *Trans Am Neurol Assoc* 1974; **99**: 253–5.

11. Caviness JN, Alving LI, Maranganore DM *et al.* The incidence and prevalence of myoclonus in Olmsted County, Minnesota. *Mayo Clin Proc* 1999; **74**: 5665–69.

12. Marsden CD, Fahn S. Problems in the dyskinesias. *Movement Disorders*. Vol. 2. London: Butterworths; 1987: 305.

13. Marsden CD, Hallett M, Fahn, S. The nosology and pathophysiology of myoclonus. *Movement Disorders*. London: Butterworths; 1982: 196.

14. Mahloudji M, Pikielny RT. Hereditary essential myoclonus. *Brain* 1967; **90**: 669.

15. Kinugawa K, Bidaihet M, Clot F *et al.* Myoclonus-dystonia: an update. *Mov Disord* 2009; **24**: 479.

16. Kurlan R, Behr J, Medved L, Shoulson I. Myoclonus and dystonia: a family study. *Adv Neurol* 1988; **50**: 385.

17. Gerschlager W, Brown P. Myoclonus. *Curr Opin Neurol* 2009; **22**: 414–18.

18. Shibaski J. AAEE minimonograph #30: Electrophysiological studies of myoclonus. *Muscle Nerve* 1988; **11**: 899–907.

19. Nirenberg MJ, Frucht SJ. Myoclonus. *Curr Treat Options Neurol* 2005; **7**: 221–30.

20. Frucht S, Louis E, Chuang C *et al.* A pilot tolerability and efficacy study of levetiracetam in patients with chronic myoclonus. *Neurology* 2001; **57**: 1112–14.

21. Andrade DM, Hamani C, Minassian BA. Treatment options for epileptic myoclonus and epilepsy syndromes associated with myoclonus. *Expert Opin Pharmacother* 2009; **10**: 1549–60.

22. Kiskiniemi M, Van Vleymen B, Hakamies L *et al.* Piracetam relieves symptoms in progressive myoclonus epilepsy: a multicentre, randomized, double blind, crossover study comparing the safety and efficacy of three dosages of oral piracetam with placebo. *J Neurol Neurosurg Psychiatry* 1998; **64**: 344–8.

23. Frucht S, Bordelon Y, Houghton WH. Marked amelioration of alcohol-responsive posthypoxic myoclonus by gamma-hydroxybutyric acid (Xyrem). *Mov Disord* 2005; **20**: 745–51.

24. Jankovic J, Pardo R. Segmetnal myoclonus. Clinical and pharmacologic study. *Arch Neurol* 1986; **43**: 1025–31.

25. Penney SE, Bruce IA, Saeed SR. Botulinum toxin is effective and safe for palatal tremor: a report of five cases and review of the literature. *J Neurol* 2006; **253**: 857–60.

Tourette syndrome and other tic disorders

Roger Kurlan and David Shprecher

Phenomenology of tics

The Tourette Syndrome Classification Study Group defines tics as brief movements (motor tics) or sounds produced by the movement of air through the nose, mouth or throat (vocal tics) [1]. As a category of movement disorders, tics are characterized by their intermittent nature (unless very severe), occurrence out of a background of normal motor activity, tendency to mimic normal movements, lack of rhythmicity, variation in intensity and form, and some degree of voluntary suppressibility.

Both motor and vocal tics can be divided into simple and complex types. Simple motor tics are abrupt and brief movements occurring in single and isolated fashion. Common examples are eyeblinks, facial twitches, head jerks and shoulder shrugs. A variant of simple motor tics, termed "dystonic tics," consists of slower, twisting or muscle tightening movements, such as torticollis-like head twisting or abdominal muscle tensing [2]. Simple vocal tics include inarticulate noises or sounds produced by the movement of air through the nose, mouth or throat. Examples include throat clearing, sniffing, coughing, humming and snorting.

Complex motor tics are distinct, coordinated patterns of sequential movements [1]. They may appear purposeful, as if performing a voluntary action, such as touching, tapping, kicking or smelling. Other examples of complex motor tics include copropraxia (obscene gestures) and echopraxia (mimicking the movements of others). A repetitive coordinated sequence of simple tics (e.g., eyeblink, shoulder shrug and arm jerk) may not appear purposeful and would be considered to represent an intermediate tic phenomenon between simple and complex motor tics.

Complex vocal tics have linguistic meaning, consisting of a partial word (syllables), word or phrase. Examples include coprolalia (obscene or insulting

words, often truncated such as "shi-"), echolalia (repeating the words of others), and palilalia (repeating one's own words; such as "Where did you go, go, go?"). Although coprolalia is the feature of Tourette syndrome (TS) most responsible for the notoriety of the condition, we find it only rarely (about 1–2%) in our TS patients. Some patients have only internal, nonverbalized obscene words, thoughts or images, termed "mental coprolalia."

Both simple and complex tics are often preceded by body or psychic sensations and irresistible urges, sometimes referred to as "sensory tics" [3] or "premonitory sensations." Such sensations are usually uncomfortable and are localized at the site of a tic. Patients often describe a need to tic in order to relieve the abnormal sensation, but it inevitably returns to induce further tics.

The phenomenology of tics is summarized in Table 17.1.

Classification of tic disorders

According to the DSM-IV, diagnostic criteria for Tourette disorder include the presence of multiple motor tics and at least one vocal tic, tic duration of at least 1 year, onset before age 18 years, and no other known cause of the tics [4]. Some clinicians use the diagnosis "Tourette's disorder" when the tics are clearly disabling and "Tourette syndrome" to describe persons who have chronic motor and vocal tics whether they are disabling or not, but generally these two diagnoses are used interchangeably. When only one tic type is present, the diagnoses chronic motor tic disorder (CMTD) or chronic vocal tic disorder (CVTD) are used. Transient tic disorder (TTD) refers to the presence of tics for a period of less than 1 year. TS, CMTD, CVTD and TTD are generally viewed as parts of a spectrum of primary tic disorders [5]. Since contraction of

Uncommon Causes of Movement Disorders, ed. Néstor Gálvez-Jiménez and Paul J. Tuite. Published by Cambridge University Press. © Cambridge University Press 2011.

Table 17.1. Phenomenology of tics.

Motor tics
Simple
Dystonic
Complex
Copropraxia
Echopraxia
Vocal tics
Simple
Complex
Coprolalia
Echolalia
Palilalia

muscles (buccal, pharyngeal, laryngeal, diaphragmatic, respiratory) is needed to move air through the nose, mouth or throat to produce vocal tics, the phenomenological separation of motor and vocal tic types may not have neurobiological significance and the distinctions likely exist for historical reasons alone. Accordingly, many clinicians consider TS, CMTD and CVTD to be the same condition [6].

Unusual phenomenology

It is clear that tics have a heterogeneous phenomenology, with motor and vocal types and simple and complex varieties. It is safe to say that motor tics can be manifested by virtually any movement the human body is capable of making and vocal tics by any noise or sound. Another aspect of the great variability of tic manifestations comes from interrelationships with the common behavioral comorbidities, obsessive-compulsive disorder (OCD) and attention deficit hyperactivity disorder (ADHD), an important feature that many clinicians are unfamiliar with [7].

About half of individuals with TS experience obsessive-compulsive symptoms. These are more commonly expressed in females. Compulsions and complex motor tics may be difficult to distinguish. In contrast to tics, compulsions are carried out in response to an obsession (e.g., repeated showering to prevent contamination), to ward off future problems (e.g., saying certain words to prevent harm from coming to a loved one), to reduce anxiety, or according to certain rules. Such rule-based (ritualistic) quality is characteristic of compulsions. Common rules relate to time of day

(e.g., bedtime rituals), order, symmetry, or number of repetitions. It is very unusual for complex tics to occur in the complete absence of simple tics, thus helping to correctly identify them. It is clear, however, that some individual actions (e.g., touching, tapping) may be difficult to classify as a tic or a compulsion and that some have characteristics of both. We call these "compulsive tics" or "compultics" [7]. An example would be shoulder shrugs that have to be done the same number of times on the right and left sides.

Some tics have qualities of impulsiveness and sometimes aggressiveness and social inappropriateness typically linked to ADHD [7,8]. We call these "impulsive tics" or "impultics" and examples include hitting oneself or others, yelling out insults, touching a hot stove, or driving toward oncoming traffic. There are even actions that overlap tics, compulsions and impulsiveness (e.g., pushing someone after they have coughed to avoid contamination) and might be considered "compulsive/impulsive tics."

These complex, sometimes socially inappropriate tic manifestations are summarized in Table 17.2. Recognizing the overlapping phenomenology of certain actions has practical importance since it appears that optimal treatment of compulsive tics involves a dual targeting of both tics and OCD and, similarly, optimal control of impulsive tics involves treatments aimed at both tic suppression and impulse control (see below) [7].

Differential diagnosis of tics

Myoclonus and choreic jerks can resemble simple tics, but these movement disorders tend not to be repetitive in the same location like tics. Simple motor tics are often accompanied by complex motor tics, allowing them to be correctly classified on the basis of "the company they keep." Similarly, the presence of vocal tics can allow the proper identification of body jerks as motor tics. As opposed to torsion dystonia, dystonic tics usually occur in brief bursts of movements, are not continuous and tend to produce abnormal postures that are less sustained. Dystonic tics are usually accompanied by other more typical motor tics and by vocal tics, revealing their nature.

In addition to differences and potential overlaps with compulsions discussed above, complex tics must be distinguished from stereotypies, which are seen in patients with autism, mental retardation, Rett syndrome, psychosis, encephalopathies, and congenital blindness and deafness. Compared to complex motor

Table 17.2. Complex, overlapping tic phenomenology in Tourette syndrome.

	Complex motor tics	Compulsive tics	Impulsive tics	Compulsive-impulsive tics
Definition	Coordinated, purposeless involuntary movements that can resemble voluntary activity	Repetitive movements performed according to rules (i.e., ritualistic), in response to an obsession or to reduce tension	Repetitive movements performed without forethought and without regard to consequences. Often socially unacceptable	Repetitive movements with qualities of both compulsive and impulsive tics
Examples	Skipping; hopping, rubbing, jumping, smelling	Touching a door a certain number of times; smelling fingers to check for contamination	Touching oneself or others; touching a hot stove; stepping into traffic	Hitting someone a certain number of times Pushing someone after they cough to avoid contamination
Treatments	Alpha-adrenergic agonists, antipsychotics	SSRIs, alpha-adrenergic agonists, antipsychotics, cognitive-behavioral therapy	Antipsychotics, alpha-adrenergic agonists, mood stabilizers, stimulants	Antipsychotics, alpha-adrenergic agonists, SSRIs, mood stabilizers, stimulants, cognitive-behavioral therapy

Reproduced from reference 7, with permission.

tics, stereotypies tend to be more stereotyped with the same movement (e.g., head nodding, body rocking, hand flapping) or vocalization (e.g., moaning, shouting) occurring over and over for prolonged periods. Stereotypies are not known to be associated with premonitory sensations and may be more difficult to suppress than tics.

Etiology and pathogenesis

The neurobiological basis for tics remains largely unexplained. Substantial scientific evidence points to the importance of genetic factors, but no specific gene loci have yet been established. Genetic transmission models tend to point to complex inheritance, likely with a variety of potential susceptibility loci contributing [9]. An underlying state of heightened basal ganglia dopamine neurotransmission has long been suspected in TS because of the predictable lessening of tics in response to dopamine receptor antagonist drugs. This observation, combined with the finding of reduced levels of homovanillic acid, the main metabolite of dopamine, in the CSF point to probable postsynaptic dopamine receptor supersensitivity. Recent neuroimaging studies in patients with TS have been inconclusive about whether there is an increase in presynaptic dopamine transporters or excessive dopaminergic innervation in the striatum [10,11]. Most evidence points to a

dysfunction in corticostriatal inhibitory circuitry, perhaps allowing the unwanted expression of stored basal ganglia motor programs as tics [12].

Community-based epidemiological studies indicate that at least transient tics occur commonly during the course of childhood development, perhaps resulting from the process of normal basal ganglia synaptogenesis [13]. We have applied the term "physiological tics" to this phenomenon [14]. Tics can be seen in association with a wide variety of conditions associated with abnormal brain development or cerebral injury. Examples include mental retardation, autism and pervasive developmental disorder. Other secondary causes of tics include neuroacanthocytosis, encephalitis, Huntington disease and traumatic brain injury. Secondary tic disorders are usually evident by the presence of neurological deficits beyond tics. In our experience, secondary causes of tic disorders are usually associated with simple rather than complex tics.

Course of tics

In TS, about 90% of cases experience the onset of tics by age 10 years. Tics tend to follow a waxing and waning course over time, with exacerbations and remissions occurring over periods of weeks or a few months. While tics tend to be exacerbated by stress, worsenings commonly occur with no environmental precipitants.

Tics typically occur in waves, with one group of tics being replaced by another group. Tic severity tends to peak between ages 10 and age 16 years (15,16). In about two-thirds of TS cases, tics either substantially lessen or fully resolve by adulthood. Thus, the overall prognosis for TS is very good.

Treatment

We recently reviewed the appropriate management of tics [17]. For individuals with mild tics, education and supportive counseling may be sufficient to avoid the need for tic-suppressing therapy. When tics are disabling, causing social problems, pain or discomfort, or interference with routine activities, it is appropriate to initiate treatment aimed at lessening tics.

We usually start with the alpha-agonist guanfacine (0.5–4 mg/day) given in a single bedtime dose or divided into two daily doses. The most common potential side-effects of this drug are sedation, irritability and dizziness. We have seen a few patients experience syncope. Overall the drug is generally well-tolerated and its side-effect spectrum is milder than those of alternative tic suppressants. Guanfacine also has beneficial effects on ADHD, so it is a good medication choice for patients having both conditions.

If the response to guanfacine is inadequate or if there are intolerable side-effects, we usually switch to or add an antipsychotic drug. The atypical antipsychotics risperidone (0.25–16 mg/day) and aripiprazole (2–30 mg/day) are the ones we usually use. Due to growing appreciation of the potential side-effects of increased appetite, weight gain and glucose intolerance (metabolic syndrome) associated with the atypical antipsychotics, there has been renewed interest in the older classical neuroleptic antipsychotic drugs. Haloperidol (0.5–10 mg/day), pimozide (0.5–10 mg/day) and fluphenazine (0.5–20 mg/day) have demonstrated tic-suppressing efficacy. For debilitating or dangerous complex tics, such as loud coprolalia or self-mutilation tics, we tend to initiate medication therapy with an antipsychotic drug in order to achieve more rapid and predictable control. Fortunately, the feared antipsychotic drug side-effect of tardive dyskinesia rarely occurs in treated TS patients. Other medications to consider include clonazepam (0.5–10 mg/day) and the recently marketed tetrabenazine (12.5–200 mg/day), although the latter drug is very expensive. Local intramuscular injections of botulinum toxin can be very helpful when there are a small number of disabling tics, such as eye-blinking/blepharospasm, neck jerking or twisting, or muscle tensing tics, and can achieve faster control than medications [18,19].

Deep brain stimulation has been reported to lessen tics in some patients with severe, medication-refractory symptoms. The best anatomical target, the optimal subject selection criteria, and the long-term safety and efficacy of this approach remain to be established. Some TS patients with self-harming behaviors have not tolerated deep brain stimulation surgery due to self-induced damage to the equipment or infection related to constant picking at the operative sites. Surgical anterior cingulotomy can be considered for patients with medication-refractory self-harming behavior or associated severe obsessive-compulsive disorder. For patients with complex phenomenology (e.g., compulsive tics, impulsive tics, compulsive/impulsive tics), a combination of tic-suppressing medications, obsessive-compulsive disorder therapies (e.g., cognitive behavioral therapy, selective serotonin reuptake inhibitors [SSRIs]) and impulse control therapies (e.g., behavior therapy, stimulants, mood stabilizers) may be needed for optimum control.

References

1. The Tourette Syndrome Classification Study Group. Definitions and classification of tic disorders. *Arch Neurol* 1993; **50**: 1013–16.

2. Jankovic J, Stone L. Dystonic tics in patients with Tourette's syndrome. *Mov Disord* 1991; **6**: 248–52.

3. Kurlan R, Lichter D, Hewitt D. Sensory tics in Tourette's syndrome. *Neurology* 1989; **39**: 731–4.

4. American Psychiatric Association. *Diagnostic and Statistical Manual of Mental Disorders*, 4th ed. Washington, DC: American Psychiatric Association; 2000.

5. Kurlan R, Behr J, Medved L, Como PG. Transient tic disorder and the clinical spectrum of Tourette's syndrome. *Arch Neurol* 1988; **45**: 1200–1.

6. Kurlan R. Tourette's syndrome: current concepts. *Neurology* 1989; **39**: 1625–30.

7. Palumbo D, Kurlan R. Complex obsessive-compulsive and impulsive symptoms in patients with Tourette's syndrome. Neuropsychiatr Dis Treat 2007; **3**: 687–93.

8. Kurlan R, Daragjati C, McDermott MP *et al.* Complex socially inappropriate behavior in Tourette's syndrome. *J Neuropsychiatry Clin Neurosci* 1996; **8**: 311–17.

9. Walkup JT, LaBuda MC, Singer HS, Brown J, Riddle MA, Hurko O. Family study and segregation analysis of Tourette syndrome: evidence for a mixed model of inheritance. *Am J Hum Genet* 1996; **59**: 684–93.

10. Meyer P, Bohnen NI, Minoshima S *et al.* Striatal pre-synaptic monoaminergic vesicles are not increased in Tourette's syndrome. *Neurology* 1999; **53**: 371–4.

11. Albin RL, Koeppe RA, Wernette K *et al.* Striatal [^{11}C] dihydrotetrabenazine and [^{11}C]mehylphenidate binding in Tourette syndrome. *Neurology* 2009; **72**: 1390–6.

12. Mink JW. Basal ganglia dysfunction in Tourette syndrome: a new hypothesis. *Pediatr Neurol* 2001; **25**: 190–8.

13. Kurlan R, McDermott MP, Deeley C. Prevalence of tics in school children and association with placement in special education. *Neurology* 2001; **57**: 1383–8.

14. Palumbo D, Maughan A, Kurlan R. Hypothesis III: Tourette's syndrome is only one of several causes of a developmental basal ganglia syndrome. *Arch Neurology* 1997; **54**: 475–83.

15. Leckman JF, Zhang H, Vitale A *et al.* Course of tic severity in Tourette syndrome: the first two decades. *Pediatrics* 1998; **102**: 14–19.

16. Goetz CG, Tanner CM, Stebbins GT, Leipzig G, Carr WC. Adult tics in Gilles de la Tourette's syndrome: description and risk factors. *Neurology* 1992; **42**: 784–8.

17. Shprecher D, Kurlan R. The management of tics. *Mov Disord* 2009; **24**(1): 15–24.

18. Jankovic J. Botulinum toxin in the treatment of tics associated with Tourette's syndrome. *Neurology* 1993; **43**(Suppl 2): A310 [Abstract].

19. Scott BL, Jankovic J, Donovan DT. Botulinum toxin injection into vocal cord in the treatment of malignant coprolalia associated with Tourette's syndrome. *Mov Disord* 1996; **11**: 431–3.

Chapter 8

Unusual gait disorders

Samuel Kim and Victor S. C. Fung

Introduction

Bipedal stance and locomotion are among the most complex skills that humans possess yet are two of the most basic motor skills required for normal function. Their complexity can be compared to that of human speech, and require higher-order sensorimotor integration of lower-order neural mechanisms [1].

Gait and balance disorders can arise as a result of a wide range of medical problems and are common modes of presentation to neurologists. Many disorders produce characteristic disturbances of gait and posture, such that disease can often be identified by the manner in which gait is altered. The diagnostic process for more unusual and challenging gait disorders begins with careful examination to characterize the phenomenology. In order to analyze abnormal gait, it is important to have an explicit understanding of the components of normal gait. We therefore begin by reviewing the characteristics and physiology of normal gait.

Normal walking

Normal gait is comprised not only of the repetitive stepping movements of the legs but also the associated movements of the trunk and arms, both of which are built upon a stable upright posture in stance and during walking. There is a coordinated series of movements in the lower limbs. Flexion of the hip and knee is associated with dorsiflexion and out-turning of the foot as each leg moves forward. The internal malleoli almost touch each other during the swing phase, with toes clearing the ground. The arms move loosely by the sides, swinging effortlessly in time with the opposite leg [2].

Gait parameters

Gait parameters provide an objective framework with which to quantitatively analyze the components of gait.

The *gait cycle* is defined as the period of time between any two identical events during walking, and is divided into *stance* and *swing phases*, which follow on from each other. *Stance phase* denotes the period when the foot is in contact with the ground, and begins with initial foot contact (heel strike) and ends with the same foot leaving the ground (push-off). This is followed by the *swing phase* that begins with push off and ends with heel strike. The times spent in the two phases are unequal and the stance phase occupies 60–65% of the cycle. There is a period when both feet are in contact with the ground, referred to as *double limb support phase*, which occupies 20–25% of the cycle.

Analysis of gait is further aided by looking at specific leg movement parameters. *Stride length* is the distance from initial heel strike to the next heel strike of the same foot, whereas *step length* is the distance between the feet as one foot is in push-off phase and the other foot is in heel strike phase. Both of these parameters vary with the speed of walking. *Stride width* is the transverse distance between the central long axes of the feet during foot-to-floor contact, with a mean value of approximately 8.0 cm. *Foot angle* is the angle formed by the long axis of the foot with the plane of progression; there is slight out-toeing in the majority at an angle of approximately 7°. *Cadence* denotes the rhythm and is measured by the number of steps per minute. With normal aging, significant differences are noted in the gait parameters, perhaps in order to adapt to a less destabilizing gait. Velocity is significantly reduced, resulting from stride length reduction rather than changes in cadence, culminating in increased stance phase (elderly, 65.5%; young adult, 62.3%) and double limb support time (elderly, 31.0%; young adults, 24.6%). In terms of balance-related parameters, foot angle is increased while stride width remains remarkably constant. However, toe clearance during swing phase does not significantly change with aging, with an average

Uncommon Causes of Movement Disorders, ed. Néstor Gálvez-Jiménez and Paul J. Tuite. Published by Cambridge University Press. © Cambridge University Press 2011.

toe clearance of about 1 cm when the horizontal velocity is maximal [3–5].

Requirements for normal walking

It is helpful to understand the physiology that underpins the phenomenology of normal gait as this assists in understanding the pathophysiology of disordered gait.

Walking is accompanied by movement processes that are automatically controlled by the brain stem and spinal cord, but virtually all levels of the nervous system are intricately involved. At the very core, walking may be broadly divided into two fundamental elements, *posture and balance* and *locomotion* [6].

Posture is a term that describes the orientation of any body segment relative to the gravitational vector, whereas *balance* is a generic term describing the dynamics of body posture to prevent falling, related to the inertial forces acting on the body and the inertial characteristics of body segments [7]. As such, postural and balance control can be defined as stabilization or maintenance of *equilibrium* of the whole body in relation to gravitational force. The term *locomotion* is used to describe the forward progression associated with walking, and may be defined as the ability to initiate and maintain rhythmic stepping that results in forward displacement [6,8].

Posture and balance (equilibrium)

Posture is the foundation on which walking is executed. It provides the mechanical support for performing movements. Maintenance of an upright body posture in humans is an automatic activity that requires minimal attention [9]. The central nervous system provides coordination between posture, equilibrium and movement by utilizing two main mechanisms. The first is *postural reactions* that occur in response to sensory information that signals postural disturbances caused by movement, received from the visual, vestibular and somatosensory systems. There is a certain degree of redundancy in the sensory system such that compensation can occur when one or more sensory inputs are lost, e.g., in a blind person walking. The second mechanism utilizes *anticipatory postural adjustments*, which usually occur in association with voluntary movements. Unlike postural reactions, anticipatory postural adjustments precede the disturbance onset, thereby dampening the effects of the forthcoming postural perturbations in a feedforward manner [10,11]. Overall, these mechanisms provide postural stability required for walking.

Locomotion

Gait initiation, culminating in a forward step, is much more than voluntary movement of the legs and requires highly integrated postural shifts and limb movements, as well as normal postural control. There is an elegant stereotyped sequence of postural shifts that is achieved by redistribution of muscle activation involved in posture control (and limb movements under automatic neural control). It begins with a lateral shift of the center of gravity onto the stance limb that allows the swing limb to be raised. Almost simultaneously, the center of gravity is accelerated forward and laterally toward the future position of the swinging foot [12,13]. Once initiated, there follow cyclical stepping movements that result in forward progression. These rhythmic leg movements are controlled by spinal pattern generators, under the continuous influence of supraspinal (brain stem locomotor centers) and sensory signals [14–16].

Disordered gait

After eliciting the history, the next step in the diagnosis of a movement disorder is to characterize the phenomenology of the abnormal movements. In the case of gait disorders, this involves analyzing the components of gait described in the previous sections. This section will concentrate on providing a framework for classifying the phenomenology of different gait disorders, rather than specific diseases, although some attention will be given to conditions that are particularly illustrative. It is beyond the scope of this chapter to discuss all aspects of specific diseases in detail. We begin with descriptions of some common gait disorders encountered in clinical practice, to allow comparison and contrasting with the more unusual gait patterns.

Phenomenology of typical gait disorders

Typical parkinsonian gait

The typical gait of Parkinson disease (PD) is characterized by small, shuffling steps that result in reduced velocity. Importantly, the stride width is normal [17,18] and the ability for tandem gait is preserved [19,20]. Turns are executed with multiple small steps, and have the appearance of turning en bloc. These changes are associated with reduced arm swing which may be unilateral, and stooped posture that is characterized by forward-flexion of the shoulders, neck and trunk. In the later stages of the disease, the gait becomes increasingly interrupted by start hesitation and freezing, which tend to be particularly problematic when encountering doorways or obstacles.

When analyzed in greater detail, gait velocity is reduced and variable, being associated with diminished stride length and cadence, while double limb support is increased. However, when speed of walking is taken into account, the cadence is higher and the stride length shorter in PD patients [21,22].

Upper-half movements are also abnormal. One of the earliest signs of parkinsonian gait is reduced or absent arm swing. The en bloc turning appearance results from turns being executed with near-simultaneous turning of head and trunk rather than being produced with normal cranial–caudal order of axial segment displacement (head turning precedes trunk rotation by approximately 220 ms in control subjects). Abnormal turning may be an earlier sign of gait and posture disturbance than walking in PD patients [23,24]. With disease progression, start hesitation and freezing become increasingly troublesome, present in approximately 7% after 2 years of disease and 28% after 5 years, and tend to be less responsive to levodopa [25,26].

Spastic gait

The spastic gait arises from pathology along the pyramidal pathways. There may be a varying combination of weakness and spasticity (velocity-dependent hypertonia), which is more marked in the antigravity muscles.

Unilateral pathology results in a spastic hemiparesis with abnormal posturing characterized by slight flexion at the hip and extension at the knee, together with plantar flexion and inversion of the foot. The gait is initiated with pronounced postural shifts, with lateral truncal flexion toward the unaffected side and hyperextension of the hip on the paretic side, both of which help to swing the paretic leg forward in an arc from the hip, i.e., circumduction. There is reduced or absent knee flexion and ankle dorsiflexion during the swing phase, with the toes often scuffing the ground before landing on the forefoot or toes instead of the heel (heel strike). In the upper limbs, there is reduced or absent arm swing on the paretic side, and the arm is held stiffly with adduction and internal rotation at the shoulder, flexion at the elbow, wrist and fingers, and pronation at the elbow.

Bilateral spinal pathology causes a spastic paraparetic gait, which is in essence a bilateral hemiparetic gait affecting only the lower limbs. The gait is slow and is achieved with great effort, with both legs circumducted in the swing phase. There is a tendency to adduct the legs, causing the legs almost to cross (scissor gait), particularly when the disorder begins in childhood.

Balance may be affected despite the fact that the primary defect lies in the stepping mechanism and in propulsion (not in support or equilibrium), because hemiparesis or paraparesis interferes with corrective postural adjustments.

Cerebellar gait

Cerebellar ataxia is characterized by an irregular staggering gait on a widened base. The steps are irregular, with some longer while others are shorter than intended, and the patient may lurch unpredictably.

Gait kinematic studies have revealed that the most consistent feature is the significant variability in gait parameters arising from imprecise movement execution (combination of dysmetria, dysrhythmia and dyssynergia, and poor balance), including step height and length, and foot rotation angles. In addition, compensatory changes occur in order to improve stability during stance and walking; step width and foot rotation angles are significantly increased, with prolonged stance and double limb support duration and reduced cadence. Remarkably, despite these changes the gait velocity and stride length remain almost normal in patients with cerebellar disease [27,28].

Tandem gait testing, which places the greatest stress on the cerebellar system and thus accentuates any subtle features of cerebellar ataxia, is the most sensitive clinical test, with some showing a step width of greater than 5 cm to be a marker of cerebellar dysfunction with tandem walking [27]. Often, anatomy determines the type of cerebellar gait pattern, with alcohol-related cerebellar degeneration of the anterior lobe resulting in a slow wide-based halting gait with irregular and lurching type of locomotion, whereas lesions of the cerebellar hemisphere produce deviation toward the ipsilateral side during walking [29].

Sensory ataxic gait

This describes a gait that results from impairment of joint position and muscle kinesthetic sense due to a lesion anywhere in the proprioceptive afferent pathway from peripheral nerve to dorsal columns. Despite the use of the term "ataxia," the overall gait pattern is more reminiscent of the gait adaptations observed in the elderly, which serve to produce a more secure and less destabilizing gait [5, 30]. The stride width is increased as in cerebellar ataxia, but the gait is slow and appears cautious due to reduced stride length and cadence. The truncal and limb movements are dampened, and each step is visually monitored [30,31]. In addition, the steps have a slapping quality that is often audible due to the feet hitting the floor forcibly (slapping gait). Visual guidance is employed as a compensatory mechanism during stance and walking, which when removed results in unmasking of the deficit, e.g., difficulty walking in the dark. This forms the basis of Romberg's test in which truncal sway is increased in both cerebellar and sensory ataxia but to a significantly greater degree in sensory ataxia, often resulting in falls if the patient is not caught.

Phenomenology of unusual gait disorders

Atypical parkinsonian disorders

Parkinsonian gait can be mimicked by a host of conditions; however, the typical gait produced by PD is virtually diagnostic. It follows that any deviation from the typical pattern is a "red flag" against the diagnosis of PD, and it serves one well to have an intimate knowledge of the clinical features of parkinsonian gait described above. A "red flag" is useful because, firstly, it alerts one to consider other possibilities and, secondly, it helps narrow the list of differential diagnosis to be considered; for example, a parkinsonian gait with a widened base raises the possibility of vascular parkinsonism. In this section, conditions that mimic PD will be discussed and also the "red flags" that serve as clues.

Lower-half parkinsonism

The term "lower-half parkinsonism" was first coined by Thompson and Marsden in their description of patients with gait disorders associated with subcortical arteriosclerotic encephalopathy (Binswanger disease), who shared a similar gait pattern with patients affected by hydrocephalus and frontal lobe lesions. It was postulated that the gait pattern resulted from interruption of the networks involved in high-level organization and execution of planned movements.

The term depicts the disproportionate lower limb parkinsonism and gait impairment with relatively preserved arm swing. However, it should also be noted that the gait is characterized by variable amount of ataxia (parkinsonism-ataxia), forming a spectrum from signs predominantly of lower-half parkinsonism but with an element of ataxia, to severe ataxia on top of lower-half parkinsonism [32].

When the gait features are studied in detail (in vascular parkinsonism, see below), they confirm the clinical observation of lower-half parkinsonism. The lower limb features are identical to those of PD apart from a widened base, with gait parameters showing similar changes in gait velocity, stride length and cadence. The upper limb parameters on the other hand show preserved (normal) arm excursion and coordination [33].

Vascular parkinsonism

Vascular parkinsonism (VP) is a recognized cause of lower-half parkinsonism, arising secondary to either a multilacunar state involving the basal ganglia or subcortical arteriosclerotic encephalopathy. The validity of the concept had been questioned by some because ischemic lesions, despite being common in the elderly, are rarely seen together with parkinsonism, and furthermore vascular lesions are common incidental findings in pathologically confirmed PD. In recent years, magnetic resonance imaging and clinicopathological studies have provided firm evidence in support of the concept of VP, with both showing that there is a higher burden of subcortical white matter lesions in patients with suspected VP than in patients with PD and controls with hypertension [33,34].

Apart from the typical gait disorder as described above, other notable features that support the diagnosis of VP include early cognitive impairment, urinary incontinence and corticospinal or pseudobulbar signs or symptoms. Tremor can be present in more than half of the patients with VP, including some degree of rest, postural or kinetic tremor, but the classic pill-rolling rest tremor of the fingers and hands is almost never seen [35,36].

Normal pressure hydrocephalus

Normal pressure hydrocephalus (NPH) is another disorder that produces lower-half parkinsonism. The lower limb gait parameters show similar features to that of VP, with markedly reduced gait velocity, stride length and step height although cadence is preserved rather than increased [37]. Arm swing is relatively preserved and balance-related measurements such as step width (140 mm vs. 50 mm) and foot rotation angles are increased as in VP resulting from disturbance of dynamic equilibrium [37,38].

Differentiation between VP and NPH is critical, as NPH may be amenable to CSF shunting procedures, particularly if the history is short and the predominant problem is that of gait disturbance rather than dementia. However, as one can appreciate from the above descriptions, the similarity of gait features in VP and NPH make clinical differentiation often quite difficult. The so called clinical hallmarks ("classical triad") of NPH often do not serve to distinguish between the two, as cognitive impairment and urinary incontinence are nonspecific, and are perhaps more commonly found in VP. Furthermore, periventricular white matter changes (due to transependymal CSF absorption) of NPH not only resemble the imaging characteristics of VP but also often affect the same locations, making it difficult to reliably differentiate between the two entities. The issue is further complicated by the fact that patients who do not satisfy the strictest definitions of NPH may still respond to CSF shunting [39].

There is no single standard for the prognostic evaluation of NPH for CSF shunting, although supplemental tests can increase predictive accuracy to greater than 90%. The 40–50 ml tap test cannot be used as an exclusionary test because of its low sensitivity (26–61%). The prognostic value increases as greater amounts of fluid are removed as in external lumbar drainage, with the highest sensitivity (50–100%) and positive predictive value (80–100%) associated with prolonged controlled lumbar drainage (500 ml/3 days). Determination of the CSF outflow resistance via an infusion test carries a higher sensitivity (57–100%) with a similar predictive value (75–92%) [40].

Frontal lobe lesions

Although Nutt *et al.* in their classification of higher-level gait disorders suggest that lower-half parkinsonism can also be caused by frontal lobe lesions, well-documented examples are rare. There are reports of "gait apraxia" resulting from focal frontal lobe lesions (lymphoma), and parkinsonian gait disturbance with neurodegenerative diseases (Alzheimer disease, corticobasal degeneration), but these suffer from lack of detailed clinical description of gait features, particularly with regard to the "upper-half" features [41,42].

Notwithstanding this, it is likely that frontal lobe lesions also result in lower-half parkinsonism, as damage to the similar afferent and efferent projections of the leg areas of the motor cortex and supplementary motor area results with all three conditions (VP, NPH, and frontal lobe lesions), and it is hypothesized that it is the interruption of these higher level neural networks that underlie lower-half parkinsonism.

Parkinson-plus syndromes

The diagnosis of Parkinson-plus syndromes (neurodegenerative diseases that mimic PD but with different pathological findings) is often quite challenging, particularly early in the course of the disease when the full spectrum of clinical features may not yet have fully evolved. There is a lack of studies examining the phenomenology or quantitative parameters of gait in different Parkinson-plus syndromes despite the attention that has been focused on other clinical features. Therefore, diagnosis requires the assistance of "red flags" that help to distinguish between different syndromes. The following discussion will concentrate mainly on distinctive postural disturbances as relevant to gait disorder and other highly characteristic features.

The features of a typical Parkinsonian gait, with reduction in amplitude of leg movements, shuffling, and difficulty turning tend to be seen relatively more commonly in progressive supranuclear palsy (PSP) than multiple system atrophy (MSA). MSA is associated with a variable degree of cerebellar features, with widened base and truncal ataxia, and the gait may therefore resemble those of VP and NPH. Of course, the presence of autonomic failure is a major diagnostic clue pointing to MSA [43]. In general, early falls, particularly backward falls, due to loss of postural and righting reflexes are a feature of both PSP and MSA but it tends to be more consistent and occur earlier in PSP. A clinical cohort study of 187 patients with PSP found vertical supranuclear gaze palsy in 94% and falls in 88% of cases, with 70% those who had falls reporting falling backward [44]. In contrast, gait disorder and postural instability tend to be less prominent in corticobasal degeneration (CBD). The most common initial symptom reported by the patients is a "clumsy, stiff, or jerky arm," and the most common presenting features are unilateral or strongly asymmetric rigidity and bradykinesia (79% and 71%, respectively) that typically affect an arm, and ideomotor apraxia (65%) [43,45]. Clinical diagnosis can be difficult due to overlap with other neurodegenerative disorders, being most often confused with PSP. When first seen, clinical diagnosis has a sensitivity of 35% that only rises to 48% at the last review, although specificity is near perfect (>99%) [46].

Abnormal postures are useful differentiating features. Compared with the stooped posture of PD, patients with PSP often have erect posture and retrocollis, whereas patients with MSA often have disproportionate antecollis, Pisa syndrome or campto-cormia. Both disproportionate antecollis and Pisa syndrome are highly specific, being seen in approximately a third of patients with MSA, whereas camptocormia is somewhat lower in sensitivity and specificity [47,48]. Asymmetric dystonia involving an extremity (typically an arm) is a prominent feature of CBD, being present in 43% at presentation. The typical picture is that of a hand tightly clenched in a fixed flexion posture with the thumb adducted and buried in the palm of the hand by the fingers, associated with tight forearm pronation, and wrist and elbow flexion [43].

Freezing, previously considered to be uncommon in Parkinson-plus syndromes, is probably at least as common, and perhaps occurs earlier than in PD [49].

Early gait disturbance with freezing in the absence of other parkinsonian features may rarely be encountered, and has been described in the literature with a confusing array of terms, including pure akinesia, primary progressive freezing gait, and primary gait ignition failure. More recently, "pure akinesia with gait freezing" (PAGF) has been proposed as a unifying term that encapsulates the salient features. The consistent clinical features are gait unsteadiness and slowness that gradually evolve into start hesitation and freezing, associated with handwriting (micrographia) and speech difficulties (hypophonia) despite relative sparing of other fine motor tasks and absent rigidity or tremor. It is noteworthy that PAGF is associated with a phenomenon that has been designated as rapid akinesia, which describes rapid stuttering or hypophonia, and rapid micrographia. PSP-tau pathology appears to be responsible for the clinical syndrome, and has been suggested as the third clinical phenotype of PSP along with Richardson syndrome (postural instability and falls, supranuclear gaze palsy and cognitive impairment) and PSP-parkinsonism (asymmetric onset, tremor, moderate initial therapeutic response to levodopa – frequently confused with PD) [50].

Vascular parkinsonism ("lower-body Parkinsonism") as described earlier in the chapter may present with similar features (gait disorder and freezing of gait with relative sparing of upper limbs), but these patients can be distinguished from PAGF by the presence of tremor, limb rigidity, or cognitive dysfunction. In addition, the phenomenology of rapid akinesia and relative lack of bradykinesia are further clues supporting the diagnosis of PAGF.

Higher-level gait disorders

The concept of *higher-level gait disorder* arises from the observation that some patients present with a gait disorder that defies explanation on the basis of impairment of lower-level nervous system such as disturbances of proprioceptive, visual, vestibular, or musculoskeletal function, or even middle level nervous system disease such as loss of pyramidal, extrapyramidal, or cerebellar function, or even still superimposition of abnormal involuntary movements [6,51]. So defined, higher-level gait disorders are more common in the older population, accounting for approximately 20% of gait disorders in elderly patients [52]. It has been suggested that the core clinical features are combinations of disequilibrium and impaired stepping, with secondary compensatory mechanisms designed to preserve balance.

The clinical classification of higher-level gait disorders is a confusing area, as gait disorders with overlapping features have been described using different terminology. Some have used the term to include lower-half parkinsonism with its potential associated causes outlined above [6,53], while others have used it to describe a gait disorder characterized by severe impairment of truncal control or postural instability that is often associated with frontal release signs, so called "frontal disequilibrium" [54].

The term *gait apraxia* has often been used to describe higher-level gait disorders because of the disproportionate difficulty in using the legs to walk when the legs are not weak. In particular, based on Liepmann's theories of apraxia for complex limb movements, some have attributed "frontal disequilibrium" to gait apraxia, defining it as "inability to properly use the lower limbs in the act of walking which cannot be accounted for by demonstrable sensory impairment or motor weakness"[55]. However, this definition has been criticized as it overlooks the critical role of truncal control that is also a fundamental requirement for walking [1]. Furthermore, some have argued that as apraxia is the inability to perform "skilled" or "learned" motor acts," apraxia of gait is perhaps a misnomer since walking is more "hard wired" [56].

Dystonic gait

The term dystonia is used to describe involuntary, sustained, stereotyped, and often repetitive muscle contractions causing twisting movements or abnormal postures [57,58]. The hallmark of a dystonic gait is abnormal posturing that becomes superimposed on otherwise relatively well-preserved components of gait. Accordingly, dystonia produces gait disturbance by disrupting stable posture of the legs, upper half, or both, or interrupting the smooth flow of limb movements. It is important to try to distinguish which abnormalities in gait and posture are caused by the underlying dystonia as opposed to alterations in gait that are compensatory or form part of a sensory trick, such as placing the palm of the hand on the anterior thigh throughout the gait cycle.

As the abnormal posturing between individuals can be highly variable, dystonic gait can sometimes appear quite bizarre and mistakenly diagnosed as a psychogenic disorder. There are several key features that, if present, support the diagnosis. A characteristic feature is that dystonic movements are repetitive, patterned and predictable, i.e., stereotyped. Therefore, when there is any doubt about the phenomenology, it is important to note whether there is any variability in the posturing and movements with repeated attempts at walking; it may well take several examinations on different occasions to be confident of the phenomenology.

Another key feature is that dystonia is activated by a voluntary task (action dystonia), and may not be present or only very subtle at rest. The activating voluntary task may range from nonspecific to highly specific. *Task specificity* is a feature of milder forms of dystonia that tends to disappear with progression, e.g., primary dystonia of childhood, particularly involving the trunk and legs, may begin as an action dystonia that is evident on walking forward but show marked improvement with walking backward or running. However, with progression over time, dystonia may be brought on by many actions, even standing [59]. One should be mindful that this phenomenon could be misinterpreted, leading to mislabeling of dystonia as psychogenic, whereas it may actually support the diagnosis of dystonia.

In childhood, dystonia most frequently manifests initially in the lower limbs, thus presenting with gait disorder in the absence of other neurological signs. The classic presentation of childhood-onset primary dystonia begins as mobile action dystonia of a leg, most commonly with sustained plantar flexion and inversion of the ankle. With time, dystonia may progress to involve the whole leg before becoming generalized [60].

The lower limb onset pattern is infrequently seen in adult-onset dystonia, where dystonia is usually confined to the upper body, particularly in the craniocervical region. When dystonia affects the foot in isolation, it is rarely on a primary basis but more commonly arises secondary to a number of conditions including parkinsonism, trauma, stroke, or a structural lesion, making it critical to seek an underlying etiology when encountered with adult-onset isolated focal lower limb dystonia. In addition, one should also be mindful of the possibility of a psychogenic disorder, although unlike primary focal lower limb dystonia that presents with mobile limb dystonia, psychogenic limb dystonia most often presents as fixed dystonia [60].

Dopa-responsive dystonia

Dopa-responsive dystonia (DRD) is an autosomal dominant disorder with reduced penetrance (~30%). It bears specific mention because it is a curable condition, and also because it can present with highly atypical features that are not easily recognized as being dystonic. It is an important diagnostic consideration in young-onset lower limb dystonia with diurnal variation, usually becoming more severe at the end of the day [61]. Early- or mid-childhood cases typically begin as gait dysfunction or dystonic foot posturing (equinovarus), whereas late-onset cases often present with parkinsonism. It is commonly accompanied by signs of pyramidal tract dysfunction, with hyperreflexia and less commonly ankle clonus. However, in recent years, it has become apparent that the clinical features are highly variable both within and between families, and the phenotype continues to be extended, including some bizarre presentations. There are case reports of spastic paraplegia, cerebellar ataxia [62], camptocormia [63,64], and also generalized hypotonia with proximal weakness [65].

It can be difficult to distinguish between DRD and *parkin* mutation resulting in juvenile parkinsonism, although presence of several clinical features is more suggestive of DRD rather than *parkin* mutation. These include clear diurnal variation, benign course and sustained responsiveness to low doses of levodopa without emergence of motor complications or other neurologic manifestations [66,67].

Gait caused by choreiform/mixed movement disorders

Pure chorea usually does not have a major impact on gait, although the involuntary movements superimposed on the normal components of gait produce dance-like movements that gave rise to its name. If severe or associated with hypotonia, chorea can give rise to truncal or limb perturbations from which the patients can usually recover without major instability.

In some diseases, chorea characteristically occurs as part of a mixed movement disorder. In these conditions, the resulting combination of chorea, dystonia and parkinsonism can give rise to bizarre gaits that can be mistakenly labeled psychogenic, with the dystonic component leading to unusual postures but the variability of the superimposed choreiform movements and parkinsonian balance impairment interfering with the stereotyped nature of the underlying dystonia and making its recognition more difficult.

Huntington disease

A variety of movement problems is seen in Huntington disease (HD), including chorea, dystonia, bradykinesia and rigidity. Each of these problems may be present concurrently, although chorea tends to predominate early in the course of the disease and tends to disappear as the disease advances, being replaced by dystonia, bradykinesia and rigidity. The abnormal gait in HD may be produced as a consequence of any one or combination of these movement problems, which likely results in different phenomenology between patients as well as within patients whose gait pattern can change with time. Particularly early on in the course of the disease, the combination of dystonia and chorea can give rise to bizarre abnormal postures that lack the typical stereotyped nature of dystonic gait because of the superimposed uncoordinated lurching due to random perturbations caused by chorea. In support of this view, a study examining the effect of chorea on gait disturbance showed no improvement in gait despite effective suppression of choreic movements [68]. In the latter stages of the disease but also in juvenile-onset cases, dystonia tends to be more prominent, producing stereotyped abnormal posturing and phasic limb movements, sometimes with prominent postural instability due to coexistent parkinsonism. In terms of gait kinematics, a study has shown reduced gait velocity and stride length in HD, and those who have falls have increased stride length variability and trunk sway in the mediolateral direction than non-fallers [69]. Subtle gait disturbance may be observed early in the disease, including difficulty with tandem walking, sudden stopping on command, and turning [68].

Neuroacanthocytosis

Neuroacanthocytosis is a genetically heterogeneous syndrome with core features of acanthocytosis, movement disorder (chorea, orofacial tics, gait impairment),

cognitive or psychiatric changes, amyotrophy often with hyper-CKemia, and normobetalipoproteinemia. Autosomal recessive chorea-acanthocytosis is most common, followed by X-linked (McLeod syndrome) and rarer autosomal dominant forms. It is important to note that this form of neuroacanthocytosis is distinct from disorders of lipoprotein (abetalipoproteinemia [Bassen-Kornzweig syndrome] and hypolipoproteinemia) in which patients develop progressive spinocerebellar ataxia, peripheral neuropathy, dorsal column sensory loss, and retinitis pigmentosa but not movement disorders [70, 72].

Despite the recessive and X-linked forms arising as a result of mutations in two different genes, the phenotypes are remarkably uniform in the two conditions. The most striking features of presentation are gait difficulties with bizarre patterns that include leg buckling and violent truncal spasms, sometimes associated with dangerous head banging. Orofacial dyskinesia is quite typical and presents in a variety of ways including, grimacing, self-mutilating tongue and lip biting, involuntary vocalizations, dysarthria or dysphagia. Chorea and dystonia are more common than parkinsonism and is present in over half of the patients. Cognitive or psychiatric changes are found in almost all patients [71–73]. In addition, variant syndromes involving the spinocerebellar pathways have been reported, with patients presenting with gait imbalance as a prominent neurological symptom [74]. McLeod syndrome, to a greater extent than chorea-acanthocytosis, is also associated with sensorimotor axonopathy (absent ankle reflexes in 90% of the patients) and myopathy [75].

As indicated by the clinical features (bizarre gait disorder comprised of dystonia and chorea, and sometimes superimposed behavioral abnormalities arising from coexistent cognitive and psychiatric impairment), neuroacanthocytosis resembles many aspects of HD. Again the combination of chorea and dystonia in the presence of psychiatric features can result in the misdiagnosis of a psychogenic disorder.

Gait disturbance due to myoclonus and asterixis

Myoclonus is a phenomenological term for shock-like involuntary movements caused by abrupt and brief muscular contractions (positive myoclonus) or inhibition (negative myoclonus, asterixis). Most myoclonic movements are due to positive myoclonus although they often coexist with variable amount of negative myoclonus which can either occur in isolation or more commonly following positive myoclonus. Positive and negative myoclonus are clinically very similar, producing sudden brief shock-like jerks, and therefore may be difficult to distinguish on clinical basis alone. A key feature of asterixis is that it causes sudden lapses in posture which is best appreciated during isometric muscle contractions (76); for example, knee buckling when standing with knees slightly flexed or flapping hands when holding the arms outstretched with the hands in dorsiflexed position. Asterixis can be confirmed neurophysiologically, as described in Lance and Adams' seminal work on action myoclonus induced by hypoxic encephalopathy, as postural lapses and falls take place during the period of electrical silence in the postural muscles (neck, trunk, proximal leg muscles), which may or may not be preceded by the spike of a myoclonic jerk [77,78].

Gait disturbance due to pure myoclonus gives rise to a jerky appearance with the unpredictable perturbations leading to variable step height and stride length and truncal jerks, as well as to reactive postural adjustments that can give an oscillatory quality to the truncal movements. If truncal or in particular lower limb muscle asterixis is present, there will be episodes of knee buckling or even falls. At times this leads to severe fear of falling and may present as an extreme cautious gait or even refusal to stand or walk. If there is coexistent cerebellar ataxia, there is significant widening of the step width and greater risk of falling due to the failure to compensate for truncal perturbations.

The combination of myoclonus and cerebellar ataxia is seen in progressive myoclonic syndromes (progressive myoclonic epilepsy (PME) and progressive myoclonic ataxia (PMA)). PMA, also known eponymously as Ramsay Hunt syndrome, is characterized by myoclonus and progressive cerebellar ataxia and sometimes infrequent tonic clonic seizures in the absence of prominent dementia, where as PME is characterized by myoclonus, tonic-clonic seizures, progressive dementia, and ataxia. Although these two syndromes share common causes, (most commonly Unverricht–Lundborg disease and mitochondrial encephalomyopathy), there are a substantial number of patients with PMA in whom no underlying cause can be identified as compared with PME, in which the majority can be accurately diagnosed during life [79,80].

Myopathic weakness

Myopathic conditions typically cause proximal muscle weakness that affects the lower limbs more than the upper limbs with disproportionately greater weakness in the extensors than the flexors. The pattern of weakness results in the characteristic waddling gait, due to poor stabilization of the weight-bearing hip, which rotates excessively with each step (Trendelenburg, gluteal gait). Extensor weakness results in difficulty walking up steps as well as rising from a sitting or supine position, requiring the support of the arms to push up. Duchenne muscular dystrophy (DMD) results in the classic myopathic waddling gait, with additional features of hyperlordosis and equinovarus, but it should be noted that any condition affecting the proximal muscles can result in a similar picture. Indeed, spinal muscular atrophy (SMA), a neurogenic disorder, can mimic the gait impairment of DMD, although a study has shown that they use different forward movement strategy despite having in common excessive pelvic tilt and lordosis; SMA patients rotated their pelvis and pulled forward their lower limb, whereas DMD patients used hip flexion and circumduction, owing to stronger hip flexion [81].

Occasionally, proximal lower limb myopathy can cause gait disturbance that is mistaken for a parkinsonian gait as there is a compensatory reduction in step height and stride length with attendant reduction in arm swing. For example, inclusion body myositis (IBM) is an important consideration in anyone who presents with quadriceps and ankle dorsiflexion weakness (which can be unilateral), particularly in those over the age of 50 years. [82–84]. Quadriceps weakness leads to gait impairment and a propensity to fall, particularly when descending stairs, as the knee may buckle when weight of the body is transferred to the affected limb.

Psychogenic gait

Based on data from various studies, gait disturbance is a relatively common mode of presentation of a psychogenic movement disorder (PMD), accounting for approximately 8–10% of patients, with only tremor and dystonia being more common [85–87]. The diagnosis of psychogenic gait disorder should not be made simply on the basis that it is bizarre and unlike anything one has seen before, as some organic gaits can have a bizarre appearance (see sections on dystonic and mixed movement disorder gaits above).

Studies have shown that there are several key features that allow phenomenological diagnosis of psychogenic gait. Psychogenic gait often shows striking slowness and momentary fluctuations during examinations, often in response to suggestion and distraction. In addition, the patients often adopt uneconomic postures that require considerable amount of energy and effort as well as balance to maintain the posture, providing information about various neurological domains that need to be intact in order for the patients to be able to achieve such strenuous postures [88]. Excessive slowing of movements (not gait) has been reported as the most common feature when those with pure psychogenic gait disorder and those with more generalized PMDs that also compromised the gait were taken together as a group. Taken separately, slowness of gait was the most common feature in patients who had combined psychogenic movement disorder and gait abnormality, whereas the buckling at the knee pattern was the most common type of gait abnormality (followed by astasia-abasia) in those with pure psychogenic gait disorder [86].

Lempert *et al.*, in their study of 37 patients with psychogenic stance and gait disorders, found six characteristic features of psychogenic disorder (present in 97% of the patients). These included (1) fluctuations of impairment; (2) excessive slowness of movements; (3) "psychogenic Romberg test" (response with constant falls toward or away from the observer irrespective of the observer's position; large-amplitude body sway, building up after a silent latency of a few seconds and an improvement of postural stability when distracted); (4) "walking on ice" gait pattern (wide based with decreased stride length and height, stiffening of the knees and ankles, some degree of antagonist innervation and shuffling of the feet); (5) uneconomic postures; and (6) sudden buckling of the knees with and without falls. Less commonly, astasia and vertical shaking tremor (up and down shaking of the body) were seen [88].

There are several tests that may aid in strengthening the diagnosis of psychogenic gait disorder. Psychogenic gait and movement disorders often improve when the patient is engaged in mental and motor distraction tasks such as serial 7's or externally paced hand tapping. Presenting a patient with a novel gait task can be instructive. Walking backwards is a good test as the physical requirements differ little from forward motion, and yet may cause the patient to walk with an altered pattern or excessive slowness. However, one has to be mindful of the possibility of a dystonic gait, which may result in an altered pattern, although the stereotyped nature of dystonic movements is a good positive diagnostic clue for dystonic gait and a pointer against a psychogenic movement disorder [89].

Recently, Okun *et al.* [90] assessed whether the "chair test" could distinguish psychogenic from organic gait based on Paul Blocq's original description of an astasia-abasia patient who effectively propelled a chair while being seated (astasia-abasia describes the paradoxical ability to use the legs normally except when standing (abasia) and walking (astasia)). Compared with their walking, 8 of the 9 patients in the psychogenic group showed improved ability to propel a chair forward when seated. In contrast, all 9 disease control patients (7 with PD) performed equally in both conditions. However, this is yet to be reproduced in a larger population using more diverse disease controls, as false-positive results might be expected in patients with dystonic conditions who are able to use the chair as a *geste antagoniste*, and in patients with "gait apraxia" who can perform normal bicycling leg movements [91].

References

1. Thompson PD, Nutt JG. Higher level gait disorders. *J Neural Transm* 2007; **114**: 1305–7.

2. Ropper AH, Brown RH. Disorders of stance and gait. In: Ropper AH, Brown RH, eds. *Adams and Victor's Principles of Neurology*. 8th ed. New York: McGraw-Hill; 2008: 100–8.

3. Murray MP, Drought AB, Kory RC. Walking patterns of normal men. *J Bone Joint Surg Am* 1964; **46**: 335–60.

4. Murray MP, Kory RC, Sepic SB. Walking patterns of normal women. *Arch Phys Med Rehabil* 1970; **51**: 637–50.

5. Winter DA, Patla AE, Frank JS, Walt SE. Biomechanical walking pattern changes in the fit and healthy elderly. *Phys Ther* 1990; **70**: 340–7.

6. Nutt JG, Marsden CD, Thompson PD. Human walking and higher-level gait disorders, particularly in the elderly. *Neurology* 1993; **43**: 268–79.

7. Winter DA. Human balance and posture control during standing and walking. *Gait Posture* 1995; **3**: 193–214.

8. Tyrrell, PJ. Apraxia of gait or higher level gait disorders: review and description of two cases of progressive gait disturbance due to frontal lobe degeneration. *J R Soc Med* 1994; **87**: 454–6.

9. Deliagina TG, Orlovsky GN. Comparative neurobiology of postural control. *Curr Opin Neurobiol* 2002; **12**: 652–7.

10. Armstrong, DM. The supraspinal control of mammalian locomotion. *J Phys* 1988; **102**: 2–13.

11. Massion, J. Postural control systems in developmental perspective. *Neurosci Biobehav Rev* 1998; **22**: 465–72.

12. Elble RJ, Moody C, Leffler K, Sinha R. The initiation of normal walking. *Mov Dis* 1994; **9**: 139–46.

13. MacKinnon CD, Winter DA. Control of whole body balance in the frontal plane during human walking. *J Biomech* 1993; **26**: 633–44.

14. Borghese NA, Bianchi L, Lacquanti F. Kinematic determinants of human locomotion. *J Physiol* 1996; **494**: 863–79.

15. Zehr EP, Duysens J. Regulation of arm and leg movement during human locomotion. *Neuroscientist* 2004; **10**: 347–61.

16. Mori S, Matsuyama K, Mori F, Nakajima K. Supraspinal sites that induce locomotion in the vertebrate central nervous system. *Adv Neurol* 2001; **87**: 25–40.

17. Murray MP, Sepic SB, Gardner GM, Downs WJ. Walking patterns of men with parkinsonism. *Am J Phys Med* 1978; **57**: 278–94.

18. Vieregge P, Stolze H, Klein C, Heberlein L. Gait quantitation in Parkinson's disease: locomotor disability and correlation to clinical scales *J Neural Transm* 1997; **104**: 237–48.

19. Bloem BR, Grimbergen YA, Cramer M, Willemsen M, Zwinderman AH. Prospective assessment of falls in Parkinson's disease. *J Neurol* 2001; **248**: 950–8.

20. Abdo WF, Borm GF, Munneke M *et al.* Ten steps to identify atypical parkinsonism. *J Neurol Neurosurg Psychiatry* 2006; **77**: 1367–9.

21. Knutsson E. An analysis of Parkinsonian gait. *Brain* 1972; **95**: 475–86.

22. Morris M, Iansek R, Matyas T, Summers J. Abnormalities in the stride length-cadence relation in parkinsonian gait. *Mov Dis* 1998; **13**: 61–9.

23. Crenna P, Carpinella I, Rabuffetti M *et al.* The association between impaired turning and normal straight walking in Parkinson's disease. *Gait Posture* 2007; **26**: 172–8.

24. Patla AE, Prentice SD, Rietdyk S, Allard F, Martin C. What guides the selection of alternate foot placement during locomotion in humans. *Exp Brain Res* 1999; **128**: 441–50.

25. Giladi N, Treves TA, Simon ES *et al.* Freezing of gait in patients with advanced Parkinson's disease. *J Neural Transm* 2001; **108**: 53–61.

26. Giladi N, McDermott MP, Fahn S *et al.* Freezing of gait in PD: prospective assessment in the DATATOP cohort. *Neurology* 2001; **56**: 1712–21.

27. Stolze H, Klebe S, Petersen G, Raethjen J *et al.* Typical features of cerebellar ataxic gait. *J Neurol Neurosurg Psychiatry* 2002; **73**: 310–2.

28. Palliyath S, Hallett M, Thomas SL. Lebiedowska MK. Gait in patients with cerebellar ataxia. *Mov Disord* 1998; **13**: 958–64.

29. Dietz V. Neurophysiology of gait disorders: present and future applications. *Electroencephalogr Clin Neurophysiol* 1997; **103**: 333–55.

30. Elble RJ, Thomas SS, Higgins C, Colliver J. Stride-dependent changes in gait of older people. *J Neurol* 1991; **238**: 1–5.

31. Lajoie Y, Barbeau H, Hamelin M. Attentional requirements of walking in spinal cord injured patients compared to normal subjects. *Spinal Cord* 1999; **37**: 245–50.

32. Thompson PD, Marsden CD. Gait disorder of subcortical arteriosclerotic encephalopathy: Binswanger's disease. *Mov Disord* 1987; **2**: 1–8.

33. Zijlmans JC, Poels PJ, Duysens J *et al.* Quantitative gait analysis in patients with vascular parkinsonism. *Mov Disord* 1996; **11**: 501–8.

34. Zijlmans JC, Thijssen HO, Vogels OJ *et al. Neurology* 1995; **45**: 2183–8.

35. Zijlmans JC, Daniel SE, Hughes AJ, Revesz T, Lees AJ. Clinicopathological investigation of vascular parkinsonism, including clinical criteria for diagnosis. *Mov Disord* 2004; **19**: 630–40.

36. Mevawalla N, Fung V, Morris J, Halliday GM. Unilateral rest tremor in vascular parkinsonism associated with a contralateral lesion of the locus ceruleus. *Mov Disord* 2009; **24**: 1242–4.

37. Stolze H, Kuhtz-Buschbeck JP, Drucke H *et al.* Gait analysis in idiopathic normal pressure hydrocephalus – which parameters respond to the CSF tap test? *Clin Neurophysiol* 2000; **11**: 1678–86.

38. Stolze H, Khutz-Buschbeck JP, Drucke J, Johnk K, Illert M, Deuschl G. Comparative analysis of the gait disorder of normal pressure hydrocephalus and Parkinson's disease. *J Neurol Neurosurg Pyshciatry* 2001; **70**: 289–97.

39. Vanneste JA. Three decades of normal pressure hydrocephalus: are we wiser now? *J Neurol Neurosurg Psychiatry* 1994; **57**: 1021–5.

40. Marmarou A, Bergsneider M, Klinge P, Relkin N, Black PM. The value of supplemental prognostic tests for the preoperative assessment of idiopathic normal-pressure hydrocephalus. *Neurosurgery* 2005; **57**(Suppl 3): S17–28.

41. Nadeau SE. Gait apraxia: further clues to localization. *Eur Neurol* 2007; **58**(3): 142–5.

42. Rossor MN, Tyrrell PJ, Warrington EK, Thompson PD, Marsden CD, Lantos P. Progressive frontal gait disturbance with atypical Alzheimer's disease and corticobasal degeneration. *J Neurol Neurosurg Psychiatry* 1999; **67**: 345–52.

43. Wenning GK, Litvan I, Jankovic J *et al.* Natural history and survival of 14 patients with corticobasal degeneration confirmed at postmortem examination. *J Neurol Neurosurg Psychiatry* 1998; **64**: 184–9.

44. Nath U, Ben-Shlomo Y, Thomson RG, Lees AJ, Burn DJ. Clinical features and natural history of progressive supranuclear palsy: a clinical cohort study. *Neurology* 2003; **60**: 910–6.

45. Rinne JO, Lee MS, Thompson PD, Marsden CD. Corticobasal degeneration: a clinical study of 36 cases. *Brain* 1994; **117**: 1183–96.

46. Litvan I, Agid Y, Goetz C *et al*. Accuracy of the clinical diagnosis of corticobasal degeneration: a clinicopathologic study. *Neurology* 1997; **48**: 119–25.

47. Wenning GK, Tison F, Ben Shlomo Y, Daniel SE, Quinn NP. Multiple system atrophy: a review of 203 pathologically proven cases. *Mov Disord* 1997; **12**: 133–47.

48. Kollensperger M, Geser F, Seppi K *et al*. Red flags for multiple system atrophy. *Mov Disord* 2008; **23**: 1093–9.

49. Muller J, Seppi K, Stefanova N, Poewe W, Litvan I, Wenning GK. Freezing of gait in postmortem-confirmed atypical parkinsonism. *Mov Disord* 2002; **17**: 1041–5.

50. Williams DR, Holton JL, Strand K, Revesz T, Lees AJ. Pure akinesia with gait freezing: a third clinical phenotype of progressive supranuclear palsy. *Mov Disord* 2007; **22**: 2235–41.

51. Fife TD, Baloh RW. Disequilibrium of unknown cause in older people. *Ann Neurol* 1993; **34**: 694–702.

52. Sudarsky L, Ronthal M. Gait disorders among elderly patients. A survey study of 50 patients. *Arch Neurol* 1983; **40**: 740–3.

53. Thompson PD. Higher level gait disorders. *Curr Neurol Neurosci Rep* 2007; **7**: 290–4.

54. Bruns L. Uber storungen des gleichgewichts bei stirnhirntumoren. *Dtsch Med Wschr* 1892; **18**: 138–43.

55. Meyer JS, Barron DW. Apraxia of gait: A clinico-physiological study. *Brain* 1960; **83**: 261–84.

56. Zadikoff C, Lang AE. Apraxia in movement disorders. *Brain* 2005; **128**(Pt 7): 1480–97.

57. Jankovic J. Dystonic disorders. In: Jankovic J, Tolosa E, eds. *Parkinson's Disease and Movement Disorders*. 5th ed. Philadelphia: Lippincott Williams and Wilkins; 2007: 321–47.

58. Berardelli A, Rothwell JC, Hallett M, Thompson PD, Manfredi M, Marsden CD. The pathophysiology of primary dystonia. *Brain* 1998; **121**(Pt 7): 1195–212.

59. Albanese A. The clinical expression of primary dystonia. *J Neurol* 2003; **250**: 1145–51.

60. Schneider SA, Edwards MJ, Grill SE *et al*. Adult-onset primary lower limb dystonia. *Mov Disord* 2006; **21**(6): 767–71.

61. Nygaard TG, Marsden CD, Duvoisin RC. Dopa-responsive dystonia. *Adv Neurol* 1988; **50**: 377–84.

62. Chaila EC, McCabe DJH, Delanty N, Costello DJ, Murphy RP. Broadening the phenotype of childhood-onset dopa-responsive dystonia. *Arch Neurol* 2006; **63**(8): 1185–8.

63. Micheli F, Pardal MM. Dopa-responsive dystonic camptocormia. *Neurology* 2007; **68**(18): 1543.

64. Van Gerpen, JA. Dopa-responsive dystonic camptocormia. *Neurology* 2006; **66**: 1779.

65. Kong CK, Ko CH, Tong SF, Lam CW. Atypical presentation of dopa-responsive dystonia: generalized hypotonia and proximal weakness. *Neurology* 2001; **57**: 1121–4.

66. Uc EY, Rodnitzky RL. Childhood dystonia. *Semin Pediatr Neurol* 2003; **10**: 52–61.

67. Tassin J, Durr A, Bonnet AM *et al*. Levodopa-responsive dystonia. GTP cyclohydrolase I or parkin mutations? *Brain* 2000; **123**: 1112–21.

68. Koller WC, Trimble J. The gait abnormality of Huntington's disease. *Neurology* 1985; **35**: 1450–4.

69. Grimbergen YAM, Knol MJ, Bloem BR, Kremer BPH, Roos RAC, Munneke M. Falls and gait disturbances in Huntington's disease. *Mov Disord* 2008; **23**: 970–6.

70. Danek A, Walker RH. Neuroacanthocytosis. *Curr Opin Neurol* 2005; **18**: 386–92.

71. Danek A, Dobson-Stone C, Velayos-Baeza A. The phenotype of chorea-acanthocytosis: a review of 106 patients with VPS13A mutations. *Mov Disord* 2005; **20**: 1678.

72. Stevenson VL, Hardie RJ. Acantocytosis and neurological disorders. *J Neurol* 2001; **248**: 87–94.

73. Hardie RJ, Pullon HW, Harding AE *et al. Brain* 1991; **114**: 13–49.

74. Tsai CH, Chen RS, Chang HC, Lu CS, Liao KK. Acanthocytosis and spinocerebellar degeneration: a new association? *Mov Disord* 1997; **12**: 456–9.

75. Jung HH. McLeod syndrome: clinical and neuroradiological aspects. *Mov Disord* 2005; **20**: 1673–94.

76. Deuschl G, Bain P, Brin M. Consensus statement of the Movement Disorder Society on Tremor. Ad Hoc Scientific Committee. *Mov Disord* 1998; **13**(Suppl 3): 2–23.

77. Lance JW, Adams RD. The syndrome of intention or action myoclonus as a sequel to hypoxic encephalopathy. *Brain* 1963; **86**: 111–36.

78. Obeso JA, Artieda J, Burleigh A. Clinical aspects of negative myoclonus. *Adv Neurol* 1995; **67**: 1–7.

79. Marsden CD, Harding AE, Obeso JA, Lu CS. Progressive myoclonic ataxia (the Ramsay Hunt syndrome). *Arch Neurol* 1990; **47**: 1121–5.

80. Marsden CD, Obeso JA. The Ramsay Hunt syndrome is a useful clinical entity. *Mov Disord* 1989; **4**: 6–12.

81. Armand S, Mercier M, Watelain E *et al*. A comparison of gait in spinal muscular atrophy, type II and Duchenne muscular dystrophy. *Gait Posture* 2005; **21**: 369–78.

82. Amato AA, Gronseth GS, Jackson CE *et al.* Inclusion body myositis: clinical and pathological boundaries. *Ann Neurol* 1996; **40**: 581–6.

83. Needham M, Mastaglia FL. Inclusion body myositis: current pathogenetic concepts and diagnostic and therapeutic approaches. *Lancet Neurol* 2007; **6**: 620–31.

84. Dabby R, Lange DJ, Trojaborg W, *et al.* Inclusion body myositis mimicking motor neuron disease. *Arch Neurol* 2001; **58**: 1253–6.

85. Ertan S, Uluduz D, Ozekmekci S *et al.* Clinical characteristics of 49 patients with psychogenic movement disorders in a tertiary clinic in Turkey. *Mov Disord* 2009; **24**: 759–62.

86. Baik JS, Lang AE. Gait abnormalities in psychogenic movement disorders. *Mov Disord* 2007; **22**: 395–9.

87. Sudarsky L. Psychogenic gait disorders. *Semin Neurol* 2006; **26**: 351–6.

88. Lempert T, Brandt T, Dieterich M, Huppert D. How to identify psychogenic disorders of stance and gait. A video study in 37 patients. *J Neurol* 199; **238**: 140–6.

89. Hayes MW, Graham S, Heldorf P, de Moore G, Morris JG. A video review of the diagnosis of psychogenic gait: appendix and commentary. *Mov Disord* 1999; **14**: 914–21.

90. Okun MS, Rodriguez RL, Foote KD, Fernandez HH. The "chair test" to aid in the diagnosis of psychogenic gait disorders. *Neurology* 2007; **13**: 87–91.

91. Gupta A, Lang AE. Psychogenic movement disorders. *Curr Opin Neurol* 2009; **22**: 430–6.

Chapter 19

Cerebellar disorders
Balancing the approach to cerebellar ataxia

Brent L. Fogel and Susan Perlman

History

The cerebellum acts to fluidly integrate multimodal sensory information to predict the effects of motor commands and implement corrections to actively shape movement based on further sensory updates [1]. Clinically, disorders of the cerebellum are most frequently associated with the symptom of ataxia, which is commonly defined as impairment of coordination in the absence of muscle weakness. Although cerebellar dysfunction can manifest in numerous ways, gait abnormalities are often one of the most sensitive signs of cerebellar dysfunction [2] and, in progressive disease, can present quite early in the course. Often patients simply complain of feelings of imbalance or may even report subjective feelings of lower extremity weakness. Observation of the patient and a thorough neurological examination are important tools for identification of an early cerebellar disorder, particularly if it involves only gait, as it can easily be confused with other common disorders. In particular, disorders involving parkinsonism (e.g., Parkinson disease or a related syndrome) and conditions featuring myelopathy, neuropathy, or both can present in a similar fashion during their early stages. Conversely, patients with early cerebellar ataxia may present with generalized complaints such as tremor, diplopia, vertigo, dizziness, muscle weakness, or simply recurrent falls. Occasionally such patients are seen for second opinions of such diagnoses as essential tremor, Parkinson disease, multiple sclerosis, cerebral palsy, and others. Basic screening tests of coordination and balance become essential tools to the physician, enabling proper classification of these patients.

Classification of disorders of the cerebellum is commonly based on etiology with the principal differentiating feature being whether the condition is hereditary, acquired, or sporadic. Often this may not be readily apparent for a given patient, so disorders can be further subdivided by age of onset, typically as early onset if before the age of 20 years [3] or as adult onset. Disease course (static versus progressive) and whether or not the condition is associated with other extracerebellar symptoms are other distinguishing features. Isolation of the disease process to the cerebellum or involvement of other structures such as the brain stem or the spinal cord is another important distinction. Defining a condition as a spinocerebellar ataxia, for example, can strongly influence the diagnostic evaluation as many of the hereditary cerebellar disorders exhibit this pattern of degeneration.

Clinical findings and diagnosis

Ataxia can arise from damage to the cerebellar, vestibular, or proprioceptive systems [4]. The effects of cerebellar ataxia are seen prominently in voluntary movements, which become dysmetric and dyssynergic, and in the muscles that coordinate speech, swallowing and eye movements, resulting in scanning dysarthria, dysphagia, ocular dysmetria, saccadic pursuit, and gaze-evoked nystagmus [4]. The effects on movement are often most noticeable in the gait, as impairment of cerebellar function diminishes the ability to dynamically regulate balance and adapt to changes in terrain leading to a postural instability with a tendency to fall, which often results in the adoption of a wide-based stance and a need for ambulatory support [2,4].

When ataxia results from damage to a single balance system in isolation, that ataxia is described as "pure." A pure cerebellar ataxia can be distinguished from a vestibular disorder by the presence of vertigo, oscillopsia, or past-pointing in the latter, and from a proprioceptive disorder by the presence of joint position/vibration sensory abnormalities and by a worsening of symptoms in the absence of visual cueing [4]. It is important to note that many of the progressive

Uncommon Causes of Movement Disorders, ed. Néstor Gálvez-Jiménez and Paul J. Tuite. Published by Cambridge University Press. © Cambridge University Press 2011.

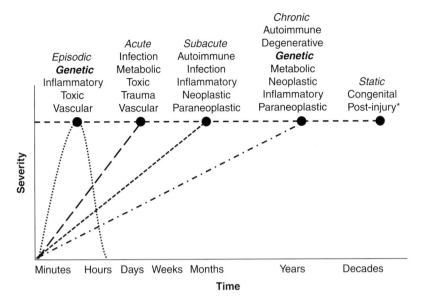

Figure 19.1. Diagnostic considerations based on rate of disease progression. Plots illustrating the various tempos of cerebellar disease are shown. Common etiologies are shown above each line. The tempo of genetic disease is shown in bold. * Nonprogressive cerebellar injury from any source.

hereditary and acquired neurodegenerative ataxias impair all of these systems to some degree so, in these cases, a pure cerebellar ataxia is the exception rather than the rule.

Natural history

The pattern of disease onset and progression can have an important influence on the diagnosis of cerebellar ataxia [4,5] (Figure 19.1). Isolated cerebellar lesions due to trauma, stroke, etc. present suddenly and severely but are essentially stable and may even show improvement to targeted therapies. In contrast, acquired or sporadic causes tend to present acutely or subacutely and subsequently progress, often at a rapid pace. The hereditary cerebellar ataxias are insidious in onset and progress slowly. It may even be difficult for a patient to precisely determine the onset of symptoms in some cases. A detailed family history is an essential component of any history although, for certain hereditary conditions, a negative family history is not uncommon due to extremely late onset of symptoms [6]. Besides probing for a family history of gait and balance disorders, as well as other neurological conditions, individuals should be asked about the occurrence of mental retardation or other developmental disorders as well as early death or disability as these clues may herald an underlying metabolic, mitochondrial, or other hereditary disorder. Ethnic origin can provide important clues as well, as some hereditary disorders are more common in certain geographical regions [3, 7, 8].

Laboratory investigations

A patient presenting with clinical evidence of a progressive cerebellar ataxia requires a thorough evaluation for an acquired cause [6] (Figure 19.2). There are two important reasons for this: (1) as a group, the acquired etiologies are much more common than the hereditary etiologies, and (2) the majority of acquired causes are treatable (or even curable) to varying degrees, whereas the treatment for the vast majority of hereditary disorders remains symptomatic. Even patients with a family history of a hereditary etiology require basic screening as it is not uncommon for both acquired and hereditary conditions to coexist in the same patient, particularly those with late-onset disease [6].

Various algorithms have been proposed to systematically evaluate acquired etiologies [6,9]. The focal point of such evaluations is neuroimaging of the brain, with magnetic resonance imaging the modality of choice [6,9]. Cerebellar insults caused by trauma, vascular lesions, tumors, or congenital abnormalities can be readily identified in this manner [10,11]. Further evaluation is directed toward the identification of underlying autoimmune, endocrine, infectious, inflammatory, metabolic, neoplastic, nutritional, and/or toxic etiologies [6, 9] (Figure 19.2). Such evaluations must be complete as, in late-onset cases, a multifactorial etiology is not an uncommon occurrence.

Among the various etiologies, inflammatory and autoimmune disease are important to consider when evaluating a patient with ataxia, as this may underlie a subset of sporadic ataxia [12]. This includes screening

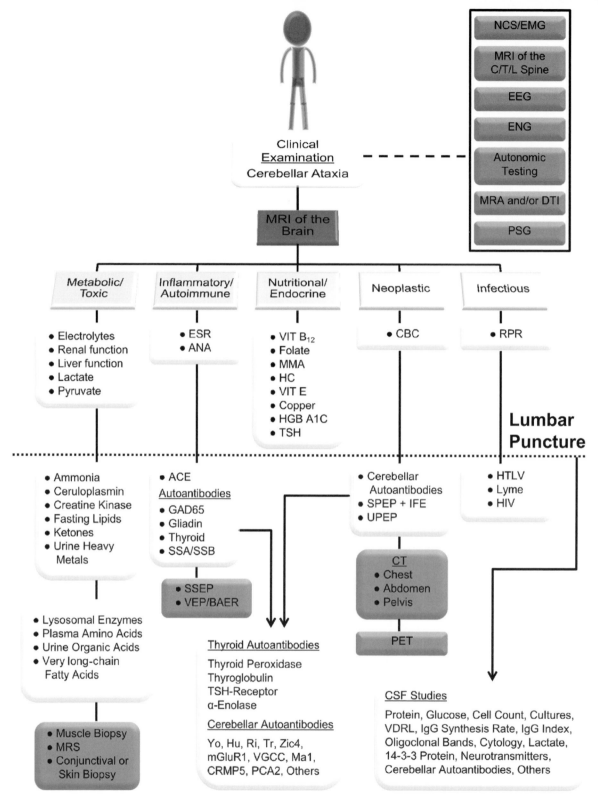

Figure 19.2. Diagnostic evaluation of an acquired cerebellar ataxia. The evaluation begins with a clinical examination. All patients with cerebellar ataxia identified clinically should have an MRI of the brain performed to assess for masses, vascular lesions/anomalies, traumatic injury, and/or structural problems in addition to evidence of neurodegeneration and/or white matter changes. Additional diagnostic studies (gray boxes) should be performed as warranted on the basis of the clinical examination (dashed line). If the MRI does not reveal the cause, then laboratory tests (white boxes) should be performed systematically as indicated. Studies are listed under the heading of the class of disorders they most often identify. Note that some tests could identify disorders in more than one class. In a complete evaluation, a patient should receive all

for collagen vascular disorders [13] and for paraneo-plastic antibodies (e.g., Yo, Hu, Tr, Ri, mGluR1, VGCC, Ma1, CRMP5, Zic4) [14]. There is also evidence supporting glutamic acid decarboxylase (GAD-65), gliadin and thyroid autoantibodies either as disease-causing or as potential markers for an underlying autoimmune process [15], so these should also be tested for.

In patients who have undergone a thorough negative work-up for acquired and hereditary causes, one should consider the diagnosis of multiple system atrophy (MSA), an α-synucleinopathy characterized by varying degrees of autonomic failure, cerebellar ataxia, and/or parkinsonism [16]. In the remaining patients who do not meet this criterion, idiopathic late-onset cerebellar ataxia (ILOCA) becomes a consideration. Although well-established in the literature, ILOCA is essentially a classification of as-yet-to-be-explained ataxias, as evidenced by the fact that about one-third eventually develop MSA [17]. It is possible that these patients, or subsets thereof, represent currently unidentified genetic ataxias [18].

Genetics

The hereditary ataxias are a diverse group of neurogenetic disorders whose members can present themselves at all stages of life, often with complex and detailed phenotypes. The one commonality among them is cerebellar ataxia, although the severity can range from mild to profound. A number of recent publications address the various classes of disorders and their differential diagnosis in great detail [3,7–9], which is beyond the scope of this chapter. Here we hope to present a flavor of the diversity of the heritable ataxias and provide a sense of the basic diagnostic evaluation.

Autosomal recessive hereditary ataxias

The autosomal recessive cerebellar ataxias are an incredibly rich and diverse group of disorders. Although typical age of onset is early, prior to age 20 years, there has been a growing recognition that milder forms of these disorders can present at essentially any age [3,8,9]. Additionally, in contrast to the autosomal dominant disorders, the precise definition of an autosomal recessive cerebellar ataxia is debatable as there is no universal classification system in wide usage. This presents a challenge as there are a number of metabolic, mitochondrial and storage disorders, or other syndromes which include ataxia as a relatively common or occasional feature yet may be better characterized by other aspects of their phenotype. Our preference here is to focus on those disorders for which cerebellar dysfunction and ataxia are key defining diagnostic features [3]. Because of the phenotypic variability seen among individual diseases associated with ataxia, as well as in late-onset presentations of well-characterized childhood diseases, we also do not include disorders defined only by a locus or by a clinical phenotype. For completeness, we refer readers to other works that discuss related disorders featuring ataxia in more detail, e.g., [8,9,19].

Currently, there are 19 autosomal recessive cerebellar ataxias with identified genes and characterized mutations (Table 19.1). As a group, the autosomal recessive hereditary cerebellar ataxias are probably of a similar prevalence to the autosomal dominant, although there is much variability between geographic regions and ethnicities [8]. Furthermore, an accurate number is difficult to determine given the difficulties in grouping the disorders as described above. It is clear, however, that Friedreich ataxia is the most common of the autosomal recessive disorders, as well as the most common hereditary ataxia worldwide, with a prevalence of approximately 1 case in 30 000–50 000 people and a carrier frequency as high as 1 in 85 [3,20]. Ataxia-telangiectasia appears to be the next most common, perhaps as high as 1 case in 40 000 individuals, but this number may vary considerably [3,8,20].

Caption for Figure 19.2. (*cont.*)

studies listed above the dotted line. Items listed below the dotted line are chosen for more in-depth evaluation of specific etiologies and not all patients may require all studies. The dotted line represents the threshold for performing a lumbar puncture in a patient undergoing an initial work-up. Suggested CSF studies are indicated (arrow). Specific cerebellar antibodies (also called paraneoplastic antibodies) and thyroid autoantibodies are also shown (arrow). Note that this is a general scheme that is appropriate for most patients, but there are additional rare causes of cerebellar ataxia that are not listed.

Abbreviations: ACE = angiotensin converting enzyme, ANA = anti-nuclear antibodies, BAER = brain stem auditory evoked response, CBC = complete blood count, C/T/L = cervical, thoracic, and/or lumbar, CSF = cerebral spinal fluid, CT = computed tomography, DTI = diffusion tensor imaging, EEG = electroencephalogram, EMG = electromyogram, ENG = electronystagmogram, ESR = erythrocyte sedimentation rate, GAD = glutamic acid decarboxylase, HC = homocysteine, HGB = hemoglobin, HIV = human immunodeficiency virus, HTLV = human T-lymphotropic virus, IFE = immunofixation electrophoresis, MMA = methylmalonic acid, MRI = magnetic resonance imaging, MRA = magnetic resonance angiography, MRS = magnetic resonance spectroscopy, NCS = nerve conduction study, PET = positron emission tomography, PSG = polysomnogram, RPR = rapid plasma reagin, SSA/SSB = Sjögren syndrome antigen, SPEP = serum protein electrophoresis, SSEP = somatosensory evoked potentials, TSH = thyroid stimulating hormone, UPEP = urine protein electrophoresis, VDRL = venereal disease research laboratory test, VEP = visual evoked potential, VIT = vitamin.

Table 19.1. Autosomal recessive spinocerebellar ataxias.

Disease	Abbreviation	Locus	Gene	Protein	Function[a]	Phenotype[b]
Class I: Friedrich ataxia-like disorders						
Friedreich ataxia	FRDA	9q13	FXN	Frataxin[c]	Mitochondrial metabolism	**CM**, DM, GFI, HL, **PN**, SCD, SCO
Ataxia with vitamin E deficiency	AVED	8q13.1-q13.3	TTPA	Alpha-tocopherol transfer protein	Vitamin E metabolism	**PN**, **PR**, TR
Abetalipoproteinemia	ABL	4q22-q24	MTP	Microsomal triglyceride transfer protein	Lipoprotein metabolism	**LM**, PN, **PR**
Refsum disease	RD	10pter-p11.2	PHYH	Phytanoyl-CoA hydroxylase	Fatty acid metabolism	**AN**, CM, HL, PN, **PR**
		6q22-q24	PEX7	Peroxin-7	Peroxisomal import	
Class II: Friedrich ataxia-like disorders with cerebellar atrophy						
Late-onset Tay–Sachs	LOTS	15q23-q24	HEXA	Hexosaminidase A	Ganglioside metabolism	CVL, DEM, **EPS**, PN, PS, **PSY**, SZ
Cerebrotendinous xanthomatosis	CTX	2q33-qter	CYP27	Sterol 27-hydroxylase	Bile acid metabolism	**CAT**, CVL, DEM, DIA, EPS, PN, PS, PSY, SZ, **TX**, WM
DNA polymerase gamma disorders[d]	POLG[d]	15q25	POLG	DNA polymerase gamma	Mitochondrial DNA metabolism	CVL, **DEM**, EPS, HL, MY, OP, PN, PSY, **SZ**, TR, WM
Spinocerebellar ataxia with axonal neuropathy	SCAN1	14q31-q32	TDP1	Tyrosyl-DNA phoshodiesterase-1	DNA repair	CVL, **PN**
Autosomal recessive cerebellar ataxia, type 1	ARCA1	6q25	SYNE1	Synaptic nuclear envelope protein-1	Cerebellar architecture	**AO**, CVL, HR, **PC**, SAC
Class III: Early-onset disorders with cerebellar atrophy						
Ataxia telangiectasia	AT	11q22.3	ATM	Ataxia-telangiectasia mutated	DNA repair	CVL, EPS, ID, NEO, **OA**, PN, RS, **TEL**
Ataxia telangiectasia-like disorder	ATLD	11q21	MRE11	Meiotic recombination-11	DNA repair	CVL, EPS, **OA**, PN, RS
Ataxia with oculomotor apraxia, type 1	AOA1	9p13.3	APTX	Aprataxin	DNA repair	CVL, DEM, EPS, GFI, **OA**, OPA, **PN**, SCO

Disease	Abbreviation	Locus	Protein	Function	Clinical features
Ataxia with oculomotor apraxia, type 2	AOA2	9q34	Senataxin	DNA repair, transcription, RNA processing	CVL, EPS, **OA, PN**, PS, TR
Autosomal recessive ataxia of Charlevoix–Saguenay	ARSACS	13q12	Sacsin	Protein folding and/or quality control	CVL, DEM, HMR, **HR**, PN, **PS**, SAC, SCD
Infantile-onset spinocerebellar ataxia	IOSCA	10q24	Twinkle, twinky	Mitochondrial DNA metabolism	CVL, DEM, **EPS**, HG, HL, OP, **PN**, SCD, SZ
Cayman ataxia	CA	19p13.3	Caytaxin	Glutamate signaling	CVL, **PC, PSY**, TR
Marinesco–Sjögren syndrome	MSS	5q31	BiP-associated protein	Protein folding and/or quality control	**CAT**, CVL, HG, MR, **MYO**, PN, PSY
Autosomal recessive cerebellar ataxia, type 2	ARCA2	1q42.2	aarF domain-containing kinase-3	CoQ_{10} synthesis, mitochondrial metabolism	CVL, **MR, PC**
Dysequilibrium syndrome	DES	9p24	Very low-density lipoprotein receptor	Intracellular signaling	CVL, HR, **MR, QG**, SZ
	CA8	8q11-q12	Carbonic anhydrase VIII	Intracellular calcium signaling	

The known autosomal recessive spinocerebellar ataxias are listed. Typical age of onset is in childhood or early adulthood, less than the age of 25 years, although many disorders can atypically present in later life. The Class III early-onset disorders typically present before age 5 years (see text for details). Gene, protein, genetic loci, function, and clinical features are as reported in reference 70 or from references indicated in the text. Excepted as noted, all pathogenic mutations produce a change in the expressed protein sequence, reduce gene expression, or involve gene deletions.

Clinical abbreviations: AN = anosmia, AO = typical age of onset greater than 25 years, CAT = cataracts, CM = cardiomyopathy, CVL = cerebellar atrophy, DEM = dementia, DIA = chronic diarrhea, DM = diabetes mellitus, EPS = extrapyramidal signs, GFI = gaze fixation instability, HG = hypogonadism, HL = hearing loss, HMR = hypermyelinated retinal fibers, HR = hyperreflexia, ID = immunodeficiency, LM = lipid malabsorption, MR = mental retardation, MY = myoclonus, MYO = myopathy, NEO = increased predisposition to cancer, OA = oculomotor apraxia, OP = ophthalmoparesis, OPA = optic atrophy, PC = pure cerebellar ataxia, PN = polyneuropathy, PR = pigmentary retinopathy, PS = pyramidal signs, PSY = psychiatric symptoms, QG = quadrupedal gait, RS = radiosensitivity, SAC = abnormal saccades, SCD = spinal cord atrophy, SCO = scoliosis, SZ = seizures, TEL = oculocutaneous telangiectasias, TR = tremor, TX = tendon xanthomas, WM = white matter changes on MRI.

[a] In many cases, the functions of these proteins are speculative and not well characterized. Proteins may also have other functions besides those listed.

[b] Phenotype represents selected clinical features that may aid in diagnosis. Clinical features of particular usefulness are highlighted in bold type. Not all features will be present in all patients. Cerebellar ataxia is a common clinical characteristic in all patients.

[c] Compound heterozygotes with a point mutation on one allele are seen in about 2% of patients [3].

[d] Includes mitochondrial recessive ataxia syndrome (MIRAS).

In those genes that have been most well studied, pathogenesis generally appears to result from a loss of specific gene function, which, in turn, impacts vital cellular pathways and appears to promote oxidative stress, contribute to genetic instability, and/or disrupt normal metabolism, leading to premature cell death [3]. This has been best studied in Friedreich ataxia where, most commonly, an intronic GAA triplet repeat expansion acts to reduce gene expression, leading to mitochondrial dysfunction, increased oxidative stress and cell damage [3,21]. Unlike the autosomal dominant disorders, Friedreich ataxia is the only autosomal recessive disorder commonly caused by a repeat expansion [3]. The other autosomal recessive ataxias are thought to arise from causes including dysfunction of various organelles such as the peroxisome (RD), the lysosome (LOTS), the mitochondria (CTX, POLG, IOSCA, ARCA2), or impairment of other basic cell functions such as DNA repair (AT, ATLD, AOA1, AOA2, SCAN1), transcription and RNA processing (AOA2), protein folding/quality control (ARSACS, MSS), lipoprotein metabolism (AVED, ABL), or signaling pathways (CA, DES) [3,8,19,22–29]. Additionally, although not yet well-studied, ARCA1 may result from impaired cerebellar structural integrity [30].

Clinically, the autosomal recessive ataxias are characterized by cerebellar or spinocerebellar involvement, commonly associated with a peripheral sensory or sensorimotor neuropathy that features posterior column involvement and/or areflexia, and often show involvement of other systems outside the nervous system [3,8]. We prefer to group the autosomal recessive cerebellar ataxias into clinical categories (Table 19.1) based on phenotypic similarities to Friedreich ataxia and to each other [3]. The first group (FRDA, AVED, ABL and RD) share the closest phenotypic characteristics with Friedreich ataxia, namely, a teenage-onset cerebellar ataxia and prominent sensory neuropathy with loss of vibration and proprioceptive sense, reduced deep tendon reflexes, and normal cerebellar imaging studies [3,8,31]. While Friedreich ataxia often is associated with the extraneurological symptoms of scoliosis, diabetes, and/or cardiomyopathy, the other disorders of the class typically lack these but do share another feature, pigmentary retinopathy [3,8,31]. The second class (LOTS, CTX, POLG, SCAN1 and ARCA1) also present phenotypically similarly to Friedreich ataxia but all have cerebellar atrophy on imaging [3,8,30]. LOTS, CTX and POLG disorders can also present with seizures, extrapyramidal signs, dementia, and psychiatric symptoms

[3,8]. POLG disorders can show ophthalmoplegia and both POLG disorders and CTX can have white matter changes on MRI [3,8]. ARCA1 is unique because of a typical onset after age 30 and an essentially pure cerebellar phenotype [30]. The third class encompasses the remaining disorders and is notable for cerebellar atrophy as well as an earlier typical age of onset, generally before the age of 5 years [3,8]. AOA1 and AOA2 are exceptions to this but are included because, along with AT and ATLD, they involve DNA repair pathways and share similar clinical features with oculomotor apraxia and extrapyramidal signs [3,8,25]. Ataxia telangiectasia is quite recognizable because of the presence of oculocutaneous telangiectasias, and there is also a predisposition to cancer [3,8,25]. ARSACS is characterized by prominent upper motor neuron signs with hyperreflexia, while ARCA2, MSS and DES feature varying degrees of mental retardation, and CA is an essentially pure cerebellar ataxia [3,8,22,24,26–28,32,33]. In contrast to the autosomal dominant cerebellar ataxias, the diversity of phenotypes for the autosomal recessive disorders lend themselves more readily for use as a diagnostic tool (Table 19.1). Furthermore, a number of serum screening tests exist for many of these disorders [3], which can cost-effectively be performed prior to initiating genetic testing.

Autosomal dominant hereditary ataxias

The autosomal dominant hereditary ataxias are often synonymous with the term "spinocerebellar ataxia" and the majority are characterized by that term, regardless of clinical phenotype. Currently, there are 32 designated autosomal dominant ataxias (encompassing at least 29 distinct disorders as a result of redundancies and misassignments) and for 18 of these the causative gene is known and disease-causing mutations have been characterized (Table 19.2). As a group, their prevalence has been estimated as high as 4 cases per 100 000 individuals worldwide, although this number varies considerably among different geographic locations and ethnic populations, and by individual disease [7,8]. SCA3 appears to be the most prevalent disorder worldwide, causing 25–30% of all autosomal dominant ataxia, with SCA1, SCA2 and SCA6 together accounting for another 30–35% [7,8]. Typically, with only a few exceptions, these are disorders of early and middle adulthood, with the typical age of onset between ages 20 and 50 years [7]. The exceptions to this are SCA6, SCA23 and SCA30, which tend to begin after age 50, and SCA18, SCA21 and SCA28, which tend to begin

Table 19.2. Autosomal dominant spinocerebellar ataxias.

Disease	Locus	Gene	Mutation[a]	Protein	Function[b]	Phenotype[c]
SCA1	6p23	ATXN1	CAG rpt	Ataxin-1	Transcription	**OP**, PN, **PS**, SAC
SCA2	12q24	ATXN2	CAG rpt	Ataxin-2	RNA processing	EPS, MY, **OP**, **PN**, SAC, TR
SCA3	14q24.3-q31	ATXN3	CAG rpt	Ataxin-3	Protein quality control	**EPS**, OP, PN, **PS**
SCA4	16q22.1[d]	nd[d]	nd	nd	nd	PN
SCA5	11q13	SPTBN2	Functional	Beta-III spectrin	Glutamate signaling, protein trafficking	PC
SCA6	19p13	CACNA1A	CAG rpt	Ca$_V$2.1	Calcium channel	**LO**, PC
SCA7	3p21.1-p12	ATXN7	CAG rpt	Ataxin-7	Transcription	OP, **PR**, PS, SAC
SCA8	13q21	ATXN8	CAG rpt	Ataxin-8	Unknown	PN, **PS**
		ATXN8OS	noncoding CUG rpt	None	Unknown	
SCA9	nd[e]	nd	nd	nd	nd	**EPS**, **OP**, PN, PS
SCA10	22q13	ATXN10	Intronic AATTCT rpt	Ataxin-10	Unknown	**SZ**
SCA11	15q15.2	TTBK2	Functional	Tau tubulin kinase-2	Tau phosphorylation	**PC**
SCA12	5q31-q33	PPP2R2B	5UTR CAG rpt	Protein phosphatase 2 regulatory subunit B, beta	Mitochondrial morphogenesis	DEM, EPS, PN, PS, **TR**
SCA13	19q13.3-q13.4	KCNC3	Functional	K$_V$3.3	Potassium channel	**MR**, PS
SCA14	19q13.4	PRKCG	Functional	Protein kinase C gamma	Intracellular signaling	DEM, MY, **PC**
SCA15	3p26-p25	ITPR1	Functional	Inositol 1,4,5-triphosphate receptor, type 1	Intracellular ligand-gated calcium channel	**PC**, TR
SCA16	na[f]	—	—	—	—	—
SCA17	6q27	TBP	CAG rpt	TATA box-binding protein	Transcription	**DEM**, **EPS**, PSY, SZ
SCA18	7q22-q32	nd	nd	nd	nd	**EO**, PN
SCA19	*1p21-q21[g]*	nd	nd	nd	nd	**DEM**, MY
SCA20	11p12.2-q12.3	nd	Gene duplication	nd	nd	**PT**
SCA21	7p21.3-p15.1	nd	nd	nd	nd	DEM, **EO**, EPS, TR
SCA22	1p21-q23[g]	nd	nd	nd	nd	**PC**
SCA23	20p13-p12.3	nd	nd	nd	nd	**LO**, PN, PS, SAC

Table 19.2. (*cont.*)

Disease	Locus	Gene	Mutation[a]	Protein	Function[b]	Phenotype[c]
SCA24	na[h]	-	-	-	-	-
SCA25	2p21-p13	nd	nd	nd	nd	**PN**
SCA26	19p13.3	nd	nd	nd	nd	**PC**
SCA27	13q34	FGF14	Functional	fibroblast growth factor-14	Synaptic function	EPS, PSY, **TR**
SCA28	18p11.22-q11.2	AFG3L2	Functional	SCA28	Mitochondrial protein quality control	**EO**, OP, PS
SCA29	3p26[i]	nd	nd	nd	nd	**EO**[i]
SCA30	4q34.3-q35.1	nd	nd	nd	nd	**LO**, **PC**, SAC
DRPLA	12p13.31	ATN1	CAG rpt	Atrophin-1	Transcription	**DEM**, **EPS**, MY, PSY, SZ
16q-ADCA[j]	16q22.1[d]	PLEKHG4[d, j]	5UTR	Puratrophin-1	Intracellular signaling, Golgi function	**PC**

The known autosomal dominant spinocerebellar ataxias (SCAs) are listed. Except as noted, typical age of onset is in adulthood, between the ages of 20 and 50 years. Gene, protein, genetic loci, mutations, function, and clinical features are as reported in references 70 and 71 or from references cited in the text.

Abbreviations: 5UTR = 5′ untranslated region, ADCA = autosomal dominant cerebellar ataxia, DRPLA = dentatorubral-pallidoluysian atrophy, na = locus is not assigned, nd = not determined, rpt = nucleotide repeat expansion.

Clinical abbreviations: DEM = dementia, EO = average age of onset < 20 years, EPS = extrapyramidal signs, LO = average age of onset >50 years, MR = mental retardation, MY = myoclonus, OP = ophthalmoparesis, PC = pure cerebellar ataxia, PN = polyneuropathy, PR = pigmentary retinopathy, PS = pyramidal signs, PSY = psychiatric symptoms, PT = palatal tremor, SAC = abnormal saccades, SZ = seizures, TR = tremor.

[a] Mutations are listed as functional if they either produce a change in the expressed protein sequence, reduce gene expression, or involve gene deletions.

[b] In many cases, the functions of these proteins are speculative and not well characterized. Proteins may also have other functions besides those listed.

[c] Phenotype represents selected clinical features that may aid in diagnosis. Clinical features of particular usefulness are highlighted in bold type. Not all features will be present in all patients and/or additional features may also be present. Cerebellar ataxia is a common clinical characteristic for all patients.

[d] The SCA4 locus on 16q22.1 overlaps with the PLEKHG4 locus defined for a hereditary autosomal dominant ataxia described in several Japanese families, but the two conditions appear to differ both phenotypically and genotypically [45].

[e] This disease name was assigned to a phenotype seen in an American family of British origin [72], but has not yet been further characterized molecularly.

[f] SCA16 was originally defined as a separate disease; however, molecular studies ultimately revealed it to be caused by mutation of the same gene as SCA15 [43].

[g] SCA19 and SCA22 may be allelic to one another [73].

[h] The phenotype that was designated SCA24 was found to be autosomal recessive [74].

[i] SCA29 is a congenital nonprogressive ataxia that has been shown to represent a genetically heterogeneous phenotype [36].

[j] During publication of this chapter a noncoding insertion and pentanucleotide repeat intergenic to the BEAN and TK2 genes was reported as the causative mutation in these patients and renamed as SCA31 [75].

before the age of 20 [7,8,34,35]. Additionally, SCA29 is defined as congenital but may not be a distinct disorder [36].

Seven of these disorders (SCA1, SCA2, SCA3, SCA6, SCA7, SCA17 and DRPLA) arise from expansion of a CAG triplet-repeat region within the gene and likely share a common pathogenesis, whereby expression of the corresponding large polyglutamine tract within the protein either exerts a toxic effect directly, through the impairment of basic cellular processes, and/or disrupts an essential function of the specific protein [7,8,37–39]. Recently, the loci of another disease, SCA8, which had originally been described as resulting from a noncoding CTG repeat expansion, was reported to be bidirectionally expressed, with the reading frame on the opposing strand expressing the repeats as CAG and generating a pure polyglutamine expansion protein [40]. The precise mechanism of

SCA8 pathogenesis remains under investigation but may be similar to the other triplet repeat disorders. Two additional disorders, SCA10 and SCA12, involve noncoding repeat expansions which may cause disease by altering gene expression or through RNA-mediated effects [8,37,41]. Repeat disorders are often more recognizable in families due to anticipation, whereby longer repeat lengths tend to be unstable and grow larger in subsequent generations, which generally results in more severe disease in the younger generations as there is a genotype–phenotype correlation with repeat length [7,8].

The majority of the remaining SCA genes are affected by a variety of genetic mutations that are predicted to disrupt the function of the corresponding protein product and thus cause disease (Table 19.2). The one potential exception currently known is SCA20, which appears to be caused through the duplication of one or more as-yet-unidentified genes [42], although exactly how this leads to disease has yet to be determined. Possible molecular etiologies of the various SCAs include impairment of transcription (SCA1, SCA7, SCA17, DRPLA), RNA processing (SCA2), protein trafficking or quality control (SCA3, SCA5, SCA28), signaling pathways (SCA5, SCA14, SCA15, 16q-ADCA), ion channel function (SCA6, SCA13), tau phosphorylation (SCA11), mitochondrial morphogenesis (SCA12), synaptic plasticity (SCA27), mitochondrial function (SCA28), and function of the Golgi apparatus (16q-ADCA) [8,37,41,43–45].

Clinically the autosomal dominant disorders are quite heterogeneous (Table 19.2). In addition to cerebellar ataxia, these disorders can present with a variety of extracerebellar findings such as dementia, retinopathy, extrapyramidal signs, spasticity, varying degrees of peripheral neuropathy and/or autonomic dysfunction, psychiatric symptoms, and/or seizures [7,8]. A classification scheme originally devised by Harding is still in wide use [37,46], and essentially can be broken down into three classes consisting of SCA with pigmentary retinopathy (ADCA Class II; SCA7), pure cerebellar ataxias (ADCA Class III; SCA5, SCA6, SCA11, SCA14, SCA15, SCA22, SCA26, SCA30, 16q-ADCA), and all others (ADCA Class I). The diagnostic utility of finding pigmentary retinopathy is well established [47] but the utility of the other classifications is less so, as the phenotypes are very generalized and include many different disorders. More specific phenotypic descriptions are also of limited usefulness, as the various disorders can show considerable overlap and

phenotype may markedly vary among individuals with the same disease, thus making diagnosis extremely difficult by clinical features alone. Assessment of the clinical phenotype can aid in diagnosis [7,8,47], especially rarer features such as the previously mentioned pigmentary retinopathy of SCA7 or the palatal tremor of SCA20 [8,47]; however, we find clinical features most useful as a guide to the selection of genetic testing. As the cost of extensive genetic testing can be substantial, we generally refrain from ordering comprehensive genetic screening panels since a good clinical examination coupled with a detailed medical and family history can often narrow the selection considerably. However, given the clinical heterogeneity of the autosomal dominant SCAs, it may often be necessary to test several genes at once and, in some cases, to test one or more genes solely on the basis of ethnic and/or geographic considerations.

Other hereditary ataxias

In addition to the autosomal dominant and recessive disorders mentioned above, it is important to include a brief discussion of the X-linked and episodic disorders because of their clinical relevance in the evaluation of the ataxic patient. While there are other classes of disorders that can also present with cerebellar ataxia, e.g., mitochondrial disorders, we will not discuss these here as ataxia is more commonly an associated feature as opposed to a defining symptom.

When faced with a late-onset cerebellar ataxia, especially in a male patient, an essential consideration is Fragile-X-associated tremor ataxia syndrome (FXTAS) [8,9,48] (Table 19.3). FXTAS is caused by a 55–200 CGG repeat expansion in the FMR1, the gene that causes Fragile X syndrome when over 200 repeats are present [8,9,48]. As many as 1 in 3000 men are affected with FXTAS and female carriers can occasionally be symptomatic [48]. All late-onset ataxic patients should therefore be assessed for a family history of male mental retardation in subsequent generations as the repeats may further expand.

The final class of disorders for discussion are the episodic ataxias, which are autosomal dominant diseases associated with ion channel mutations that generally present with recurrent ataxia associated with vertigo [8,9,49] (Table 19.3). In contrast to the other autosomal dominant spinocerebellar ataxias, episodic ataxias are not always progressive [49]. Two of the progressive ataxias, SCA6 and SCA13, are also caused by

Table 19.3. X-linked and episodic hereditary ataxias.

Disease	Locus	Gene	Protein	Function[a]	Phenotype[b]
X-linked hereditary ataxia					
Fragile X-associated tremor ataxia syndrome (FXTAS)	Xq27.3	FMR1[c]	Fragile X mental retardation protein	mRNA translation	CVL, DEM, EPS, **LO**, PN, **TR**, WM
Autosomal dominant episodic ataxias					
EA1	12p13	KCNA1	$K_V1.1$	Potassium channel	**MIN**, **MYK**, STR
EA2	19p13	CACNA1A[d]	$Ca_V2.1$	Calcium channel	**HRS**, **NYS**, STR, SZ, VTG
EA3	1q42	nd	nd	nd	**TIN**, **VTG**
EA4	nd	nd	nd	nd	**NYS**, **VTG**
EA5	2q22-q23	CACNB4	Beta-4 subunit of $Ca_V2.1$	Calcium channel	**HRS**, NYS, **SZ**, VTG
EA6	5p13	SLC1A3	Glial high-affinity glutamate transporter	Glutamate reuptake	**HMP**, **SZ**, VTG
EA7	19q13	nd	nd	nd	**HRS**, STR, **VTG**

The known X-linked and episodic autosomal dominant spinocerebellar ataxias are listed. Except as noted, typical age of onset is in childhood or early adulthood, prior to age 20 years. Gene, protein, genetic loci, function, and clinical features are as reported in reference 70 or from references cited in the text. Genetic mutations, except as noted, either produce a change in the expressed protein sequence, reduce gene expression, or involve gene deletions.
Abbreviations: nd = not determined.
Clinical Abbreviations: CVL = cerebellar atrophy, DEM = dementia, EPS = extrapyramidal signs, HMP = hemiplegia, HRS = attacks last hours, LO = average age of onset >50 years, MIN = attacks last seconds to minutes, MYK = myokymia, NYS = nystagmus, PN = polyneuropathy, STR = attack triggered by emotional stress, SZ = seizures, TIN = tinnitus, TR = tremor, VTG = vertigo, WM = white matter changes on MRI.
[a] Proteins may also have other functions besides those listed.
[b] Phenotype represents selected clinical features that may aid in diagnosis. Clinical features of particular usefulness are highlighted in bold type. Not all features will be present in all patients and/or additional features may also be present. Cerebellar ataxia is a common clinical characteristic for all patients. Patients with episodic features can also have varying degrees of progressive ataxia.
[c] FXTAS is caused by expansion of noncoding CGG repeats in the FMR1 gene to between 55 and 200 copies. This is called a premutation as expansions over 200 cause Fragile X syndrome [8,9,48].
[d] Mutations of this gene also cause SCA6 and familial hemiplegic migraine [8, 49].

mutations in ion channels, and, interestingly, mutations in the SCA6 gene CACNA1A, distinct from the CAG repeat, cause one of the episodic ataxias, EA2 [8,9,49]. Onset of the episodic ataxias is typically in childhood or early adulthood [8,9,49]. Seven different disorders are described, although only four (EA1, EA2, EA5 and EA6) have identified genes with known causative mutations [8,49].

Evaluation for genetic causes

Given the complexity of the hereditary cerebellar ataxias, diagnostic evaluation can be daunting. While the generation of a comprehensive protocol for systematic evaluation is difficult, there are several effective examples in the literature [3,9,20,31]. We propose a more fluid framework for shaping and guiding the genetic evaluation (Figure 19.3). The keys to a successful

outcome are a detailed medical history, family history, and clinical neurological examination. Often this will provide the most important clues to direct the investigation toward a solution within a structured framework. We do not recommend an evaluation be undertaken without such framework as the time and cost involved in genetic testing can be substantial and an evaluation lacking structure could easily overlook a quick solution or neglect to include important differentials. With the advent of genetic screening panels and the time pressures of the clinic, it is sadly often easier for clinicians to "test everything" rather than select tests based on clinical criteria and judgment, a practice we feel does a great disservice to the patient in terms of cost and time. We therefore would suggest a practice of referral to a specialty center for complete diagnostic work-up if time or resources are not available for a detailed systematic evaluation. Recent technological

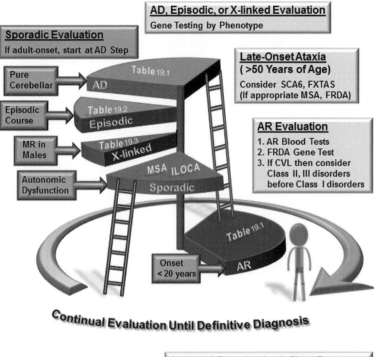

Figure 19.3. Diagnostic evaluation for suspected genetic causes of cerebellar ataxia. Prior to initiating this evaluation, all patients are to be screened for acquired causes of cerebellar ataxia (Figure 19.2). This algorithm is designed for patients with either (1) a positive family history for cerebellar ataxia or (2) sporadic onset and an appropriate clinical phenotype. The design is a "staircase" where platforms represent diagnostic evaluations and vertical distance represents phenotypic similarity between classes of disorders. If family history is consistent with an autosomal recessive (AR) phenotype the evaluation begins there (AR evaluation), if inheritance is autosomal dominant (AD), episodic, or X-linked then those evaluations are conducted first (ladder and steps). The appropriate tables in this chapter for phenotype and genetic considerations are indicated. The two sporadic disorders for consideration, idiopathic late-onset cerebellar ataxia (ILOCA) and multiple system atrophy (MSA) are also shown. These are, in general, diagnoses of exclusion; see the text for details. Text in white boxes refers to specific diagnostic strategies or testing. Special consideration is given for genetic testing in cerebellar ataxia of late-onset. Text in gray boxes represents important clinical clues to specific evaluations in a patient with sporadic cerebellar ataxia. If the evaluations at a particular step are unsuccessful then the evaluation is carried to the next clinically appropriate step along the staircase. If the evaluation is completed without successful resolution, it may be reinitiated with a different focus or reexamined periodically to determine whether new genetic testing options have become available that would be relevant to the patient (ladder and arrow). Abbreviations: CVL = cerebellar atrophy on magnetic resonance imaging, FRDA = Friedreich ataxia, FXTAS = fragile X-associated tremor ataxia syndrome, MR = mental retardation, SCA = spinocerebellar ataxia. See Table 19.1 for abbreviations used for autosomal recessive ataxia blood tests.

advances suggest that we may soon be able to rapidly, accurately and cheaply sequence individual genomes [50], which may render the need for such testing algorithms obsolete, but until that time we would advocate the use of judicious and systematic testing protocols.

Pathology and neuroimaging

The term most commonly applied to the pattern of degeneration seen in the majority of cerebellar ataxias is olivopontocerebellar atrophy (OPCA) [17]. OPCA is applied to individuals showing atrophy of the cerebellum, the brain stem (especially the pons) and the cervical spinal cord [17,51]. This pattern is caused by extensive neurodegeneration that extends beyond the cerebellar cortex to involve the pontine, inferior olivary, arcuate, and pontobulbar nuclei, resulting in demyelination and gliosis [17]. T2-weighted hyperintensities can be seen diffusely in the middle cerebellar peduncles [51] and in

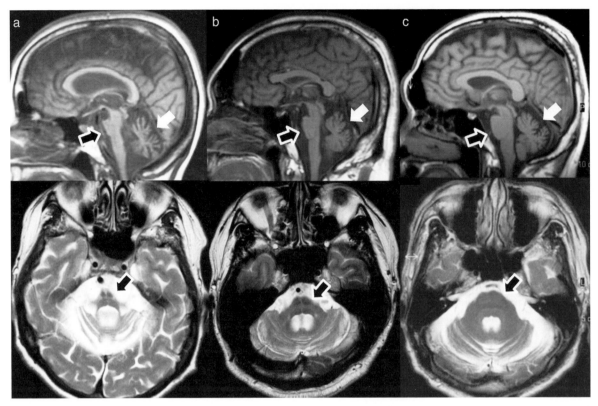

Figure 19.4. Imaging cerebellar ataxia. Magnetic resonance imaging is shown for three patients with (a) spinocerebellar ataxia type 2 (SCA2), (b) multiple system atrophy (MSA), and (c) spinocerebellar ataxia type 6 (SCA6). Panels (a) and (b) represent the cerebellar-plus syndrome, also called olivopontocerebellar atrophy (OPCA), whereas panel (c) represents a pure cerebellar atrophy. In the sagittal T1-weighted images (upper panels), note significant cerebellar atrophy (closed white arrows) in all three panels with atrophy of the pons (open white arrows) in panels (a) and (b) but not panel (c), which is normal. In the axial T2-weighted images (lower panels) note atrophy of the pons with a loss of transverse fibers, the so-called "cross sign," (open white arrows) in panels (a) and (b) while (c) is normal.

a cruciform pattern within the pons due to a loss of the transverse fibers [51] – the so-called "cross sign," which is commonly associated with multiple system atrophy but is not specific for the disease [17,52,53]. Although often descriptively linked with many of the hereditary autosomal dominant ataxias, OPCA is not specific for this and can be seen in other acquired or sporadic ataxias including multiple system atrophy, metabolic conditions, mitochondrial disease, or even prion disorders [11,17]. For this reason, the term "cerebellar-plus syndrome" has been suggested instead of OPCA [11,17]. Examples of these findings are shown in Figure 19.4. In addition to a cerebellar-plus syndrome, many of the hereditary ataxias can demonstrate a pattern of cerebellar atrophy without brain stem or spinal cord involvement [3,51]. Friedreich ataxia commonly shows a distinct pattern with isolated spinal cord atrophy [51], which can aid diagnosis [3]. In adults and children, pattern recognition approaches may prove useful for

differentiating among cases with atypical features such as white matter abnormalities or basal ganglia involvement, but diagnosis often requires further confirmatory investigations [3,54]. In adults, MRI characteristics may be useful in aiding the differentiation of the hereditary spinocerebellar ataxias at advanced stages, but earlier in the course this is less helpful due to similarities in the disorders at that stage [53]. Preliminary evidence suggests that diffusion tensor imaging may ultimately be a more useful modality in differentiating these etiologies [52].

Management

Many of the acquired causes of ataxia have treatments that either are definitive or have been shown to be effective, a fact that further illustrates the need for insuring that such processes are not contributing to the disease process. Some of these treatments are straightforward (e.g., supplementation for nutritional deficiencies), but the management of more complicated disorders (e.g., autoimmune, endocrine, inflammatory, or neoplastic) can often be quite detailed and may require the enlistment of a specialist in that particular field. Depending on the degree of cerebellar injury, the goal of treatment is generally not to restore premorbid function, as the majority of neuronal damage is generally irreversible, but rather to halt the degenerative progression, making the condition more amendable to symptomatic and rehabilitative treatments [5].

Specific treatments of important consideration are immunomodulating therapies (corticosteroids, plasmapheresis, intravenous immunoglobulin, etc.) for inflammatory and autoimmune disease [5] and treatment of the underlying neoplasm in paraneoplastic disease. Specialty care is essential in paraneoplastic cases as immunomodulating treatments are rarely effective, with the most definitive treatment being removal of the inciting tumor [14].

For some of the metabolic cerebellar ataxias, supplementation of a missing nutrient or restriction of a toxic substance can have significant symptomatic benefit, generally by arresting the neurodegenerative process. In this way, AVED can be treated with supplementation of vitamin E, ABL with lipid-soluble vitamins and dietary modification, RD with dietary restriction of foods high in phytanic acid, CTX with chenodeoxycholic acid to replace bile acids, and ARCA2 with coenzyme Q_{10} [3, 22].

Treatment of the other hereditary ataxias is generally symptomatic as definitive or curative treatments are currently not yet available. However, it must be emphasized that these symptomatic treatments can dramatically improve quality of life for these individuals and should be offered to all ataxic patients regardless of etiology. Foremost among these are physical, occupational and speech therapies with the key goals of preventing falls, maximizing functional capabilities and minimizing the risks associated with dysphagia [5,6,55]. Falls can be reduced with therapies designed to teach gait and with balance retraining, assessments for appropriate assistive devices and/or orthotics, and a home safety evaluation. Functionality can be maximized through the teaching and performance of home exercise regimens that incorporate stretching, cardiovascular health, muscle conditioning, and strengthening of the core muscles in the abdomen, pelvis and back. Dysphagia complications can be minimized through proper evaluation and dietary modifications. In addition, it is important

that patients maintain a healthy lifestyle and diet to benefit both cardiovascular and neurological health [55–57].

For those patients with hereditary cerebellar ataxia, genetic counseling should be provided for both patients and their families. We find educating patients about their disease and its heritability to be extremely beneficial from a psychological and psychosocial perspective as the majority of patients and their loved ones crave understanding of the cause of their disease [5]. Utilization of ataxia support groups (especially online services for severely affected patients) can also yield enormous benefits, even in acquired or sporadic cases, by helping patients realize they are not alone in their disease and that others share their symptoms, if not their exact cause. Genetic testing of at-risk adult family members should also be discussed, particularly for young adults of reproductive age with potential autosomal dominant or X-linked disorders, as *in vitro* fertilization and preimplantation genetic techniques may be capable of preventing transmission [58]. The psychological impact of potentially abnormal genetic testing results on healthy individuals must always be considered, although there is recent evidence that suggests such concerns need not be prohibitive [59]; however, more studies will be needed to fully address this question.

There are currently no medications approved by the FDA for the treatment of these disorders in the United States, but a number of medications have shown varying degrees of success in treating the symptoms of ataxia, cerebellar tremors and central nystagmus [5,6]. For ataxia, amantadine and buspirone are generally the first-line agents [5,6], although the effects tend to be mild so that these medications are best suited as an adjuvant to physical therapies in patients with less advanced disease. Response to these medications tends to be patient-dependent so a failure of response to one medication does not predict whether any others will be beneficial. For the episodic ataxias, acetazolamide may be beneficial in symptomatic treatment, especially with EA1 and EA2 [9,49].

Antioxidant therapy is a mainstay of neuroprotective treatments for the hereditary ataxias, as most are presumed to exert some or all of their damaging effects via oxidative stress damage [60]. Aside from an effective role as supplementation in deficiency disorders (e.g., AVED or CoQ_{10} deficiency) [60], antioxidants, especially vitamin E and coenzyme Q_{10}, have been widely used in many neurodegenerative ataxias. The best-studied

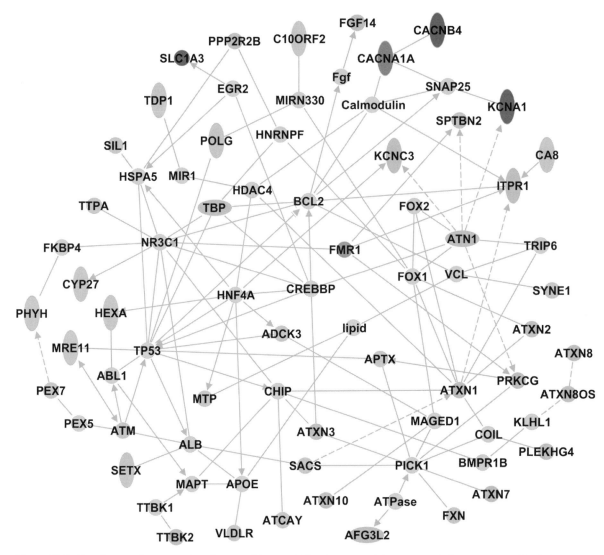

Figure 19.5. Hereditary ataxia gene products form a social network. The 19 autosomal dominant cerebellar ataxia genes (blue), the 21 autosomal recessive cerebellar ataxia genes (green), the 1 X-linked cerebellar ataxia gene (pink), and the 4 episodic ataxia genes (red) discussed in this chapter were analyzed using Ingenuity pathway analysis software (http://www.ingenuity.com) and representative relationships are shown. CACNA1A causes both an autosomal dominant and an episodic ataxia and is therefore depicted in purple. Additional gene products that bridge the various ataxia gene products are shown in orange. The relationships between genes are shown as direct (solid lines) or indirect (dashed lines). Not all known interactions are shown and proteins may be further connected by interactions not depicted here. All interactions are from the Ingenuity database or from additional references [40,68,69]. (See the color plate section for a color version of this figure.)

disorder is Friedreich ataxia, for which various studies have employed vitamin E, *N*-acetylcysteine, coenzyme Q_{10} and idebenone [60,61]. The most complete studies have utilized the coenzyme Q analog idebenone and, taken together, have suggested a protective effect against some features of cardiomyopathy and potential for a slowing of the neurological decline using intermediate to high doses [60,61].

Conclusions and future directions

The most active areas for future developments in the cerebellar ataxias lie in the identification of new causative genes and biomarkers to aid in the diagnosis of hereditary disorders, research into the molecular and cellular mechanisms of pathology to identify new therapeutic targets, and studies of new drugs or other strategies for the treatment of the disease in both animal models and human patients. Some examples of molecules being studied as potential therapeutic agents include histone deacetylase inhibitors as a means of correcting transcriptional dysregulation [62–64], small interfering RNAs to silence expression of disease genes [64,65], and drugs that promote the autophagy of toxic intracellular protein aggregates [64,66].

Our understanding of the pathways underlying the hereditary ataxias is also expanding. Although a unifying feature of these disorders is dysfunction of the cerebellum, in many instances the expression of these disease genes is much more widespread. One possible explanation is a shared mechanism of pathogenesis, but the diversity of gene products involved implies that this may not be the complete answer. Alternative possibilities are that these genes contribute to essential pathways specific to the cerebellum or that there is important interplay between the various gene products within the cerebellum. Most likely, the true answer is a combination of these explanations, depending on the proteins in question, as they need not be mutually exclusive. For example, as has been shown previously for subsets of these proteins [67], in Figure 19.5 we demonstrate that it is possible to create a social network uniting the genes responsible for all the hereditary ataxias. While there are a number of direct interactions between the various ataxia gene products, the majority of linkage extends through one or more additional factors, suggesting that there may be specific cerebellar pathways that are impacted by disruption of these genes. Ultimately, it may be possible to define the cellular pathways responsible for the clinical appearance of cerebellar ataxia that could yield new therapies and new diagnostic tools.

In this chapter we have attempted to outline the diversity of etiologies that can underlie the finding of cerebellar ataxia. In this way we hope to highlight cerebellar ataxia as a symptom of a final diagnosis and not the diagnosis itself. All patients with ataxia require a thorough investigation for an underlying cause to ensure (1) that any treatable causes are expediently identified, and (2) that any contributing components to a multifactorial process are dealt with appropriately to minimize cerebellar injury. The remaining patients represent the hereditary and sporadic cases that encompass one of the great challenges of modern medicine: the caring for patients with chronic progressive neurological disease. Much of medical training focuses on curative treatments and it is often both difficult and frustrating for physicians and patients to be faced with a disease that will not readily yield to available therapies. It is important for all to remember that the absence of a cure is never the absence of treatment. The majority of these disorders do not shorten lifespan, so rehabilitative services and neuroprotective treatments offer enormous benefits in maximizing mobility and maintaining good quality of life for these patients. Education becomes a vital component and patients must be recruited into the process and empowered with the responsibility for actively promoting their well-being through nutrition, exercise and routine preventive health maintenance. Although the day-to-day care of these patients can be managed by general practitioners, an annual visit with a specialist in the field of cerebellar disorders and ataxia is often useful as advances in the field occur at a rapid pace and the advent of new technologies and new research discoveries yields better diagnostic tools for patients with unknown disorders, as well as additional information regarding new potential treatments and/or clinical trials for patients with established disease.

Acknowledgments

The authors wish to acknowledge all the excellent work in this field that could not be directly cited due to space constraints, necessitating a need to refer readers to comprehensive reviews for specific topics.

References

1. Manto M. Mechanisms of human cerebellar dysmetria: experimental evidence and current conceptual bases. *J Neuroeng Rehabil* 2009; **6**: 10.

2. Morton SM, Bastian AJ. Mechanisms of cerebellar gait ataxia. *Cerebellum* 2007; **6**(1): 79–86.

3. Fogel BL, Perlman S. Clinical features and molecular genetics of autosomal recessive cerebellar ataxias. *Lancet Neurol* 2007; **6**(3): 245–57.

4. Perlman SL. Ataxias. *Clin Geriatr Med* 2006; **22**(4): 859–77, vii.

5. Perlman SL. Symptomatic and disease-modifying therapy for the progressive ataxias. *Neurologist* 2004; **10**(5): 275–89.

6. Fogel BL, Perlman S. An approach to the patient with late-onset cerebellar ataxia. *Nat Clin Pract Neurol* 2006; **2**(11): 629–35; quiz 1 p following 35.

7. Schols L, Bauer P, Schmidt T, Schulte T, Riess O. Autosomal dominant cerebellar ataxias: clinical features, genetics, and pathogenesis. *Lancet Neurol* 2004; **3**(5): 291–304.

8. Finsterer J. Ataxias with autosomal, X-chromosomal or maternal inheritance. *Can J Neurol Sci* 2009; **36**(4): 409–28.

9. Brusse E, Maat-Kievit JA, van Swieten JC. Diagnosis and management of early- and late-onset cerebellar ataxia. *Clin Genet* 2007; **71**(1): 12–24.

10. Fogel BL, Salamon N, Perlman S. Progressive spinocerebellar ataxia mimicked by a presumptive cerebellar arteriovenous malformation. *Eur J Radiol Extra* 2009; **71**(1): e1–e2.

11. Brunberg JA. Ataxia. *AJNR Am J Neuroradiol* 2008; **29**(7): 1420–2.

12. Hadjivassiliou M, Boscolo S, Tongiorgi E *et al.* Cerebellar ataxia as a possible organ-specific autoimmune disease. *Mov Disord* 2008; **23**(10): 1370–7.

13. Berlit P. Neuropsychiatric disease in collagen vascular diseases and vasculitis. *J Neurol* 2007; **254**(Suppl 2): II87–9.

14. Toothaker TB, Rubin M. Paraneoplastic neurological syndromes: a review. *Neurologist* 2009; **15**(1): 21–33.

15. Irani S, Lang B. Autoantibody-mediated disorders of the central nervous system. *Autoimmunity* 2008; **41**(1): 55–65.

16. Gilman S, Wenning GK, Low PA JQ *et al.* Second consensus statement on the diagnosis of multiple system atrophy. *Neurology* 2008; **71**(9): 670–6.

17. Berciano J, Boesch S, Perez-Ramos JM, Wenning GK. Olivopontocerebellar atrophy: toward a better nosological definition. *Mov Disord* 2006; **21**(10): 1607–13.

18. Kerber KA, Jen JC, Perlman S, Baloh RW. Late-onset pure cerebellar ataxia: differentiating those with and without identifiable mutations. *J Neurol Sci* 2005; **238**(1–2): 41–5.

19. Palau F, Espinos C. Autosomal recessive cerebellar ataxias. *Orphanet J Rare Dis* 2006; **1**: 47.

20. Anheim M, Fleury M, Monga B G *et al.* Epidemiological, clinical, paraclinical and molecular study of a cohort of 102 patients affected with autosomal recessive progressive cerebellar ataxia from Alsace, Eastern France: implications for clinical management. *Neurogenetics* 2010; **11**(1): 1–12.

21. Pandolfo M, Pastore A. The pathogenesis of Friedreich ataxia and the structure and function of frataxin. *J Neurol* 2009; **256**(Suppl 1): 9–17.

22. Lagier-Tourenne C, Tazir M, Lopez LC N *et al.* ADCK3, an ancestral kinase, is mutated in a form of recessive ataxia associated with coenzyme Q_{10} deficiency. *Am J Hum Genet* 2008; **82**(3): 661–72.

23. Suraweera A, Lim Y, Woods R *et al.* Functional role for senataxin, defective in ataxia oculomotor apraxia type 2, in transcriptional regulation. *Hum Mol Genet* 2009; **18**(18): 3384–96.

24. Hakonen AH, Goffart S, Marjavaara S *et al.* Infantile-onset spinocerebellar ataxia and mitochondrial recessive ataxia syndrome are associated with neuronal complex I defect and mtDNA depletion. *Hum Mol Genet* 2008; **17**(23): 3822–35.

25. Lavin MF, Gueven N, Grattan-Smith P. Defective responses to DNA single- and double-strand breaks in spinocerebellar ataxia. *DNA Repair (Amst)*. 2008; **7**(7): 1061–76.

26. Ozcelik T, Akarsu N, Uz E *et al.* Mutations in the very low-density lipoprotein receptor VLDLR cause cerebellar hypoplasia and quadrupedal locomotion in humans. *Proc Natl Acad Sci U S A*. 2008; **105**(11): 4232–6.

27. Moheb LA, Tzschach A, Garshasbi M *et al.* Identification of a nonsense mutation in the very low-density lipoprotein receptor gene (VLDLR) in an Iranian family with dysequilibrium syndrome. *Eur J Hum Genet* 2008; **16**(2): 270–3.

28. Boycott KM, Bonnemann C, Herz J *et al.* Mutations in VLDLR as a cause for autosomal recessive cerebellar ataxia with mental retardation (dysequilibrium syndrome). *J Child Neurol* 2009; **24**(10): 1310–5.

29. Buschdorf JP, Chew LL, Soh UJ, Liou YC, Low BC. Nerve growth factor stimulates interaction of Cayman ataxia protein BNIP-H/Caytaxin with peptidyl-prolyl isomerase Pin1 in differentiating neurons. *PLoS One* 2008; **3**(7): e2686.

30. Gros-Louis F, Dupre N, Dion P *et al.* Mutations in SYNE1 lead to a newly discovered form of autosomal recessive cerebellar ataxia. *Nat Genet* 2007; **39**(1): 80–5.

31. Schulz JB, Boesch S, Burk K *et al.* Diagnosis and treatment of Friedreich ataxia: a European perspective. *Nat Rev Neurol* 2009; **5**(4): 222–34.

32. Turkmen S, Guo G, Garshasbi M *et al.* CA8 mutations cause a novel syndrome characterized by ataxia and mild mental retardation with predisposition to quadrupedal gait. *PLoS Genet* 2009; **5**(5): e1000487.

33. Vermeer S, Meijer RP, Pijl BJ *et al.* ARSACS in the Dutch population: a frequent cause of early-onset cerebellar ataxia. *Neurogenetics* 2008; **9**(3): 207–14.

34. Mariotti C, Brusco A, Di Bella D *et al.* Spinocerebellar ataxia type 28: a novel autosomal dominant cerebellar ataxia characterized by slow progression and ophthalmoparesis. *Cerebellum* 2008; **7**(2): 184–8.

35. Storey E, Bahlo M, Fahey M, Sisson O, Lueck CJ, Gardner RJ. A new dominantly inherited pure cerebellar ataxia, SCA 30. *J Neurol Neurosurg Psychiatry* 2009; **80**(4): 408–11.

36. Jen JC, Lee H, Cha YH, Nelson SF, Baloh RW. Genetic heterogeneity of autosomal dominant nonprogressive congenital ataxia. *Neurology* 2006; **67**(9): 1704–6.

37. Duenas AM, Goold R, Giunti P. Molecular pathogenesis of spinocerebellar ataxias. *Brain* 2006; **129**(Pt 6): 1357–70.

38. Orr HT, Zoghbi HY. Trinucleotide repeat disorders. *Annu Rev Neurosci* 2007; **30**: 575–621.

39. Soong BW, Paulson HL. Spinocerebellar ataxias: an update. *Curr Opin Neurol* 2007; **20**(4): 438–46.

40. Ikeda Y, Daughters RS, Ranum LP. Bidirectional expression of the SCA8 expansion mutation: one mutation, two genes. *Cerebellum* 2008; **7**(2): 150–8.

41. Dagda RK, Merrill RA, Cribbs JT *et al.* The spinocerebellar ataxia 12 gene product and protein phosphatase 2A regulatory subunit Bbeta2 antagonizes neuronal survival by promoting mitochondrial fission. *J Biol Chem* 2008; **283**(52): 36241–8.

42. Knight MA, Hernandez D, Diede SJ *et al.* A duplication at chromosome 11q12.2–11q12.3 is associated with spinocerebellar ataxia type 20. *Hum Mol Genet* 2008; **17**(24): 3847–53.

43. Iwaki A, Kawano Y, Miura S *et al.* Heterozygous deletion of ITPR1, but not SUMF1, in spinocerebellar ataxia type 16. *J Med Genet* 2008; **45**(1): 32–5.

44. Maltecca F, Magnoni R, Cerri F, Cox GA, Quattrini A, Casari G. Haploinsufficiency of AFG3L2, the gene responsible for spinocerebellar ataxia type 28, causes mitochondria-mediated Purkinje cell dark degeneration. *J Neurosci* 2009; **29**(29): 9244–54.

45. Hellenbroich Y, Bernard V, Zuhlke C. Spinocerebellar ataxia type 4 and 16q22.1-linked Japanese ataxia are not allelic. *J Neurol* 2008; **255**(4): 612–3.

46. Harding AE. Classification of the hereditary ataxias and paraplegias. *Lancet* 1983; **1**(8334): 1151–5.

47. Maschke M, Oehlert G, Xie TD *et al.* Clinical feature profile of spinocerebellar ataxia type 1–8 predicts genetically defined subtypes. *Mov Disord* 2005; **20**(11): 1405–12.

48. Hall DA, Berry-Kravis E, Jacquemont S *et al.* Initial diagnoses given to persons with the fragile X associated tremor/ataxia syndrome (FXTAS). *Neurology* 2005; **65**(2): 299–301.

49. Jen JC. Hereditary episodic ataxias. *Ann N Y Acad Sci* 2008; **1142**: 250–3.

50. Pushkarev D, Neff NF, Quake SR. Single-molecule sequencing of an individual human genome. *Nat Biotechnol* 2009; **27**(9): 847–50.

51. Mascalchi M. Spinocerebellar ataxias. *Neurol Sci* 2008; **29**(Suppl 3): 311–3.

52. Prakash N, Hageman N, Hua X, Toga AW, Perlman SL, Salamon N. Patterns of fractional anisotropy changes in white matter of cerebellar peduncles distinguish spinocerebellar ataxia-1 from multiple system atrophy and other ataxia syndromes. *Neuroimage* 2009; **47**(Suppl 2): T72–81.

53. Dohlinger S, Hauser TK, Borkert J, Luft AR, Schulz JB. Magnetic resonance imaging in spinocerebellar ataxias. *Cerebellum* 2008; **7**(2): 204–14.

54. Poretti A, Wolf NI, Boltshauser E. Differential diagnosis of cerebellar atrophy in childhood. *Eur J Paediatr Neurol* 2008; **12**(3): 155–67.

55. Perlman SL. Cerebellar ataxia. *Curr Treat Options Neurol* 2000; **2**(3): 215–24.

56. Warnberg J, Gomez-Martinez S, Romeo J, Diaz LE, Marcos A. Nutrition, inflammation, and cognitive function. *Ann N Y Acad Sci* 2009; **1153**: 164–75.

57. Gidding SS, Lichtenstein AH, Faith MS *et al.* Implementing American Heart Association pediatric and adult nutrition guidelines: a scientific statement from the American Heart Association Nutrition Committee of the Council on Nutrition, Physical Activity and Metabolism, Council on Cardiovascular Disease in the Young, Council on Arteriosclerosis, Thrombosis and Vascular Biology, Council on Cardiovascular Nursing, Council on Epidemiology and Prevention, and Council for High Blood Pressure Research. *Circulation* 2009; **119**(8): 1161–75.

58. Spits C, Sermon K. PGD for monogenic disorders: aspects of molecular biology. *Prenat Diagn* 2009; **29**(1): 50–6.

59. Green RC, Roberts JS, Cupples LA *et al.* Disclosure of APOE genotype for risk of Alzheimer's disease. *N Engl J Med* 2009; **361**(3): 245–54.

60. Pandolfo M. Drug Insight: antioxidant therapy in inherited ataxias. *Nat Clin Pract Neurol* 2008; **4**(2): 86–96.

61. Schulz JB, Di Prospero NA, Fischbeck K. Clinical experience with high-dose idebenone in Friedreich ataxia. *J Neurol* 2009; **256**(Suppl 1): 42–5.

62. Butler R, Bates GP. Histone deacetylase inhibitors as therapeutics for polyglutamine disorders. *Nat Rev Neurosci* 2006; **7**(10): 784–96.

63. Kazantsev AG, Thompson LM. Therapeutic application of histone deacetylase inhibitors for central nervous system disorders. *Nat Rev Drug Discov* 2008; **7**(10): 854–68.

64. Underwood BR, Rubinsztein DC. Spinocerebellar ataxias caused by polyglutamine expansions: a review of therapeutic strategies. *Cerebellum* 2008; **7**(2): 215–21.

65. Jagannath A, Wood M. RNA interference based gene therapy for neurological disease. *Brief Funct Genomic Proteomic* 2007; **6**(1): 40–9.

66. Sarkar S, Rubinsztein DC. Small molecule enhancers of autophagy for neurodegenerative diseases. *Mol Biosyst* 2008; **4**(9): 895–901.

67. Lim J, Hao T, Shaw C *et al.* A protein-protein interaction network for human inherited ataxias and disorders of Purkinje cell degeneration. *Cell* 2006; **125**(4): 801–14.

68. Parfitt DA, Michael GJ, Vermeulen EG *et al.* The ataxia protein sacsin is a functional co-chaperone that protects against polyglutamine-expanded ataxin-1. *Hum Mol Genet* 2009; **18**(9): 1556–65.

69. Asai H, Hirano M, Shimada K *et al.* Protein kinase C{gamma}, a protein causative for dominant ataxia, negatively regulates nuclear import of recessive-ataxia-related aprataxin. *Hum Mol Genet* 2009; **18**(19): 3533–43.

70. Online Mendelian Inheritance in Man, OMIM. McKusick-Nathans Institute of Genetic Medicine, Johns Hopkins University (Baltimore, MD) and National Center for Biotechnology Information, National Library of Medicine (Bethesda, MD). www.ncbi.nlm.nih.gov/omim/.

71. HGNC Database. HUGO Gene Nomenclature Committee (HGNC), EMBL Outstation – Hinxton, European Bioinformatics Institute, Wellcome Trust Genome Campus, Hinxton, Cambridge, CB10 1SD, UK. www.genenames.org.

72. Higgins JJ, Pho LT, Ide SE, Nee LE, Polymeropoulos MH. Evidence for a new spinocerebellar ataxia locus. *Mov Disord* 1997; **12**(3): 412–7.

73. Schelhaas HJ, Verbeek DS, Van de Warrenburg BP, Sinke RJ. SCA19 and SCA22: evidence for one locus with a worldwide distribution. *Brain* 2004; **127**(Pt 1): E6; author reply E7.

74. Swartz BE, Burmeister M, Somers JT, Rottach KG, Bespalova IN, Leigh RJ. A form of inherited cerebellar ataxia with saccadic intrusions, increased saccadic speed, sensory neuropathy, and myoclonus. *Ann N Y Acad Sci* 2002; **956**: 441–4.

75. Sato N, Amino T, Kobayashi K *et al.* Spinocerebellar ataxia type 31 is associated with "inserted" pentanucleotide repeats containing (TGGAA)n. *Am J Hum Genet*. 2009; **85**(5): 544–57.

Chapter 20

Stiff person syndrome

Daniel S. Sa

History

In 1956, Drs. Frederick Moersch (1889–1975) and Henry Woltman (1889–1964) at the Mayo Clinic in Rochester published the first report of patients with an unusual condition of muscular rigidity and spasms which at the time was called stiff-man syndrome. Years later, it has been suggested to call it stiff person syndrome as the disease entity obviously affects women and children [1].

Their original description detailed 14 patients collected over decades. That description was enlarged and enriched over the years, including Gordon's first suggestion of an inhibitory failure, and Lorish expanding on diagnostic features [2,3].

The condition they described is one of rigidity, predominantly affecting axial and proximal limb muscles with frequent associated muscle spasms that can be triggered by a variety of stimuli. It is usually progressive and symmetric.

Dr. Henry Woltman became the first full-time neurologist at the Mayo Clinic in 1917, becoming Chair of Neurology in 1930 when he succeeded Walter Sheldon. Dr. Frederick Moersch was a medical student under Henry Woltman at University of Minnesota and joined the Mayo Clinic in 1920.

Neurologic education at that institution included daily conferences in which unusual or instructive cases were discussed, a daily occurrence usually set for 13:30, occasionally associated with brain cutting sessions directed by Dr. James Kernohan (1896–1981). These initial case discussions spearheaded an interest in what was then an unknown, nameless syndrome. It now carries their name as the eponym Moersch–Woltman syndrome, or more aptly described a stiff person syndrome (SPS). It took almost seven years until an effective treatment was first attempted, reported by Howard in 1963 with diazepam [4]. After multiple other empirical, poorly understood attempts at treatment, nearly four decades later, the first appropriately controlled trial was reported [5].

These long delays in the discovery of appropriate treatments are due in great part to poor understanding of its pathophysiological basis. Indeed, it took more than two decades from its original description until the work of Solimena reported conclusive findings about the pathogenesis of the condition, with the discovery of antibodies against glutamic acid decarboxylase in 1988 [6].

Clinical findings

Stiff person syndrome is quite rare and, like any rare disease, is probably underdiagnosed and is clearly poorly understood and studied. Epidemiological information is largely unavailable, and suggested incidence/prevalence numbers are just that, an estimation and, for that matter, probably an underestimation.

It has been suggested that SPS has a prevalence as low as one in one million. There has been no reported race predominance to this day, and ages have varied widely across the spectrum from babies to the elderly, the most common presenting decades being the third to the fifth, ranging from 7 to 71 years of age [7–9]. Although autoimmune diseases frequently affect women more than men, not all series in SPS reflect that. Some series suggest that incidence and severity are quite similar between men and women – hence the name change to SPS – but the disparity is great, from an early study in 1967 suggesting a male to female preponderance of 2:1 and other studies suggesting a female to male preponderance of up to 70% women, 30% men [2,10–12]. It should be noted here that, further complicating the already quite limited epidemiological data, most series do not clearly differentiate between the three recognizable types: autoimmune, paraneoplastic and sporadic [12].

The disease and its symptoms usually start insidiously, progressing slowly over years; it might also occasionally evolve in a more abrupt fashion, over a few weeks. More abrupt onset and progression should raise suspicion for a paraneoplastic phenomenon, although that is not always the case. The most common presenting complaints seems to be episodic achiness and tightness of the axial musculature, although more suggestive symptoms such as persistent progressive stiffening of the back or a limb, which may be worse under pressure or time constraints, usually develop over time. Although essentially all body parts have been described as affected, even sometimes in isolation as in stiff limb syndrome, back and lower limbs seem to be more frequently affected and reported. Associated feelings of pain or dull aches are frequently described by the patients, and may evolve from being episodic as in the presenting symptoms to more constant, uncomfortable sensations.

Physicians have described or reported their findings over the years using a quite varied nomenclature, the most common descriptions being stiffness, rigidity, hypertonia and increased tone.

Beyond the slow evolution of stiffness and related problems, there are frequently superimposed, severe and painful spasms of the involved muscles that may last hours to occasionally days. Interestingly, an "aura" type phenomenon preceding the spasms has been described, and in one report seemed to be quite common, although such complaints have been rarely reported since [13]. Examination may find hardened muscles on palpation, and even abnormal joint positions caused by such "stiffening."

A multitude of triggers have been described over the years, usually sudden environmental changes, including noise, touch, passive or voluntary movement. The involuntary movements are typically relieved by sleep. This clear association with sudden changes and movements has been noted to cause behavioral changes in patients, who tend to voluntarily move more slowly, afraid that more abrupt movements could cause such severe painful spasms. Additional examination findings include an increase in the normal curvature of the lumbar spine, or hyperlordosis. Signs of other autoimmune diseases, which are frequently associated with SPS, can be seen, such as diabetic changes, anemia and vitiligo.

Multiple other complaints, secondary to the hypertonicity or related to chronic disease, have been reported, including depression and sleep difficulties, as sleep improvement is observed only after the patient finally falls asleep. Patients have been frequently subject to psychiatric evaluations, given the elusive and rare nature of the disease as well as its intermittent symptoms.

Late in the course of the disease, most body muscles can be affected, although trismus is usually conspicuously absent. Joint deformities secondary to the continuous hypertonicity eventually ensue, and dislocations are frequently reported. Muscular and bone fractures/ruptures seem rare but have been reported. Furthermore, any surgical incision has an increased risk of post-operative dehiscence.

Variants of the disease have been reported, including stiff baby syndrome, further detailed below, stiff limb syndrome, jerking stiff person syndrome, and progressive encephalitis with rigidity and myoclonus [12].

Stiff baby syndrome

It is unclear whether the cases reported in children as stiff baby syndrome all relate to the same entity because the clinical presentation is different as will be noted. Such cases have frequently been considered and reported under a broad definition of hyperekplexia, or startle syndrome, even though hyperekplexias are different, inherited disorders related to glycine neurotransmission [14]. Stiff person syndrome has no known genetic predisposition other than an HLA association.

As a general rule, the attacks in babies are more prominent, and the examination between attacks is closer to normal, with less rigidity, and sometimes a normal examination. The pattern of muscular involvement is different as well, with more prominent involvement of distal musculature, which is usually obvious during the attacks. Opisthotonus is reportedly common, and startle, as well as stress, are very common precipitants of these events, similar to what is seen in adults.

Diagnosis is frequently complicated in babies by a more limited history and examination, as well as a potentially broader differential diagnosis including seizures, intoxication or withdrawal, neuromuscular disorders, and other situations. Particularly for research purposes, clinical differentiation and proper classification should be reserved for cases where the presence of anti-GAD (glutamic acid decarboxylase) antibodies has been confirmed.

Natural history

The disease follows a variable course, although almost invariably progressive, with few reported stabilizations. Disease duration, according to available literature, has also varied, from 6 to 28 years, although that data is limited, and such duration might be related to death or simply to loss to follow-up [3].

Complications of this disease are common and highly variable, and may occur at any stage of the disease. This can be further impacted by associated conditions, particularly whether or not each specific SPS is related to an autoimmune, paraneoplastic or sporadic condition.

In general, complications are responsible for the mortality and morbidity and are discussed in more detail in the Complications section.

Infants with stiff baby syndrome are at particularly high risk of sudden infant death and require monitoring. Sudden death has also been reported in older individuals, but usually related to atypical cases, with encephalomyelitis signs.

Patients who develop clearer encephalomyelitic signs, sometimes called stiff person-plus syndrome, often follow a relentless subacute course with death frequently reported within 3 years from symptom onset. Signs of encephalomyelitis, with prominent gray matter involvement have been recorded in pathological reports [15].

Multiple complications may also occur in relation to baclofen pump failure. Marked, abrupt exacerbations of the disease have been reported due to baclofen pump failure, just as in any other diseases associated with increased tone and baclofen use. At least one death has been reported. In addition, rare malfunctions of the baclofen pump have been associated with excessive release of baclofen intrathecally, resulting in death or permanent disability [16,17].

Psychiatric morbidity from this disease is common. The unpredictability of symptoms and the linkage to stressful events only serve to exacerbate the situation. In addition, GABA mechanisms subserve many of the brain's emotional centers, which may contribute significantly to the psychiatric symptomatology.

Musculoskeletal complications are common, particularly in later stages of the disease. Joint deformity, joint dislocation, joint contracture, skeletal fracture and muscle rupture have been reported.

The natural history can also be affected by the presence or absence of the multiple diseases that have been associated with SPS, including diabetes mellitus, breast cancer, epilepsy, ataxia, thyroiditis and vitiligo.

Differential diagnosis

Once the disease is suspected, the differential diagnosis is relatively straightforward, though somewhat more complicated in very young patients.

Trauma and spasms from multiple sclerosis can usually be ruled out by careful history and physical examination, as should be the case for myopathies including myotonias. Hyperekplexias and drug intoxication should be evident from family history, screening tests and evolution of the clinical picture, and other conditions such as encephalomyelitis and tetanus should be accompanied by other changes suggesting the underlying diagnosis.

Dystonia, myoclonus, Isaac syndrome and psychogenic disorders might rarely be a consideration, but such differentiation should be readily apparent on clinical grounds, rarely requiring ancillary tests in antibody-negative cases.

Additional considerations, usually readily apparent during history taking or examination include:

- Parkinson disease, multiple system atrophy, progressive supranuclear palsy, toxic parkinsonism as in carbon monoxide or manganese, among others
- Myelopathies due to a variety of causes
- Radiation-induced damage, peripheral or central
- Congenital, acquired and hereditary spasticities
- Ankylosing spondylitis

Laboratory investigations

Routine laboratory tests are generally unremarkable, unless comorbidities such as diabetes mellitus or thyroid disease are present.

The absence of antibodies in the serum certainly does not rule out SMS, but the presence of anti-GAD autoantibodies strongly supports that diagnosis. There are several accepted ways to measure anti-GAD antibodies: immunocytochemistry and western blotting were the first methods used. Immunocytochemistry allows the detection of antigens in tissue section, whereas western blotting visualizes protein antigens that have been separated by size. ELISA and radioimmunoassay (RIA) use antigen specific binding to attach enzyme-linked or radioactively labeled substrates to the antibodies in serum.

ELISA and RIA, which are comparatively more recent, quantitatively assess the amount of anti-GAD antibody a patient has produced, which can be considered an advantage of such methods. Amphiphysin antibodies, less common than anti-GAD, have also shown a strong association with SPS, and frequently with associated neoplasms (see below) [18,19].

Electromyography (EMG) should be considered part of the routine work-up, as it frequently supports the clinical diagnosis. It is also included in current diagnostic criteria [18].

Careful EMG studies will frequently reveal continuous action potentials during rest, predominantly over the axial musculature, as would be seen in voluntary movements. Bursts of 5–6 Hz activity with a 50–60 ms duration are frequently interspersed with spasms.

Patterns of relatively continuous firing of normal motor units or continuous motor unit activity can be observed simultaneously affecting agonist and antagonist muscles. This abnormal firing pattern can be abolished by multiple centrally and peripherally acting agents including general anesthesia, diazepam and neuromuscular blockade.

Chest CT may be considered given reports of associated thymomas, as well as small-cell lung cancer, particularly when anti-amphiphysin antibodies are identified [12].

Mention should be made that an underlying cancer is found in approximately 5% of cases, although it is impossible by clinical features alone to distinguish paraneoplastic from non paraneoplastic cases [12]. The presence of amphiphysin antibodies, however, should prompt a more thorough investigation designed to identify an underlying tumor [19,20].

Brain imaging would be required in case corticospinal findings are present on examination. EEG may also be considered based on history suggestive of seizures. CSF analysis should always be considered in patients with a presentation that is consistent with stiff person syndrome to rule out alternative causes, particularly in babies. Oligoclonal bands have been reported in approximately two-thirds of patients with antibody-positive SPS [21].

Additional tests would include anti-pancreatic islet cell antibodies for diabetes mellitus and anti-amphiphysin antibodies in paraneoplastic cases, frequently associated with breast cancer and small-cell lung cancer [22]. Rarely, in the appropriate setting, genetic testing could be considered, as SCA1 has been reported as presenting with similar features to SPS [23].

Establishing a diagnosis

Multiple diagnostic criteria have been proposed and modified over the years, but basic criteria can be summarized as follows [18,24]:

1. Muscular rigidity in the limbs and axial muscles, prominent in the abdominal and thoracolumbar paraspinals.
2. Continuous co-contraction of agonist and antagonists muscles, clinically and electrophysiologically.
3. Episodic spasms precipitated by unexpected noises, other sensory stimuli or emotional stress.
4. Absence of any other neurological disease that could explain the symptoms.
5. Positive anti-GAD or anti-amphiphysin antibodies by immunocytochemistry, western blot or radioimmunoassay.

Genetics

There are no convincing reports of SPS affecting different members of the same family, and there is no well-described genetic predisposition. An association with certain human leukocyte antigen (HLA) types has been described [25–28].

Pathology/pathophysiology

All the evidence points to a central mechanism at the origin of the spasms and other abnormalities, from their disappearance with sleep to response to nerve blocks, general anesthesia and other central nervous system-depressing drugs [18].

The majority of symptoms in SPS, particularly stiffness and spasms, suggest abnormalities in inhibitory modulation of spinal cord reflexes; as expected, gamma-aminobutyric acid (GABA) changes and antibodies against glutamic acid decarboxylase were eventually documented [6]. The abnormalities in modulation seem to have an immunological substrate, as has become evident by the observation of common associations with antibodies, particularly anti-GAD and anti-amphiphysin [18,29].

In normal subjects, regular discharges from spinal motor neurons are frequently controlled, avoiding excessive or continuous activity through inhibitory inputs in the motor pathways. This is usually accomplished by the action of glycine from spinal interneurons, as well as GABA-mediated inhibition from the cortex, brain stem and cerebellum; such neurons involved in GABA inhibition are called GABAergic. GABA can be formed from glutamate, through GAD, or directly from the Krebs cycle through GABA-transaminase.

Glutamate is a generally excitatory amino acid, synthesized from glucose via the Krebs cycle, that can be used and released at synaptic clefts; as mentioned, it can also be transformed to GABA or glutamine through the action of the enzyme GAD, which is generally localized in the synaptic nerve terminal as well as in pancreatic beta cells. GAD itself is nearly ubiquitous in the CNS, and is rate limited by the availability of glutamate.

The importance of GAD in SPS is evident by the very common association of its antibodies with the disease; GAD is the protein antigen that is specifically bound by the anti-GAD autoantibodies found in a substantial number of SMS patients [6]. It seems reasonable that if GAD function is inhibited significantly, then the effects or availability of GABA are decreased, and muscles may become hyperexcitable, continuously stimulated by the motor neurons.

The precise prevalence of such antibodies is unknown, obviously subject to the use of more or less stringent research diagnostic criteria, but has varied from 60% to 90% of patients throughout the literature [6,10,11,22,24,25,30–32]. However, GAD antibodies have also been reported in a vast number of seemingly unrelated diseases/syndromes, including cerebellar abnormalities, seizures, myelopathies and other forms of cortical dysfunction, as well as nonneurological problems including type I diabetes mellitus and autoimmune polyendocrine syndromes. Furthermore, GAD antibodies alone seem insufficient to cause SPS, and well-documented cases exist without such antibodies; a few do not even have the anti-amphiphysin antibodies [33]. It is also not known whether the antibodies have a causative role or are epiphenomena, the consequence of a process that leads to impairment of neurotransmission [34].

This large body of data concerning the heterogeneity of GAD antibody associations makes clear that such antibodies are only a part of the pathophysiology of stiff person syndrome.

Postsynaptic GABA-related mechanisms such as synaptobrevins, reported in association with tetanus as well, and gephyrin and GABA-transaminase have been postulated as alternative or supplemental causative factors [29,35–39].

Management

As expected, similarly to the case of other rare/uncommon neurological disorders, the treatment of SPS is based on anecdotal reports and small case series, and properly randomized trials are lacking.

Despite the clear immunological abnormalities reported in these patients, immunomodulation has shown variable results. Anecdotal reports over the years have included prednisone, intravenous immunoglobulin, plasmapheresis and more recently rituximab [11,18,25,39,40].

A study by Dalakas and colleagues, funded by the National Institute of Neurological Disorders and Stroke (NINDS), suggested the effectiveness of intravenous immunoglobulin (IVIg) for both stiffness and sensitivity to outside stimuli in people with SPS [5]. In that crossover study, 16 patients with SPS defined by clinical criteria and the presence of GAD65 received either IVIg or placebo for 3 months, followed by a 1-month washout period and a crossover to the alternative therapy [5].

Patients treated with IVIg showed a statistically significant decrease in both stiffness and spasms, which clearly worsened when such patients crossed to the placebo group. Eleven of the 14 patients who finished the study became less stiff and more mobile, and were able to walk unassisted, resume work activities, or remain upright without fear of falling. It should be mentioned here that the study obviously did not address long-term use of IVIg and was also unable to provide appropriate blinding as is frequently the case with aggressive therapies such as IVIg [5]. Despite such study weaknesses, the American Association of Neuromuscular and Electrodiagnostic Medicine (AANEM), in a consensus statement, considers the evidence for IVIg in stiff person syndrome category I, where evidence exists to support its use, though it acknowledges that there is very little evidence to provide information on optimal doses and duration of therapy [41].

Symptomatic benefit has been more consistently achieved with drugs that could be loosely categorized as muscle relaxants, benzodiazepines being considered the drug of choice by most, but baclofen (oral formulation or intrathecal pump), tizanidine, dantrolene and barbiturates as well as propofol have also been reported as efficacious [25,30,31,39,42–44]. Anticonvulsants such as tiagabine, levetiracetam and gabapentin have also been reported [44–50].

Excessive sedation is frequently a problem, as the high benzodiazepine doses employed are frequently associated with drowsiness and sleepiness, impairing function in their own right.

Unfortunately, such medications are usually required on a continuous basis and at high doses, with all its side-effects, as attempts to taper or discontinue it almost invariably produce recurrence or exacerbation of symptoms.

Consideration can also be given to therapy with botulinum toxin injections carefully placed in the most affected muscles, but this approach will frequently be limited by the widespread distribution of the disease, which would require massive doses, well beyond FDA-approved doses, which are clearly unsafe. As mentioned, careful selection of a single limb that could present functional gain can be considered, as opposed to widespread injections, by someone well familiarized with such therapy.

Physical therapy, common in most neurological disorders, should be used sparingly, preferably after a response is achieved with pharmacological therapy, as the exercises and even passive motion are known to exacerbate or trigger spasms.

Conclusions

Like most uncommon/rare neurological disorders, SPS is relatively poorly understood, and management is based mostly on anecdotal reports, as proper randomized studies are nearly impossible to conduct unless multiple centers become involved. Therefore, review of the literature should be extremely critical, and decisions on each patient should be carefully considered on an individual basis, recognizing the limitations of the current available data, and inherent risk of the potential treatment options as well as the disease itself.

Future studies are clearly necessary to better understand and treat this debilitating condition.

References

1. Moersch FP, Woltman HW. Progressive fluctuating muscular rigidity and spasm ('stiff-man syndrome'): report of a case and some observations in 13 other cases. *Mayo Clin Proc* 1956; **31**: 421–7.

2. Gordon EE, Januszko DM, Kaufman L. A critical survey of stiff-man syndrome. *Am J Med* 1967; **42**: 582–99.

3. Lorish TR, Thorsteinsson G, Howard FM. Stiff man syndrome updated. *Mayo Clin Proc* 1989; **64**: 629–36.

4. Howard FM. A new and effective drug in the treatment of stiff-man syndrome: preliminary report. *Mayo Clin Proc* 1963; **38**: 203–12.

5. Dalakas M, Fujii M, Li M, Lutfi B, Kyhos J, McElroy B. A randomized controlled trial of high-dose intravenous immunoglobulin in the treatment of patients with stiff person syndrome. *N Engl J Med* 2001; **345**: 1870–6.

6. Solimena M, Folli F, Denis-Donini S et al. Autoantibodies to glutamic acid decarboxylase in a patient with stiff-man syndrome, epilepsy and type I diabetes mellitus. *N Engl J Med* 1988; **318**: 203–12.

7. Kugelmass N. Stiff-man syndrome in a child. *NY State J Med* 1961; **61**: 2483–7.

8. Trethowan WH, Allsop JL, Turner B. The stiff-man syndrome. *Arch Neurol* 1960; **3**: 114–22.

9. Isaacs H. Stiff-man syndrome in a black girl. *J Neurol Neurosurg Psychiatry* 1979; **42**: 988–94.

10. Dalakas MC, Fujii M, Li M, McElroy B. The clinical spectrum of anti-GAD antibody positive patients with stiff-person syndrome. *Neurology* 2000; **55**: 1531–5.

11. Blum P, Jankovic J. Stiff person syndrome: an autoimmune disease. *Mov Disord* 1991; **6**: 12–20.

12. Grant R, Graus F. Paraneoplastic movement disorders. *Mov Disord* 2009; **24**: 1715–14.

13. Meinck HM, Ricker K, Hulser PJ et al. Stiff man syndrome: clinical and laboratory findings in eight patients. *J Neurol* 1994; **241**: 157–66.

14. Tohier C, Roze JC, David A, Veccierini MF, Renaud P, Mouzard A. Hyperkeplexia or stiff baby syndrome. *Arch Dis Child* 1991; **66**(4): 460–1.

15. Brown P, Marsden CD. The stiff-man and stiff-man plus syndromes. *J Neurol* 1999; **246**: 648–52.

16. Meinck HM, Tronnier V, Rieke K, Wirtz CR, Flugel D, Schwab S. Intrathecal baclofen pump for stiff man syndrome: pump failure may be fatal. *Neurology* 1994; **44**: 2209–10.

17. Bardutzky J, Tronnier V, Schwab S, Meinck HM. Intrathecal baclofen for stiff-person syndrome: life-threatening intermittent catheter leakage. *Neurology* 2003; **60**: 1976–8.

18. Gershanik OS. Stiff-person syndrome. *Parkinsonism Relat Disord* 2009; **15**(Suppl 3): S130–S134.

19. Pittock SJ, Lucchinetti CF, Parisi JE et al. Amphiphysin autoimmunity: paraneoplastic accompaniments. *Ann Neurol* 2005; **58**: 96–107.

20. Grimaldi LM, Martino G, Braghi S et al. Heterogeneity of autoantibodies in stiff man syndrome. *Ann Neurol* 1993; **34**: 57–64.

21. Dalakas MC, Li M, Fujii M, Jacobowitz DM. Stiff person syndrome: quantification, specificity, and intrathecal synthesis of GAD65 antibodies. *Neurology* 2001; **57**(5): 780–4.

22. Solimena M, Folli F, Morello F et al. Autoantibodies to GABAergic neurons and pancreatic beta cells in stiff-man syndrome. *N Engl J Med* 1990; **322**: 1555–60.

23. Singhal S, Gontu V, Choudhary P, Auer D, Bajaj N. Spinocerebellar ataxia type 1 mimicking stiff person syndrome. *Mov Disord* 2009; **24**: 2158–60.

24. Barker RA, Revesz T, Thom M et al. Review of 23 patients affected by the stiff man syndrome: clinical subdivision

into stiff trunk (man) syndrome, stiff limb syndrome, and progressive encephalomyelitis with rigidity. *J Neurol Neurosurg Psychiatry* 1998; **655**: 633–640.

25. Hattan E, Angle MR, Chalk C. Unexpected benefit of propofol in stiff-person syndrome. *Neurology* 2008; **70**: 1641–2.

26. Pugliese A, Gianani R, Eisenbarth GS *et al.* Genetics of susceptibility and resistance to insulin dependent diabetes mellitus in stiff man syndrome. *Lancet* 1994; **344**: 1027–8.

27. Pugliese A, Solimena M, Awdeh ZL *et al.* Association of HLA DQB180201 with stiff man syndrome. *J Clin Endocrinol Metab* 1993; **77**: 1550–3.

28. Williams AC, Nutt JG, Hare T. Autoimmunity in stiff man syndrome. *Lancet* 1988; **2**: 222.

29. Geis C, Beck M, Jablonka S *et al.* Stiff person syndrome associated anti-amphiphysin antibodies reduce GABA associated $[Ca^{2+}]_i$ rise in embryonic motor neurons. *Neurobiol Dis* 2009; **36**: 191–9.

30. Meinck HM. Stiff man syndrome. *CNS Drugs* 2001; **15**: 515–26.

31. Dalakas MC. Stiff person syndrome: advances in pathogenesis and therapeutic interventions. *Curr Treat Options Neurol* 2009; **11**(2): 102–10.

32. Baekkeskov S, Aanstoot H-J, Christgau S *et al.* Identification of the 64 K autoantigen in insulin dependent diabetes mellitus as the GABA synthesizing enzyme glutamic acid decarboxylase. *Nature* 1990; **347**: 151–6.

33. Duddy ME, Baker MR. Stiff person syndrome. *Front Neurol Neurosci* 2009; **26**: 147–65.

34. Levy LM, Dalakas MC, Floeter MK. The stiff-person syndrome: an autoimmune disorder affecting neurotransmission of gamma: aminobutyric acid. *Ann Intern Med* 1999; **131**(7): 522–30.

35. Butler MH, Hayashi A, Ohkoshi N *et al.* Autoimmunity to gephyrin in stiff-man syndrome. *Neuron* 2000; **26**: 307–12.

36. Lernmark A. Glutamic acid decarboxylase: gene to antigen to disease. *J Intern Med* 1996; **240**(5): 259–77.

37. Ziegler B, Strebelow M, Rjasanowski I, Schlosser M, Ziegler M. A monoclonal antibody-based characterization of autoantibodies against glutamic acid decarboxylase in adults with latent autoimmune diabetes. *Autoimmunity* 1998; **28**(2): 61–8.

38. Murinson BB, Guarnaccia JB. Stiff person syndrome with amphiphysin antibodies: distinctive features of a rare disease. *Neurology* 2008; **71**: 1955–8.

39. Hayashi A, Nakamagoe K, Ohkoshi N, Hoshino S, Shoji S. Double filtration plasma exchange and immunoadsorption therapy in a case of stiff-man syndrome with negative anti-GAD antibody. *J Med* 1999; **30**(5–6): 321–7.

40. Baker MR, Das M, Isaacs J, Fawcett PR, Bates D. Treatment of stiff person syndrome with rituximab. *J Neurol Neurosurg Psychiatry* 2005; **76**: 999–1001.

41. Donofrio PD, Berger A, Brannagan TH 3rd *et al.* Consensus statement: the use of intravenous immunoglobulin in the treatment of neuromuscular conditions. Report of the AANEM ad hoc committee. *Muscle Nerve* 2009; **40**(5): 890–900.

42. Stayer C, Tronnier V, Dressnandt J *et al.* Intrathecal baclofen therapy for stiff man syndrome and progressive encephalomyelopathy with rigidity and myoclonus. *Neurology* 1997; **49**: 1591–7.

43. Propofol for stiff-person syndrome: learning new tricks from an old dog. *Neurology* 2008; **70**: 1584–5.

44. Lockman J, Burns TM. Stiff person syndrome. *Curr Treat Options Neurol* 2007; **9**: 234–40.

45. Shimber WR, Patel NB, Sullivan KL, Hauser RA, Zesiewicz TA. Levetiracetam for stiff person syndrome: report of two cases. *Clin Neuropharmacol* 2008; **31**: 301–2.

46. Holmoy T. Long term effect of gabapentin in stiff limb syndrome: a case report. *Eur Neurol* 2007; **58**: 251–2.

47. Vasconcelos OM, Dalakas MC. Stiff person syndrome. *Curr Treat Options Neurol* 2003; **5**: 79–90.

48. Secchi G, Barrocu M, Piluzza MG, Cocco GA, Deiana GA, Sau GF. Levetiracetam in stiff person syndrome. *J Neurol* 2008; **255**: 1721–5.

49. Ruegg SJ, Steck AJ, Fuhr P. Levetiracetam improves paroxysmal symptoms in a patient with stiff person syndrome. *Neurology* 2004; **62**: 338.

50. Murinson BB, Rizzo M. Improvement of stiff person syndrome with tiagabine. *Neurology* 2001; **57**: 366.

Hereditary spastic paraplegias

Ramon Lugo, Matthew Bower, Taranum Khan and Néstor Gálvez-Jiménez

Introduction

Hereditary spastic paraplegias (HSPs) are a heterogeneous group of diseases of which the prominent features are increased muscle tone and weakness of the lower extremities. HSPs can be inherited in autosomal dominant (AD), autosomal recessive (AR), or X-linked patterns. Age of onset and disease progression can vary markedly, even within the same family. The prevalence of HSP differs with geographical area and type of inheritance. It ranges from 0.6/100 000 to 9.6/100 000 according to various studies [1,2]. HSP was originally described by the German neurologist Adolph Strumpell in 1883 and the French neurologist Maurice Lorrain in1888. Anita Harding described the original classification scheme in 1983 [3,4]. The elucidation of the genetic basis of HSP has led to significant revisions in the classification of HSP. This chapter will focus on the classification, genetics and clinical aspects of the spastic paraplegias.

Classification

The spastic paraplegias were originally classified by Anita Harding as "pure" or uncomplicated (uHSP) and complicated HSP (cHSP) on the basis of clinical features (see Table 21.1) [3,4]. Uncomplicated HSP is characterized by the presence of increased tone of the lower extremities with absence of other neurological symptoms, although some degree of dysfunction of vibratory sense and urinary incontinence is permitted. Furthermore, uHSP is divided into Type I and Type II based upon age of onset. Type I uHSP is characterized by onset before the age of 35 years and a slow disease progression. Type II uHSP generally presents after age 35 years and is characterized by a faster disease progression, marked muscle weakness and sensory loss. Complicated forms of HSP present with these same core findings in addition to variable findings of cognitive impairment, dementia, cerebellar symptoms, amyotrophy, peripheral neuropathy, deafness, epilepsy, retinal symptoms, cataracts and extrapyramidal signs.

The great variability of symptoms of HSP within the same family complicated early attempts to comprehensively classify HSP. Currently, HSP is classified by mode of inheritance. Approximately 70% of uHSP is inherited in an autosomal dominant pattern, with 40% of these families having mutations in the SPG4 (*SPAST*) gene [5]. Advances in molecular biology suggest entirely new classification schemes. In one sense, classification by genetic mechanism suggests that a single clinical entity may in fact be subdivided into dozens of genetic forms of HSP. On the other hand, molecular biology suggests that some of these distinct genetic forms of HSP can be grouped by distinct molecular mechanisms such as mitochondrial dysfunction or axonal transport.

Clinical manifestations

Hereditary spastic paraplegia is characterized by increased muscle tone of the lower extremities. The onset of can range from age 2 to 82 years, and the progression is insidious. Age of onset, symptoms at presentation and disease progression can all vary even within the same family. Some studies have suggested genetic anticipation, with earlier onset of symptoms in subsequent generations. While this raises the possibility that some forms of HSP could be related to trinucleotide repeat expansion disorders, others have argued that earlier diagnosis could easily be attributed to heightened surveillance in younger generations [6–8].

In the pure form, HSP is characterized by progressive lower extremity spasticity with or without posterior column dysfunction (proprioception and vibratory sense loss) and urinary incontinence. Mild cognitive

---

Uncommon Causes of Movement Disorders, ed. Néstor Gálvez-Jiménez and Paul J. Tuite. Published by Cambridge University Press. © Cambridge University Press 2011.

Table 21.1. Modified Anita Harding classification [3,4].

Pure spastic paraplegia
Autosomal dominant: age of onset usually before age 35 years (type I)
Autosomal dominant: age of onset usually after age 35 years (type II)
Autosomal recessive
X-linked recessive
Complicated forms of spastic paraplegia
With amyotrophy
Spastic quadriparesis
Sjögren–Larsson syndrome
With macular degeneration and mental retardation
With optic atrophy
With extrapyramidal features
With cerebellar features
With motor or sensory neuropathy
With disordered skin pigmentation
With thin corpus callosum
With white matter lesions in brain
With seizures
With dystonia
With thalamic cerebellar degeneration
With dementia

Table 21.2. Diagnostic criteria for HSP.

Clinical features	
Obligatory	• Family history
	• Progressive gait disturbance
	• Spasticity of the lower limbs
	• Hyperreflexia of lower limbs
	• Extensor plantar responses
Common	• Paresis of lower limbs
	• Sphincter disturbances
	• Mild dorsal column disturbance
	• Pes cavus
	• Hyperreflexia of upper limbs
	• Mild terminal dysmetria
	• Loss of ankle jerks
Uncommon	• Paresis of upper limbs
	• Distal amyotrophy
Diagnostic alerts (consider alternative diagnoses)	• Paresis greater than spasticity
	• Prominent ataxia
	• Prominent amyotrophy
	• Prominent upper limb involvement
	• Peripheral neuropathy
	• Asymmetry
	• Retinal pigmentation
	• Extrapyramidal signs

Modified from McDermott *et al.* [7].

impairment has been suggested in some patients with this form of the disease [9,10]. Most often patients present with progressive gait dysfunction. Specifically, patients may complain of falls while climbing stairs due to weakness of foot dorsiflexion. The symptoms are usually symmetric, with the spasticity being more prominent than muscle weakness. As the disease progresses, weakness becomes more prominent, especially in the hip flexors and tibialis anterior muscles. Gait analysis often shows significantly slowed, cautious gait with considerably increased gait width and stride variation. Delay in walking is frequently noted with childhood-onset forms of HSP. Additional clinical findings include decreased range of motion with increased knee flexion and maximum ankle angle deviations leading to equinovarus foot position [11]. Suggested diagnostic criteria are included in Table 21.2.

On examination, there is spasticity of the lower extremities, particularly in the hamstring, quadriceps and ankles, with sparing of the upper extremities. Deep tendon reflexes in lower extremities are increased with absent ankle jerks [12–14]. Increased deep tendon reflexes may be noted in the upper extremities. In some families the phenotype is complicated by the asymptomatic absence of vibratory and joint position sense, pes cavus, bladder hyperreflexia, mild ataxia of upper extremities and distal muscle wasting [7].

Differential diagnosis

It is important to exclude treatable causes of spasticity, such as vitamin B_{12} and vitamin E deficiency, copper myelopathy, disorders of very long-chain fatty acid metabolism, disorders of amino acids, dopa-responsive dystonia, structural spinal cord disorders and neurosyphilis [7,15]. Other conditions that might differ in prognosis should also be evaluated, including multiple sclerosis and familial/sporadic motor neuron disease.

Table 21.3. Evaluation of differential diagnoses.

Differential diagnosis	Investigation
Cervical/lumbar spondylosis	MRI spine
Neoplasm: primary or secondary	MRI brain, spine
Arnold–Chiari malformation	MRI brain, spine
Diplegic cerebral palsy	MRI brain, birth history
Spinal cord arteriovenous malformation	MRI/spinal angiography
Progressive multiple sclerosis	MRI, CSF analysis, evoked responses
Motor neuron disease	EMG
Spinocerebellar ataxias	Gene testing
Adrenoleukodystrophy, adrenomyeloneuropathy	MRI brain, very long-chain fatty acids
Metachromatic leukodystrophy	MRI brain, arylsulfatase
Krabbe leukodystrophy	MRI, galactocerebrosidase
Subacute combined degeneration of the cord	Vitamin B_{12}
Arginase deficiency	Plasma arginine, aminoaciduria
Neurolathyrism	History of *Lathyrus sativus*
Abetalipoproteinemia	Lipoprotein electrophoresis
Dopa-responsive dystonia	L-Dopa trial, gene testing
Vitamin E deficiency	Serum vitamin E level
Neurosyphilis	Syphilis serology
Human T-lymphotropic virus type 1 (HTLV1) infection (tropical spastic paraparesis)	Serum/CSF HTLV-1 antibodies
AIDS	HIV testing, CD4 count

Modified from McDermott *et al.* [7].

Usually, patients with uHSP do not have a shortened life span [16]. One study described increased frequency of restless legs syndrome in patients with HSP [17]. Table 21.3 summarizes the differential diagnosis.

Pathology, neuroradiological and neurophysiological findings

The most prominent neuroradiological feature is atrophy of the cervical and thoracic spinal cord [18], with signal alterations in the corticospinal tracts and the posterior columns. Some forms of cHSP show a prominent thinning of the corpus callosum, cerebellar and cerebral atrophy and white matter lesions on brain MRI [9,16,19–22]. One study showed significant generalized brain atrophy in both forms of HSP when compared with healthy controls [23].

Most patients have normal electromyography/nerve conduction studies (EMG/NCS) unless there is

a subclinical peripheral neuropathy. Peripheral neuropathy has been described with and without chronic painless cutaneous ulcers [24]. Somatosensory and cortical evoked potentials often demonstrate a delay of conduction from the lower extremities but they are usually normal in the upper extremities [25]. This is consistent with clinical observations that symptoms are generally more pronounced in the lower extremities.

On pathological evaluation, muscle biopsy is usually normal. However, in SPG7 muscle biopsies have demonstrated ragged red fibers and cytochrome oxidase *c*-negative fibers [8,14–16,26–28]. An autopsy on an autosomal recessive patient showed frontotemporal and cerebellar atrophy, thinning of the corpus callosum and atrophy of both thalami [29]. In addition, atrophy of the spinal cord, in particular of the ventral roots, was found. Severe atrophy of the corticospinal tracts was also present. Interestingly, in this report, loss of motor neurons in the lumbar cord as well as neuronal loss on

Clarke's nucleus, with degeneration of the fasciculus gracilis on the spinal cord was found. Postmortem comparisons of HSP patients versus controls have been made and showed that patients have a significantly decreased number of axons in the corticospinal tracts, especially on the lumbar area [30].

Gene testing

Given that HSP represents at least 48 discrete genetic entities (and likely many remain to be discovered), genetic testing can both simplify and complicate the diagnostic process. The vast majority of mutations associated with HSP can be detected by sequencing-based assays. There are some important exceptions. Large-scale genetic duplications or deletions, which cannot be detected by standard sequencing, are frequently seen in SPG1, SPG2 and SPG4. Laboratories have developed technologies to look for these rearrangements, but they may not always be offered as part of the standard testing. A more extensive discussion of genetic testing issues can be found at the genetests website (www.genetests.org).

Potential benefits of gene testing:

- Genetic testing can provide a precise diagnosis.
- In the future, treatments or interventions may be based upon the specific genetic mechanism of the disease.
- A genetic diagnosis simplifies the process of evaluating other family members to confirm or exclude the diagnosis.
- A genetic diagnosis allows unaffected family members the choice of whether or not they want to have predictive genetic testing.

Potential limitations of gene testing:

- A substantial number of individuals with clinical findings and family history consistent with HSP will have normal gene test results. In some cases, this may suggest an incorrect diagnosis. More likely this is due to the incomplete understanding of the genetic basis of HSP.
- Some individuals may harbor genetic variations of uncertain significance. As many of the HSP genes are only recently discovered, the full extent of normal and pathological variation has not been described. These variants can be confusing for both the patient and the clinician. In some cases, other affected family members can be evaluated to see whether the novel variant is

segregating with the disease phenotype in the family.

- At the time of writing, genetic testing is an expensive endeavor. Panels of genetic tests often cost several thousand US dollars. This may change as "next-generation" sequencing technologies are adopted in diagnostic laboratories in the near future.

Pathogenesis and molecular basis of the disease

At least 48 distinct genetic loci have now been implicated in the causation of HSP. At the molecular level, neuronal cell recognition, signaling, vesicular sorting, mitochondrial dysfunction, intracellular trafficking and transport defects have been found to be the most common culprits leading to defective axonal development or affecting axonal transport with later degeneration [26,31]. The three most common abnormal proteins – atlastin-1, REEP1 and spastin – affect the endoplasmic reticulum network and vesicular transport [31,32].

The causative gene has been identified at 22 of the 48 mapped HSP loci. A comprehensive review of each type of HSP is beyond the scope of this chapter (see Tables 21.4, 21.5 and 21.6). Several of the more common forms of HSP are discussed in detail below. Readers interested in additional information are referred to the genetests website (www.genetests.org).

SPG1

SPG1 was the first gene discovered causing a form of X-linked cHSP [33]. The protein product, L1 cell adhesion molecule (L1 CAM) is a cell surface transmembrane glycoprotein in the immunoglobulin superfamily [26,34,35]. Mutation of this gene may also cause MASA syndrome (mental retardation, aphasia, shuffling gait and adducted thumbs), X-linked hydrocephalus and X-linked agenesis of the corpus callosum. These disorders are grouped together as L1 disease or CRASH syndrome (corpus callosum hypoplasia, retardation, adducted thumbs, spastic paraplegia, shuffling gait and hydrocephalus). Use of the term CRASH is now discouraged as it may carry a negative connotation for patients and families. In the case of the SPG1 phenotype, it is characterized by absence of cerebellar involvement, variable mental retardation and absence of extensor hallucis longus among other musculoskeletal abnormalities [11].

Table 21.4. Autosomal dominant forms of HSP.

Locus	Gene	Type	Proportion	Specific clinical features	Protein	Protein function	Final common pathway
SPG3A	ATL1	U	10% of AD	Childhood onset, slow progression	Atlastin	Morphogenesis of endoplasmic reticulum (ER) and Golgi	Axonal transport/membrane trafficking
SPG4	SPAST	U	40% of AD	Most common form of AD pure HSP	Spastin	Microtubule severing protein involved in retrograde axonal transport	Axonal transport/membrane trafficking
SPG6	NIPA1	U		Adult onset	NIPA1	Mg transport	Axonal transport/membrane trafficking
SPG8	KIAA0196	U		Adult onset	Strumpellin	Link membrane to intracellular cytoskeleton	Short, abnormally branched motor neurons
SPG9		C		Cataracts, short stature, neuropathy, skeletal defects			
SPG10	KIF5A	C/U		Childhood onset with distal muscle wasting	Kinesin family member 5A	Anterograde microtubule-dependent axonal transport	Axonal transport/membrane trafficking
SPG12		U		Average onset age 14 years with rapid progression			
SPG13	HSPD1	U		Adult onset with upper extremity involvement	Heat shock protein 60	Mitochondrial heat shock protein	Mitochondrial function
SPG17	BSCL2	C		Slow progression, distal amyotrophy	Seipin	Acts at interface of ER and lipid droplets	ER network disruption and vesicular transport
SPG19		U		Mean onset 47 years with slow progression			

Locus	Gene	Type	Proportion	Clinical features	Protein name		
SPG29		C		Hearing impairment, hiatal hernia, vomiting			
SPG31	*REEP1*	U	3–8% of AD	Variable onset uncomplicated	Receptor expression-enhancing protein 1	Localized to mitochondria	Mitochondrial function
SPG33	*ZFYVE27*	U		Adult onset	Protrudin	Promotes membrane trafficking to promote neurite outgrowth	Axonal transport/membrane trafficking
SPG36		C		Onset early adulthood, demeylination			
SPG37		U		Adult onset with slow progression			
SPG38		U		Onset teenage years			
SPG40		U		Adult onset			
SPG41		U					
SPG42	*SLC33A1*	U		Onset 4–42 years, one nonpenetrant carrier reported	Acetyl-CoA Carrier 1	Acetyl-CoA transport	

Locus: Unique designation for each chromosomal location associated with a unique form of HSP. *Gene*: If the specific gene at the locus has been identified, the official HUGO is provided. If the gene has not been identified, the entry is blank. *Type*: C = complicated, U = uncomplicated, C/U = both presentations described. *Proportion*: if known, the proportion of patients with the type and inheritance pattern that is explained by mutations in the particular gene.

Table 21.5. Autosomal recessive forms of HSP.

Locus	Gene	Type	Proportion	Specific clinical features	Protein	Protein function	Final common pathway
SPG5A	CYP7B1	U		Variable onset, posterior column and bladder dysfunction	Cytochrome p450-7B1	Alternate pathways for cholesterol degradation	Cholesterol metabolism
SPG7	SPG7	C/U	5% of AR	Variable onset, optic atrophy, neuropathy, dysarthria, dysphagia	Paraplegin	mitochondrial assembly	Mitochondrial function
SPG11	SPG11	C/U		TCC, MR, dysarthria, nystagmus, neuropathy	Spastizin	Present in ER and endosomes	Axonal transport/membrane trafficking
SPG14		C		Mild cognitive delay, distal motor neuropathy			
SPG18				Early onset with agenesis or hypoplasia of corpus callosum, cognitive delays			
SPG15	ZFYVE26	C		Thin corpus callosum (TCC), pigmented maculopathy, distal amyotrophy, dysarthria, cognitive delay	Spastizin	Present in ER and endosomes	ER network disruption and vesicular transport
SPG20	SPG20	C		Childhood onset, spastic quadriparesis, cerebellar signs, short stature	Spartin	Mitochondrial, nuclear, and cytoplasmic localization	Axonal transport/membrane trafficking
SPG21	SPG21	C		Early adult onset, TCC, dementia, extra pyramidal signs	Maspardin	Vesicular transport of endosomal and Golgi apparatus	Axonal transport/membrane trafficking
SPG23		C		Pigmentary abnormalities, peripheral neuropathy			
SPG24		C		Spastic dysarthria and pseudobulbar signs			

Locus	Gene	Type	Clinical features	Protein	Function	
SPG25		C	Spinal disc herniations			
SPG26		C	Intellectual impairment, dysarthria, distal amyotrophy			
SPG27		C/U	Dysarthria			
SPG28		U	Onset 6–15 years			
SPG30		C	Sensory neuropathy, ataxia			
SPG32		C	Childhood onset, slow progression, TCC, cerebellar atrophy			
SPG35	FA2H	C	Childhood onset Seizures, cognitive decline, foot drop	Fatty acid-2 hydroxylase	Hydroxylation of sphingolipids in myelin	Myelin formation
SPG39	PNPLA6	C	Distal muscle wasting, spinal cord atrophy	Neuropathy target esterase		
SPG43		C	Childhood onset, amyotrophy			
SPG44	GJC2	U	Adult onset			
SPG45		C	Childhood onset, cognitive delay			
SPG46		C	Childhood onset, TCC, cognitive delay			
SPG48	KIAA0415	U	Onset in adulthood	KIAA0415	DNA helicase	DNA repair

Locus: Unique designation for each chromosomal location associated with a unique form of HSP. *Gene*: If the specific gene at the locus has been identified, the official HUGO is provided. If the gene has not been identified, the entry is blank. *Type*: C = complicated, U = uncomplicated, C/U = both presentations described. *Proportion*: if known, the proportion of patients with the type and inheritance pattern that is explained by mutations in the particular gene.

Table 21.6. X-linked forms of HSP.

Locus	Gene	Type	Specific clinical features	Protein	Protein function	Final common pathway
SPG1	*L1CAM*	C	Affects males, intellectual disability, normal MRI, allelic to more severe "MASA" syndrome and X-linked aqueductal stenosis	L1 cell adhesion molecule		Embryonic development of corticospinal tracts
SPG2	*PLP1*	C	Affects males, can be a later onset uncomplicated form with normal lifespan or early onset complicated form with nystagmus and ataxia. Allelic with the more severe Pelizaeus–Merzbacher disease	Myelin proteolipid protein	Myelination	Myelination
SPG16		C/U	Motor aphasia, reduced vision, mild cognitive delay			
SPG22		C	Proposed-Allan–Herndon–Dudley syndrome			
SPG34		U	Childhood onset with slow progression			

Locus: Unique designation for each chromosomal location associated with a unique form of HSP. *Gene*: If the specific gene at the locus has been identified, the official HUGO is provided. If the gene has not been identified, the entry is blank. *Type*: C = complicated, U = uncomplicated, C/U = both presentations described.

L1 CAMs are signaling molecules that have been found in neurons and Schwann cells. These molecules have been found to be concentrated on the axonal growth cones during development [34]. It is theorized that they are involved in directing growth of the axon based on axonotropic signals [14,15,35,36]. Mice lacking L1 CAM have failure of the corticospinal tracts to cross at the level of the medulla [26]. The disruption of early development of the corticospinal tracts might explain the early onset of symptoms in affected patents.

SPG2

The product of the X-linked *PLP1* gene is the myelin proteolipid protein. Mutations on *PLP1* can give rise to two diseases: HSP (either complicated or uncomplicated) and Pelizaeus–Merzbacher disease (PMD) [26,35]. Besides the spastic paraplegia, HSP phenotype patients also have nystagmus, ataxia, cognitive impairment, tremor and slow growth. Patients lacking normal *PLP1* gene expression show axonal degeneration of the distal corticospinal tracts and fasciculus gracilis [6,26]. Brain MRI studies may reveal white matter changes [15,35,36]. The defect of myelination and oligodendrocyte structure caused by *PLP1*

mutations may affect axonal signaling and/or transport. Accumulation of membranous dense bodies and mitochondria has been observed, suggesting impaired axonal transport [15,26].

SPG3

SPG3 accounts for approximately 10% of dominant uHSP [15,27]. Childhood onset of uHSP symptoms is common. SPG3 is caused by mutations in the *ATL1* gene, which encodes the atlastin protein. This protein is a member of the dynamin GTPases. These types of proteins play an important role in vesicle trafficking [26,27]. Furthermore, these proteins have been implicated in the maintenance of cytoskeleton and distribution of mitochondria.

SPG4

This is the most common type of autosomal dominant HSP, accounting for approximately 40% of cases [5]. The product of this gene is called spastin. The spastin protein has an AAA domain, which is involved in several cellular functions [37]. Spastin is able to sever and disassemble microtubules [26,27,34,38]. It is suggested that loss of function of spastin may impair maintenance of cytoskeleton and organelle trafficking, especially in mitochondria [27]. The majority of people with SPG4 retain the ability to walk independently or with mild support. However, there is a great variability, with some patients being almost asymptomatic and others bedridden. Cognitive decline and dementia are also seen in some families with the disease [39]. The disease progression is much faster if the onset of symptoms is after age 35 years [8].

SPG5

SPG5 is an autosomal recessive form of HSP caused by mutations in the *CYP7B1* gene [40–42]. *CYP7B1* mutations have been described in both pure and complex forms of SPG5. In these patients, age at onset ranged from 4 to 47 years. In advanced stages, most of the patients have severe handicap, being wheelchair-bound or requiring a walking aid. Brain involvement was not thought to be the norm but a recent study revealed abnormal MRI brain white matter changes in 3 of 23 studied patients [43].

Cholesterol is converted in mammals into bile acids. *CYP7B1* has been found to encode the enzyme oxysterol, which is involved in the alternative acidic pathway of the bile acid synthesis from cholesterol. It has been hypothesized that loss of function of *CYP7B1* leads to abnormal oxysterol levels.

SPG6

SPG6 is an autosomal dominant form of HSP linked to chromosome 15q and caused by mutations in the *NIPA1* gene (nonimprinted in Prader-Willi/Angelman syndrome 1) [44,45]. The onset is usually in adolescence or early adulthood, with a mean age of onset of 22 years. It is a slowly progressive form of uHSP [7,27]. The function of the NIPA1 protein is unknown. It has been suggested that the protein could function as a receptor, as a transporter or in membrane trafficking [26]. Patients with Prader–Willi or Angelman syndrome, who are most often missing one copy of this gene, do not develop HSP symptoms. This suggests a "gain of function" type of mutation is responsible for HSP6 rather than haploinsufficiency [26,27].

SPG7

SPG7 is an autosomal recessive form of HSP mapped to chromosome 16. The causative gene encodes the paraplegin protein, which is known to be associated with mitochondria. SPG7 can present as either cHSP or uHSP [15]. The complicated phenotype is remarkable for dysarthria, optic disc pallor, dysphagia, axonal neuropathy, and evidence of vascular lesions, cerebral and cerebellar atrophy [7,15,26,27]. This protein is homologous to several yeast mitochondrial proteins that have chaperone-like activity in the inner membrane of the mitochondria [7]. Some patients have shown ragged red fibers and cytochrome *c* oxidase-negative fibers on muscle biopsy [7,14,15,26,34]. In affected neurons, the dysfunctional mitochondria are aggregated in the presynaptic terminal. In a normal neuron, young mitochondria are transported from neuron soma to the axon terminal, while the reverse is true for old mitochondria. This process is dependent on dyneins and kinesins, both of which require ATP to function. With dysfunctional mitochondria, this process is impaired [46].

SPG10

Kinesin heavy chain (KIF5A) is a molecule responsible of organelle and macromolecule locomotion along the microtubules in anterograde direction [14,15,26,27]. Mutations in the *KIF5A* gene cause an early-onset form of uHSP or cHSP associated with distal muscle atrophy [1]. The KIF5A protein acts as a "motor" using ATP to move organelles and macromolecules along microtubules.

SPG11, SPG 15

SPG11 and SPG15 are recessive forms of HSP characterized by overlapping clinical phenotypes. They are both characterized by early-onset spastic paraplegia complicated by cognitive deficits followed by peripheral neuropathy and amyotrophy. Thin corpus callosum (TCC), peripheral neuropathy with hand muscle atrophy and cerebellar ataxia are common features. These two clinical entities account for 35% of autosomal recessive HSP with TCC. In one study they accounted for 59% of AR HSP cases with TCC and cognitive impairment [47]. TCC is more consistently seen in SPG11, as opposed to SPG15. Kjellin syndrome was originally described as an autosomal recessive form of HSP complicated by findings of TCC and retinal degeneration. Recent research has demonstrated that SPG11 and SPG15 mutations are the underlying cause of Kjellin syndrome, with retinal degeneration occurring as a later complication in the disease process [48–52].

SPG20

SPG20 is an autosomal recessive form of cHSP with distal muscle atrophy and dysarthria also known as Troyer syndrome [15,27,28]. The product of this gene is spartin. It has been described in the Amish population of the United States. One study found that native spartin is located inside the mitochondria, while the mutant spartin loses this mitochondrial localization, further supporting the importance of mitochondria in axonal maintenance and in the pathophysiology of HSP.

SPG48

The recent discovery that mutations in the *KIAA0415* gene cause an uncomplicated recessive form of HSP (SPG48) introduces yet another molecular pathway to the already complicated HSP story [53]. Mutations in this gene were discovered as part of a screen for DNA damage repair genes. Mutations in DNA damage repair have already been implicated in several forms of the degenerative disease spinocerebellar ataxia.

Treatment

Unfortunately, there is no specific treatment either to improve or stop the progression of this disease. The mainstay of treatment consists of physical therapy to improve strength and mobility and to avoid contractures. Antispasmodics such as baclofen (oral or via pump), dantrolene or benzodiazepines are used. Oxybutin is given for bladder symptoms. Onabotulinum neurotoxin type A has been used to improve spasticity in HSP. In a case series, it was concluded that patients treated earlier in the disease perceived the most benefit from onabotulinum neurotoxin type A, especially when the muscle strength is preserved [54]. Surgical treatment to lengthen tendons and improve mobility has also been used.

Nocodazole as a specific treatment for SPG4 is a promising agent, which is being evaluated as a potential treatment for HSP. This agent acts by destabilizing microtubules in vitro. It has been shown to suppress the mutant phenotypes observed in a *Drosophila* model [26].

Future directions

Genetics and molecular biology have greatly advanced our understanding of the causes of HSP. Among the 22 known genes associated with HSP, there is a consistent theme of axonal transport, mitochondrial maintenance, disruptions in the development and myelination of axons. While a large number of pathways have been implicated, it is important to note that more than half of the putative genes associated with HSP have not yet been identified. This suggests that many more molecular and cellular pathways may be identified.

From a patient perspective, these advances are meaningless unless they translate into effective interventions or cures. Future research will focus on how to identify individuals at risk and intervene before symptoms develop.

References

1. Salinas S, Proukakis C, Crosby A *et al.* Hereditary spastic paraplegia: clinical features and pathogenetic mechanism. *Lancet Neurol* 2008; **7**: 1127–38.

2. Kjersti Erichsen A, Koht J, Stray-Pedersen A *et al.* Prevalence of hereditary ataxia and spastic paraplegia in Southeast Norway: a population based study. *Brain* 2009; **132**: 1577–88.

3. Harding AE. Hereditary "pure" spastic paraplegia: a clinical and genetic study of 22 families. *J Neurol Neurosurg Psychiatry* 1981; **44**(10): 871–83.

4. Harding AE. Classification of the hereditary ataxias and paraplegias. *Lancet* 1983; **1**(8334): 1151–5.

5. Lindsey JC, Lusher ME, McDermott CJ *et al.* Mutation analysis of the spastin gene (SPG4) in patients with hereditary spastic paraparesis. *J Med Genet.* 2000; **37**(10): 759–65.

6. Fink JK, Hedera P. Hereditary spastic paraplegia: genetic heterogeneity and genotype-phenotype correlation. *Semin Neurol* 1999; **19**: 301–9.

7. McDermott CJ, White K, Bushby K *et al.* Hereditary spastic paraparesis: a review of new developments. *J Neurol Neurosurg Psychiatry* 2000; **69**: 150–60.

8. Tallaksen CM, Dürr A, Brice A. Recent advances in hereditary spastic paraplegia. *Curr Opin Neurol* 2001; **14**: 457–63.

9. Uttner IP, Baumgartner A, Sperfeld AD, Kassubek J. Cognitive performance in pure and complicated hereditary spastic paraparesis: a neuropsychological and neuroimaging study. *Neurosci Lett* 2007; **419**: 158–61.

10. Tallaksen CM, Guichart-Gomez E, Verpillat P *et al.* Subtle cognitive impairment but no dementia in patients with spastin mutations. *Arch Neurol* 2003; **60**: 1113–8.

11. Klebe S, Stolze H, Kopper F *et al.* Gait analysis of sporadic and hereditary spastic paraplegia. *J Neurol* 2004; **251**: 571–8.

12. Strong MJ, Gordon PH. Primary lateral sclerosis, hereditary spastic paraplegia and amyotrophic lateral sclerosis: Discrete entities or spectrum? *Amyotroph Lateral Scler* 2005; **6**: 8–16.

13. Fink JK. Advances in hereditary spastic paraplegia. *Curr Opin Neurol* 1997; **10**: 313–8.

14. Fink JK. Advances in hereditary spastic paraplegias. *Exp Neurol* 2003; **184**: 106–10.

15. Crosby AH, Proukakis C. Is the transportation highway the right road for hereditary spastic paraplegia? *Am J Hum Genet*. 2002; **71**: 1009–16.

16. Fink JK. Hereditary spastic paraplegia. *Neurol Clin* 2002; **20**: 711–726.

17. Sperfeld AD, Unrath A, Kassubek J. Restless legs syndrome in hereditary spastic paraparesis. *Eur Neurol* 2007; **57**: 31–35.

18. Sperfeld AD, Baumgartner A, Kassubek J. Magnetic resonance investigation of upper spinal cord in pure and complicated hereditary spastic paraparesis. *Eur Neurol* 2005; **54**(4): 181–5.

19. Okubo S, Ueda M, Kamiya T *et al*. Neurological and radiological progression in hereditary spastic paraplegia with thin corpus callosum. *Acta Neurol Scand* 2000; **102**: 196–9.

20. Brockmann K, Simpson MA, Faber A *et al*. Complicated hereditary paraplegia with thin corpus callosum and childhood onset. *Neuropediatrics* 2005; **36**: 274–8.

21. Hedera P, Eldevik OP, Maly P *et al*. Spinal cord magnetic resonance imaging in autosomal dominant hereditary spastic paraplegia. *Neuroradiology* 2005; **47**: 730–4.

22. Franca MC, D'Abreu A, Maurer-Morlli CV *et al*. Prospective neuroimaging study in hereditary spastic paraplegia with thin corpus callosum. *Mov Disord* 2007; **22**: 1556–62.

23. Kassubek J, Sperfeld, AD. Baumgartner A, Huppertz HJ, Riecker A, Juengling FD. Brain atrophy in pure and complicated hereditary spastic paraparesis: a quantitative 3D MRI study. *Eur J Neurol* 2006; **13**: 880–6.

24. Shady W, Smith CML. Sensory neuropathy in hereditary spastic paraplegia. *J Neurol Neurosurg Psychiatry* 1994; **57**: 693–8.

25. Schulte T, Miterski B, Bornke C, Przuntek H, Epplen JT, Schols L. Neurophysiological findings in SPG4 patients differ from other types of spastic paraplegias. *Neurology* 2003; **60**: 1529–32.

26. Soderblom C, Blackstone C. Traffic accidents: molecular genetic insights into pathogenesis of hereditary spastic paraplegias. *Pharmacol Ther* 2009; **109**: 42–56.

27. Fink JK. The hereditary spastic paraplegias: nine genes and counting. *Arch Neurol* 2003; **60**: 1045–9.

28. McDermott CJ, Shaw PJ. Hereditary spastic paraplegia. *Int Rev Neurobiol* 2002; **53**: 191–204.

29. Nomura H, Koike F *et al*. Autopsy case of autosomal recessive hereditary spastic paraplegia with reference to muscular pathology. *Neuropathology* 2001; **21**: 212–7.

30. DeLuca GC, Ebers GC, Esiri MM. The extent of axonal loss in the long tracts in hereditary spastic paraplegia. *Neuropathol Appl Neurobiol* 2004; **30**: 576–84.

31. Park SH, Zhu PP, Parker RL *et al*. Hereditary spastic paraplegia proteins REEP1, spastin, and atlastin-1 coordinate microtubule interactions with the tubular ER network. *J Clin Invest*. 2010; **120**(4): 1097–110.

32. Hewamadduma C, McDermott CJ, Kirby J *et al*. New pedigrees and novel mutations expand the phenotype of REEP1-associated hereditary spastic paraplegia. *Neurogenetics* 2009; **10**: 105–10.

33. Jouet M, Rosenthal A, Armstrong G *et al*. X-linked spastic paraplegia (SPG1), MASA syndrome and X-linked hydrocephalus result from mutations in the L1 gene. *Nat Genet* 1994; **7**(3): 402–7.

34. Casari G, Rugarli E. Molecular basis of inherited spastic paraplegias. *Curr Opin Gen Dev* 2001; **11**: 336–42.

35. Züchner S. The genetics of hereditary spastic paraplegia and implications for drug therapy. *Expert Opin Pharmacother* 2007; **8**: 1433–9.

36. Kobayashi H, Garcia CA, Alfonso G *et al*. Molecular genetics of familial spastic paraplegia: a multitude of responsible genes. *J Neurol Sci* 1996; **137**: 131–8.

37. Rugarli EI, Thomas, L. Translating m-AAA protease function in mitochondria to hereditary spastic paraplegia. *Trends Mol Med* 2006; **12**: 262–9.

38. Roehl White S, Evans KJ, Lary J *et al*. Recognition of C-terminal amino acids in tubulin by pore loops in Spastin is important for microtubule severing. *J Cell Biol* 2007; **176**: 995–1005.

39. Murphy S, Gorman G, Beetz C *et al*. Dementia in SPG4 hereditary spastic paraplegia, clinical, genetic and neuropathological evidence. *Neurology* 2009; **73**: 378–84.

40. Goizet C, Boukhris A, Durr A *et al*. CYP7B1 mutations in pure and complex forms of hereditary spastic paraplegia type 5. *Brain* 2009; **132**: 1589–600.

41. Biancheri R, Ciccolella M, Rossi A *et al*. White matter lesions in spastic paraplegia with mutations in SPG5/CYP7B1. *Neuromuscul Disord* 2009; **19**: 62–5.

42. Tsaousidou MK, Ouahchi K, Warner TT *et al*. Sequence alterations within CYP7B1 implicate defective cholesterol homeostasis in motor-neuron degeneration. *Am J Hum Genet* 2008; **82**: 510–15.

43. Biancheri R, Ciccolella M, Rossi A *et al*. White matter lesions in spastic paraplegia with mutations in SPG5/CYP7B1. *Neuromuscul Disord* 2009; **19**(1): 62–5.

44. Goytain A, Hines RM, El-Husseini A *et al*. NIPA1 (SPG6), the basis for autosomal dominant form of hereditary spastic paraplegia, encodes a functional Mg transporter. *J Biol Chem* 2007; **282**(11): 8060–8.

45. Tsang HTH, Edwards TL, Wang X *et al*. The hereditary spastic paraplegia proteins NIPA1, spastin, and spartin

are inhibitors of mammalian BMP signaling. *Hum Mol Genet* 2009; **18**(20): 3805–21.

46. Ferreirinha F, Quattrini A, Pirozzi M *et al.* Axonal degeneration in paraplegin deficient mice is associated with abnormal mitochondria and impairment of axonal transport. *J Clin Invest* 2004; **113**: 231–42.

47. Stevanin G, Azzedine H, Denora P *et al.* Mutations in SPG11 are frequent in autosomal recessive spastic paraplegia with thin corpus callosum, cognitive decline and lower motor neuron degeneration. *Brain* 2008; **131**: 772–84.

48. Orlen H, Melberg A, Raininko R *et al.* SPG11 mutations cause Kjellin syndrome, a hereditary spastic paraplegia with thin corpus callosum and central retinal degeneration. *Am J Med Gen* 2009; **150B**: 984–92.

49. Pippucci T, Panza E, Pompilli E *et al.* Autosomal recessive hereditary spastic paraplegia with thin corpus callosum: a novel mutation in the SPG11 gene and further evidence for genetic heterogeneity. *Eur J Neurol* 2009; **15**: 121–6.

50. Schule R, Schlipf N, Synofzik M *et al.* Frequency and phenotype of SPG11 and SPG15 in complicated hereditary spastic paraplegia. *J Neurol Neurosurg Psychiatry* 2009; **80**: 1402–4.

51. Goizet C, Boukhris A, Maltete D *et al.* SPG15 is the second most common cause of hereditary spastic paraplegia with thin corpus callosum. *Neurology* 2009; **73**: 1111–9.

52. Hanein S, Martin E, Boukhris A *et al.* Identification of the SPG15 gene, encoding Spastizin, as a frequent cause of complicated autosomal-recessive spastic paraplegia, including Kjellin syndrome. *Am J Hum Genet* 2008; **82**: 992–1002.

53. Słabicki M, Theis M, Krastev DB *et al.* A genome-scale DNA repair RNAi screen identifies SPG48 as a novel gene associated with hereditary spastic paraplegia. *PLoS Biol* 2010; **8**(6): e1000408.

54. Hecht MJ, Stolze H, Auf dem Brinke M *et al.* Botulinum neurotoxin type A injections reduce spasticity in mild to moderate hereditary spastic paraplegia: report of 19 cases. *Mov Disord* 2008; **23**: 228–33.

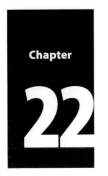

Cramps, contractures and myalgias

Twilight zone between movement disorders and neuromuscular diseases

Michelle M. Dompenciel and Virgilio D. Salanga

History

Myalgias, stiffness and muscle cramps are common complaints encountered by neurologists and primary care physicians. The significance of these symptoms ranges from benign conditions, such as benign cramp-fasciculation syndrome, to devastating neurological conditions like motor neuron disorders. That is why it is essential to perform a thorough history and physical examination when evaluating a patient with suspected muscle disease. There has been substantial uncertainty regarding the classification and definition of muscle cramps, mainly due to the use of this term to designate many symptoms related to muscle diseases such as myalgias, contractures or even muscle stiffness. Several authors have addressed this subject and have proposed newer classifications to describe the cramping syndromes. Some have classified the diverse cramping syndromes on the basis of their origin, dividing them into muscle disorders, disorders of the peripheral nervous system, or conditions of uncertain origin. Other authors have classified them on the basis of their pathogenesis (myogenic, motor neurons or peripheral nerves, or central disorders); and others have proposed a classification according to their electromyographic distinctiveness, based on the different characteristics on needle EMG of true cramps, tetany, contractures and dystonia. Using these classifications when evaluating patients helps differentiate among the different causes and helps the clinician focus on the specific disorder underlying the muscle cramps.

Clinical findings

A cramp is commonly described as an episodic and involuntary muscle contraction, generally associated with pain, which tends to occur when a muscle is in the shortened position and contracting, due to motor neuron hyperactivity causing a sustained muscle spasm.

This is the definition of a true cramp, which is usually preceded clinically by fasciculations or muscle twitching due to the repetitive contractions of motor units. On electromyography (EMG), it is defined as a usually stable and high-frequency discharge (20–150 Hz) that is generated by the motor neuron axon, therefore making it not a muscle phenomenon. Cramps are commonly mistaken clinically with contractures, making the use of EMG essential since contractures are typically electrically silent on needle EMG, which is not the case in cramps. Contractures do not occur at rest and usually develop during exercise and are typically related to the occurrence of muscle damage, leading to myoglobinuria and renal failure due to acute tubular necrosis. Contractures can be painful, painless, or compensating for other aching processes. Examples of painless contractures include those conditions related to spasticity or prolonged muscle immobility, whereas painful contractures are usually caused by metabolic myopathies. Patients with prominent spasticity due to damage to the descending motor pathways frequently complain of muscle stiffness, muscle cramps and spasms. Muscle diseases associated with contractures include inherited disorders of glucose metabolism, paramyotonia congenita (sodium channelopathy), hypothyroid myopathy, and rippling muscle disease, among others.

Some of the disorders of glycolytic or glycogenolytic enzyme defects are associated with myalgias and painful muscle cramps only during forceful exercise, such as in myophosphorylase (McArdle) and phosphofructokinase (Tarui) deficiencies (Table 22.1). In McArdle disease, symptoms develop within minutes of exercise and resolve with rest, and patients have the characteristic hand-cramp posture after the forearm exercise test for lactate production and after performing repetitive gripping movements. This hand posture may clinically be similar to myotonia or a focal dystonia. In Tarui

Uncommon Causes of Movement Disorders, ed. Néstor Gálvez-Jiménez and Paul J. Tuite. Published by Cambridge University Press. © Cambridge University Press 2011.

Table 22.1. Specific muscle disorders associated with myalgias and muscle cramps.

Myotonic dystrophy	Glycogen metabolism disorders
Channelopathies	Lactate dehydrogenase deficiency
Calcium channel disease	Myophosphorylase deficiency
Hypokalemic periodic paralysis	Phosphofructokinase deficiency
Sodium channel disease	Muscle phosphoglycerate mutase deficiency
Paramyotonia congenital	Phosphoglycerate kinase deficiency
Hyperkalemic periodic paralysis	Phosphorylase b kinase deficiency
Chloride channel disease	Lipid metabolism disorders
Myotonia congenital	Carnitine palmitoyltransferase II deficiency
Becker disease	Myotonia congenital with cramps
Thomsen disease	Drug-induced or malignancy related

disease, the clinical findings and muscle biopsy results are similar to those seen in McArdle disease, comprising exercise intolerance, progressive weakness and painful contractures, but differentiated by genetic testing. In McArdle deficiency there is improved exercise tolerance after a "warm-up" period of nonexhausting exercise, also known as "second-wind phenomenon."

Another example is rippling muscle disease, which is a rare disorder characterized by painful muscle stiffness, contractures and rippling movement in muscles that have been stretched by either voluntary contraction or percussion. They also exhibit myoedema in conjunction with the rippling muscle movements, which are electrically silent on electromyography. In hypothyroid myopathy there is also myoedema and an overlap of symptoms to include myalgia, contractures, muscle cramps, and more importantly the slowness of muscle contraction and relaxation. The latter can be clinically confused, when severe, with dystonia due to the muscle stiffness with slowed movements. This phenomenon is worsened by exposure to cold and clinically is seen as a slow return phase of the Achilles reflex after percussion, along with myoedema. However, it is important to understand that both hypo- and hyperthyroidism can cause muscle disease symptoms. There have been case reports of patients found to have hypothyroidism that presented initially with nonspecific symptoms of myalgias, muscle cramps, and stiffness with symptom improvement after thyroxine replacement. It has been reported that the incidence of musculoskeletal symptoms in hypothyroidism is likely close to 30–80% [1].

Several other entities can be confused with muscle cramps such as myotonia, muscle stiffness/tightness, and even focal dystonias. That is why careful consideration of the patient's symptoms may help separate the etiology into a true cramp, focal dystonia, contracture, or even tetany. Tetany is defined as a continuous tonic spasm of a muscle due to motor unit hyperactivity associated clinically with sensory hyperactivity leading to paresthesias, usually associated with metabolic derangements; once these are corrected, the tetany and sensory symptoms should resolve. Myotonia is a phenomenon of impaired relaxation of the muscle after forceful voluntary contraction due to repetitive depolarization of the muscle membrane. Patients typically complain of muscle stiffness and difficulty releasing their handgrip after a handshake, which typically improves after repeated contractions and should not be confused with contractures. In some cases there is reported worsening of symptoms when exposed to cold temperatures. On needle EMG, myotonic discharges are spontaneous discharges of a muscle fiber, characterized by a waxing and waning of amplitude and frequency with a firing rate between 20 and 150 Hz, frequently described as a "revving engine" sound on the speaker. These discharges are typically seen in disorders such as myotonic dystrophy, myotonia congenita (chloride channelopathy), paramyotonia congenita (sodium channelopathy), hypokalemic periodic paralysis (calcium channelopathy), and acquired myotonia related to drugs or malignancy, among others.

Focal dystonias can easily be mistaken for cramps or spasms. They are characterized by directional and sustained agonist and antagonistic muscle contractions that produce abnormal postures or repetitive movements. Patients may refer to spasmodic twisting of the neck or face or of an extremity that remains in a persistent posture even after a skilled motor act, as seen in writer's cramp (occupational cramp), which is now considered as a focal dystonia. Electromyograms confirm this by the co-contraction of agonist and antagonistic muscles consistent with the definition of dystonia. Occupational cramps can also be associated clinically with tremors or myoclonic movements, and it is with cautious attentions to these details that we can best differentiate these entities clinically and clarify the overlap between movement disorders and neuromuscular diseases.

Myalgias, like fatigue, are nonspecific symptoms usually associated with myopathic processes. They are related to metabolic or inflammatory muscle diseases such as tubular aggregate myopathy, mitochondrial myopathy, intracellular acidosis, X-linked myalgia and cramps (Becker dystrophy variant), drug-induced conditions (chloroquine, lipid-lowering drugs, zidovudine/AZT, etc.), hypothyroid myopathy, inflammatory myopathies (dermatomyositis, polymyositis), among others, and may even occur after a viral illness.

The etiology of cramps is very broad and to further simplify their categorization Parisi et al. recommended a new classification for muscle cramps [2]. They propose that muscle cramps should be classified on the basis of site of pathogenesis [2], particularly into one of these basic groups: paraphysiological cramps, idiopathic cramps, and symptomatic cramps. Paraphysiological cramps are defined by the occurrence of cramps in otherwise healthy patients related to specific physiological circumstances related to pregnancy or exercise, such as low levels of magnesium, hydroelectrolyte disturbances, or hyperexcitability of nerve terminal branches due to continued muscle use. Idiopathic cramps can be either sporadic or inherited and are not associated with sensory, pyramidal, cerebellar, or cognitive abnormalities. Examples of such are familial nocturnal cramps for the inherited forms and cramp-fasciculation syndrome and myokymia-hyperhidrosis syndrome for the sporadic forms of idiopathic cramps. In contrast, symptomatic cramps comprise an assortment of conditions ranging from central and peripheral nervous system diseases, muscle diseases, endocrine-metabolic conditions, cardiovascular diseases, hydroelectrolyte disturbances, to toxic and psychiatric causes (Table 22.2). In the cramp-fasciculation syndrome patients report painful muscle cramps, myalgias, muscle stiffness and fasciculations without muscle atrophy or progressive weakness on neurological examination. It has been stipulated that this is a benign process due to peripheral nerve hyperexcitability [3].

However, there have been case reports of evolution from benign fasciculations and cramps to motor neuron disease, proposing an anterior horn cell dysfunction in the pathogenesis of this syndrome, preceding motor neuron cell death [4,5].

Another condition associated with muscle stiffness and muscle spasms is stiff person syndrome (SPS), a rare autoimmune disease that exhibits severe and intermittent stiffness of the axial musculature and proximal limbs, along with painful muscle spasms that are typically triggered by external stimuli. The muscle stiffness particularly affects the abdominal, neck and thoracolumbar regions, sometimes causing unnatural and painful positions such as seen in an opisthotonus posture. This form is associated with autoantibodies to glutamic acid decarboxylase (GAD). There is another clinically distinct form of SPS associated with amphiphysin antibodies presenting with a pattern of stiffness affecting the arms and neck muscles, as opposed to the variant associated with anti-GAD antibodies affecting more the thoracolumbar musculature [6]. This variant associated with amphiphysin antibodies is much rarer and has been associated with breast and lung cancers.

Laboratory investigations

When evaluating a patient with possible muscle disease it is essential to distinguish between negative and/or positive symptoms. Negative symptoms include weakness, fatigue, exercise intolerance and muscle atrophy; whereas positive symptoms comprise myalgias, contractures, cramps, muscle stiffness and myoglobinuria. In addition to these symptoms, it is important to inquire whether fasciculations and weakness are present, which would imply damage to motor neurons. If there is evidence of concurrent upper motor neuron involvement, the clinical suspicion of amyotrophic lateral sclerosis comes to question. A thorough neurological evaluation is warranted and should include careful attention to the presence of fasciculations, weakness, muscle spasms, myokymia and even dystonic postures. Family history should be sought as well to decide on molecular genetic studies. Sensory abnormalities should also be sought to further clarify whether there is a peripheral neuropathic or radicular process associated with muscle cramps. It has been shown that nerve root compression can cause muscle cramps, fasciculations and even myokymia in the distribution of the muscles supplied by that root. That is why testing should include imaging studies to exclude

Table 22.2. Etiology of muscle cramps.

Metabolic/endocrine disorders	Central and peripheral nervous system
Hypo- and hyperthyroidism	Motor neuron disease
Hypo- and hyperparathyroidism	Sequelae of poliomyelitis
Uremia and dialysis	Radiculopathy/plexopathies
Cirrhosis	Peripheral neuropathy
Hypoadrenalism	Multiple sclerosis
Pregnancy	Parkinson disease
Hydroelectrolyte disorders	Muscle diseases
Hypomagnesemia	Metabolic myopathy
Dehydration	Mitochondrial myopathy
Heat cramps, perspiration	Inflammatory myopathy
Diuretic therapy	Myotonic disorders
Hypo- and hypercalcemia	Channelopathies
Hypo- and hyperkalemia	Dystrophic myotonias
Hypo- and hypernatremia	Toxic/medications
Idiopathic cramps	Statins, diuretics, clofibrate
Familial nocturnal cramps	Cardiovascular
Idiopathic nocturnal cramps	Venous/arterial diseases
Myokymia-hyperhidrosis syndrome	Hypertension
Exercise-related	Psychiatric disorders

structural lesions as such seen in degenerative disk disease or when upper motor neuron signs are present in the examination.

Electromyography is very useful in distinguishing between cramps, contractures and dystonia, as well as helping to establish the diagnosis in certain conditions as discussed earlier. It also aids in evaluating for the presence of myotonic discharges, myopathic or neuropathic units, active denervation, fasciculations or anterior horn cell instability, myokymia, neuromyotonia and cramps, which in combination with the neurological examination can further reduce the differential diagnosis. It also helps in the selection of muscles that have been affected and later deciding on biopsy. In myophosphorylase (McArdle) and phosphofructokinase (Tarui) deficiencies, nerve conduction studies are usually normal. In some of these patients the CMAP (compound muscle action potential) may show a decrementing response on repetitive nerve stimulation. Needle EMG may show positive waves and fibrillation potentials, as well as myotonic discharges with myopathic units and early recruitment. Since symptoms are typically provoked by exercise, after an attack the motor unit potentials (MUPs) may be abnormal in

configuration and show a reduction in number. EMG is also very helpful in diseases like myotonic dystrophy type 1 due to the presence of myotonic discharges and myopathic motor units, as described earlier. This condition is characterized by distal rather than proximal extremity muscle weakness with facial muscle weakness, myotonia, diminished intellect, gonadal atrophy, cardiomyopathy and several endocrinopathies, among others. Other EMG findings typically seen in muscle diseases include myokymia, which consists of continuous twitching muscle movements that resemble fasciculations. Myokymia is typically seen in Isaac syndrome. The phenomenon is seen in this condition in distal limbs and also may include the face, jaw and trunk muscles. Patients also present with muscle stiffness and cramps, which may persist during sleep. Myokymia is generated by bursts of continuous motor unit activity, which are captured on needle EMG. Besides myokymic discharges, Isaac syndrome may present with neuromyotonic discharges and fasciculations on needle EMG. The condition is thought to be autoimmune related.

In terms of laboratory testing, CK (creatine kinase) levels are very useful in the evaluation of suspected

Table 22.3. Conditions related to elevated creatine kinase (CK).

Motor neuron diseases	Medications
Amyotrophic lateral sclerosis	Lipid-lowering drugs
Post-polio syndrome	Zidovudine (AZT)
Spinal muscular atrophy	Chloroquine
Myopathies	Ciclosporin
Inflammatory	Trauma/vigorous exercise
Dermatomyositis	Channelopathies
Polymyositis	Metabolic/endocrine disorders
Metabolic	Hypothyroidism
Drug-induced	Hypoparathyroidism
Congenital	Idiopathic causes
Muscular dystrophies	Increased muscle mass
Postviral illness	Medications

muscle disease. Refer to Table 22.3 for conditions related with elevation of CK. Most of the glycogen metabolism disorders (Table 22.1) typically present with elevated creatine kinase levels, some of them with normal levels between attacks. Medication side-effects and toxic causes should be considered as part of the initial evaluation as well. Additional blood tests include thyroid function tests, parathyroid hormone levels, HIV testing, serum electrolytes, hematologic evaluation, aldolase, liver enzymes, lactate dehydrogenase (LDH), paraneoplastic evaluation, immunological markers (Jo-1 antibodies and evaluation for systemic lupus erythematosus and rheumatoid arthritis), heavy-metal testing, urine analysis (myoglobinuria) and serum immunofixation/urine electrophoresis, among others. Several glycogen storage disorders are usually associated with myoglobinuria provoked by exercise, such as those listed in Table 22.1. The presence of hemolytic anemia should be sought because its presence raises the possibility of phosphofructokinase deficiency (Tarui), due to the defect in the erythrocyte phosphofructokinase enzyme. If a patient presents with severe axial muscle stiffness and leg muscle spasms triggered by external stimuli, anti-GAD antibodies should be ordered for the possibility of SPS, as discussed earlier. However, if the muscle stiffness affects primarily the neck and arm musculature, it is recommended that amphiphysin antibodies be ordered for evaluation of the SPS variant. If this is found, then a search for possible breast or lung cancer must be made because of their association with this condition [6].

Forearm exercise testing can be considered when metabolic myopathies are of concern. Lactate and ammonia venous levels are obtained at baseline and compared with subsequent levels measured at 1, 2, 4, 6 and 10 minutes of isometric handgrip contractions. It is expected to find 3-fold to 5-fold elevated levels of lactate and ammonia in normal individuals within 5 minutes of exercise, with a return to baseline levels within 30 minutes. Levels of both ammonia and lactate should increase together if the test is to be considered done satisfactorily. In phosphofructokinase (Tarui) deficiency, myophosphorylase (McArdle) deficiency, phosphorylase b kinase deficiency, lactate dehydrogenase deficiency and phosphoglycerate kinase (type IX glycogenosis) deficiency, the elevation of venous lactate levels is not seen. Forearm ischemic testing is not considered useful in conditions of fat metabolism because it is usually normal.

Pathology

Muscle biopsy should be considered to help confirm a diagnosis, although there are genetic tests available that help establish carrier status, if such is the case. In McArdle disease, the enzyme that is deficient (myophosphorylase) is responsible for breaking down glycogen, leading to exercise intolerance. Muscle biopsy usually reveals variation in muscle fiber size, and may show myofiber necrosis after a myoglobinuric episode. The light -microscopic features consist of the presence of linear or crescent-shaped vacuoles of glycogen accumulations in the subsarcolemmal areas [7].

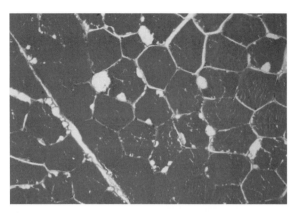

Figure 22.1. McArdle disease (myophosphorylase deficiency). (Courtesy of Dr. Richard Prayson.) (See the color plate section for a color version of this figure.)

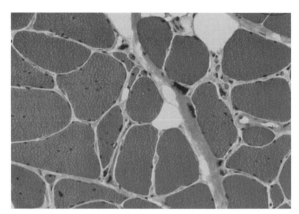

Figure 22.2. Myotonic dystrophy. (Courtesy of Dr. Richard Prayson.) (See the color plate section for a color version of this figure.)

Refer to Figure 22.1 for the hematoxylin–eosin stained section showing subsarcolemmal vacuoles seen in McArdle disease. Myophosphorylase activity is absent or significantly reduced in histochemical staining from all nonregenerating muscle fibers. Tarui disease is distinguished from McArdle disease by deficient phosphofructokinase in histochemical staining. Carnitine palmitoyltransferase II deficiency is an autosomal recessive vacuolar myopathy showing foci of muscle necrosis during attacks, presenting with generalized weakness, myoglobinuria, muscle stiffness and contractures. However, muscle biopsy usually appears normal between attacks.

Muscle biopsy from patients with myotonic dystrophy type 1 usually show central nuclear migration within most muscle fibers with widespread muscle fiber atrophy, without particular fiber-type grouping. Even though these features can be seen in several other muscle diseases, the combination of these findings with histochemical studies revealing selective type 1 fiber atrophy makes myotonic dystrophy type 1 distinctive [7]. Refer to Figure 22.2 for the hematoxylin-eosin stained section showing prominent variation in muscle fiber size with nuclear bag formations and increased central nuclei in a patient diagnosed with myotonic dystrophy.

Tubular aggregates are typically seen in channelopathies such as hyperkalemic and hypokalemic periodic paralyses. Histochemical staining reveals these tubular aggregates in subsarcolemmal regions of red-staining granular material on trichrome staining. Patients present with episodic muscle weakness and feeling of muscle heaviness as a result of exercise secondary to specific ion channel dysfunction, which

may last up to 24 hours in hypokalemic periodic paralysis patients. The distinction between these channelopathies relies on specific channel protein mutation analysis, as described in Table 22.1. If muscle biopsy shows nonspecific findings but there is a high suspicion for a muscle disease, molecular genetic studies are warranted. We will consider some examples of the diseases discussed previously, in terms of available genetic studies.

Genetics

Most of the glycogen storage disorders discussed earlier are inherited in an autosomal recessive trait, except for phosphoglycerate kinase deficiency, which is an X-linked disorder located on chromosome Xq13. McArdle disease is due to mutations in the gene for muscle phosphorylase on chromosome 11q13 responsible for breaking down the glycogen molecule and releasing glucose 1-phosphate, and several distinct mutations have been discovered. It has been postulated that the sodium–potassium ATPase pump concentrations are reduced in this disorder, resulting in exercise-induced increased extracellular potassium. This causes depolarization of the muscle membrane, inactivating sodium channels and further reducing membrane excitability. In Tarui disease there is deficiency of phosphofructokinase enzyme activity, which is the rate-limiting step in glycolysis, in muscles and a partial deficiency of this enzyme in erythrocytes, leading specifically to hemolytic anemia. This mutation has been localized to chromosome 12q13.

In some conditions there are trinucleotide repeats such as seen in myotonic dystrophy type 1. The mutation was mapped to chromosome 19q13.3 involving the *DMPK* (myotonin protein kinase) gene demonstrating a CTG trinucleotide unstable expansion. This molecular diagnostic test is 100% accurate. Patients with milder symptoms have fewer CTG repeats and genetic anticipation has been documented in this disease, in which increased number of repeats is associated with earlier onset and greater disease severity.

Within the muscle channelopathies, both hyperkalemic and hypokalemic periodic paralyses are inherited in an autosomal dominant trait. The hyperkalemic periodic paralysis attacks are triggered by rest following exercise, fasting, potassium-rich foods and stress. Mutations in the *SCN4A* gene have been documented in this disorder, affecting the normal function of sodium channels. In hypokalemic periodic paralysis, attacks usually last days, often precipitated by carbohydrate-rich foods, viral illness, certain medications and vigorous exercise. Mutations in the *CACNA1S* and *SCN4A* genes have been described, causing disruption transport of normal calcium and sodium ions, respectively, due to alteration of the normal structure of these ion channels.

Management

The treatment for some of the conditions discussed depends on the etiology. Identifying and understanding the cause of the muscle cramps, myalgias, or contractures is essential in order to decide on treatment. It is important also to consider that most of these conditions are associated with other organ-tissue damage and adequate patient referral becomes vital, mostly in cases of cardiac or respiratory failure. In the majority of cases, symptomatic treatment is the only feasible option. Quinine, an antimalarial agent, has been used for many years for the symptomatic treatment of muscle cramps, although some studies question its effectiveness. Several side-effects have been linked to the use of this medication, such as hematologic and renal complications (thrombocytopenia, hemolytic uremic syndrome), hepatotoxicity, blindness, ventricular arrhythmias, and even stimulation of insulin secretion leading to hypoglycemia, among others. Several alternatives to the use of quinine in idiopathic nocturnal leg cramps have been established. Some studies suggest that the use of verapamil, vitamin E, clonazepam, gabapentin, or carisoprodol showed documented efficacy and tolerability in patients with nocturnal leg muscle cramps [8]. Baclofen is another commonly used medication for the treatment of muscle cramps and muscle stiffness, particularly in patients who suffer from motor neuron disease or multiple sclerosis. Carbamazepine and phenytoin have been used to improve muscle cramps and even tonic spasms associated with multiple sclerosis. For dialysis-related muscle cramps, the use of L-carnitine has been a source of debate, but some studies suggest that it may offer some benefit if the intravenous infusion is given toward the end of dialysis [9]. However, some of these treatment options fail to prove significant improvement in most of the conditions discussed earlier in this chapter.

In most of the channelopathies and glycogen storage disorders mentioned, the most basic recommendation is lifestyle modification, such as avoidance of strenuous exercise, fasting, or ingestion of specific foods. Vissing *et al.* performed a single-blind, randomized, placebo-controlled crossover study in 12 patients with McArdle disease who showed improved exercise tolerance after the ingestion of sucrose before exercise. The authors also were able to demonstrate that this treatment may protect these patients from developing exercise-induced rhabdomyolysis [10]. Although there is no specific medical treatment for glycogen storage disorders, patients should be advised on a mild exercise program and to avoid vigorous activity.

In patients with muscle channelopathies, sometimes antiepileptic and/or antiarrhythmic medications are used to alleviate symptoms of severe myotonia and muscle stiffness. In the hyperkalemic periodic paralysis channelopathy, most patients benefit from avoiding potassium-rich foods and vigorous exercise. These patients may also benefit from the use of thiazide diuretics and carbonic anhydrase inhibitors. Patients with hypokalemic periodic paralysis channelopathy may benefit from daily oral potassium supplements to prevent attacks.

Some of the diseases discussed ultimately lead to physical disability, requiring special equipment and/or the need of an orthopedist. When patients develop musculoskeletal contractures due to long-standing duration of symptoms, botulinum toxin becomes a feasible option. In patients with myotonic dystrophy, for example, as the patient becomes weaker distally, ankle–foot orthosis may be needed for foot drop. Treatment is mostly supportive and prevention of contractures becomes essential in limiting disability, so it is important to refer patients for passive stretching physical therapy. Once more, antiepileptics, antiarrhythmics and even acetazolamide can help these patients in the treatment of myotonic attacks.

More invasive treatment is needed for certain auto-immune diseases such as stiff person syndrome. The use of intravenous immunoglobulins has been shown to be effective in the treatment of SPS GAD-associated antibodies. However, in the variant linked with amphiphysin antibodies, there is evidence to suggest that plasmapheresis with steroid treatment is a better option [6]. In some cases related to malignancy, the treatment of the primary process (i.e., breast or lung cancer) may show improvement of muscle cramps and muscle stiffness.

Conclusions

Despite the availability of sophisticated diagnostic testing, the most important aspect when evaluating a patient with suspected muscle disease who presents with nonspecific symptoms (i.e., muscle cramps, contractures, and myalgias) is a thorough physical and neurological examination. This should serve as a guide in developing a differential diagnosis and focusing the clinical evaluation and performance of confirmatory diagnostic testing. Additional testing, such as electromyography, may help the clinician to distinguish between cramps, contractures and dystonia, and to further classify these conditions and avoid clinical confusion due to the significant overlap of movement disorders and neuromuscular diseases. We have discussed the various treatments available for some of the diseases discussed in this chapter, most of them only symptomatic, but it is necessary to

recognize that gene therapy is a strong consideration in the near future.

References

1. George G. Case Report: Hypothyroidism presenting as puzzling myalgias and cramps in 3 patients. *J Clin Rheumatol* 2007; **13**: 273–5.

2. Parisi L, Pierelli F *et al.* Muscular cramps: proposals for a new classification. *Acta Neurol Scand* 2003; **107**: 176–86.

3. Tahmoush AJ, Alonso RJ *et al.* Cramp, fasciculation syndrome: a treatable hyperexcitable peripheral nerve disorder. *Neurology* 1991; **41**: 1021–3.

4. Fleet WS, Watson RT. From benign fasciculations and cramps to motor neuron disease. *Neurology* 1986; **36**: 997–8.

5. De Carvalho M, Swash, M. Cramps, muscle pain, and fasciculations: not always benign? *Neurology* 2004; **63**: 721–3.

6. Murinson BB, Guarnaccia JB. Stiff-person syndrome with amphiphysin antibodies. *Neurology* 2008; **71**: 1955–8.

7. Prayson RA. *Neuropathology: Foundations in Diagnostic Pathology*. New York: Elsevier; 2005.

8. Guay DR. Clinical Review: Are there alternatives to the use of quinine to treat nocturnal leg cramps? *Consult Pharm* 2008; **23**: 141–56.

9. Lynch KE, Feldman HI *et al.* Effects of L-carnitine on dialysis-related hypotension and muscle cramps: a meta-analysis. *Am J Kidney Dis* 2008; **52**: 962–71.

10. Vissing J, Haller R. The effect of oral sucrose on exercise tolerance in patients with McArdle's disease. *N Engl J Med* 2003; **349**: 2503–9.

Chapter 23

Movement disorders in neurometabolic diseases

David Grabli, Karine Auré, Marie Vidailhet and Emmanuel Roze

Introduction

Correct identification and classification of movement disorders is crucial for diagnosis of underlying inherited metabolic disorders (IMDs). The brain networks involved in movement disorders are often damaged in this setting. Movement disorders are thus a frequent presenting manifestation of IMDs and are generally present throughout the disease course. Identification of movement disorders is challenging in patients with IMD, as (i) movement disorders may be the only presenting symptom, yet early correct diagnosis of treatable IMDs is crucial; (ii) IMDs generally involve more than one neuronal system, leading to atypical or complex movement disorders; and (iii) a given IMD can cause a variety of movement disorders, while a given movement disorder can occur in a variety of IMDs. A few basic principles can help the clinician pointing to the possibility of an IMD in the patient presenting with a movement disorder:

1. The diagnostic approach should first focus on the search for treatable diseases (see Table 23.1).
2. Movement disorders in IMDs differ in certain respects from the corresponding primary disorder. For example, dystonia secondary to an IMD is often associated with parkinsonism (leading to hypokinetic and rigid dystonia) and involves facial and bulbar muscles more frequently and more severely than in primary dystonia. The pattern of movement disorders may vary with age at onset and the disease duration. As it is well-documented in Lesch–Nyhan disease [1], GM1 gangliosidosis type 3 [2] and glutaric aciduria type 1 [3], young patients tend to have an axial hypotonia/hyperkinetic limb pattern, whereas fixed dystonia and akineto-rigid parkinsonism predominate in older patients.

3. Movement disorders are usually part of a multisystem disease in IMDs. Other neurological and extraneurological features should be carefully sought, as they can provide useful diagnostic clues.
4. Etiological diagnosis is based on a few relevant findings, including the abrupt or insidious nature of onset (see Figure 23.1), associated clinical features, and brain MRI abnormalities (see Figures 23.2 and 3).

This review describes a simple clinical diagnostic approach to IMDs in patients with movement disorders. Forms of IMD frequently associated with movement disorders are described in detail, while rarer etiologies are briefly listed in Table 23.2.

Disorders of metal metabolism

Wilson disease

Wilson disease is due to altered copper metabolism. Changes in the basal ganglia and liver lead to neurological and hepatic manifestations. About 50% of patients initially present with neurological disorders [4] of which three main types have been described: (a) a pseudosclerotic form, affecting patients with disease onset after age 20 years, in which progressive slow tremor predominates, resting and/or postural tremor starts in one limb and may spread to the whole body, and high-amplitude proximal tremor ("wing-beating tremor") is typically present; (b) dystonic or juvenile forms, with onset before age 20 years and in which severe dystonic postures predominate; the dystonia is characterized by orofacial muscle involvement, leading to the classical *risus sardonicus* expression; and (c) parkinsonian forms, in which the dominant feature is akineto-rigid parkinsonism. The various movement disorders (tremor, dystonia and parkinsonism) can

Uncommon Causes of Movement Disorders, ed. Néstor Gálvez-Jiménez and Paul J. Tuite. Published by Cambridge University Press. © Cambridge University Press 2011.

Table 23.1. Treatable metabolic disorders and current treatments. An overview of treatable IMDs causing MD, together with current treatments. The main treatments are shown in bold type.

Disease	Treatment
Wilson disease	**Oral zinc, D-penicillamine and trientine**
Monoamine metabolism disorders	**Levodopa**, anticholinergic drugs, dopamine agonists **5-HTTP, BH₄ or phenylalanine restricted diet, depending on the enzyme deficiency**
Biotin-responsive basal ganglia disease	**Biotin 5–10 mg/kg daily**
Pyruvate dehydrogenase deficiency	**Vitamin B₁, ketogenic diet**
Cerebral glucose transporter (Glut1) deficiency	**Ketogenic diet**
Glutaric aciduria type 1	**Lysine- and tryptophan-restricted diet, carnitine**
Propionic aciduria	**Branched-chain amino acid-restricted diet**
Gaucher disease	Enzyme therapy (imiglucerase): effective on systemic but not neurological symptoms

BH₄, tetrahydrobiopterin; 5-HTTP, 5-hydroxytryptophan.

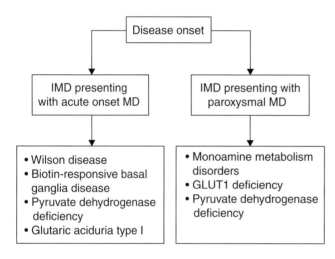

Figure 23.1. Diagnostic approach, according to manifestations at onset. The diagnostic approach to movement disorders (MDs) in patients with inherited metabolic disorders (IMDs), according to the acute or paroxysmal presentation at onset.

be combined, and choreic movements are also occasionally observed. In addition, cerebellar dysfunction, psychiatric disorders and mild cognitive disorders are common. Almost all patients have dysarthria and swallowing disorders due to parkinsonism, dystonia and/or a cerebellar syndrome. Seizures, pyramidal signs, myoclonia and oculomotor abnormalities are occasionally observed [5]. Diagnosis is based on low serum ceruloplasmin and copper levels, elevated urinary copper levels, and Kayser–Fleischer ring identification. Molecular analysis of the *ATP7B* gene can confirm the diagnosis. Brain MRI may show diffuse, generally symmetrical brain atrophy and lesions (often revealed by T2 hyperintensity) in the striatum, thalamus, brain stem, cerebellum (see Figure 23.3d) and/or white matter [6].

Neurodegeneration with brain iron accumulation

Neurodegeneration with brain iron accumulation (NBIA) encompasses a group of rare inherited disorders characterized by cerebral iron accumulation and neurodegeneration [7]. Movement disorders such as dystonia, chorea and parkinsonism are frequent presenting features of NBIA and are consistently present throughout the disease course. Recent advances in genetic testing have improved the classification and extended the phenotypic spectrum of NBIA. The main forms of NBIA comprise (i) pantothenate kinase-associated neurodegeneration caused by mutations in the *PANK2* gene and accounting for about two-thirds

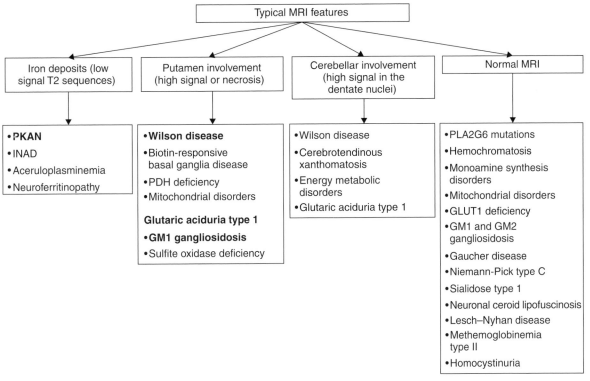

Figure 23.2. Diagnostic approach, according to typical MRI features. A simple diagnostic approach to IMDs causing movement disorders, according to typical MRI presentations. PKAN, pantothenate kinase-associated neurodegeneration; INAD, infantile neuroaxonal dystrophy, PDH, pyruvate dehydrogenase.

of cases of NBIA; (ii) aceruloplasminemia due to mutations in the *CP* gene, (iii) neuroferritinopathy caused by mutations in the *FTL* (ferritin light chain) gene, (iv) infantile neuroaxonal dystrophy (INAD) caused by mutations in the *PLA2G6* gene, also characterized by iron accumulation in 50–75% of patients; and (iv) idiopathic NBIA. No clear evidence of brain iron deposition has been found in hemochromatosis, which is not therefore included in the NBIA spectrum.

Pantothenate kinase-associated neurodegeneration

Pantothenate kinase-associated neurodegeneration (PKAN; or NBIA type 1) is caused by mutation of the *PANK2* (pantothenate kinase) gene. Clinically, PKAN is subdivided into classical and atypical forms [8]. The classical form predominates and has a relatively uniform phenotype. The disease usually starts before age 6 years and progresses rapidly to loss of walking ability after an average of 15 years. The most common presenting symptoms are gait disorders and postural difficulties, although upper limb impairment and global psychomotor retardation have also been described

[8,9]. Dystonia – a fairly consistent feature during the disease course – often involves the cranial and limb musculature, while axial dystonia predominates later on. Severe generalized dystonia is frequent in PKAN patients, and life-threatening *status dystonicus* can occur. Facial, bulbar and oromandibular muscle involvement is more prominent in PKAN than in primary dystonia [8,10]. Other frequent motor features include dysarthria, parkinsonism and signs of corticospinal tract involvement. In addition to motor impairment, two-thirds of patients with classical PKAN have clinical or electric pigmentary retinopathy [8]. Cognitive deficits are inconsistent and heterogeneous, ranging from no impairment to severe global retardation [11]. Interestingly, periods of subacute marked deterioration alternate with longer periods of clinical stability [8].

Atypical PKAN is more heterogeneous, with older age at onset (average 14 years). The disease course is protracted, and most patients are still able to walk on reaching adulthood. Speech disorders, including palilalia and dysarthria, are frequent presenting symptoms

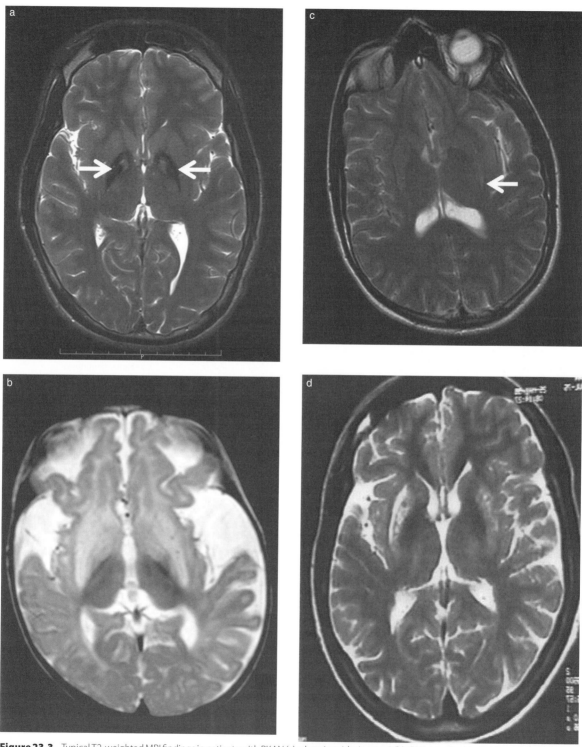

Figure 23.3. Typical T2-weighted MRI findings in patients with PKAN (a), glutaric aciduria type 3 (b), GM1 gangliosidosis (c) and Wilson disease (d). (a) Typical "eye-of-the-tiger" sign in a patient with PKAN (white arrows). (b) Typical features of glutaric aciduria type 1. Note the bilateral signal increase in the putamen, caudate and pallidum, and the enlargement of the anterior temporal and sylvian CSF spaces. (c) A patient with GM1 gangliosidosis. Note the subtly increased signal intensity and atrophy of the posterior putamen (white arrow). (d) High T2 signal of the putamen in a patient with Wilson disease.

Table 23.2. Miscellaneous inherited metabolic disorders causing movement disorders. An overview of miscellaneous inherited metabolic diseases that may cause movement disorders, albeit infrequently. The main clinical features, imaging findings, laboratory tests and treatments are described.

Disease	Movement disorders	Other features	MRI findings	Laboratory tests	Treatment
Cerebrotendinous xanthomatosis	Oromandibular dystonia, parkinsonism	Cerebellar syndrome, spastic paraparesis, dementia, psychiatric features, xanthoma, juvenile cataract	High signal intensity in the dentate nucleus	High serum cholestanol	Chenodeoxycholic acid
Methemoglobinemia type II	Generalized dystonia, choreoathetosis	Mental retardation, strabismus, cyanosis, microcephaly	Cortico-subcortical atrophy	Increased methemoglobinemia in arterial blood. Low cytochrome b_5 reductase activity in erythrocytes and leukocytes/fibroblasts	Symptomatic
β-Mannosidase deficiency	Tourette syndrome	Mental retardation, behavioral problems, hearing loss, recurrent airway infection, angiokeratoma, facial dysmorphism, skeletal deformation, hepatosplenomegaly	Cortico-subcortical atrophy	Decrease in beta-mannosidase activity in leukocytes or fibroblasts	Symptomatic
Sulfite oxidase deficiency	Generalized dystonia	Seizures, hypotonia, mental retardation, ectopia lentis	Cortico-subcortical, cystic encephalomalacia, cystic changes and calcifications in the basal ganglia	Urinary sulfite	Symptomatic
Hepatic cirrhosis, dystonia, polycythaemia and hypermanganesemia	Generalized dystonia	Liver cirrhosis	High T1 signal in the basal ganglia (manganese deposits)	High blood level of manganese	Chelation therapy with disodium calcium edetate and iron supplementation
Fatty acid-2 hyroxylase deficiency	Generalized dystonia with bulbar and facial involvement	Gait disorders, lower-limb spasticity, cerebellar ataxia	High T2 signal in periventricular regions	Screening for mutations in the *FA2H* gene	Symptomatic

Table 23.2 (cont.)

Disease	Movement disorders	Other features	MRI findings	Laboratory tests	Treatment
Creatine synthesis deficiency (GAMT deficiency)	Dystonia or other hyperkinetic movement disorders	Mental retardation with severe language retardation, seizures, autistic syndrome	High T2 signal in the globus pallidus, decreased creatine peak on MR spectroscopy	Elevated urinary guanidinoacetate, reduced plasma creatine, decreased GAMT enzymatic activity and screening for GAMT mutations	Oral creatine, diet with low protein, low arginine and high ornithine
Dopamine transporter (DAT) deficiency	Early-onset dopa dystonia-parkinsonism with no response to L-dopa	Pyramidal tract features, developmental retardation	Normal	High HVA level in CSF, screening for mutations in DAT gene	Symptomatic
Homocystinuria	Generalized dystonia (focal onset involving the face, masseter or larynx), chorea, Parkinsonism (rare)	Mental retardation, lens dislocation, marfanoid habitus, thromboembolic events	Cortico-subcortical atrophy	Homocystinuria	Pyridoxine supplementation, methionine-restricted diet and betaine supplementation

MRI, magnetic resonance imaging; GAMT, guanidinoacetate methyltransferase; HVA, homovanillic acid; CSF, cerebrospinal fluid.

(39% of 23 patients in Hayflick's series) [8]. Although atypical PKAN is less severe and more slowly progressive than the typical form, 75% of patients have dystonia, rigidity and parkinsonism, while pigmentary retinopathy is infrequent. Other atypical and less-frequent presenting manifestations include pure akinesia, mild gait freezing and tourettism, bulbar motor neuron disease, and psychiatric manifestations such as obsessive-compulsive disorder.

PKAN is highly likely if the "eye-of-the-tiger" sign (bilateral areas of hyperintensity within a hypointense region of the internal globus pallidus) is observed on T2-weighed brain MRI (see Figure 23.3a). This sign is present in virtually all *PANK2*-mutated patients [8,10]. Although highly suggestive of PKAN, the "eye-of-the-tiger" sign was recently described in patients with neuroferritinopathy, another form of NBIA. Diagnostic confirmation is based on molecular analysis of the *PANK2* gene.

Infantile neuroaxonal dystrophy

Infantile neuroaxonal dystrophy (INAD) is associated with mutations in the *PLA2G6* gene. INAD is characterized by childhood onset and rapidly progressive loss of motor and cognitive skills, with axial hypotonia, limb spasticity, bulbar dysfunction, cerebellar ataxia, optic atrophy and strabismus [12,13]. Movement disorders are frequent but occur somewhat later. In a cohort of 14 children, severe dystonia was present in 80% of children under 3 years of age and in all those over 9 years old. Almost all early-onset INAD patients die before age 20 years. Evidence of iron accumulation in the pallidum (GP) and substantia nigra is found on T2-weighed MRI in 50% of patients. The MRI pattern differs from that of PKAN, as the hypointensity is not restricted to the medial GP and the "eye-of-the tiger" sign is lacking [12–14]. Other diagnostic signs include cerebellar atrophy and hyperintensity on T2-weighed MRI.

Diagnosis is based on molecular analysis of the *PLA2G6* gene. Recently, the phenotypic spectrum of *PLA2G6* mutations was extended to cover a recessive form with adult onset combining dystonia-parkinsonism with a partial response to L-dopa, cognitive decline and psychiatric features [15].

Neuroferritinopathy

Neuroferritinopthy is caused by mutations in the ferritin light-chain gene (*FTL1*). In the largest published series, age at onset was about 40 years on average and ranged from 13 to 63 years [16]. Movement disorders are the usual presenting symptom and remain prominent throughout the disease course. Focal-onset chorea is present in 50% of patients at onset, and limb dystonia in 40% of patients. Atypical presenting features include blepharospasm, writer's cramp, parkinsonism, ballistic limb movement with abrupt onset, and palatal tremor. The initial movement disorder remains predominant, with marked asymmetry, throughout the disease course. In contrast to primary dystonia, oromandibular dyskinesia and pharyngolaryngeal involvement are frequent and patients often develop speech disorders characterized by dysarthria and hypophonia. Brain MRI shows iron deposits within the basal ganglia, red nucleus, dentate nucleus and cortex, with cystic degeneration in advanced cases. Serum ferritin assay showing low levels is a useful screening test, and the diagnosis is confirmed by molecular analysis of the *FTL1* gene.

Aceruloplasminemia

Hereditary aceruloplasminemia is a rare disorder caused by mutations in the ceruloplasmin (*CP*) gene. The disease usually starts during the fourth to sixth decades. The main presenting clinical features are movement disorders with predominant orofacial involvement, including parkinsonism, dystonia, chorea and tremor (both resting and dystonic) [17]. Other features include cerebellar ataxia, retinal degeneration and cognitive and psychiatric disorders. Diabetes mellitus and microcytic anemia with high serum ferritin levels are always present in the disease course and often precede neurological involvement. T2- and T2*-weighed sequences show diffuse hypointensity within the basal ganglia, thalamus, dentate nucleus and cortex, without cavitation [13]. Low serum ceruloplasmin levels are a highly suggestive sign, but firm diagnosis requires molecular analysis of the *CP* gene.

Hemochromatosis

The relationship between movement disorders and hereditary hemochromatosis (HH), an inherited disorder of iron metabolism, is controversial [18]. Except for a few case reports [19], there is no clear evidence of brain iron accumulation in HH, and movement disorders are not a classical presenting manifestation. However, certain case reports and association studies raise the possibility of a causal association between HH and parkinsonism, cerebellar ataxia, dementia, myoclonus, dystonia, or action tremor [20].

Monoamine disorders

Disorders of biogenic amine metabolism can result in various clinical manifestations, among which movement disorders are almost always prominent. Diurnal fluctuations and a marked response to levodopa, when present, are key diagnostic clues in all of these disorders. Clinical features can be classified according to the type of neurotransmitter deficit, namely, (a) dopamine deficiency, with focal, segmental or generalized dystonia, parkinsonism, and oculogyric crises; (b) serotonin deficiency, with hypersomnia, hyperphagia, depression and temperature instability; (c) norepinephrine deficiency, with ptosis, myosis, excessive diaphoresis, hypotension, bradyarrhythmia, temperature instability and retrograde ejaculation; and (d) additional nonspecific manifestations such as mental retardation, behavioral disorders and epilepsy. The two main phenotypes are chronic progressive encephalopathy and dopa-responsive dystonia (DRD).

Chronic progressive encephalopathy (CPE) can be due to deficiencies in various enzymes, including enzymes involved in tetrahydrobiopterin synthesis (GTP cyclohydrolase I [GTPCHI; recessive form], pyruvoyl-tetrahydropterin synthase [PTPS], and dihydropteridine reductase [DHPR]), tyrosine hydroxylase [TH], and amino acid decarboxylase [21,22]. Onset occurs usually in the first months of life, with marked hypotonia, psychomotor retardation and signs of monamine deficiency (see above). Left untreated, the disorder progresses relentlessly to severe disability and death. Early detection and treatment can permit survival into adulthood, some patients living near-normal lives, depending on the underlying enzyme defect.

Dopa-responsive dystonia (DRD) is mostly due to GTPCHI deficiency (dominant form) but can occasionally result from PTPS, TH or sepiapterin reductase deficiency [23]. It is typically characterized by childhood-onset dystonia with initial involvement of one limb (often a lower limb) and gradual generalization (often asymmetric) and deterioration [24]. Postural tremor is frequently present throughout the disease course. Parkinsonism, axial hypotonia, oculogyric crises, cerebellar features and a restless-leg-like syndrome are occasionally observed. Diurnal fluctuations of motor status are highly suggestive of DRD. These patients have a marked and sustained response to low-dose levodopa throughout their lives. Some patients may experience levodopa-induced dyskinesias that resolve when the levodopa daily dose is reduced; these dyskinesias appear to be more frequent in DRD patients with defects other than GTPCHI deficiency. Atypical phenotypes include adult-onset generalized dystonia, dystonia that remains focal over decades, exercise-induced dystonia, task-specific dystonia, myoclonus-dystonia, isolated parkinsonism, and spastic paraparesis. The common feature of these atypical forms is marked levodopa responsiveness.

Diagnosis is based on early detection of hyperphenylalaninemia in neonates (only present in recessive GTPCHI, DHPR and PTPS), CSF neurotransmitter assays, measurement of enzyme activities, and molecular analysis of the corresponding genes [23].

Disorders of energetic metabolism and related diseases

Biotin-responsive basal ganglia disease

Biotin-responsive basal ganglia disease (BBGD) is very rare but treatable [25]. All cases begin in infancy or the teen years. Onset is subacute, frequently triggered by episodes of fever, vomiting or diarrhea. These patients have subacute encephalitic manifestations of unknown origin. Without treatment, the encephalopathy persists, with loss of developmental milestones, inability to swallow, loss of speech, tetraparesis or hemiparesis with frequent dystonia of an upper extremity, and seizures. Akinetic mutism ensues, together with severe extrapyramidal and pyramidal dysfunction. Severe nonfluctuating dystonia with choreoathetosis and severe rigidity at rest are often present, along with an opisthotonic posture. Some patients have only intermittent dystonia of the extremities. Brain MRI findings are characteristic in all cases of BBGD, including mild forms. They consist of central destruction of the caudate heads, and partial or complete loss of the putamen. White matter patchiness may be seen during the disease course. All laboratory investigations, including specific metabolic examinations, are normal. A deficiency in biotin transporter encoded by the *SLC19A3* gene is responsible.

Pyruvate dehydrogenase deficiency

Pyruvate dehydrogenase (PDH) is a ubiquitous mitochondrial enzyme connecting anaerobic to aerobic metabolism by converting pyruvate to acetyl-CoA. PDH deficiency results in early-onset encephalopathy with X-linked recessive transmission. Newborns usually have severe lactic acidosis, and subsequently develop significant neurologic defects similar to those observed in patients with the Leigh syndrome. Children with later-onset forms may present with paroxysmal neurological episodes, often precipitated by fever or exercise and frequently associated with psychomotor retardation and pyramidal tract signs. Cases with intermittent ataxia have been reported, occasionally responding to thiamine supplementation and a ketogenic diet [26]. Other patients have episodes of paroxysmal dystonia. These may be very frequent, last from a few minutes to an hour, and can affect the face, the tongue and the four limbs [27]. Choreiform movements of the tongue, face and upper and lower limbs, associated with stereotypic tapping of the fingers and feet, have been described in adult-onset forms. Brain MRI can show bilateral lytic lesions of the putamen. A disproportionate increase in the CSF lactate concentration may suggest the diagnosis, which is confirmed by PDH activity assay. Residual enzyme activity is associated with slower disease progression.

GLUT-1 deficiency syndrome

Glucose transport across the blood-brain barrier is exclusively mediated by GLUT-1. Heterozygous mutations in the *GLUT1* gene limit brain glucose availability and lead to cerebral energy failure. Importantly, GLUT-1 deficiency syndrome is treatable. The phenotypic spectrum includes complex associations of action dystonia, chorea, cerebellar signs, seizures, mental retardation and acquired microcephaly. Based on early clinical descriptions, three main phenotypes have been described [28], namely, (a) the classic form, with carbohydrate-responsive symptoms (aggravation by fasting, improvement after carbohydrate intake); (b) a predominant ataxia and dystonia syndrome without seizures; and (c) paroxysmal exercise-induced dyskinesia (PED) with seizures. *GLUT1* gene mutations were recently identified in both familial and apparently sporadic cases of PED [29,30]. Age at onset in PED patients ranges from 3 to 30 years. Paroxysmal dyskinesia manifests in the form of choreoathetotic and/or dystonic movements. They are exclusively induced by exercise and consistently affect the legs, leading to walking difficulties and falls. They may also involve the face. The episodes resolve after an average of 15 minutes but may last several hours. Precipitating factors include prolonged exercise, and stress. Eating and rest are alleviating factors. PED tend to become less severe with age.

Diagnosis is based on a low CSF glucose level after 12 hours fasting, a low CSF/serum glucose concentration ratio. Impaired glucose uptake by erythrocytes may also be present. Search for mutations in GLUT1 gene can confirm diagnosis.

Mitochondrial diseases

Mitochondrial diseases are the most frequent metabolic disorders but are probably the more difficult to diagnose. They are suspected on the basis of converging clinical, biochemical and morphologic arguments. Identification of the precise genetic cause is rare, given the dual genetic origin of the mitochondrial respiratory chain. Striatal neurons show increased sensitivity to energy failure due to respiratory chain defects. This accounts for the high incidence of movement disorders. In Leigh syndrome, characterized by basal ganglia necrosis, all types of movement disorders (tremor, chorea, myoclonia, tics, etc.) can be observed. The most frequent is multifocal (or generalized), slowly progressive dystonia [31]. Diffuse cortical myoclonus is typical in the MERRF syndrome (myoclonic epilepsy with ragged red fibers), linked to a mitochondrial DNA point mutation, but is also observed in other genetic forms (due to other mitochondrial DNA mutations or mutation of nuclear genes encoding mitochondrial proteins or proteins involved in mitochondrial DNA maintenance). The myoclonic jerks are often associated with progressive myoclonic epilepsy and/or ataxia. Some patients also have parkinsonism due to mitochondrial DNA mutations [32] and especially polymerase-gamma mutations [33]. Finally, a mitochondrial disorder should be suspected in young patients with hyperglycemic chorea-ballism. Multisystem involvement and increased lactate levels in serum and CSF are good diagnostic clues in mitochondrial disorders.

Organic acidurias
Glutaric aciduria type I

Glutaric aciduria type I is due to glutaryl-CoA dehydrogenase deficiency. Typical cases are characterized by early progressive macrocephaly and/or hypotonia, preceding an acute encephalopathic crisis occurring before age 2 years, with sudden onset of movement disorders. Progressive forms are occasionally observed. The clinical picture is usually one of generalized dystonia superimposed on baseline axial hypotonia, which remains the dominant feature throughout the disease course [3]. With aging, this disorder tends to evolve from mobile to fixed dystonia and to be associated with akineto-rigid parkinsonism. Chorea, athetosis and myoclonic dystonia are occasionally observed. Prominent facial involvement is an early and near-constant feature, resulting in swallowing disorders and speech disturbances consisting of a combination of hyperkinetic dysarthria and speech apraxia. Brain MRI can show signal abnormalities in the putamen, caudate, pallidum and ventricles that are associated with movement disorders; extrastriatal abnormalities include widening of the anterior temporal and sylvian CSF spaces (Figure 23.3b), pseudocysts, signal changes in the substantia nigra, nucleus dentatus, thalamus, tractus tegmentalis centralis and supratentorial white matter, as well as signs of delayed maturation. Diagnosis is based on identification of glutaric aciduria by means of chromatography–mass spectrometry of organic acids in urine, measurement of GCDH activity, and molecular analysis of the *GCDH* gene.

Patients with other forms of organic aciduria, including propionic aciduria, methylmalonic aciduria, L-hydroxyglutaric aciduria and hydroxybutyric aciduria, can develop similar acute-onset movement disorders, which may be transient (following acute periods of decompensation) and are not generally the main manifestation.

Lysosomal disorders
GM1 gangliosidosis

GM1 gangliosidosis is due to beta-galactosidase deficiency. The late-onset form, type 3, is characterized by a protracted clinical course with early-onset progressive generalized dystonia, often associated with akineto-rigid parkinsonism [2]. Onset occurs at a median age of 6 years, and usually before age 20 years. Dystonia is an early manifestation and remains prominent throughout the disease course, with major facial involvement. Akineto-rigid parkinsonism is frequent and also gradually worsens with aging. Choreoathetoid movements can also be present, mostly in the early stages of the disease. These patients typically have swallowing

disorders and severe speech disturbances, with combined hyperkinetic dysarthria and speech apraxia. A pyramidal syndrome and mental retardation are usually mild when present. Mild skeletal dysplasia and short stature are good diagnostic clues. Brain MRI can show abnormalities of the posterior putamen (Figure 23.3c). The diagnosis is based on measurement of beta-galactosidase activity and molecular analysis of the *GLB1* gene.

GM2 gangliosidosis

GM2 gangliosidosis (GM2g) is due to a deficiency in beta-hexosaminidase A, A and B, or their cofactor, GM2 activator. Movement disorders, including tremor, generalized or focal dystonia, chorea and parkinsonism, are present in 30–50% of late-onset juvenile and adult forms but rarely dominate the clinical picture [34,35]. They are usually part of a more complex multisystem neurological disorder. A combination of movement disorders and more common manifestations resulting from cerebellar and motor neuron dysfunction is suggestive of late-onset GM2g. Psychotic manifestations, mental impairment, seizures, mild pyramidal signs, painful sensory polyneuropathy, dysautonomia, vertical supranuclear palsy and visual disturbances can also be observed. Progressive swallowing and speech disorders (mostly ataxic and/or hyperkinetic dysarthria) are near-constant features. Brain MRI can show cerebellar atrophy, either alone or associated with mild global brain atrophy. Neurophysiological examination can reveal abnormalities consistent with anterior horn cell disease or axonal sensory polyneuropathy. Diagnosis is based on measurement of beta-hexosaminidase activity and molecular analysis of the *HEXA*, *HEXB* or *GM2A* genes.

Niemann–Pick C disease

Niemann Pick C disease (NPC) is due to dysfunction of proteins involved in transport within the endosomal/lysosomal system, affecting intracellular lipid trafficking and lysosomal lipid storage. The first neurological manifestations usually occur between the ages of 10 and 30 years, but later onset is possible. Movement disorders are present in 50–60% of NPC patients, typically in the form of progressive generalized dystonia [36]. Mild parkinsonism, chorea or myoclonus may be isolated or associated with dystonia. Movement disorders are rarely the presenting or predominant neuropsychiatric manifestation and are typically associated with cognitive, psychiatric or cerebellar disorders. Vertical supranuclear palsy and hepatomegaly or splenomegaly are frequent and are key diagnostic signs. Progressive swallowing and speech disorders (mostly ataxic and/or hyperkinetic dysarthria) are also frequent. Epilepsy, cataplexy and deafness are occasionally observed. Brain MRI can show cerebellar, cortical or brain stem atrophy. Diagnosis is based on biochemical detection of altered LDL-cholesterol trafficking or LDL-induced cholesterol ester formation, and on molecular analysis of the *NPC1* and *NPC2* genes.

Neuronal ceroid lipofuscinosis

Neuronal ceroid lipofuscinoses are a heterogeneous group of progressive neurodegenerative diseases characterized by lysosomal accumulation of autofluorescent lipopigments (ceroid lipofuscin). Onset typically occurs in the first years of life and the key clinical features are cognitive deterioration, epilepsy and retinopathy. Movement disorders observed in this setting include myoclonus, parkinsonism and dystonia [37,38]. Adult-onset forms are very rare and are not always associated with visual impairment.

Sialidosis type I

Sialidosis type 1 is due to lysosomal sialidase deficiency. Onset typically occurs in the second or third decade of life. The main manifestation is diffuse myclonus of cortical origin that predominates on action and is usually associated with ataxia and visual deterioration [39]. Macular cherry-red spots on funduscopy are a key diagnostic sign.

Gaucher disease

Gaucher disease is due to glucocerebrosidase deficiency resulting from mutations in the *GBA* gene. Type 3 is typically characterized by progressive myoclonic epilepsy, ataxia, cognitive impairment and spasticity. Horizontal supranuclear gaze palsy is an early manifestation and a good diagnostic sign. Note that heterozygous mutations of the *GBA* gene are also a risk factor for Parkinson disease [40].

Lesch–Nyhan disease

Lesch–Nyhan disease is due to hypoxanthine-guanine phosphoribosyltransferase deficiency. The phenomenon underlying the associated neurological disorders appears to be dopamine pathway dysfunction, possibly due to alteration of the molecular pathways that govern early development of dopaminergic neurons [41]. The picture at onset is one of early psychomotor retardation with major hypotonia in the first year of life. Movement disorders appear between 6 and 12 months of life and are characterized by generalized dystonia superimposed on a baseline of axial hypotonia [1]. Major orofacial involvement results in swallowing disturbances and speech disorders, with hyperkinetic dysarthria and speech apraxia. Other motor manifestations can include chorea, athetosis, ballism and a pyramidal syndrome. Self-harm, mainly involving the lips, tongue and fingers, is present in almost all patients and is the key diagnostic sign. Additional neurological manifestations include mild to moderate cognitive dysfunction (particularly attention deficit), anxiety, depression and mild behavioral disturbances [42]. Gout and kidney stones are frequent systemic manifestations, due to hyperuricemia. Patients with residual enzymatic activity have a milder dystonic phenotype and tend not to harm themselves; these forms are referred to as the Lesch–Nyhan variant and can be difficult to diagnose. The main diagnostic signs are clinical manifestations and hyperuricemia. Confirmation is obtained by enzymatic activity assay and molecular analysis of the *HPRT* gene.

Treatment

Symptomatic drug therapy of movement disorders in patients with IMDs is the same as in other clinical settings. In addition to physical therapy, anticholinergic drugs, benzodiazepines, baclofen, dopaminergic treatments, tetrabenazine, antiepileptic medications and atypical neuroleptics (mainly clozapine) are widely used on an empirical basis. Given the possibility of dopa-responsive dystonia in patients with no firm etiological diagnosis, treatment should always start with a levodopa trial in case of dystonia or Parkinsonism. In addition, patients with IMDs often have complex encephalopathies with cognitive deficits or behavioral disorders. There is a higher risk of adverse effects, which should be carefully monitored. Botulinum toxin injections are also used in focal movement disorders and, when a focal target can be identified, in generalized movement disorders [43].

Bilateral high-frequency stimulation of the internal pallidum (GP-HFS) was recently shown to be effective in patients with severe forms of primary dystonia [44,45] and also in choreoathethoid cerebral palsy [46]. Although progressive lesions in IMD often involve the basal ganglia, GP-HFS has been tried in a few IMD patients with severe and otherwise untreatable movement disorders. The results are encouraging, but controlled studies are needed and the best candidates for this modality (based on clinical or imaging features) remain to be identified. A sustained benefit of GP-HFS was seen in five out of six PKAN patients reported in the literature [47] as well as in one patient with GM$_1$ gangliodisosis [48] and in another patient with bilateral striatal necrosis due to mitochondrial DNA deletion [49]. In Lesch–Nyhan disease, GP-HFS using two targets within the GPi (sensorimotor and limbic) was beneficial in terms of both self-harm and dystonia [50]. As in primary movement disorders, patients with hyperkinetic dystonia may benefit more from GP-HFS than those with fixed postures. Although encouraging, these results should be considered cautiously, as a positive publication bias is likely. Further studies are thus needed to assess the place of functional surgery in patients with movement disorders secondary to inherited metabolic disorders.

References

1. Jinnah HA, Visser JE, Harris JC et al. Delineation of the motor disorder of Lesch–Nyhan disease. *Brain* 2006 May; **129**(Pt 5): 1201–17.

2. Roze E, Paschke E, Lopez N et al. Dystonia and parkinsonism in GM1 type 3 gangliosidosis. *Mov Disord* 2005; **20**(10): 1366–9.

3. Gitiaux C, Roze E, Kinugawa K et al. Spectrum of movement disorders associated with glutaric aciduria type 1: a study of 16 patients. *Mov Disord* 2008; **23**(16): 2392–7.

4. Ala A, Walker AP, Ashkan K, Dooley JS, Schilsky ML. Wilson's disease. *Lancet* 2007; **369**(9559): 397–408.

5. Machado A, Chien HF, Deguti MM et al. Neurological manifestations in Wilson's disease: report of 119 cases. *Mov Disord* 2006; **21**(12): 2192–6.

6. Sinha S, Taly AB, Ravishankar S et al. Wilson's disease: cranial MRI observations and clinical correlation. *Neuroradiology* 2006; **48**(9): 613–21.

7. Gregory A, Polster BJ, Hayflick SJ. Clinical and genetic delineation of neurodegeneration with brain iron accumulation. *J Med Genet*. 2009; **46**(2): 73–80.

8. Hayflick SJ. Unraveling the Hallervorden–Spatz syndrome: pantothenate kinase-associated neurodegeneration is the name. *Curr Opin Pediatr* 2003; **15**(6): 572–7.

9. Pellecchia MT, Valente EM, Cif L et al. The diverse phenotype and genotype of pantothenate kinase-associated neurodegeneration. *Neurology* 2005; **64**(10): 1810–2.

10. Hartig MB, Hortnagel K, Garavaglia B et al. Genotypic and phenotypic spectrum of PANK2 mutations in patients with neurodegeneration with brain iron accumulation. *Ann Neurol* 2006; **59**(2): 248–56.

11. Freeman K, Gregory A, Turner A, Blasco P, Hogarth P, Hayflick S. Intellectual and adaptive behaviour functioning in pantothenate kinase-associated neurodegeneration. *J Intellect Disabil Res* 2007; **51**(Pt 6): 417–26.

12. Kurian MA, Morgan NV, MacPherson L et al. Phenotypic spectrum of neurodegeneration associated with mutations in the PLA2G6 gene (PLAN). *Neurology* 2008; **70**(18): 1623–9.

13. McNeill A, Birchall D, Hayflick SJ et al. T2* and FSE MRI distinguishes four subtypes of neurodegeneration with brain iron accumulation. *Neurology* 2008; **70**(18): 1614–9.

14. Gregory A, Westaway SK, Holm IE et al. Neurodegeneration associated with genetic defects in phospholipase A(2). *Neurology* 2008; **71**(18): 1402–9.

15. Paisan-Ruiz C, Bhatia KP, Li A et al. Characterization of PLA2G6 as a locus for dystonia-parkinsonism. *Ann Neurol* 2009; **65**(1): 19–23.

16. Chinnery PF, Crompton DE, Birchall D et al. Clinical features and natural history of neuroferritinopathy caused by the FTL1 460InsA mutation. *Brain* 2007; **130**(Pt 1): 110–9.

17. McNeill A, Pandolfo M, Kuhn J, Shang H, Miyajima H. The neurological presentation of ceruloplasmin gene mutations. *Eur Neurol* 2008; **60**(4): 200–5.

18. Aamodt AH, Stovner LJ, Thorstensen K, Lydersen S, White LR, Aasly JO. Prevalence of haemochromatosis gene mutations in Parkinson's disease. *J Neurol Neurosurg Psychiatry* 2007; **78**(3): 315–7.

19. Dekker MC, Giesbergen PC, Njajou OT et al. Mutations in the hemochromatosis gene (HFE), Parkinson's disease and parkinsonism. *Neurosci Lett* 2003; **348**(2): 117–9.

20. Demarquay G, Setiey A, Morel Y, Trepo C, Chazot G, Broussolle E. Clinical report of three patients with hereditary hemochromatosis and movement disorders. *Mov Disord* 2000; **15**(6): 1204–9.

21. Pearl PL, Capp PK, Novotny EJ, Gibson KM. Inherited disorders of neurotransmitters in children and adults. *Clin Biochem* 2005; **38**(12): 1051–8.

22. Manegold C, Hoffmann GF, Degen I et al. Aromatic L-amino acid decarboxylase deficiency: clinical features, drug therapy and follow-up. *J Inherit Metab Dis* 2009; **32**(3): 371–80.

23. Clot F, Grabli D, Cazeneuve C et al. Exhaustive analysis of BH$_4$ and dopamine biosynthesis genes in patients with dopa-responsive dystonia. *Brain* 2009; **132**(Pt 7): 1753–63.

24. Trender-Gerhard I, Sweeney MG *et al.* Autosomal-dominant GTPCH1-deficient DRD: clinical characteristics and long-term outcome of 34 patients. *J Neurol Neurosurg Psychiatry* 2009; **80**(8): 839–45.

25. Ozand PT, Gascon GG, Al Essa M *et al.* Biotin-responsive basal ganglia disease: a novel entity. *Brain* 1998; **121**(Pt 7): 1267–79.

26. Bindoff LA, Birch-Machin MA, Farnsworth L, Gardner-Medwin D, Lindsay JG, Turnbull DM. Familial intermittent ataxia due to a defect of the E1 component of pyruvate dehydrogenase complex. *J Neurol Sci* 1989; **93**(2–3): 311–8.

27. Head RA, de Goede CG, Newton RW *et al.* Pyruvate dehydrogenase deficiency presenting as dystonia in childhood. *Dev Med Child Neurol* 2004; **46**(10): 710–2.

28. Brockmann K. The expanding phenotype of GLUT1-deficiency syndrome. *Brain Dev* 2009; **31**(7): 545–52.

29. Schneider SA, Paisan-Ruiz C, Garcia-Gorostiaga I *et al.* GLUT1 gene mutations cause sporadic paroxysmal exercise-induced dyskinesias. *Mov Disord* 2009; **24**(11): 1684–8.

30. Suls A, Dedeken P, Goffin K *et al.* Paroxysmal exercise-induced dyskinesia and epilepsy is due to mutations in SLC2A1, encoding the glucose transporter GLUT1. *Brain* 2008; **131**(Pt 7): 1831–44.

31. Macaya A, Munell F, Burke RE, De Vivo DC. Disorders of movement in Leigh syndrome. *Neuropediatrics* 1993; **24**(2): 60–7.

32. Yamamoto M, Ujike H, Wada K, Tsuji T. Cerebrospinal fluid lactate and pyruvate concentrations in patients with Parkinson's disease and mitochondrial encephalomyopathy, lactic acidosis, and stroke-like episodes (MELAS). *J Neurol Neurosurg Psychiatry* 1997; **62**(3): 290.

33. Luoma PT, Eerola J, Ahola S *et al.* Mitochondrial DNA polymerase gamma variants in idiopathic sporadic Parkinson disease. *Neurology* 2007; **69**(11): 1152–9.

34. Oates CE, Bosch EP, Hart MN. Movement disorders associated with chronic GM2 gangliosidosis. Case report and review of the literature. *Eur Neurol* 1986; **25**(2): 154–9.

35. Nardocci N, Bertagnolio B, Rumi V, Angelini L. Progressive dystonia symptomatic of juvenile GM2 gangliosidosis. *Mov Disord* 1992; **7**(1): 64–7.

36. Sevin M, Lesca G, Baumann N *et al.* The adult form of Niemann–Pick disease type C. *Brain* 2007; **130**(Pt 1): 120–33.

37. Berkovic SF, Carpenter S, Andermann F, Andermann E, Wolfe LS. Kufs' disease: a critical reappraisal. *Brain* 1988; **111**(Pt 1): 27–62.

38. Nijssen PC, Brusse E, Leyten AC, Martin JJ, Teepen JL, Roos RA. Autosomal dominant adult neuronal ceroid lipofuscinosis: parkinsonism due to both striatal and nigral dysfunction. *Mov Disord* 2002; **17**(3): 482–7.

39. Federico A, Battistini S, Ciacci G *et al.* Cherry-red spot myoclonus syndrome (type I sialidosis). *Dev Neurosci* 1991; **13**(4–5): 320–6.

40. Neumann J, Bras J, Deas E *et al.* Glucocerebrosidase mutations in clinical and pathologically proven Parkinson's disease. *Brain* 2009; **132**(Pt 7): 1783–94.

41. Ceballos-Picot I, Mockel L, Potier MC *et al.* Hypoxanthine-guanine phosphoribosyl transferase regulates early developmental programming of dopamine neurons: implications for Lesch–Nyhan disease pathogenesis. *Hum Mol Genet* 2009 1; **18**(13): 2317–27.

42. Schretlen DJ, Ward J, Meyer SM *et al.* Behavioral aspects of Lesch–Nyhan disease and its variants. *Dev Med Child Neurol* 2005; **47**(10): 673–7.

43. Adam OR, Jankovic J. Treatment of dystonia. *Parkinsonism Relat Disord* 2007; **13**(Suppl 3): S362–8.

44. Vidailhet M, Vercueil L, Houeto JL *et al.* Bilateral deep-brain stimulation of the globus pallidus in primary generalized dystonia. *N Engl J Med* 2005; **352**(5): 459–67.

45. Kupsch A, Benecke R, Muller J *et al.* Pallidal deep-brain stimulation in primary generalized or segmental dystonia. *N Engl J Med* 2006; **355**(19): 1978–90.

46. Vidailhet M, Yelnik J, Lagrange C *et al.* Bilateral pallidal deep brain stimulation for the treatment of patients with dystonia-choreoathetosis cerebral palsy: a prospective pilot study. *Lancet Neurol* 2009; **8**(8): 709–17.

47. Mikati MA, Yehya A, Darwish H, Karam P, Comair Y. Deep brain stimulation as a mode of treatment of early onset pantothenate kinase-associated neurodegeneration. *Eur J Paediatr Neurol* 2009; **13**(1): 61–4.

48. Roze E, Navarro S, Cornu P, Welter ML, Vidailhet M. Deep brain stimulation of the globus pallidus for generalized dystonia in GM1 Type 3 gangliosidosis: technical case report. *Neurosurgery* 2006; **59**(6): E1340; discussion E.

49. Aniello MS, Martino D, Petruzzella V *et al.* Bilateral striatal necrosis, dystonia and multiple mitochondrial DNA deletions: case study and effect of deep brain stimulation. *Mov Disord* 2008; **23**(1): 114–8.

50. Cif L, Biolsi B, Gavarini S, *et al.* Antero-ventral internal pallidum stimulation improves behavioral disorders in Lesch–Nyhan disease. *Mov Disord* 2007; **22**(14): 2126–9.

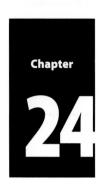

Chapter

24

Mitochondrial disorders

Mary Vo and Claire Henchcliffe

History, background and terminology

Mitochondria, first described as "sarcosomes" in 1857, are essential intracellular organelles whose main functions involve cellular respiration through the oxidative phosphorylation pathway, fatty acid oxidation, the Krebs cycle, pyruvate oxidation, and amino acid metabolism. Primary mitochondrial diseases impede the oxidative phosphorylation pathway, compromising mitochondrial function and cellular respiration. This disproportionately affects tissues that are more dependent on aerobic respiration, and therefore has marked effects on the central nervous system and skeletal muscle. Mitochondrial dysfunction was originally implicated in human disease as early as 1959, and mitochondrial movement disorders have been described at an increasing rate over the past three decades.

The genetics of mitochondrial diseases is complex. The majority of mitochondrial proteins are encoded by mitochondrial DNA (mtDNA), discovered in the 1960s. The remainder of the mitochondrial respiration machinery is encoded by nuclear DNA. Therefore, mitochondrial diseases may arise as a consequence of mutations in either mtDNA or nuclear DNA. Clinical diagnosis is complicated by individual mtDNA mutations producing multiple phenotypes, and by specific clinical features being attributable to several different mutations. To date, hundreds of mtDNA mutations have been linked to clinical syndromes, and characterization of the genotype–phenotype relationship is a highly active ongoing area of research. A unique feature of mitochondrial genetics is heteroplasmy, defined as the presence of the wild-type mtDNA and at least one other population of mutated mtDNA. Heteroplasmy, and the proportion of mutant mtDNA present, impacts upon the expression and clinical phenotype, further complicating clinical presentations.

In this chapter we discuss primary mitochondrial diseases that lead to movement disorders, such as neurogenic muscular weakness, ataxia and retinitis pigmentosa (NARP), Leber hereditary optic neuropathy (LHON), Leigh syndrome, and others. Certain more common movement disorders, including Parkinson disease, are now known to be at least partly associated primarily or secondarily with mitochondrial dysfunction, either due to endogenous factors or to possible environmental exposures, and these are well discussed elsewhere [1].

Clinical findings

Mitochondrial diseases lead to a variety of unusual and highly variable movement disorders, presenting either alone or in combination with each other. These include ataxia, myoclonus, parkinsonism, chorea and dystonia [2]. Diagnosis can therefore be challenging, but when evaluating an unusual movement disorder, careful assessment may reveal other signs that provide clues to a mitochondrial etiology. For example, myopathy is a common feature of mitochondrial disease. This can manifest as ophthalmoplegia, chronic progressive weakness, isolated myopathy (with or without exercise intolerance) or severe encephalomyopathy beginning in infancy or early childhood. Other clues to a mitochondrial etiology include coexistence of seizures, strokes or stroke-like episodes, neuropathy, sensorineural hearing loss, migraine, cognitive deficits and dementia. Furthermore, mitochondrial disease may also be associated with systemic complications such as diabetes, retinopathy, cardiomyopathy or deafness.

Given the variability in clinical symptoms, mitochondrial diseases have been classified according to groupings of certain core features: for example, NARP and MERRF (myoclonic epilepsy with ragged red fibers), in which ataxia may also occur. However, the

Uncommon Causes of Movement Disorders, ed. Néstor Gálvez-Jiménez and Paul J. Tuite. Published by Cambridge University Press. © Cambridge University Press 2011.

precise phenotype may vary, and the relationship of each disorder to any given underlying mutation is complex, depending upon several factors including threshold mutation burden, heteroplasmy and location of the mutation. We therefore discuss clinical manifestations separately for each condition later in this chapter.

Incidence and natural history

A recent study of a northern English population reports the minimum incidence of all mitochondrial disease to be 9.2 per 100 000, and estimates that an additional 16.5 per 100 000 children and young adults are at risk for developing mitochondrial disease [3]. However, this figure may be significantly higher in pediatric populations, as certain mitochondrial encephalomyopathies have infantile onset and early childhood fatalities from this cause are likely underdiagnosed [4]. One study reported the minimum birth prevalence as 13.1 per 100 000 with onset at any age, making mitochondrial encephalomyopathies more common than inborn errors of metabolism [5]. Regardless of the age of onset, mitochondrial disease is typically progressive. Mitochondrial disorders may manifest at any stage of life. Mitochondrial diseases due to nuclear gene mutations are more likely to manifest in infancy or early childhood, whereas those attributable to mtDNA mutations may emerge in adulthood [6].

Laboratory investigations

Impairment of mitochondrial respiration entails an increase in reducing equivalents (NAD/NADH$^+$), reduced ATP formation, increased monovalent oxygen reduction, and impairment of several metabolic pathways (including the Krebs cycle and β-oxidation). This results in elevated postprandial hyperketonemia (β-hydroxybutyrate and acetoacetate), and elevated lactate:pyruvate ratio, the latter causing hyperlactatemia. Fasting and 1-hour postprandial serum lactate, pyruvate and ketone bodies should be measured. Persistent hyperlactatemia (lactate >2.5 mmol/l, lactate/pyruvate ratio >20) and paradoxical hyperketonemia (ketone bodies >2) postprandially suggest respiratory chain deficiency, and may be used to screen for mitochondrial disease. Lumbar puncture is commonly performed when mitochondrial disorders are suspected as elevated lactate in cerebrospinal fluid (CSF) may also be observed. Additionally, spectrophotometric enzyme assays and functional studies may be performed on tissue to further delineate deficiencies in particular respiratory chain components [7].

Magnetic resonance imaging (MRI) in patients with mitochondrial disease yields highly variable results, and standard clinical sequences may be normal in some cases. Most MRI abnormalities in patients with mitochondrial disease are nonspecific, although certain MRI findings such as T2/FLAIR hyperintense and T1 hypointense signal in bilateral deep gray structures are suggestive of mitochondrial disease. Cerebral and cerebellar atrophy may be evident, but again are nonspecific. However, elevated lactate levels may be detected by magnetic resonance spectroscopy and can be helpful in determining a mitochondrial etiology of an unusual movement disorder [8]. Abnormal cerebral parenchymal and ventricular CSF lactate concentration, resulting from impaired oxidative phosphorylation (favoring glycolysis and leading to lactate accumulation), is demonstrated in Figure 24.1 in two subjects with a mitochondrial disorder.

Muscle biopsy can provide critical data during work-up of possible mitochondrial disorders, as myopathy is often a feature of mitochondrial disease. Subsarcolemmal or intramyofibrillary collections of abnormal mitochondria known as ragged red fibers (RRF) (Figure 24.2) are observed in some mitochondrial myopathies, and are best revealed by Gomori trichrome stains of muscle biopsy tissue. Histochemical enzyme reactions for mitochondrial enzymes such as succinyl dehydrogenase (SDH) and cytochrome-c oxidase (COX) may also reveal subsarcolemmal accumulation of mitochondria. COX contains subunits encoded by both mitochondrial and nuclear DNA, and muscle fibers affected by mitochondrial myopathy appear pale with this particular histochemical stain. Normal muscle shows more deeply stained type I oxidative muscle fibers interspersed between the paler type II glycolytic fibers. The presence of a sporadic staining pattern after COX reaction, with the majority of muscle fibers being COX deficient, is described as a mosaic pattern, and suggests heteroplasmic mtDNA disease. In contrast, a global decrease in COX activity suggests a nuclear mutation in one of the structural proteins. However, there are many cases of mitochondrial myopathy with normal COX staining, and such testing should therefore be performed in conjunction with SDH histochemistry [9]. However, the findings of muscle biopsy analysis and histochemical enzyme reactions must be interpreted with caution and in the appropriate clinical context.

Although rarely performed, neuropathological studies have demonstrated variable abnormal findings

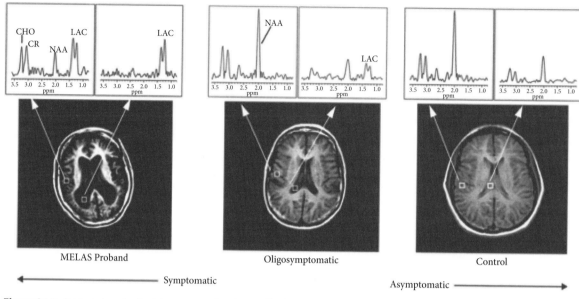

Figure 24.1. Increased cerebral lactate concentration detected by ¹H magnetic resonance spectroscopy in mitochondrial encephalomy-opathy, lactic acidosis, and stroke-like episodes (MELAS). Lactate concentrations (LAC) are demonstrated in parenchyma (left in each panel) and CSF (right in each panel). The left panel is from study of a subject with symptomatic MELAS. The middle panel is from the study of an oligosymptomatic relative. The right panel is from an asymptomatic control subject. Also denoted are CHO (total choline), CR (total creatine), and NAA (*N*-acetylaspartate) resonances. (Reproduced from reference 8 with permission. Copyright © 2004 Wolters Kluwer Health. All rights reserved.)

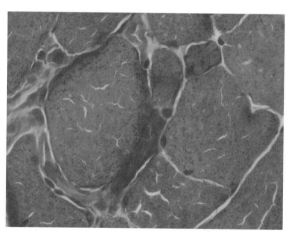

Figure 24.2. A typical ragged red fiber in mitochondrial disease demonstrated by modified Gomori trichrome staining of a skeletal muscle biopsy. (Courtesy of Dr. Ehud Lavi, Weill Cornell Medical College, New York NY.) (See the color plate section for a color version of this figure.)

including cystic cavitation, neuron necrosis, demyelination, vascular proliferation and gliosis in various areas of the brain.

Genetic testing can provide a definitive diagnosis, but deciding what genes to test, and interpreting the results, is difficult. The genotype–phenotype relationships for many mitochondrial disorders are complex. Increased awareness of mitochondrial disease in the medical community and technological advancements have driven the wide availability of certain genetic, histochemical and biochemical tests. In selected patients, histochemical enzyme testing, functional enzymatic analysis and DNA sequence analysis may help elucidate a diagnosis of mitochondrial disease [10]. Genetic tests for multiple mutations (for example ATPase 6 leading to NARP, or mutations in ND1–6 and cytochrome *b* leading to LHON) are now commercially available in diagnostic laboratories. Moreover, recent literature has implicated multiple *POLG* mutations in a variety of human diseases, especially adult-onset mitochondrial disease, and diagnostic evaluation with *POLG* gene analysis is now also commercially available [11]. The genetics of mitochondrial movement disorders is discussed in the next section.

Genetics

mtDNA is comprised of a 16.6 kb double-stranded circular structure, present in approximately 2–10 copies per mitochondrion [12]. It consists of 37 genes, 13 of which encode for a minority of the subunit components of complexes I, III, IV and V, as well as the two rRNAs and 22 tRNAs central to mitochondrial protein synthesis (Figure 24.3). The remaining 74 polypeptides of the oxidative phosphorylation system are encoded

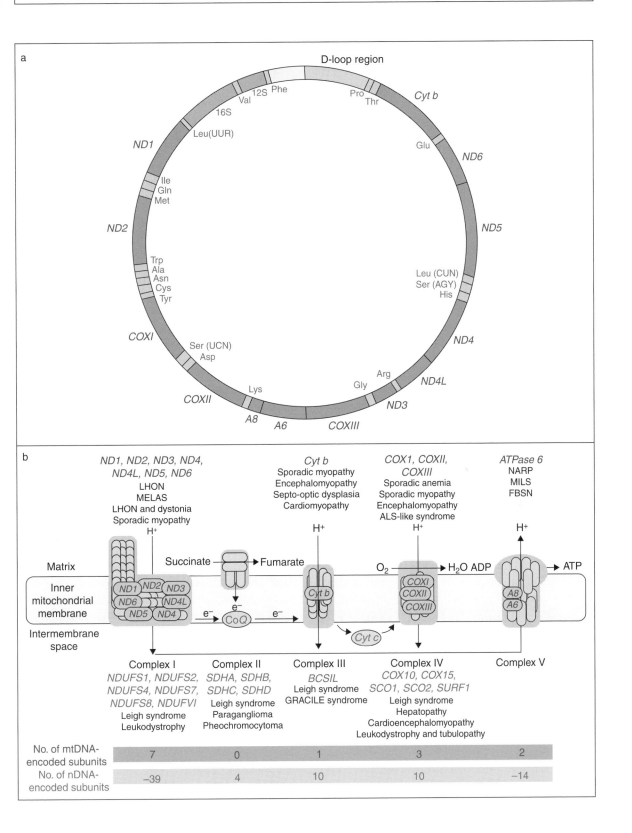

by the nuclear DNA. mtDNA is more susceptible to mutations for a variety of reasons. Compared with nuclear DNA, mtDNA possesses higher replicative error rates, lacks extensive DNA repair mechanisms, and is also exposed to reactive oxygen species in the inner mitochondrial membrane. In addition to point mutations, mtDNA may sustain large deletions and rearrangements.

Either mtDNA or nuclear DNA mutations can affect mitochondrial function by impairing electron transport chain (ETC) function. The proteins critical for ETC functions are located in the mitochondrial inner membrane [12] and make up four complexes that produce ATP via a series of electron transfers to oxygen (Figure 24.3). As electrons are shuttled along the ETC, hydrogen ions are transported across the mitochondrial membrane into the intermembrane space via proton pumps within Complexes I, III and IV in a series of redox reactions. The resultant electrochemical gradient fuels Complex V, ATP synthase, to produce ATP in a reaction coupled to proton transfer back into the matrix. Many mitochondrial diseases are found to be due to defects in complexes I and II, as opposed to the remaining ETC machinery. A possible explanation is that complexes I and II function in parallel and deficiencies in one can be partially compensated by residual function of the other, whereas defects in complexes III to V, which function in series, would result in terminal failure of the electron transport chain and subsequent cell death.

The genotype–phenotype relationship in mitochondrial disease is complex, in that a particular mtDNA mutation may produce multiple phenotypes, and a specific clinical feature may be attributed to several different mutations. The expression of mutated mtDNA depends on a variety of factors including the type of mutation, the degree of heteroplasmy and the energy requirements of tissue.

Mitochondria are strictly maternally inherited, with 100 000 per mature oocyte. Nevertheless, only a small proportion of mitochondria are passed on from one generation to the next, in a phenomenon known as mitochondrial bottlenecking [13]. Each cell can contain anywhere from 100 to 100 000 mitochondria and usually harbors multiple subpopulations of mtDNA, a phenomenon known as heteroplasmy. The degree of heteroplasmy determines overall mitochondrial function in a cell and the severity of clinical manifestation [14]. Homoplasmy occurs if all mitochondria within a cell share identical mtDNA. The majority of known missense mtDNA mutations are homoplasmic, whereas mutations that severely impair the oxidative phosphorylation pathway are generally heteroplasmic [15].

Over multiple mitotic divisions replicative segregation can occur, in which mutated and wild-type mtDNA from a heteroplasmic parent cell separate unevenly and result in a high concentration of mutated mtDNA. The result is generally two homoplasmic populations (one with very few or no mutated mtDNA and the other containing exclusively mutated mtDNA) and cells with varying degrees of heteroplasmy. If a mutated mtDNA is present in a substantial proportion within heteroplasmic cells, a threshold of expression may be reached beyond which the pathological phenotype is expressed [15]. Neurons are especially susceptible to the deleterious effects of mtDNA mutations due to their low replication potential, high mutation accumulation, and high metabolic requirements, and within the CNS the highest mtDNA levels are in the substantia nigra, caudate and putamen.

As previously noted, nuclear DNA mutations may also lead to mitochondrial disorders. Human mitochondrial DNA polymerase is the sole genetic proofreading mechanism of the mitochondria. It is a heterotrimer consisting of one catalytic subunit encoded by *POLG1* (encoding mitochondrial DNA polymerase-gamma)

Caption for Figure 24.3 (cont.)

Figure 24.3. The mitochondrial genome in human disease. Panel (a) depicts a map of the human mitochondrial genome. Protein-coding genes (red): complex I (*ND*); cytochrome *c* oxidase (*COX*); cytochrome *b* subunit of complex III (*Cyt b*); adenosine triphosphate (ATP) synthase (*A6*, *A8*). Protein-synthesis genes (blue): 12S and 16S ribosomal RNAs, 22 transfer RNAs; D-loop region. Panel (b) depicts subunits of the respiratory chain: nuclear DNA encoded (blue); mtDNA encoded (red). Protons (H⁺) are pumped by Complexes I, III and IV from matrix to the intermembrane space, and return via Complex V activity, resulting in ATP synthesis. Coenzyme Q (CoQ) and cytochrome *c* (Cyt *c*) function in electron transfer. Mitochondrial disorders are denoted beneath. Genes responsible for a subset of specific respiratory-chain disorders are also shown beneath corresponding protein complexes, as follows: *ATPase 6*, ATP synthase 6; *BCS1L*, cytochrome *b–c* complex assembly protein (Complex III); *NDUF*, NADH dehydrogenase–ubiquinone oxidoreductase; *SCO*, synthesis of cytochrome oxidase; *SDHA, SDHB, SDHC, SDHD*: succinate dehydrogenase subunits; *SURF1*: surfeit gene 1. Disorders included are as follows: ALS, amyotrophic lateral sclerosis; FBSN, familial bilateral striatal necrosis; LHON, Leber hereditary optic neuropathy; MELAS: mitochondrial encephalomyopathy, lactic acidosis, and stroke-like episodes; MILS, maternally inherited Leigh syndrome; NARP, neuropathy, ataxia, and retinitis pigmentosa; GRACILE, growth retardation, aminoaciduria, lactic acidosis, and early death. (Reproduced from reference [12] with permission. Copyright © 2003 Massachusetts Medical Society. All rights reserved.) (See the color plate section for a color version of this figure.)

and two smaller accessory subunits encoded by *POLG2*. Emerging literature has implicated POLG mutations in a variety of syndromes involving movement disorders including, but not limited to, autosomal dominant progressive external ophthalmoplegia (PEO) with ataxia; autosomal recessive peripheral neuropathy, parkinsonism, mitochondrial neurogastrointestinal encephalopathy (MNGIE); juvenile spinocerebellar ataxia-epilepsy syndrome (SCAE); myoclonus, epilepsy, myopathy, sensory ataxia (MEMSA); sensory ataxic neuropathy, dysarthria and ophthalmoparesis (SANDO); and mitochondrial recessive ataxia syndrome (MIRAS) [16,17]. Other mutations affecting the replication fork may also contribute to mitochondrial disease. In particular, mutations affecting Twinkle helicase are thought to impair the enzyme's ability to effectively unwind and expose the double-stranded mtDNA [11] and can lead to infantile-onset spinocerebellar ataxia (IOSCA).

Movement disorders in defined mitochondrial syndromes

As noted above, mitochondrial disease may manifest in a broad range of clinical manifestations as the expression of a mutation depends on a variety of factors including heteroplasmy and threshold of mutation. One clinical syndrome may be caused by more than one mtDNA mutation, and a particular mtDNA mutation may also give rise to a number of different phenotypes. A better understanding of clinicogenetic correlates continues to evolve, but the major syndromes are described individually below as they are currently understood.

Autosomal recessive mitochondrial ataxic syndrome

This recently described progressive syndrome is characterized by migraine and epilepsy in early stages but progresses to sensory and cerebellar ataxia, and ophthalmoplegia. Status epilepticus is a common feature, especially in those with myoclonic epilepsy. POLG mutations G1399A (A467T), G1491C (Q487H), and G2243C (W748S) are associated. MRI reveals abnormalities in the central cerebellum, olivary nucleus, occipital cortex and thalami [17]. Muscle biopsies demonstrate COX deficiency and depletion of mtDNA.

Chronic progressive external ophthalmoplegia

Chronic progressive external ophthalmoplegia (CPEO) may present at any age, and entails progressive symmetric weakness of extraocular muscles without diplopia, often in combination with other features including peripheral neuropathy, ataxia, tremor, depression, cataracts, pigmentary retinopathy, deafness, rhabdomyolysis and hypogonadism. CPEO may also occur with severe sensory ataxia and neuropathy in a syndrome called sensory ataxic neuropathy, dysarthria, and ophthalmoplegia (SANDO) or mitochondrial recessive ataxia syndrome (MIRAS). This syndrome often involves involuntary movement, myoclonus, epileptic seizures and cognitive impairment. SANDO is due to multiple nuclear DNA deletions, and is also associated with A467T (typically presenting in the teens) or W748S/E1143 mutations in POLG1, which induce conformational changes interfering with interaction with the accessory subunit (POLG2). A recent study in patients who met clinical criteria for SANDO characterized additional POLG mutations, G737R and R1138C, thus it is likely that the full genetic spectrum for SANDO remains to be defined [18]. Diagnosis of this disorder hinges on POLG analysis, as other diagnostic tests are highly inconsistent, and muscle biopsies may demonstrate COX-deficient ragged-red and ragged blue fibers, or may be normal in appearance. Mitochondrial copy numbers may be diminished or normal due to compensatory mitochondrial amplification and mitochondrial proliferation [19,20]. Finally, parkinsonism with PEO has also been observed in a large family with autosomal dominant transmission due to *POLG1* mutations [21].

Deafness dystonia syndrome (Mohr–Tranebjaerg syndrome)

This is an X-linked, recessive neurodegenerative disorder first described in 1960 that typically presents with sensorineural hearing loss in childhood with subsequent development of dystonia, spasticity, cognitive deterioration and cortical blindness [22,23]. Histopathology revealed degeneration of spiral ganglion cells while the organ of Corti, hairs cells, stria vascularis and spiral ligament were intact [24]. PET and MRI studies may show multifocal degeneration of the striatum and parietal and bilateral occipital lobes. Degeneration of the optic nerves and retina has also been seen. The DFN-1 gene mutation leading to deafness dystonia syndrome is located on chromosome X21–22 and impairs the function of chaperone protein DDP-1/TIMM8a to bind to TIMM13. This complex is essential in the translocation of nuclear-encoded precursor proteins across the mitochondrial intermembrane space into the mitochondrial matrix [25]. Other components of the protein import machinery including DDP2/TIMM8b, TIMM10, TIMM9a, TIMM 9b and TIMM13 may also be impaired. The highest concentrations of DDP-1 protein are found in the brain. Although the function of this protein has yet to be elucidated, the yeast homologue (Tim8p) is a zinc-binding protein involved in the transport of molecules to the inner mitochondrial membrane [26].

Familial ataxia with coenzyme Q_{10} deficiency

Coenzyme Q_{10} (CoQ_{10}) is a component of the mitochondrial electron transport chain, a potent antioxidant, and membrane stabilizer. Deficiency is a rare but treatable cause of ataxia [27], which may occur without other symptoms, although CoQ_{10} deficiency may also cause generalized muscle weakness, pyramidal signs, neuropathy and seizures. The mode of inheritance and genetic basis remain to be characterized. CoQ_{10} levels in serum can be normal or low, pyruvate and lactate levels are normal, and brain MRI typically reveals cerebellar atrophy. Diagnosis depends upon finding low CoQ_{10} levels in muscle upon biopsy. Ragged red fibers are present in the myopathic form of this disorder but not in the ataxic form. CoQ_{10} supplementation (up to 3000 mg daily) improves ataxia, strength and seizures in some patients.

Infantile-onset spinocerebellar ataxia

Recessively inherited infantile-onset spinocerebellar ataxia (IOSCA) can arise due to mutations in the Twinkle gene, which also leads to PEO and rare forms of mitochondrial depletion syndromes.

Kearns–Sayre syndrome

This aggressive mitochondrial disorder comprises CPEO, pigmentary retinopathy, progressive proximal limb myopathy, cerebellar ataxia, cardiomyopathy and mental retardation. Extraocular muscle weakness can quickly progress to complete ophthalmoparesis. Although Kearns–Sayre syndrome (KSS) may manifest

at any age, it is most common before age 20 years and is fatal by the fourth decade. KSS is caused by a large-scale mtDNA deletion between ND5 and ATPase 8 genes. The exact location of the deleted segment is variable, but it leads to failure of mitochondrial tRNA synthesis [28]. Interestingly, KSS and PEO are caused by the same large-scale deletions, yet KSS is a multi-system disease, while PEO is limited to skeletal muscle pathology. This exemplifies the complex genotype–phenotype relationship seen in mitochondrial disease and highlights the fact that we have yet to understand many of the nuances that affect mitochondrial genetic expression and function.

Leber hereditary optic neuropathy

Leber hereditary optic neuropathy (LHON) typically presents with painless optic nerve atrophy causing sudden-onset blindness in mid-life, and it can be associated with dystonia or ataxia in a subset of cases. Pathology occurs in the retinal ganglion cells (RGCs) and there may be bilateral striatal necrosis in some cases [29]. Most cases of LHON are due to three mutations: G3460A (ND1 protein); G11778A (ND4 protein); and T14484C (ND6 protein), associated with a mitochondrial complex I defect. Rarer mutations such as G3635A, G10680A, T3394C and A4148G have also been found to cause LHON in certain ethnic groups [30,31] and often have other clinical features including dystonia, cerebellar ataxia [32], peripheral neuropathy, horizontal nystagmus, dysarthria, short stature, cognitive dysfunction and dilated cardiomyopathy. In particular, mutations at G3460A, G11778A, G14459A and T14596A (ND6 protein) are associated with LHON and dystonia [33–35]. Conventional neuroimaging is unrevealing in most cases. Visual evoked potentials are also normal and are usually obtained to rule out retinal pathology [36]. Research has revealed a strong correlation between smoking and vision loss in individuals who harbor these mutations, especially in combination with heavy alcohol intake [29]. Certain individuals may benefit from early institution of antioxidants and immunosuppression to mitigate disability [37,38].

Leigh syndrome (subacute necrotizing encephalopathy)

Leigh syndrome is characterized by optic atrophy, ophthalmoplegia, nystagmus, ataxia, dystonia, spasticity, seizures and developmental delay or regression that is frequently fatal in childhood. Chorea may also be observed but is not typical. Mutations in the E1α subunit gene of the pyruvate dehydrogenase complex (PDC) [39], electron chain complexes I, III, and IV, ATP synthetase and mitochondrial electron assembly proteins lead to impaired oxidative phosphorylation [40]. Mutations in PDC may occur in either the X-linked E1 or the E2 subunit, affecting this critical enzyme of the Krebs cycle. The condition presents according to severity of enzyme depletion between the prenatal and early childhood period. Presentation in early childhood includes intermittent incoordination or ataxia, particularly during concurrent illnesses. Episodic or progressive dystonia may also occur. However, common features are developmental delay or regression, encephalopathy, seizures, dysmorphic features, oculomotor abnormalities, respiratory compromise and lethargy. Treatment involves cofactor supplementation with thiamine, lipoic acid and carnitine. A recent study of several individuals within a family affected by Leigh syndrome or a Leigh-like syndrome implicates heteroplasmic mutations of T14487C leading to impaired function of complex IV [41]. A heteroplasmic mutation at position T8993G that encodes for ATPase 6 protein was observed in several cases of Leigh syndrome and has also been associated with NARP (discussed below) [42]. Maternally inherited Leigh syndrome (MILS) has typical onset between 3 and 12 months, and characteristics include developmental delay, hypotonia, spasticity, chorea, ataxia, peripheral neuropathy and hypertrophic cardiomyopathy.

There is lactic acidosis with elevated levels in the CSF more than serum, elevated plasma alanine and hypocitrullinemia. Brain MRI of individuals with Leigh syndrome reveals progressive hypointense signal changes on T1-weighted sequences and corresponding hyperintensities on T2 and FLAIR sequences, mainly affecting the lentiform nuclei and caudate, although dorsal aspects of the pons and medulla, periaqueductal region, red nucleus and cerebellum may also frequently be involved [43,44]. Magnetic resonance spectroscopy has revealed significant lactate peaks in patients harboring the T8993G mutation and associated complex III defect [44]. Pathology may show cystic cavitation, spongiform necrosis, demyelination, vascular proliferation and gliosis [45]. Anticholinergics and neuroleptics to treat dystonia in Leigh syndrome have been tried with varying success. Botulinum toxin injections may be of use if only a few isolated muscle groups are affected [46].

Mitochondrial recessive ataxia syndrome

Mitochondrial recessive ataxia syndrome (MIRAS) is due to POLG1 mutation, and was originally characterized as W748S in cis with E1143G, as one of the most common causes of inherited ataxia in Finland with a carrier frequency of 1:125. It is now known to occur in other countries; it may be of juvenile or adult onset, and the mutations lead to a heterogeneous group of phenotypes including peripheral neuropathy, seizures, mild cognitive impairment, involuntary movements and psychiatric symptoms.

Maternally inherited diabetes, deafness with cerebellar ataxia

A mutation in mitochondrial tRNA(Leu) at position 3243, in addition to causing Leigh syndrome and a combined MERFF/PEO phenotype, has been associated with ataxia in combination with deafness and diabetes (maternally inherited diabetes, deafness with cerebellar ataxia: MIDD).

Myoclonic encephalopathy, lactic acidosis and stroke-like episodes

Over 80% of cases of myoclonic encephalopathy, lactic acidosis and stroke-like episodes (MELAS) are caused by the A3243G tRNA mutation, but to date there are more than 30 mtDNA mutations (mostly affecting ND1–4 proteins of complex I) associated with MELAS [47]. Common manifestations of MELAS include generalized seizures, dystonia, migraines, hearing loss, retinitis pigmentosa, moderate limb weakness as a result of mitochondrial myopathy, ophthalmoplegia and ptosis. Patients have stroke-like episodes that can lead to hemiparesis, hemianopsia and cortical blindness. However, MELAS is also a rare cause of ataxia, and in one reported case, hyperglycemic chorea-ballism was a presenting feature. Almost all cases present before age 40 years, with the majority presenting in childhood, and have a relapsing-remitting course hallmarked by encephalopathy with seizures or stroke-like episodes, ultimately leading to severe neurologic disability.

Diagnostic criteria include the presence of lactic acidosis, elevated CSF lactate concentration and RRF in muscle tissue obtained by biopsy (seen in more than 90% of cases). MRI studies demonstrate transient stroke-like lesions predominantly in the gray matter, which cross vascular territories. Additionally, parietal and occipital cortices may also be abnormal.

The affected areas are hyperintense on T2 and FLAIR sequences, and bright on DWI sequences, with a high or normal apparent diffusion coefficient (ADC). Magnetic resonance spectroscopy demonstrates lactate peaks and reduction of N-acetyl aspartate (NAA) both in lesions and in seemingly unaffected regions of brain that may precede DWI abnormalities [8].

Myoclonic epilepsy with ragged red fibers

Myoclonic epilepsy with ragged red fibers (MERRF) manifests with myoclonus, progressive ataxia, epilepsy, spasticity, optic neuropathy, deafness, peripheral neuropathy, myocardiopathy, diabetes, hypertension, short stature and multiple lipomas, and has a childhood onset [48]. The presence of lactic acidosis aids in diagnosis, and in addition to ragged red fibers (Figure 24.2), and COX deficiency is characteristic. Most cases are associated with the G8344A mutation of the tRNA(Lys) gene, which impairs mitochondrial protein synthesis and respiratory chain function. Defects in muscle Complex I and IV activity have been demonstrated. This same mutation also leads to Leigh syndrome, and other disorders, including a report of one case of action myoclonus with spasmodic dysphonia. MERRF has also recently been reported as a result of a mitochondrial tRNA(Pro) gene mutation. The A3243G tRNA(Leu) mtDNA mutation, in addition to causing MELAS, may also lead to a syndrome encompassing features of both MELAS and MERRF [49]. An overlap syndrome has similarly been recognized from the G12127A mitochondrial tRNA(His) gene mutation, and from a mutation in ND5. Atrophy of the superior cerebellar peduncles and the cerebellum may be demonstrated on brain MRI scans, in addition to generalized atrophy and basal ganglia calcifications. At autopsy, gliosis and neuronal loss have been noted in the inferior olivary nucleus and dentate nuclei of the cerebellum. Piracetam, levetiracetam and clonazepam have been used successfully to attenuate myoclonus in MERRF [46].

Neuropathy, ataxia and retinitis pigmentosa

Closely related to Leigh syndrome, neuropathy, ataxia and retinitis pigmentosa (NARP) is characterized by the aforementioned features but may also include dementia, seizures, and developmental delay. NARP is associated with a point mutation at T8993G and less commonly at T9176C, both within the ATPase6 gene. The former has also been associated with Leigh syndrome. Patients with NARP are found to have 70–90% mutated mtDNA. However, those with >90% heteroplasmy may demonstrate features of a much more severe disease, maternally inherited Leigh syndrome (MILS). This is one of several examples where the degree of heteroplasmy may affect phenotypic expression [50]. Leukoencephalopathy has been noted on MRI in affected individuals although bilateral T2 hyperintensities in the basal ganglia as well as pontocerebellar atrophy have also been noted. MR spectroscopy may reveal increased lactate in the frontal and occipital lobe [51].

Management

Early recognition and symptomatic management of patients with mitochondrial disease require a multidisciplinary approach, and appropriate treatment and counseling can greatly improve quality of life. Treatment approaches can be addressed broadly as falling into two categories: (1) symptom-specific, such as familiarly used medications for myoclonus, parkinsonism, chorea or dystonia (as discussed for individual disorders in the preceding sections); and (2) nonspecific, such as use of antioxidants, alternative energy sources, supplementation with cofactors, or restriction of other factors (recently reviewed in reference 52 and discussed briefly in the later section "Mitochondrial therapy").

Specific symptomatic therapy

Studies of interventions for symptomatic relief in many cases are hampered by symptomatic heterogeneity and low numbers of study participants. Indeed, it is not clear that specific movement disorders associated with mitochondrial disease respond typically to drugs in common use. In one study of levetiracetam for myoclonus, either the few subjects with mitochondrial disorders did not respond to the drug or their symptoms actually worsened [53]. However, there are other case reports of successful reduction of myoclonus by levetiracetam in mitochondrial disease [54], supporting cautious and carefully monitored empirical use of these medications according to the treating clinician's judgment. Botulinum toxin A injections have been successful in treating dystonia in mitochondrial disorders, such as in Leigh syndrome [55]. However, this has not been systematically studied, and should be pursued with great caution, weighing pros and cons, given the potential side-effects in the context of systemic neurologic and muscle disease. Finally, certain medications that impede oxidative phosphorylation should be avoided. In particular, valproic acid is known to interfere with this pathway and may precipitate clinical deterioration when used to treat seizures in patients with Leigh syndrome, MELAS or MERRF.

Other, nonpharmacologic, interventions may also be helpful. Resistance exercise training may be beneficial in patients with myopathic symptoms as it is proposed to activate satellite cells to induce wild-type mtDNA expression, thereby lowering the burden of mutant mtDNA [56]. Trials using a 12-week program to improve aerobic capacity are ongoing, and it seems worthwhile to pursue physical, occupational, and speech therapy despite lack of formal evidence from large clinical trials. Patients with mitochondrial disease, especially those with bulbar weakness, may be at risk for respiratory compromise and aspiration and may benefit where appropriate from swallowing evaluations, periodic pulmonary function testing, and nocturnal oximetry in select cases. Percutaneous endoscopic gastrostomy (PEG) placement should be considered in those with marked bulbar weakness and subsequent high risk of aspiration [57].

"Mitochondrial therapy"

Overall, there are very limited treatment options for patients affected by mitochondrial disease, and there is as yet no convincing evidence that any single medication or supplement is effective for treatment. CoQ_{10}, α-lipoic acid and creatine, among others, have been tested as potential neuroprotectants in mitochondrial disorders: these are reviewed by Rodriguez and colleagues [58]. At the time of writing, a phase III clinical trial is testing CoQ_{10} 10 mg/kg up to 400 mg daily in children with mitochondrial disorders (NCT00432744). However, large doses of CoQ_{10} may be required in some cases to achieve therapeutic concentration, and dose ranges in neurodegenerative disease and CoQ_{10} deficiency have been explored up to 3000 mg daily [59]. Riboflavin, succinate, L-carnitine, α-lipoic acid and vitamins C, E and K have been tested in mitochondrial disorders, with varying success [60]. Finally, gene therapy, mentioned briefly below, is an exciting future possibility in mitochondrial disorders [61].

Conclusions

Mitochondrial diseases are an unusual but significant cause of movement disorders. Although they may be difficult to recognize due to heterogeneous clinical presentations, association of a movement disorder with particular features, such as myopathy, deafness, and others, should raise the index of clinical suspicion and in the appropriate context this should lead to targeted testing for a mitochondrial etiology. Our understanding of mitochondrial disease is evolving as more novel mutations are being reported in association with various syndromes. In turn, multiple treatment approaches are being explored to offer relief to affected patients, including specific drugs targeting symptomatology, as well as use of nutritional supplements such as CoQ_{10}. Moreover, novel genetic approaches are now being investigated and are currently in preclinical stages. Examples include replacing affected mtDNA with constructed nuclear DNA [62], delivering cytosolic tRNA into the mitochondria [63], and selective degradation of mutant mtDNA using zinc fingers targeted specifically to the mutant sequence [64]. Although far from clinical use, they provide hope for a more fundamental treatment of potentially devastating mitochondrial disease. Finally, understanding these mitochondrial movement disorders may also yield critical information that will impact upon treatment of more common disorders in which mitochondrial function is disrupted, such as Parkinson disease.

References

1. Henchcliffe C, Beal MF. Mitochondrial biology and oxidative stress in Parkinson disease pathogenesis. *Nat Clin Pract Neurol* 2008; **4**: 600–9.

2. Finsterer J. Mitochondrial disorders, cognitive impairment and dementia. *J Neurol Sci* 2009; **283**: 143–8.

3. Schaefer A, McFarland R, Blakely E *et al.* Prevalence of mitochondrial DNA disease in adults. *Ann Neurol* 2008; **63**: 35–9.

4. Chinnery P, Johnson M, Wardell T *et al.* The epidemiology of pathogenic mitochondrial DNA mutations. *Ann Neurol* 2000; **48**: 188–93.

5. Skladal D, Halliday J, Thorburn D. Minimum birth prevalence of mitochondrial respiratory chain disorders in children. *Brain* 2003; **126**: 1905–12.

6. DiMauro S, Schon E. Mitochondrial disorders in the nervous system. *Annu Rev Neurosci* 2008; **31**: 91–123.

7. Robinson B. Lactic acidemia and mitochondrial disease. *Mol Genet Metab* **89**: 3–13.

8. Kaufmann P, Shungu D, Sano M *et al.* Cerebral lactic acidosis correlates with neurological impairment in MELAS. *Neurology* 2004; **62**: 1297–302.

9. Sciacco M, Bonilla E, Schon E *et al.* Distribution of wild-type and common deletion forms of mtDNA in normal

and respiration-deficient muscle fibers from patients with mitochondrial myopathy. *Hum Mol Genet* 1994; **3**: 13–19.

10. Taylor R, Schaefer A, Barron M *et al.* The diagnosis of mitochondrial muscle disease. Neuromuscul Disord 2004; **14**: 237–45.

11. Hudson G, Chinnery P. Mitochondrial DNA polymerase-gamma and human disease. *Hum Mol Genet* 2006; **15**(Spec No 2): R244–52.

12. DiMauro S, Schon EA. Mitochondrial respiratory-chain diseases. *N Engl J Med*, 2003; **348**: 2656–68.

13. Wai T, Teoli D, Shoubridge E. The mitochondrial DNA genetic bottleneck results from replication of a subpopulation of genomes. *Nat Genet* 2008; **40**: 1484–8.

14. Cree L, Samuels D, de Sousa Lopes S *et al.* A reduction of mitochondrial DNA molecules during embryogenesis explains the rapid segregation of genotypes. *Nat Genet* 2008; **40**: 249–54.

15. Simon D, Johns D. Mitochondrial disorders: clinical and genetic features. *Annu Rev Med* 1999; **50**: 111–27.

16. Graziewicz M, Longley M, Copeland W. DNA polymerase gamma in mitochondrial DNA replication and repair. *Chem Rev* 2006; **106**: 383–405.

17. Winterthun S, Ferrari G, He L *et al.* Autosomal recessive mitochondrial ataxic syndrome due to mitochondrial polymerase gamma mutations. *Neurology* 2005; **64**: 1204–8.

18. Milone M, Brunetti-Pierri N, Tang L *et al.* Sensory ataxic neuropathy with ophthalmoparesis caused by POLG mutations. *Neuromuscul Disord* 2008; **18**: 626–32.

19. Bohlega S, Tanji K, Santorelli F *et al.* Multiple mitochondrial DNA deletions associated with autosomal recessive ophthalmoplegia and severe cardiomyopathy. *Neurology* 1996; **46**: 1329–34.

20. Van Goethem G, Dermaut B, Löfgren A *et al.* Mutation of POLG is associated with progressive external ophthalmoplegia characterized by mtDNA deletions. *Nat Genet* 2001; **28**: 211–12.

21. Hudson G, Schaefer AM, Taylor RW *et al.* Mutation of the linker region of the polymerase gamma-1 (POLG1) gene associated with progressive external ophthalmoplegia and Parkinsonism. *Arch Neurol* 2007; **64**: 553–7.

22. Mohr J, Mageroy K. Sex-linked deafness of a possibly new type. *Acta Genet Stat Med* 1960; **10**: 54–62.

23. Tranebjaerg L, Schwartz C, Eriksen H *et al.* A new X linked recessive deafness syndrome with blindness, dystonia, fractures, and mental deficiency is linked to Xq22. *J Med Genet* 1995; **32**: 257–63.

24. Merchant S, McKenna M, Nadol JJ *et al.* Temporal bone histopathologic and genetic studies in Mohr-Tranebjaerg syndrome (DFN-1). *Otol Neurotol* 2001; **22**: 506–11.

25. Roesch K, Curran S, Tranebjaerg L *et al.* Human deafness dystonia syndrome is caused by a defect in assembly of the DDP1/TIMM8a-TIMM13 complex. *Hum Mol Genet* 2002; **11**: 477–86.

26. Binder J, Hofmann S, Kreisel S *et al.* Clinical and molecular findings in a patient with a novel mutation in the deafness-dystonia peptide (DDP1) gene. *Brain* 2003; **126**: 1814–20.

27. Lamperti C, Naini A, Hirano M *et al.* Cerebellar ataxia and coenzyme Q$_{10}$ deficiency. *Neurology* 2003; **60**: 1206–8.

28. Schon E, DiMauro S. Mitochondrial mutations: genotype to phenotype. *Novartis Found Symp* 2007; **287**: 214–25; discussion 226–33.

29. Kirkman M, Yu-Wai-Man P, Korsten A *et al.* Gene-environment interactions in Leber hereditary optic neuropathy. *Brain* 2009; **132**: 2317–26.

30. Yang J, Zhu Y, Tong Y *et al.* Confirmation of the mitochondrial ND1 gene mutation G3635A as a primary LHON mutation. *Biochem Biophys Res Commun* 2009; **386**: 50–4.

31. Liang M, Guan M, Zhao F *et al.* Leber's hereditary optic neuropathy is associated with mitochondrial ND1 T3394C mutation. *Biochem Biophys Res Commun* 2009; **383**: 286–92.

32. Johns D. Seminars in medicine of the Beth Israel Hospital, Boston. Mitochondrial DNA and disease. *N Engl J Med* 1995; **333**: 638–44.

33. Novotny EJ, Singh G, Wallace D *et al.* Leber's disease and dystonia: a mitochondrial disease. Neurology 1986; **36**: 1053–60.

34. Watanabe Y, Odaka M, Hirata K. Case of Leber's hereditary optic neuropathy with mitochondrial DNA 11778 mutation exhibiting cerebellar ataxia, dilated cardiomyopathy and peripheral neuropathy. *Brain Nerve* 2009; **61**: 309–12.

35. Bonnet C, Augustin S, Ellouze S *et al.* The optimized allotopic expression of ND1 or ND4 genes restores respiratory chain complex I activity in fibroblasts harboring mutations in these genes. *Biochim Biophys Acta* 2008; **1783**: 1707–17.

36. Man P, Turnbull D, Chinnery P. Leber hereditary optic neuropathy. *J Med Genet* 2002; **39**: 162–9.

37. Perez F, Anne O, Debruxelles S *et al.* Leber's optic neuropathy associated with disseminated white matter disease: a case report and review. *Clin Neurol Neurosurg* 2009; **111**: 83–6.

38. Sala G, Trombin F, Beretta S *et al.* Antioxidants partially restore glutamate transport defect in Leber hereditary optic neuropathy cybrids. *J Neurosci Res* 2008; **86**: 3331–7.

39. Matthews P, Marchington D, Squier M *et al.* Molecular genetic characterization of an X-linked form of Leigh's syndrome. *Ann Neurol* 1993; **33**: 652–5.

40. Loeffen J, Smeitink J, Triepels R *et al.* The first nuclear-encoded complex I mutation in a patient with Leigh syndrome. *Am J Hum Genet* 1998; **63**: 1598–608.

41. Wang J, Brautbar A, Chan A *et al.* Two mtDNA mutations 14487T>C (M63V, ND6) and 12297T>C (tRNA Leu) in a Leigh syndrome family. *Mol Genet Metab* 2009; **96**: 59–65.

42. Santorelli F, Shanske S, Macaya A *et al.* The mutation at nt 8993 of mitochondrial DNA is a common cause of Leigh's syndrome. *Ann Neurol* 1993; **34**: 827–34.

43. Lee H, Tsai C, Chi C *et al.* Leigh syndrome: clinical and neuroimaging follow-up. *Pediatr Neurol* 2009; **40**: 88–93.

44. Saneto R, Friedman S, Shaw D. Neuroimaging of mitochondrial disease. *Mitochondrion* 2008; **8**: 396–413.

45. Leigh D. Subacute necrotizing encephalomyelopathy in an infant. *J Neurol Neurosurg Psychiatry* 1951; **14**: 216–21.

46. Horvath R, Hudson G, Ferrari G *et al.* Phenotypic spectrum associated with mutations of the mitochondrial polymerase gamma gene. *Brain* 2006; **129**: 1674–84.

47. Ruiz-Pesini E, Lott M, Procaccio V *et al.* An enhanced MITOMAP with a global mtDNA mutational phylogeny. *Nucleic Acids Res* 2007; **35**: D823–8.

48. Shibasaki H, Yamashita Y, Neshige R *et al.* Pathogenesis of giant somatosensory evoked potentials in progressive myoclonic epilepsy. *Brain* 1985; **108**: 225–40.

49. Mongini T, Doriguzzi C, Chiadò-Piat L *et al.* MERRF/ MELAS overlap syndrome in a family with A3243G mtDNA mutation. *Clin Neuropathol* 21: 72–6.

50. Holt I, Harding A, Petty R *et al.* A new mitochondrial disease associated with mitochondrial DNA heteroplasmy. *Am J Hum Genet* 1990; **46**: 428–33.

51. Haas R, Dietrich R. Neuroimaging of mitochondrial disorders. Mitochondrion 2004; **4**: 471–90.

52. Finsterer J. Treatment of mitochondrial disorders. *Eur J Paediatr Neurol* 14: 29–44.

53. Lim LL, Ahmed A. Limited efficacy of levetiracetam on myoclonus of different etiologies. *Parkinsonism Relat Disord* 2005; **11**: 135–7.

54. Mancuso M, Galli R, Pizzanelli C *et al.* Antimyoclonic effect of levetiracetam in MERRF syndrome. *J Neurol Sci* 2006; **243**: 97–9.

55. Leung TF, Hui J, Yeung WL *et al.* A Chinese girl with Leigh syndrome: effect of botulinum toxin on dystonia. *J Paediatr Child Health* 1998; **34**: 480–2.

56. Murphy J, Blakely E, Schaefer A *et al.* Resistance training in patients with single, large-scale deletions of mitochondrial DNA. *Brain* 2008; **131**: 2832–40.

57. Sanaker P, Husebye E, Fondenes O *et al.* Clinical evolution of Kearns–Sayre syndrome with polyendocrinopathy and respiratory failure. *Acta Neurol Scand Suppl* 2007; **187**: 64–7.

58. Rodriguez MC, MacDonald JR, Mahoney DJ *et al.* Beneficial effects of creatine, CoQ$_{10}$, and lipoic acid in mitochondrial disorders. *Muscle Nerve* 2007; **35**: 235–42.

59. Spindler M, Beal MF, Henchcliffe C. Coenzyme Q$_{10}$ effects in neurodegenerative disease. *Neuropsychiatr Dis Treat* 2009; **5**: 597–610.

60. Chinnery P, Ma*JAMA*a K, Turnbull D *et al.* Treatment for mitochondrial disorders. *Cochrane Database Syst Rev* 2006; CD004426.

61. Kyriakouli D, Boesch P, Taylor R *et al.* Progress and prospects: gene therapy for mitochondrial DNA disease. *Gene Ther* 2008; **15**: 1017–23.

62. Manfredi G, Fu J, Ojaimi J *et al.* Rescue of a deficiency in ATP synthesis by transfer of MTATP6, a mitochondrial DNA-encoded gene, to the nucleus. *Nat Genet* 2002; **30**: 394–9.

63. Mahata B, Mukherjee S, Mishra S *et al.* Functional delivery of a cytosolic tRNA into mutant mitochondria of human cells. *Science* 2006; **314**: 471–4.

64. Minczuk M, Papworth M, Miller J *et al.* Development of a single-chain, quasi-dimeric zinc-finger nuclease for the selective degradation of mutated human mitochondrial DNA. *Nucleic Acids Res* 2008; **36**: 3926–38.

Nonhereditary chorea

Francisco Cardoso

Introduction

Chorea is a hyperkinetic syndrome characterized by brief, abrupt, involuntary movements resulting from a continuous flow of random muscle contractions. The pattern of movement may sometimes appear playful, conveying a feeling of restlessness to the observer. When choreic movements are more severe, assuming a flinging, sometimes violent, character, they are called ballism. Regardless of its etiology, overall chorea has the same motor features, although the muscle tone varies depending on the underlying etiology [1]. As several basal ganglia circuits are often involved in conditions associated with chorea, non-motor features such as subcortical cognitive decline, obsessions, compulsions, attention deficit and others are often present in choreic syndromes.

There are genetic causes of chorea, described in other chapters of this book, and nongenetic causes of chorea, listed in Table 25.1. The latter include vascular choreas, autoimmune choreas, metabolic and toxic choreas, and drug-induced choreas. Although there are very few community-based studies available regarding the prevalence and incidence of choreas as a whole, there is information regarding the situation in tertiary care centers. According to a recent study from Pennsylvania, Sydenham chorea (SC) accounts for almost 100% of acute cases of chorea seen in children [2]. In contrast, the situation is quite distinct in adult patients. Although no published data are available, it is likely that levodopa-induced chorea in Parkinson disease (PD) patients is the most common cause of chorea seen by neurologists. One study of consecutive patients seen at a tertiary hospital found that stroke accounted for 50% of all cases, drug abuse was identified in one-third of the patients, and the remaining patients had chorea related to AIDS and other infections as well as metabolic problems [3].

The aim of this chapter is to provide an overview of the main causes of nonhereditary choreas, discussing their clinical features, etiology and pathogenesis, and management.

Autoimmune choreas

Sydenham chorea

Sydenham chorea (SC), the most common form of autoimmune chorea worldwide, is a major feature of acute rheumatic fever (ARF), a nonsuppurative complication of group A β-hemolytic *Streptococcus* infection. Despite the decline of ARF, it remains the most common cause of acute chorea in children in the United States and a major public health problem in developing areas of the world. Clinically, it is characterized by a combination of chorea, other movement disorders, behavioral abnormalities and cognitive changes [1,2,4].

Clinical features

The usual age at onset of SC is 8–9 years, but there are reports on patients who developed chorea during the third decade of life. In most series, there is a female preponderance [5]. Typically, patients develop this disease 4–8 weeks after an episode of group A beta-hemolytic streptococcal pharyngitis. It does not occur after streptococcal infection of the skin. The chorea spreads rapidly and becomes generalized, but 20% of patients remain with hemichorea [5,6]. Patients display motor impersistence, particularly noticeable during tongue protrusion and ocular fixation. The muscle tone is usually decreased; in severe and rare cases (8% of all patients seen at the Movement Disorders Clinic of the Federal University of Minas Gerais, Brazil), this is so pronounced that the patient may become bedridden (chorea paralytica).

Uncommon Causes of Movement Disorders, ed. Néstor Gálvez-Jiménez and Paul J. Tuite. Published by Cambridge University Press. © Cambridge University Press 2011.

Table 25.1. Nongenetic causes of chorea.

Immunologic
- Sydenham chorea and variants (chorea gravidarum and contraceptive-induced chorea)
- Systemic lupus erythematosus
- Anti-phospholipid antibody syndrome
- Paraneoplastic syndromes
- Acute disseminated encephalomyelopathy
- Celiac disease

Drug-related
- Amantadine
- Amphetamine
- Anticonvulsants
- Carbon monoxide
- CNS stimulants (methylphenidate, pemoline, cyproheptadine)
- Cocaine
- Dopamine agonists
- Dopamine-receptor blockers
- Ethanol
- Levodopa
- Levofloxacin
- Lithium
- Sympathomimetics
- Theophylline
- Tricyclic antidepressants
- Withdrawal emergent syndrome

Infections
- AIDS related (toxoplasmosis, progressive multifocal leukoencephalopathy, HIV encephalitis)
- Bacteria
  - Diphtheria
  - Scarlet fever
  - Whooping cough
- Encephalitis
  - B19 parvovirus
  - Japanese encephalitis
  - Measles
  - Mumps
  - West Nile River encephalitis
  - Others
- Parasites
  - Neurocysticercosis
- Protozoan
  - Malaria
  - Syphilis

Endocrine-metabolic dysfunction
- Adrenal insufficiency
- Hyper/hypocalcemia
- Hyper/hypoglycemia
- Hypomagnesemia
- Hypernatremia
- Liver failure

Vascular
- Post-pump chorea (cardiac surgery)
- Stroke
- Subdural hematoma

Miscellaneous
- Anoxic encephalopathy
- Cerebral palsy
- Kernicterus
- Multiple sclerosis
- Normal maturation (less than 12 months old)
- Nutritional (e.g., B_{12} deficiency)
- Posttraumatic (brain injury)

Patients often display other neurologic and non-neurologic symptoms and signs. There are reports of common occurrence of tics in SC. It is, however, virtually impossible to distinguish simple tics from fragments of chorea. Even vocal tics, found in 70% or more of patients with SC in one study, are not a clear-cut diagnosis as in other hyperkinetic disorders [7]. In a cohort of 108 SC patients carefully followed up at our unit, we have identified vocalizations in just 8% of subjects. We have avoided the term "tic" because there was no premonitory sign or complex sound and, conversely, the vocalizations were associated with severe cranial chorea. Taken together, these findings suggest that involuntary sounds present in a few patients with SC result from choreic contractions of the upper respiratory tract muscles rather than true tics [8,9]. There is evidence that many patients with active chorea have hypometric saccades, and a few of them also show oculogyric crisis.

Dysarthria is common and there is also impairment of verbal fluency. In fact, a case–control study of patients described a pattern of decreased verbal fluency that reflected reduced phonetic, but not semantic, output [10]. This result is consistent with dysfunction of the dorsolateral prefrontal-basal ganglia circuit. Recently studying adults with SC, we have extended this finding, showing that many functions dependent on the prefrontal area are impaired in these patients. The conclusion of this study is that SC should be included among the causes of dysexecutive syndrome [11]. Prosody is also affected in SC. One investigation of 20 patients with SC has shown decreased vocal tessitura and increased duration of speech [12,13]. Interestingly, these findings are similar to those observed in Parkinson disease [14]. In a recent survey of 100 patients with rheumatic fever, half of whom had chorea, we found that migraine was more frequent in SC (21.8%) than in normal controls (8.1%, $p = 0.02$) [15]. This is similar to what has been described in Tourette syndrome [16]. In the older literature, there are also references to papilledema, central retinal artery occlusion and seizures in a few patients with SC.

Attention has also been drawn to behavioral abnormalities. Swedo and colleagues found obsessive-compulsive behavior in 5 of 13 SC patients, three of whom met criteria for obsessive-compulsive disorder, whereas no patient of the rheumatic fever group presented with obsessive-compulsive behavior [17]. In another study of 30 patients with SC, Asbahr and colleagues demonstrated that 70% of the subjects presented with obsessions and compulsions, whereas 16.7% of them met criteria for obsessive-compulsive disorder. None of 20 patients with ARF without chorea had obsessions or compulsions [18]. These results, however, were roughly replicated by a more recent study that found that patients with ARF without chorea had more obsessions and compulsions than did healthy controls [19]. This study also tackled the issue of hyperactivity and attention deficit disorder in SC and found that 45% of their 22 patients met criteria for this condition. Recently, Maia and colleagues investigated behavioral abnormalities in 50 healthy subjects, 50 patients with rheumatic fever without chorea, and 56 patients with SC [20]. The authors found that obsessive-compulsive behavior, obsessive-compulsive disorder and attention deficit and hyperactivity disorder were more frequent in the SC group (19%, 23.2%, 30.4%) than in the healthy controls (11%, 4%, 8%) or in the patients with ARF without chorea (14%, 6%, 8%). In this study,

the authors demonstrated that obsessive-compulsive behavior displays little degree of interference in the performance of the activities of daily living. Another study compared the phenomenology of obsessions and compulsions of patients with SC with subjects diagnosed with tic disorders. The authors demonstrated that the symptoms observed among the SC patients were different from those reported by patients with tic disorders but were similar to those previously noted among samples of pediatric patients with primary obsessive-compulsive disorder [21]. A recent investigation comparing healthy controls with patients with rheumatic fever showed that obsessive-compulsive behavior is more commonly seen in patients with SC with relatives who also have obsessions and compulsions [22]. This study makes clear that there is interplay between genetic factors and environment in the development of behavioral problems in SC. We recently reported that although rarely, SC may induce psychosis or trichotillomania during the acute phase of the illness [23,24].

An investigation demonstrated that the peripheral nervous system is not targeted in SC [25]. Finally, it must be kept in mind that SC is a major manifestation of rheumatic fever. From 60% to 80% of patients display cardiac involvement, particularly mitral valve dysfunction, in SC, whereas the association with arthritis is less common, seen in 30% of patients; however, in approximately 20% of patients, chorea is the sole finding [5,26]. A prospective follow-up of patients with SC with and without cardiac involvement in the first episode of chorea suggests that the heart remains spared in those without lesion at the onset of the rheumatic fever [27].

Diagnosis

The current diagnostic criteria for SC are a modification of the Jones criteria: chorea with acute or subacute onset and lack of clinical and laboratory evidence of an alternative cause. The diagnosis is further supported by the presence of additional major or minor manifestations of rheumatic fever [10,28,29]. Of note, according to the current criteria, the diagnosis of SC is still possible in the absence of any other feature of rheumatic fever.

The UFMG Sydenham Chorea Rating Scale (USCRS), the first validated scale to rate SC, provides a detailed quantitative description of the performance of activities of daily living, behavioral abnormalities, and motor function of patients with SC. It comprises 27 items, and each one is scored from 0 (no symptom or sign) to 4 (severe disability or finding) [30]. It is important to emphasize that the USCRS is not intended to be used as a diagnostic tool but rather to assess patients already with an established diagnosis of SC.

Several conditions may present with clinical manifestations similar to those of SC [1]. The most important differential diagnosis is systemic lupus erythematosus (SLE), which will be discussed later in this chapter. From a clinical point of view, the majority of subjects with SLE will have other nonneurologic manifestations such as arthritis, pericarditis, and other serositis as well as skin abnormalities. Moreover, the neurologic picture of SLE tends to be more complex and may include psychosis, seizures, other movement disorders, and even mental status and consciousness level changes. Only in rare instances will chorea, with a tendency for spontaneous remissions and recurrences, be an isolated manifestation of SLE. The difficulty in distinguishing these two conditions is increased by the finding that at least 20% of patients with SC display recurrence of the movement disorder. Eventually, patients with SLE will develop other features, meeting diagnostic criteria for this condition [1]. Primary anti-phospholipid antibody syndrome is differentiated from SC by the absence of other clinical and laboratory features of RF as well as the usual association with repeated abortions, venous thrombosis, other vascular events and the presence of typical laboratory abnormalities. Encephalitides can cause chorea, either as a result of direct viral invasion or by means of an immune-mediated postinfectious process. However, this usually happens in younger children; the clinical picture is more diversified to include seizures, pyramidal signs and impairment of the psychomotor development. There are also laboratory abnormalities suggestive of the underlying condition. Drug-induced choreas are readily distinguished by careful history demonstrating a temporal relationship between onset of the movement disorder and exposure to the agent.

Children and young adults with chorea should undergo complete neurologic examination and diagnostic testing to determine the etiology and assess the various causes of chorea. As there is no specific biological marker of SC, the aim of the diagnostic work-up in patients suspected to have rheumatic chorea is threefold: (1) to identify evidence of recent streptococcal infection or acute-phase reaction; (2) to search for cardiac injury associated with RF; and (3) to rule out alternative causes. Tests of acute-phase reactants such as erythrocyte sedimentation rate, C-reactive protein,

leukocytosis; other blood tests such as rheumatoid factor, mucoproteins, protein electrophoresis; and supporting evidence of preceding streptococcal infection (increased anti-streptolysin-O, anti-DNAse-B, or other anti-streptococcal antibodies; positive throat culture for group A streptococci; recent scarlet fever) are much less helpful in diagnosing SC than in other forms of rheumatic fever because of the usual long latency between the infection and onset of the movement disorder. Elevated anti-streptolysin-O titer may be found commonly in populations with a high prevalence of streptococcal infection. Furthermore, the anti-streptolysin-O titer declines if the interval between infection and rheumatic fever is greater than 2 months. Anti-DNase-B titers, however, may remain elevated up to 1 year after streptococcal pharyngitis. Heart evaluation (i.e., Doppler echocardiography) is mandatory because the association of SC with carditis is found in up to 80% of patients. Cardiac lesions are the main source of serious morbidity in SC. Serologic studies for SLE and primary anti-phospholipid antibody syndrome must be ordered to rule out these conditions. EEG has little importance in the evaluation work-up of these patients, showing nonspecific generalized slowing acutely or after clinical recovery. Spinal fluid analysis is usually normal, but it may show a slight increased lymphocyte count. In general, neuroimaging will help rule out vascular and other structural causes such as moyamoya disease. CT scan of the brain invariably fails to display abnormalities. Similarly, head MRI is often normal, although there are case reports of reversible hyperintensity in the basal ganglia area. In one study, Giedd and colleagues [31] showed increased signal in just 2 of 24 patients, although morphometric techniques revealed mean values for the size of the striatum and pallidum larger than controls. Unfortunately, these findings are of little help on an individual basis because there was an extensive overlap between controls and patients. PET and SPECT imaging may prove to be useful tools in the evaluation, revealing transient increases in striatal metabolism during the acute phase of the illness, a finding confirmed by a recent study [31–35]. This contrasts with other choreic disorders (such as Huntington disease) that are associated with hypometabolism. Of note, however, a recent investigation showed hyperperfusion in two patients with SC, whereas the remaining five had hypometabolism [36]. It is possible that the inconsistencies in these studies reflect heterogeneity of the population of patients [37]. In our own unit, we have observed a correlation between hypermetabolism of the basal ganglia on SPECT during acute SC, whereas patients with persistent chorea often display hypometabolism in the basal ganglia. Increasing interest is now directed to autoimmune markers that may eventually be useful for diagnosis. The test of anti-neuronal antibodies, however, is not commercially available, being performed only for research purposes. Preliminary evidence, moreover, suggests that these antibodies are not specific for SC. Similarly, the low sensitivity and specificity of the alloantigen D8/17 renders it unsuitable as a diagnostic test.

Etiology and pathogenesis

Taranta and Stollerman established the casual relationship between infection with group A β-hemolytic streptococci and the occurrence of SC [38]. Based on the assumption of molecular mimicry between streptococcal and central nervous system antigens, it has been proposed that the bacterial infection in genetically predisposed subjects leads to formation of cross-reactive antibodies that disrupt the basal ganglia function. Several studies have demonstrated the presence of such circulating antibodies in 50–90% of patients with SC [39,40]. A specific epitope of streptococcal M proteins that cross-reacts with basal ganglia has been identified [41]. In one study it was demonstrated that all patients with active SC have antibasal ganglia antibodies demonstrated by ELISA and western blot. In subjects with persistent SC (duration of disease greater than 2 years despite best medical treatment), the positivity was about 60% [42]. Recently it was determined that neuronal tubulin is the target of anti-neuronal antibodies [43]. It must be emphasized that the biological value of the anti-basal ganglia antibodies remains to be determined. One study suggests that they may interfere with neuronal function, however. Kirvan and colleagues demonstrated that IgM of one patient with SC induced expression of calcium-dependent calmodulin in a culture of neuroblastoma cells [44]. Our finding that there is a linear correlation between the increase of intracellular calcium levels in PC12 cells and antibasal ganglia antibody titer in the serum from SC patients further strengthens the hypothesis that these antibodies have a pathogenic value [45].

Although some investigations suggest that susceptibility to rheumatic chorea is linked to human leukocyte antigen-linked antigen expression [46], there are studies failing to identify any relationship between SC and human leukocyte antigen class I and II alleles [47]. An investigation has shown, however, that there is an association between HLA-DRB1*07 and recurrent streptococcal pharyngitis and rheumatic heart disease [48]. The genetic marker for ARF and related conditions would be the B-cell alloantigen D8/17 [49]. Despite repeated reports of the group that developed the essay claiming its high specificity and sensitivity [50,51], findings of other authors suggest that the D8/17 marker lacks specificity and sensitivity [1]. Another suggested genetic risk factor for development of ARF but not SC is polymorphisms within the promoter region of the tumor necrosis factor-alpha gene [52].

Because of the difficulties with the molecular mimicry hypothesis to account for the pathogenesis of SC, studies have addressed the role of immune cellular mechanisms in this condition. Investigating sera and CSF samples of patients of the Movement Disorders Clinic of the Federal University of Minas Gerais, Church and colleagues found elevation of cytokines that take part in the T_H2 (antibody-mediated) response, interleukins 4 (IL-4) and 10 (IL-10), in the serum of acute SC patients in comparison to persistent SC patients [53]. They also described IL-4 in 31% of the CSF of acute SC, whereas just IL-4 was raised in the CSF of persistent SC. The authors concluded that SC is characterized by a T_H2 response. However, as they found an elevation of IL-12 in acute SC and, more recently, we described an increased concentration of chemokines CXCL9 and CXCL10 in the serum of patients with acute SC [54], it can be concluded that T_H1 (cell-mediated) mechanisms may also be involved in the pathogenesis of this disorder.

Currently, the weight of evidence suggests that the pathogenesis of SC is related to circulating cross-reactive antibodies. It has been demonstrated that streptococcus-induced antibodies can be associated with a form of acute disseminated encephalomyelitis characterized by a high frequency of dystonia and other movement disorders as well as basal ganglia lesions on neuroimaging [55]. Anti-neural and anti-nuclear antibodies have also been found in patients with Tourette syndrome, but their relationship with prior streptococcal infection remains equivocal [56].

Management

In the past, physicians emphasized the need of bed rest for the treatment of SC. Currently there is no place for this measure. Quarantine to prevent contamination of others is usually unnecessary, because SC results from autoimmune and not direct bacterial attack against CNS [57].

The first aim of the treatment of SC is to provide control of chorea and behavioral problems often associated with this condition. Regardless of the choice of agent for symptomatic control, the physician should attempt a gradual decrease of the dosage of the medication (25% reduction every 2 weeks) after the patient remains free of the symptom for at least one month. Another important point is that in some patients symptoms are so mild that they do not cause meaningful disability. In these cases, it is possible not to introduce any pharmacologic intervention, since spontaneous remission of SC is the rule [29,58]. The second aim is prophylaxis of new bouts of ARF. Although it remains unproven whether prophylaxis of streptococcal infection prevents recurrences of SC [59], clearly it decreases the development of new cardiac lesions, which are the source of the most important disability in rheumatic fever.

There are no controlled studies of symptomatic treatment of SC and the reader must be aware that all the recommendations of this item are off-label use of the cited drugs [57]. The first choice of the authors is valproic acid with an initial dosage of 250 mg per day, which is increased during a 2-week period to 250 mg three times a day. If the response is not satisfactory, dosage can be increased gradually up to 1500 mg per day. As this drug has a rather slow onset of action, we usually wait 2 weeks before concluding that the regimen is ineffective. This is usually well-tolerated, although some patients may develop dyspepsia and diarrhea in the beginning of the treatment. Chronic exposure may be associated with action tremor of the hands and, more rarely, liver toxicity. An open-label study demonstrated that carbamazepine (15 mg/kg per day) is as effective as valproic acid (20–25 mg/kg per day) in inducing remission of chorea [1,60,61]. If the patient fails to respond to valproic acid, or, as first-line treatment, in patients who present with chorea paralytica, the next option is to prescribe neuroleptics. Risperidone, a relatively potent dopamine D2 receptor blocker, is usually effective in controlling the chorea. The usual initial regimen is 1 mg twice a day. If, 2 weeks later, the chorea is still troublesome, the dose can be increased to 2 mg twice a day. Haloperidol and pimozide are also occasionally used in the management of chorea in SC. However, they are less well tolerated than risperidone. Dopamine D2 receptor blockers must be used with great caution in patients with SC. After the observation of development of parkinsonism, dystonia, or both in patients treated with neuroleptics, we performed a case–control study,

comparing the response to these drugs in patients with SC and Tourette syndrome. We demonstrated that 5% of 100 patients with chorea developed extrapyramidal complications, whereas these findings were not seen among patients with tics matched for age and dosage of neuroleptics [60]. Other potential side-effects of these agents are sedation, depression and tardive dyskinesia. There are no published guidelines concerning the discontinuation of antichoreic agents. Our policy is to attempt a gradual decrease of the dosage (25% reduction every 2 weeks) after the patient remains free of chorea for at least 1 month. Finally, the most important measure in the treatment of patients with SC is secondary prophylaxis.

Because of the presumably autoimmune origin of SC, there have been attempts to treat patients with rheumatic chorea with corticosteroids. This is, however, a controversial area. Despite mention of the effectiveness of prednisone in suppressing chorea, this drug is only used when there is associated severe carditis. We recently reported that methylprednisolone 25 mg/kg per day in children and 1 g/day in adults for 5 days followed by 1 mg/kg per day of prednisone is an effective and well-tolerated treatment for patients with SC refractory to conventional treatment with antichoreic drugs and penicillin [61]. At least one other group has replicated our findings of good response to steroids in selected patients with SC [62]. In one of the few randomized controlled trials in SC, the authors compared oral prednisone (2 mg/kg per day) with placebo in a double-blind fashion. Simultaneous use of haloperidol was allowed. They concluded that steroid accelerates the recovery but the rate of remission and recurrence is similar in both groups [63]. This study, however, has some limitations: haloperidol use was not controlled in both groups; it remains uncertain whether the development of side-effects such as weight gain and moon face in the steroid group could have compromised the blinding of the study (this is of particular concern considering the high dosage of prednisone); the authors used a nonvalidated scale to rate the severity of chorea. The current recommendation is to reserve steroids for patients with persistent disabling chorea refractory to antichoreic agents or those who develop unacceptable side-effects with other agents. Finally, there is one open, controlled study of a small number of patients, reporting that plasma exchange or intravenous immunoglobulin are as effective as oral prednisone to control severity of chorea in SC [64]. Surprisingly, the authors report the lack of side-effects in all groups.

Because of the lack of additional studies to confirm the safety and effectiveness of these treatments, their high cost and the existence of alternative efficacious therapeutic options, plasmapheresis and immunoglobulin are presently considered as investigational, not having a place in routine medical practice.

Other autoimmune choreas

Other immunologic causes of chorea are systemic lupus erythematosus (SLE), PAPS (primary anti-phospholipid antibody syndrome), vasculitis and paraneoplastic syndromes. SLE and PAPS are classically described as the prototypes of autoimmune choreas [65]. However, several reports show that chorea is seen in no more than 1–2% of large series of patients with these conditions [66,67]. A recent PET study confirmed the concept that there is hypometabolism of the basal ganglia in chorea associated with SLE [68]. Autoimmune chorea has rarely been reported in the context of paraneoplastic syndromes associated with CV2/CRMP5 antibodies in rare patients with small-cell lung carcinoma, malignant thymoma and, less frequently, with breast cancer [69–71]. As these disorders are relatively rare, this means that chorea caused by them is an uncommon finding. Chorea associated with SLE or PAPS has been treated with immunosuppressive measures, especially IV methylprednisolone following a dosage regimen as described for SC, as well as IV immunoglobulin [72]. As it is accepted that neurological complications, including chorea, in PAPS are related to ischemic events, anti-platelet agents and even anticoagulants are often prescribed to treat chorea in this condition [73]. These recommendations are, however, based on reports of open-label studies involving small numbers of patients as well as clinical experience of physicians [1]. Recently there has been a report of the association of generalized chorea with bilateral basal ganglia lesions of Sjögren syndrome [74].

Vascular choreas

A study in a tertiary referral center showed that cerebrovascular disease was the most common cause of nongenetic chorea, accounting for 21 out of 42 cases [3]. Conversely, chorea is an unusual complication of acute vascular lesions, seen in less than 1% of patients with acute stroke. Vascular hemichorea or hemiballism, is usually related to ischemic or hemorrhagic lesions of the basal ganglia and adjacent white matter in the territory of the middle or the posterior cerebral

artery [75]. In contrast to classical textbook concepts of hemiballism, the majority of patients with vascular chorea have lesions outside the subthalamus [76]. Although spontaneous remission is the rule, treatment with antichoreic drugs such as neuroleptics or dopamine depletors may be necessary in the acute phase. A few patients with vascular chorea may remain with persistent movement disorder. In this circumstance, they can be effectively treated with stereotactic surgery such as thalamotomy or posteroventral pallidotomy [77,78].

An uncommon cause of chorea is moyamoya disease, an intracranial vasculopathy that presents with ischemic lesion or, less commonly, hemorrhagic stroke of the basal ganglia [79]. Another rare form of vascular chorea is "post-pump chorea" (PPC) – a complication of extracorporeal circulation. The pathogenesis of this movement disorder is believed to be related to vascular insult of the basal ganglia during the surgical procedure. The current evidence supports the notion that the long-term prognosis of PPC is rather poor. In one series of 8 patients, for example, 5 subjects had persistent chorea and one of them died. In another study there was a clear distinction of those 8 patients with onset at earlier age (median 4.3 months), all of whom recovered fully, from 11 other, older patients (median age 16.8 months). Among the latter, 4 died and only one of the survivors had a complete neurologic recovery [80]. Finally, it is possible that polycythemia vera, a rare cause of chorea, induces the hyperkinesia via a vascular mechanism [81].

Drug-induced choreas

Chorea can derive from exposure to a variety of drugs, and drug-induced chorea is probably the most commonly encountered type of chorea in neurological practice and in the community [82]. A list of drugs considered to cause chorea can be found elsewhere [1,82]. Certain drugs seem to require preexisting basal ganglia dysfunction to induce chorea, whereas others appear to be more universally choreogenic. Examples of the former are oral contraceptives, which are particularly likely to induce chorea in patients with previous choreic episodes such as SC, chorea with SLE, or chorea gravidarum [83,84], and levodopa, which only induces chorea in patients with idiopathic Parkinson disease or other parkinsonian disorders [85]. Dopamine antagonists, on the other hand, are capable of inducing dyskinesias without preexisting basal ganglia abnormality. In one study of 100 consecutive patients with tardive dyskinesia, we demonstrated that, in contrast to a traditional notion, chorea is rarely seen in association with use of Dopamine antagonists [86]. The most prevalent types of drug-induced choreas result from treatment of PD patients with levodopa. Levodopa-induced chorea develops in more than 40% of PD patients depending on age and the duration and dose of levodopa treatment. Furthermore, a variety of other agents have been associated with chorea in retrospective studies or anecdotal case reports. These include both tricyclic antidepressants and the SSRIs [87–89]. Phenytoin may also induce involuntary movements including orofacial chorea, particularly when other antiepileptic drugs are administered [90]. There are occasional reports of choreic dyskinesias induced by other antiepileptic drugs, such as carbamazepine [91] and lamotrigine [92]. Chronic exposure to amphetamines and other stimulants may induce orofacial dyskinesias and choreic movements of the trunk and extremities [93,94]. The onset of chorea in association with intrathecal infusion of methotrexate [95] was recently reported. The mainstay of the treatment of drug-induced choreas is the withdrawal of the offending agent. The management of levodopa-related chorea and other movement disorders is beyond the scope of the chapter.

Infectious choreas

Sydenham chorea could be considered as a form of infectious chorea since it is induced by group A beta-hemolytic streptococci; however, in a strict sense the term is limited to instances where chorea results from injury to the brain directly produced by a microorganism. Human immunodeficiency virus (HIV) and its complications are the most often reported infectious cause of chorea. In one series of 42 consecutive patients with nongenetic chorea, for instance, AIDS was found to be the cause in 12% of the subjects [3]. In HIV-positive patients, chorea is the result of either the direct action of the virus or other mechanisms such as opportunistic infections (toxoplasmosis, syphilis and others) or drugs [96]. However, with the advent of highly active antiretroviral therapy, there has been a decline of HIV-related neurologic complications, including movement disorders. Other infections related to chorea are new variant Creutzfeldt–Jakob disease, tuberculosis, syphilis and herpes simplex encephalitis [97–100].

Chorea in metabolic and toxic encephalopathy

Chronic acquired hepatolenticular degeneration was the first well-characterized metabolic cause of chorea. Originally described in the context of alcoholic hepatopathy, it can occur in any form of acquired liver disease. The clinical picture is heterogeneous since patients may present with a variable combination of neurologic and hepatic manifestations. In most instances, there is a combination of different movement disorders, but a few subjects may present with isolated chorea. MRI of the brain shows not only images compatible with cavitations in the basal ganglia (hyperintense signal on T2 and hypointense on T1) but also hyperintense T1 signal in the pallidum, putamen and upper brain stem. The latter has been interpreted as caused by deposition of manganese [101].

More recently, there is growing interest in the association of chorea and nonketotic hyperglycemia in type II diabetes mellitus – a condition particularly common among patients of Asian ethnic background. Unlike the usual neurological manifestations of nonketotic hyperglycemia, patients do not show change in the level of consciousness but develop unilateral or generalized chorea-ballism. The MRI findings are characteristic, with hyperintense signal of the pallidum on T1 possibly reflecting microhemorrhages of the pallidum, although others suggest that inflammation may also play a role in the pathogenesis [102,103]. Once glycemic control is achieved, there is gradual remission of chorea [104,105].

A few patients with hyperthyroidism may develop generalized chorea or even ballism related to this endocrine dysfunction. The lack of structural changes in the brain, appearance with onset of thyrotoxicosis and remission with endocrine control suggest that the basal ganglia dysfunction is induced by hormones [106,107]. Other possible metabolic causes of chorea are even rarer and include hypoglycemia, renal failure and ketogenic diet [1].

Miscellaneous choreas

Focal choreic limb movements or hemichorea can be a rare presenting symptom of primary or secondary brain neoplasms involving the basal-ganglia, subthalamic nucleus or adjacent areas. This type of presentation has been described most often for primary CNS lymphoma but may occur with any type of subcortical tumor or even nonneoplastic structural disease disrupting striato-pallido-thalamo-cortical motor circuitry [108,109]. Brain imaging is therefore mandatory in any new-onset focal or hemichoreic syndrome. Uncommon causes of chorea recently reported include giant tumefactive perivascular spaces [110], intracranial sewing needles [111] and psychiatric diseases [112]. Finally, although there is a decline of the frequency of cerebral palsy, a recent multicenter study demonstrated that pallidal deep brain stimulation is an effective treatment for chorea and dystonia related to this condition [113]. Despite the fact that the results of this study are preliminary, it is an important investigation considering the limited current treatment options of chorea and dystonia associated to cerebral palsy.

References

1. Cardoso F, Seppi K, Mair KJ, Wenning GK, Poewe W. Seminar on choreas. *Lancet Neurol* 2006; **5**: 589–602.

2. Zomorrodi A, Wald ER. Sydenham's chorea in western Pennsylvania. *Pediatrics* 2006; **117**: e675–9.

3. Piccolo I, Defanti CA, Soliveri P *et al.* Cause and course in a series of patients with sporadic chorea. *J Neurol* 2003; **250**: 429–35.

4. Cardoso F. Chorea. In: Hallett M, Poewe W, eds. *Therapeutics of Parkinson's Disease and Other Movement Disorders*. Philadelphia: Wiley; 2008: 212–27.

5. Cardoso F, Silva CE, Mota CC. Sydenham's chorea in 50 consecutive patients with rheumatic fever. *Mov Disord* 1997; **12**: 701–3.

6. Nausieda PA, Grossman BJ, Koller WC, Weiner WJ, Klawans HL. Sydenham's chorea: an update. *Neurology* 1980; **30**: 331–4.

7. Mercadante MT, Campos MC, Marques-Dias MJ *et al.* Vocal tics in Sydenham's chorea. *J Am Acad Child Adolesc Psychiatry* 1997; **36**: 305–6.

8. Jankovic J. Differential diagnosis and etiology of tics. *Adv Neurol* 2001; **85**: 15–29.

9. Teixeira Jr AL, Cardoso F, Maia DP *et al.* Frequency and significance of vocalizations in Sydenham's chorea. *Parkinsonism Relat Disord* 2009; **15**: 62–3.

10. Cunningham MC, Maia DP, Teixeira AL Jr, Cardoso F. Sydenham's chorea is associated with decreased verbal fluency. *Parkinsonism Relat Disord* 2006; **12**(3): 165–7.

11. Beato R, Maia D, Teixeira A, Cardoso F. Executive functioning in adult patients with Sydenham's chorea. *Mov Disord* 2010; **25**(7): 853–7.

12. Cardoso F, Oliveira PM, Reis CC *et al.* Prosody in Sydenham chorea – I: Tessitura. *Mov Disord* 2006; **21**: S359–60.

13. Cardoso F, Oliveira PM, Reis CC *et al.* Prosody in Sydenham chorea – II: Duration of statements. *Mov Disord* 2006; **21**: S360.

14. Azevedo LL, Cardoso F, Reis C. Acoustic analysis of prosody in females with Parkinson's disease: comparison with normal controls. *Arq Neuropsiquiatr* 2003; **61**: 999–1003.

15. Teixeira AL Jr, Meira FC, Maia DP, Cunningham MC, Cardoso F. Migraine headache in patients with Sydenham's chorea. *Cephalalgia* 2005; **25**(7): 542–4.

16. Kwack C, Vuong KD, Jankovic J. Migraine headache in patients with Tourette syndrome. *Arch Neurol* 2003; **60**: 1595–8.

17. Swedo SE, Leonard HL, Garvey M *et al.* Pediatric autoimmune neuropsychiatric disorders associated with streptococcal infections: clinical description of the first 50 cases. *Am J Psychiatry* 1988; **155**: 264–71.

18. Asbahr FR, Negrao AB, Gentil V *et al.* Obsessive-compulsive and related symptoms in children and adolescents with rheumatic fever with and without chorea: a prospective 6-month study. *Am J Psychiatry* 1998; **155**: 1122–4.

19. Mercadante MT, Busatto GF, Lombroso PJ *et al.* The psychiatric symptoms of rheumatic fever. *Am J Psychiatry* 2000; **157**: 2036–8.

20. Maia DP, Teixeira AL Jr, Quintao Cunningham MC, Cardoso F. Obsessive compulsive behavior, hyperactivity, and attention deficit disorder in Sydenham chorea. *Neurology* 2005; **64**: 1799–801.

21. Asbahr FR, Garvey MA, Snider LA *et al.* Obsessive-compulsive symptoms among patients with Sydenham chorea. *Biol Psychiatry* 2005; **57**: 1073–6.

22. Hounie AG, Pauls DL, do Rosario-Campos MC *et al.* Obsessive-compulsive spectrum disorders and rheumatic fever: a family study. *Biol Psychiatry* 2007; **61**: 266–72.

23. Kummer A, Maia DP, Cardoso F, Teixeira, AL. Trichotillomania in acute Sydenham's chorea. *Aust NZ J Psychiatry* 2007; **41**: 1013–4.

24. Teixeira AL Jr, Maia DP, Cardoso F. Psychosis following acute Sydenham's chorea. *Eur Child Adolesc Psychiatry* 2007; **16**(1): 67–9.

25. Cardoso F, Dornas L, Cunningham M, Oliveira JT. Nerve conduction study in Sydenham's chorea. *Mov Disord* 205; **20**: 360–3.

26. Vijayalakshmi IB, Mithravinda J, Deva AN. The role of echocardiography in diagnosing carditis in the setting of acute rheumatic fever. *Cardiol Young* 2005; **15**: 583–8.

27. Panamonta M, Chaikitpinyo A, Auvichayapat N *et al.* Evolution of valve damage in Sydenham's chorea during recurrence of rheumatic fever. *Int J Cardiol* 2007; **119**(1): 73–9.

28. Guidelines for diagnosis of rheumatic fever, Jones criteria, 1992 update. Special Writing Group of the Committee of Rheumatic Fever, Endocarditis, and Kawasaki Disease of the Council on Cardio-Vascular Disease of the Young of the American Heart Association. Guidelines for the diagnosis of rheumatic fever. *JAMA* 1992; **268**: 2069–73.

29. Cardoso F, Vargas AP, Oliveira LD, Guerra AA, Amaral SV. Persistent Sydenham's chorea. *Mov Disord* 1999; **14**: 805–7.

30. Teixeira AL Jr, Maia DP, Cardoso F. UFMG Sydenham's chorea rating scale (USCRS): reliability and consistency. *Mov Disord* 2005; **20**: 585–91.

31. Giedd JN, Rapoport JL, Kruesi MJ *et al.* Sydenham's chorea: magnetic resonance imaging of the basal ganglia. *Neurology* 1995; **45**: 2199–202.

32. Goldman S, Amrom D, Szliwowski HB *et al.* Reversible striatal hypermetabolism in a case of Sydenham's chorea. *Mov Disord* 1993; **8**: 355–8.

33. Weindl A, Kuwert T, Leenders KL *et al.* Increased striatal glucose consumption in Sydenham's chorea. *Mov Disord* 1993; **8**: 437–44.

34. Lee PH, Nam HS, Lee KY, Lee BI, Lee JD. Serial brain SPECT images in a case of Sydenham chorea. *Arch Neurol* 1999; **56**: 237–40.

35. Barsottini OG, Ferraz HB, Seviliano MM, Barbieri A. Brain SPECT imaging in Sydenham's chorea. *Braz J Med Biol Res* 2002; **35**: 431–6.

36. Ho L. Hypermetabolism in bilateral basal ganglia in Sydenham chorea on F-18 FDG PET-CT. *Clin Nucl Med* 2009; **34**: 114–6.

37. Citak EC, Gukuyener K, Karabacak NI *et al.* Functional brain imaging in Sydenham's chorea and streptococcal tic disorders. *J Child Neurol* 2004; **19**: 387–90.

38. Taranta A, Stollerman GH. The relationship of Sydenham's chorea to infection with group A streptococci. *Am J Med* 1956; **20**: 1970.

39. Husby G, Van De Rijn U, Zabriskie JB, Abdin ZH, Williams RC Jr. Antibodies reacting with cytoplasm of subthalamic and caudate nuclei neurons in chorea and acute rheumatic fever. *J Exp Med* 1976; **144**: 1094–110.

40. Cardoso F. Chorea gravidarum. *Arch Neurol* 2002; **59**: 868–70.

41. Bronze MS, Dale JB. Epitopes of streptococcal M proteins that evoke antibodies that cross-react with human brain. *J Immunol* 1993; **151**: 2820–8.

42. Church AJ, Cardoso F, Dale RC *et al.* Anti-basal ganglia antibodies in acute and persistent Sydenham's chorea. *Neurology* 2002; **59**: 227–31.

43. Kirvan CA, Cox CJ, Swedo SE, Cunningham MW. Tubulin is a neuronal target of autoantibodies in Sydenham's chorea. *J Immunol* 2007; **178**: 7412–21.

44. Kirvan CA, Swedo SE, Heuser JS, Cunningham MW. Mimicry and autoantibody-mediated neuronal cell signaling in Sydenham chorea. *Nat Med* 2003; **9**: 914–20.

45. Teixeira AL Jr, Guimaraes MM, Romano-Silva MA, Cardoso F. Serum from Sydenham's chorea patients modifies intracellular calcium levels in PC12 cells by a complement-independent mechanism. *Mov Disord* 2005; **20**: 843–5.

46. Ayoub EM, Barrett DJ, Maclaren NK, Krischer JP. Association of class II human histocompatibility leukocyte antigens with rheumatic fever. *J Clin Invest* 1986; **77**: 2019–26.

47. Donadi EA, Smith AG, Louzada-Junior P, Voltarelli JC, Nepom GT. HLA class I and class II profiles of patients presenting with Sydenham's chorea. *J Neurol* 2000; **247**: 122–8.

48. Haydardedeoglu FE, Tutkak H, Kose K, Duzgun N. Genetic susceptibility to rheumatic heart disease and streptococcal pharyngitis: association with HLA-DR alleles. *Tissue Antigens* 2006; **68**: 293–6.

49. Feldman BM, Zabriskie JB, Silverman ED, Laxer RM. Diagnostic use of B-cell alloantigen D8/17 in rheumatic chorea. *J Pediatr* 1993; **123**: 84–6.

50. Eisen JL, Leonard HL, Swedo SE *et al.* The use of antibody D8/17 to identify B cells in adults with obsessive-compulsive disorder. *Psychiatry Res* 2001; **104**: 221–5.

51. Harel L, Zeharia A, Kodman Y *et al.* Presence of the d8/17 B-cell marker in children with rheumatic fever in Israel. *Clin Genet* 2002; **61**: 293–8.

52. Ramasawmy R, Fae KC, Spina G *et al.* Association of polymorphisms within the promoter region of the tumor necrosis factor-alpha with clinical outcomes of rheumatic fever. *Mol Immunol* 2007; **44**: 1873–8.

53. Church AJ, Dale RC, Cardoso F *et al.* CSF and serum immune parameters in Sydenham's chorea: evidence of an autoimmune syndrome? *J Neuroimmunol* 2003; **136**(1–2): 149–53.

54. Teixeira AL Jr, Cardoso F, Souza AL, Teixeira MM. Increased serum concentrations of monokine induced by interferon-gamma/CXCL9 and interferon-gamma-inducible protein 10/CXCL-10 in Sydenham's chorea patients. *J Neuroimmunol* 2004; **150**(1–2): 157–62.

55. Dale RC, Church AJ, Cardoso F *et al.* Poststreptococcal acute disseminated encephalomyelitis with basal ganglia involvement and auto-reactive antibasal ganglia antibodies. *Ann Neurol* 2001; **50**: 588–95.

56. Morshed SA, Parveen S, Leckman JF *et al.* Antibodies against neural, nuclear, cytoskeletal, and streptococcal epitopes in children and adults with Tourette's syndrome, Sydenham's chorea, and autoimmune disorders. *Biol Psychiatry* 2001; **50**: 566–77.

57. Cardoso F. Sydenham's chorea. *Curr Treat Options Neurol* 2008; **10**: 230–5.

58. Tumas V, Caldas CT, Santos AC, Nobre A, Fernandes RM. Sydenham's chorea: clinical observations from a Brazilian movement disorder clinic. *Parkinsonism Relat Disord* 2007; **13**: 276–83.

59. Korn-Lubetzki I, Brand A, Steiner I. Recurrence of Sydenham chorea: implications for pathogenesis. *Arch Neurol* 2004; **61**: 1261–4.

60. Teixeira AL, Cardoso F, Maia DP, Cunningham MC. Sydenham's chorea may be a risk factor for drug induced parkinsonism. *J Neurol Neurosurg Psychiatry* 2003; **74**: 1350–1.

61. Cardoso F, Maia D, Cunningham MC, Valenca G. Treatment of Sydenham chorea with corticosteroids. *Mov Disord* 2003; **18**: 1374–7.

62. Barash J, Margalith D, Matitiau A. Corticosteroid treatment in patients with Sydenham's chorea. *Pediatr Neurol* 2005; **32**: 205–7.

63. Paz JA, Silva CA, Marques-Dias MJ. Randomized double-blind study with prednisone in Sydenham's chorea. *Pediatr Neurol* 2006; **34**: 264–9.

64. Garvey MA, Snider LA, Leitman SF, Werden R, Swedo SE. Treatment of Sydenham's chorea with intravenous immunoglobulin, plasma exchange, or prednisone. *J Child Neurol* 2005; **20**: 424–9.

65. Quinn N, Schrag A. Huntington's disease and other choreas. *J Neurol* 1998; **245**: 709–16.

66. Asherson RA, Cervera R. The antiphospholipid syndrome: multiple faces beyond the classical presentation. *Autoimmun Rev* 2003; **2**: 140–51.

67. Avcin T, Benseler SM, Tyrrell PN, Cucnik S, Silverman ED. A followup study of antiphospholipid antibodies and associated neuropsychiatric manifestations in 137 children with systemic lupus erythematosus. *Arthritis Rheum* 2008; **59**: 206–13.

68. Krakauer M, Law I. FDG PET brain imaging in neuropsychiatric systemic lupus erythematosus with choreic symprtoms. *Clin Nucl Med* 2009; **34**: 122–3.

69. Grant R, Graus F. Paraneoplastic movement disorders. *Mov Disord* 2009; **24**: 1715–24.

70. Martinková J, Valkovic P, Benetin J. Paraneoplastic chorea associated with breast cancer. *Mov Disord* 2009; **24**: 2296–7.

71. Honnorat J, Cartalat-Carel S et al. Onco-neural antibodies and tumor type determine survival and neurological symptoms in paraneoplastic neurological syndromes with Hu or CV2/CRMP5 antibodies. *J Neurol Neurosurg Psychiatry* 2009; **80**: 412–6.

72. Lazurova I, Macejova Z, Benhatchi K et al. Efficacy of intravenous immunoglobulin treatment in lupus erythematosus chorea. *Clin Rheumatol* 2007; **26**: 2145–7.

73. Levine SR, Brey RL. Neurological aspects of antiphospholipid antibody syndrome. *Lupus* 1996; **5**: 347–53.

74. Min JH, Youn YC. Bilateral basal ganglia lesions of primary Sjogren syndrome presenting with generalized chorea. *Parkinsonism Relat Disord* 2009; **15**: 398–9.

75. Park SY, Kim HJ, Cho YJ, Cho JY, Hong KS. Recurrent hemichorea following a single infarction in the contralateral subthalamic nucleus. *Mov Disord* 2009; **24**: 617–8.

76. Ghika-Schmid F, Ghika J, Regli F, Bogousslavsky J. Hyperkinetic movement disorders during and after acute stroke: the Lausanne Stroke Registry. *J Neurol Sci* 1997; **146**: 109–16.

77. Cardoso F, Jankovic J, Grossman RG, Hamilton WJ. Outcome after stereotactic thalamotomy for dystonia and hemiballismus. *Neurosurgery* 1995; **36**: 501–7.

78. Choi SJ, Lee SW, Kim MC et al. Posteroventral pallidotomy in medically intractable postapoplectic monochorea: case report. *Surg Neurol* 2003; **59**: 486–90.

79. Gonzalez-Alegre P, Ammache Z, Davis PH, Rodnitzky RL. Moyamoya-induced paroxysmal dyskinesia. *Mov Disord* 2003; **18**: 1051–6.

80. Medlock MD, Cruse RS, Winek SJ et al. A 10-year experience with post-pump chorea. *Ann Neurol* 1993; **34**: 820–6.

81. Kumar H, Masiowski P, Jog M. Chorea in the elderly with mutation positive polycythemia vera: a case report. *Can J Neurol Sci* 2009; **36**: 370–2.

82. Wenning GK, Kiechl S, Seppi K et al. Prevalence of movement disorders in men and women aged 50–89 years (Bruneck Study cohort): a population-based study. *Lancet Neurol* 2005; **4**: 815–20.

83. Miranda M, Cardoso F, Giovannoni G, Church A. Oral contraceptive induced chorea: another condition associated with anti-basal ganglia antibodies. *J Neurol Neurosurg Psychiatry* 2004; **75**: 327–8.

84. Karageyim AY, Kars B, Dansuk R et al. Chorea gravidarum: a case report. *J Matern Fetal Neonatal Med* 2002; **12**: 353–4.

85. Fahn S. The spectrum of levodopa-induced dyskinesias. *Ann Neurol* 2000; **47**: S2–S9.

86. Stacy M, Cardoso F, Jankovic J. Tardive stereotypy and other movement disorders in tardive dyskinesias. *Neurology* 1993; **43**: 937–41.

87. Miller LG, Jankovic J. Neurologic approach to drug-induced movement disorders: a study of 125 patients. *South Med J* 1990; **83**: 525–32.

88. Fox GC, Ebeid S, Vincenti G. Paroxetine-induced chorea. *Br J Psychiatry* 1997; **170**: 193–4.

89. Bharucha KJ, Sethi KD. Complex movement disorders induced by fluoxetine. *Mov Disord* 1996; **11**: 324–6.

90. Harrison MB, Lyons GR, Landow ER. Phenytoin and dyskinesias: a report of two cases and review of the literature. *Mov Disord* 1993; **8**: 19–27.

91. Bimpong-Buta K, Froescher W. Carbamazepine-induced choreoathetoid dyskinesias. *J Neurol Neurosurg Psychiatry* 1982; **45**: 560.

92. Zaatreh M, Tennison M, D'Cruz O, Beach RL. Anticonvulsants-induced chorea: a role for pharmacodynamic drug interaction? *Seizure* 2001; **10**: 596–9.

93. Stork CM, Cantor R. Pemoline induced acute choreoathetosis: case report and review of the literature. *J Toxicol Clin Toxicol* 1997; **35**: 105–8.

94. Morgan JC, Winter WC, Wooten GF. Amphetamine-induced chorea in attention deficit-hyperactivity disorder. *Mov Disord* 2004; **19**: 840–2.

95. Necioğlu Orken D, Yldrmak Y, Kenangil G *et al.* Intrathecal methotrexate-induced acute chorea. *J Pediatr Hematol Oncol* 2009; **31**: 57–8.

96. Cardoso F. HIV-related movement disorders: epidemiology, pathogenesis and management. *CNS Drugs* 2002; **16**: 663–8.

97. Kalita J, Ranjan P, Misra UK, Das BK. Hemichorea: a rare presentation of tuberculoma. *J Neurol Sci* 2003; **208**: 109–11.

98. McKee D, Talbot P. Chorea as a presenting feature of variant Creutzfeldt-Jakob disease. *Mov Disord* 2003; **18**: 837–8.

99. Ozben S, Erol C, Ozer F, Tiras R. Chorea as the presenting feature of neurosyphilis. *Neurol India* 2009; **57**: 347–9.

100. Fernández Cooke E, Simón de Las Heras R, Muñoz González A, Allende Martinez L, Camacho Salas A. Choreoathetosis after Herpes simplex encephalitis. *An Pediatr (Barc.)* 2009; **71**: 153–6.

101. Jog MS, Lang AE. Chronic acquired hepatocerebral degeneration: case reports and new insights. *Mov Disord* 1995; **10**: 714–22.

102. Cherian A, Thomas B, Baheti NN, Chemmanam T, Kesavadas C. Concepts and controversies in nonketotic hyperglycemia-induced hemichorea: further evidence from susceptibility-weighted MR imaging. *J Magn Reson Imaging* 2009; **29**: 699–703.

103. Wang JH, Wu T, Deng BQ *et al.* Hemichorea-hemiballismus associated with nonketotic hyperglycemia: a possible role of inflammation. *J Neurol Sci* 2009; **284**: 198–202.

104. Chu K, Kang DW, Kim DE, Park SH, Roh JK. Diffusion-weighted and gradient echo magnetic resonance findings of hemichorea-hemiballismus associated with diabetic hyperglycemia: a hyperviscosity syndrome? *Arch Neurol* 2002; **59**: 448–52.

105. Lin JJ, Chang MK. Hemiballism-hemichorea and nonketotic hyperglycaemia. *J Neurol Neurosurg Psychiatry* 1994; **57**: 748–50.

106. Ristic AJ, Svetel M, Dragasevic N, Zarkovic M, Koprivsek K, Kostic VS. Bilateral chorea-ballism associated with hyperthyroidism. *Mov Disord* 2004; **19**: 982–3.

107. Yu JH, Weng YM. Acute chorea as a presentation of Graves disease: case report and review. *Am J Emerg Med* 2009; **27**: 369.e1–369.e3.

108. Poewe WH, Kleedorfer B, Willeit J, Gerstenbrand F. Primary CNS lymphoma presenting as a choreic movement disorder followed by segmental dystonia. *Mov Disord* 1988; **3**: 320–5.

109. Moore FG. Bilateral hemichorea-hemiballism caused by metastatic lung cancer. *Mov Disord* 2009; **24**: 1405–6.

110. Zacharia TT. Giant tumefactive perivascular spaces manifesting as chorea bilaterally. *J Neuroimaging* 2009 Nov 3. doi: 10.1111/j.1552-6569.2009.00448.x.

111. Alp R, Ilhan Alp S, Ure H. Two intracranial sewing needles in a young woman with hemi-chorea. *Parkinsonism Relat Disord* 2009; **15**: 795–6.

112. Ertan S, Uluduz D, Ozekmekçi S *et al.* Clinical characteristics of 49 patients with psychogenic movement disorders in a tertiary clinic in Turkey. *Mov Disord* 2009; **24**: 759–62.

113. Vidailhet M, Yelnik J, Lagrange C *et al.* Bilateral pallidal deep brain stimulation for the treatment of patients with dystonia-choreoathetosis cerebral palsy: a prospective pilot study. *Lancet Neurol* 2009; **8**: 709–17.

Chapter 26

Neuroacanthocytosis

Ruth H. Walker

History

The term neuroacanthocytosis (NA) refers to a group of syndromes in which nervous system abnormalities occur together with acanthocytosis, i.e., contracted and deformed erythrocytes that show spikelike protrusions (Figure 26.1). This description has been used to refer to a number of genetically distinct disorders, hence use of the term can be somewhat confusing and imprecise.

There are two broad groups of NA disorders. The present chapter refers to those in which there is neurodegeneration of the basal ganglia, resulting in the development of movement disorders, with prominent cognitive impairment and psychiatric features. The "core" NA syndromes can now be classified as autosomal recessive chorea-acanthocytosis (ChAc), due to mutation of *VPS13A* [1–3], and X-linked McLeod syndrome (MLS), due to mutation of the *XK* gene on the X chromosome [4]. Despite being caused by distinct genes, whose functions appear to be unrelated, these two disorders share a number of similarities, including central and peripheral nervous system manifestations, hepatosplenomegaly and acanthocytosis. This striking phenotypic overlap has resulted in confusion in the literature. In this chapter the two disorders are discussed together, with emphasis upon the distinctive features of each.

It could be argued that "chorea-acanthocytosis" is an inaccurate term as neither chorea nor acanthocytosis is a necessary or invariant feature of the disorder. However, we find this term preferable as it is now associated with a single genetically defined disorder, whereas "neuroacanthocytosis" has historically been a diagnostically imprecise term.

The second group of NA conditions is due to inherited disorders of lipoproteins, namely, abetalipoproteinemia (Bassen–Kornzweig syndrome) and hypobetalipoproteinemia, the hallmarks of which are

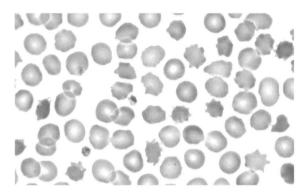

Figure 26.1. Acanthocytes in peripheral blood smear from a patient with McLeod syndrome. (Courtesy of Dr Hans H. Jung, Department of Neurology, University Hospital Zurich, Zurich, Switzerland.)

peripheral neuropathy and ataxia caused by dorsal column degeneration, due to vitamin E malabsorption. These patients do not have involuntary movements and cognitive impairment is not observed. Acanthocytosis in these patients is attributed to impaired lipid absorption from the gastrointestinal tract, which affects erythrocyte membrane composition.

The basal ganglia NA syndromes were first described in the 1960s and were known initially by the eponym "Levine–Critchley syndrome" [5–7]. The subjects reported by Critchley conform to the typical phenotype of autosomal recessive ChAc, and genetic studies of unaffected relatives from the family reported from eastern Kentucky support this diagnosis [8]. However, the inheritance pattern and clinical features of the family described by Levine do not fit so clearly with ChAc or X-linked recessive MLS inheritance, and genetic confirmation has not been possible for the subjects described in the initial reports or their descendants; hence the use of this eponym remains imprecise.

Uncommon Causes of Movement Disorders, ed. Néstor Gálvez-Jiménez and Paul J. Tuite. Published by Cambridge University Press. © Cambridge University Press 2011.

A series of 19 cases of NA was subsequently described [9], and was the definitive work on NA for many years. However, with the development of molecular methods, it has transpired that this is a heterogeneous series consisting of cases of ChAc, MLS and pantothenate kinase-associated neurodegeneration (PKAN) [10]. Reports of cases of NA in the literature without further diagnosis at the protein or molecular level should be interpreted as referring to either ChAc or MLS, although in some cases clinical information may indicate the specific disorder.

In addition, there are a small number of conditions in which acanthocytosis is seen in about 10% of cases, such as PKAN [11] and Huntington disease-like 2 (HDL2) [12] (Figure 26.2). Occasional rare cases or families are reported where acanthocytes are present in concert with other neurological features, such as paroxysmal dyskinesias [13] or mitochondrial disease [14].

All of these disorders are exceedingly rare but they are also very likely to be underdiagnosed. Estimates suggest that there are probably a few hundred cases of MLS and around one thousand ChAc cases worldwide. ChAc appears to be more prevalent in Japan, likely due to a genetic founder effect [2], and clusters have been found elsewhere in geographically isolated communities, e.g., French-Canadian [15,16]. PKAN and HDL2 are addressed in detail elsewhere in this volume and will not be considered further here.

Clinical findings

The protean neurological and psychiatric manifestations of the NA syndromes mean that the initial diagnosis can be obscure; however, with time, the full spectrum of disease manifests in the majority of patients [17–19]. In both ChAc and MLS, the co-occurrence of seizures and peripheral sensorimotor neuropathy and areflexia, along with the movement disorder, suggests the diagnosis.

The neurological features of ChAc develop in young adulthood, somewhat unusually for recessive disorders in which the protein product of the mutant gene is completely absent. McLeod syndrome presents during middle age, although subjects may be identified by laboratory evaluation, e.g., if they donate blood or undergo routine medical screening, prior to development of neurological abnormalities [17].

Psychiatric and cognitive features

The initial presentation in either ChAc or MLS may be subtle cognitive or psychiatric symptoms, and in retrospect patients may have developed related psychiatric complaints several years before the neurological manifestations. In ChAc these may present during adolescence [20]. Features of both disorders may include obsessive-compulsive behaviors, personality changes and self-neglect, depression, and psychosis. Administration of neuroleptics for psychiatric disease may confound the recognition that the subsequent movement disorder is due to a neurodegenerative process, in particular in ChAc, as orofacial or lingual dystonia may be ascribed to tardive dystonia.

Seizures

About 50% of patients develop seizures at some point in the disease course for both conditions. These typically originate in the temporal lobe [15]. In some cases, seizures may precede the appearance of movement disorders by as much as a decade [15,21].

Movement disorders

A variety of movement disorders can be seen in the NA syndromes, most typically chorea but also dystonia, parkinsonism and tics [17,19]. Prominent tics can suggest the diagnosis of Tourette syndrome [22]. Severe orofaciolingual dystonia with self-mutilating lip- and tongue-biting is typical of ChAc. Patients often place objects in the mouth such as sticks or cloth, which may function either as a mechanical obstruction to jaw closure or as a sensory trick to reduce dystonia. Dystonic protrusion of the tongue induced by eating is a pathognomic finding in ChAc that is often prominent and extremely disabling [23]. Other features of self-mutilation, such as finger-biting and head-scratching, suggest a behavioral compulsion as the etiology of these features rather than the movement disorder [24]. Orofacial dystonia and self-mutilation are not typical of MLS.

In both disorders severe, repetitive truncal flexion and extension can occur and can cause significant morbidity. The gait is often shambling as in Huntington disease, or may demonstrate bizarre-appearing knee-buckling with dystonic leg posturing.

Peripheral neuromuscular symptoms

Neuropathy and myopathy cause hypotonia and peripheral weakness and can be very debilitating feature, particularly in MLS. Myopathy was initially thought to be a relatively benign feature of MLS, but has recently been recognized as being a significant cause

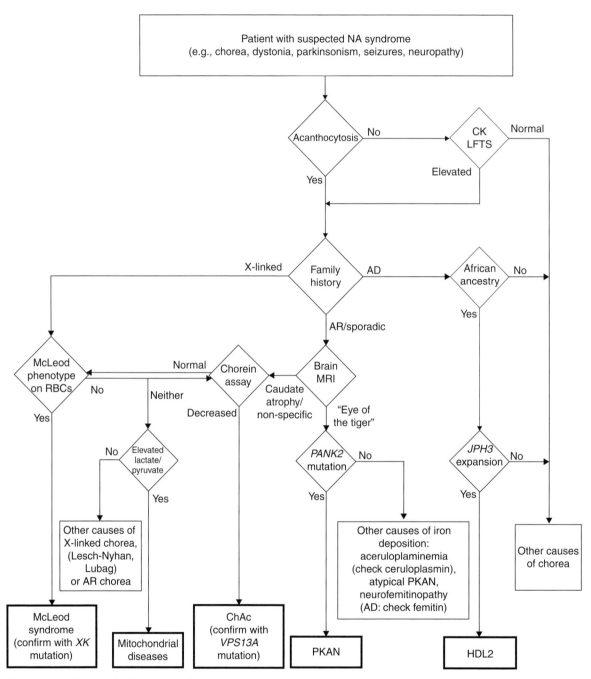

Figure 26.2. Flow chart for the diagnosis of NA syndromes. This diagram presents suggested guidelines for the diagnosis of NA but should not supersede clinical judgment. AR, autosomal recessive; AD, autosomal dominant; ChAc, chorea-acanthocytosis; CK, creatine kinase; HDL2, Huntington disease-like 2; LFTs, liver function tests; PKAN, pantothenate kinase-associated neurodegeneration, RBC, red blood cell. (Reproduced with permission from reference 18. © Wolters Kluwer Health 2007.)

of functional impairment [25]. It may predispose to rhabdomyolysis [26]. Deep tendon reflexes are absent in the majority of NA patients, along with peripheral sensory loss.

Nerve conduction studies in NA syndromes show axonal loss, although occasionally demyelination can be seen [9,27]. Electromyographic findings of myopathy may be seen at later stages.

Nonneurological features

Hepatosplenomegaly can be seen in both syndromes [17]. Fulminant hepatic failure has been reported but is unusual, and liver disease does not typically result in significant morbidity. Splenomegaly may be related to the mild hemolytic anemia that is typically found due to the acanthocytosis; there are no other appreciable effects of this hematological abnormality.

Cardiomyopathy is seen only in MLS, although without specific features on either clinical evaluation or pathological examination [28].

Natural history

Both NA syndromes show slow neurological deterioration over a few decades, with the progression of ChAc appearing to be somewhat faster than that of MLS. These disorders are progressive and eventually fatal. Sudden death may be due to seizure, autonomic dysfunction, or cardiac disease in MLS. Alternatively, there may be gradually progressive, generalized debility, as seen in other neurodegenerative conditions such Huntington or Parkinson diseases, with patients succumbing to aspiration pneumonia or other systemic infections.

Laboratory investigations

A standard procedure has been developed for acanthocyte determination on peripheral blood smear [29]. A negative screen does not exclude an NA syndrome, however [30]. Electron-microscopic examination of glutaraldehyde-fixed blood is helpful if it is available. The significance of acanthocytosis, the cause of variability over time, and its relationship to disease progression and neurological manifestations are not at present understood.

In both MLS and ChAc, muscle creatine kinase (CK) and liver enzymes are elevated in serum, and may be more informative as diagnostic markers than peripheral blood smear. Both MLS and ChAc may be detected incidentally presymptomatically by the elevation of CK or liver enzymes [17]. Recognition of the neurological syndrome may avoid the need for invasive and nondiagnostic tests such as muscle, bone marrow, or liver biopsy.

Chorea-acanthocytosis

ChAc can be definitively diagnosed by demonstrating the absence of chorein, the protein product of the mutant gene, in peripheral blood by western blot [31]. Analysis of the VPS13A gene is challenging and time-consuming due to the large gene size and heterogeneity of mutation sites [1–3], and availability of this test is limited to a small number of research laboratories.

McLeod syndrome

McLeod syndrome was named after the Harvard dental student Hugh McLeod, in whom the abnormal erythrocyte antigen pattern was first described in the 1960s, following screening of new students at Harvard for novel blood antigens [32]. This antigen pattern is referred to as "McLeod phenotype," and was initially thought to be of no clinical significance, apart from the requirement for matched blood transfusions. The delay in recognition of the association with neurological abnormalities ("McLeod syndrome") is likely to have been due, in part, to the interval of several decades before individuals found to have this erythrocyte phenotype develop neurological abnormalities. Dr. McLeod left his body for medical research and his tissues have been incorporated into recent studies [25].

The diagnostic procedure of choice in MLS is phenotyping of Kx and Kell blood group antigens. A panel of Kell antibodies is required to confirm or refute the diagnosis of MLS, and this testing is usually available in regional blood centers. The typical finding is absent Kx and depressed expression of all Kell antigens. This must not be confused with a finding of "Kell negative," which does not rule out the diagnosis of MLS [33]. Molecular genetic diagnosis is available on a research basis only.

Neuroimaging

Neuroimaging demonstrates bilateral atrophy of the caudate nuclei that corresponds with disease progression and may be reported as being similar to that seen in Huntington disease. Voxel-based morphometry of MRI scans in ChAc shows specific involvement of the head of the caudate nucleus [20,34].

Genetics

The genes responsible for the NA syndromes have been identified, but the molecular pathophysiology is not known for either MLS or ChAc.

Chorea-acanthocytosis

Chorea-acanthocytosis is an autosomal recessive disorder caused by mutations of VPS13A located at 9q21.

This is a large gene, consisting of 73 exons, and has been identified as a member of the VPS13 family involved in vacuolar protein sorting [1–3]. A wide variety of mutations have been found, including both large and small deletions, insertions, nonsense and missense mutations. There is no particularly vulnerable portion of the gene, making screening for mutations challenging. All mutations to date appear to result in absence of chorein, thus there do not appear to be any partial manifestations of the disease, e.g., with partially functional chorein. Heterozygous carriers do not appear to be affected, although this has been debated [35]. Homozygosity for mutations is relatively uncommon, except in isolated communities where consanguinity is probable. No clear phenotype–genotype correlation has been identified, with siblings showing significant phenotypic heterogeneity [18].

The protein product, chorein, is widely expressed throughout the brain and various internal organs [36]. Its function is not known, but it may be involved in protein sorting and membrane structure. Absence of chorein in ChAc appears to have critical effects only in brain, peripheral nerve and muscle, with lesser effects upon liver and spleen.

McLeod syndrome

The McLeod protein, XK, is located in the cell membrane and probably has transport functions. In erythrocytes it is linked to the Kell protein via two disulfide bonds [32,33]. This complex carries the antigens of the Kell blood group, the third most important blood group system in humans. The Kx antigen (expressed by XK) is absent in McLeod syndrome and expression of other 23 Kell system antigens (on the Kell protein) is severely depressed [32,33]. Since Kell protein is involved in enzymatic cleavage of endothelins, it is conceivable that these molecules are transported by XK; however, Kell is not present in brain, as XK is [37,38].

Occasional patients have been identified who have minimal neurological abnormalities, despite the presence of the typical erythrocyte phenotype [39]. This is likely to be due to the mutant McLeod protein being partially functional but having a conformational change that impairs protein migration to the cell surface. Apart from this observation, there is no clear phenotype–genotype correlation, and siblings tend to show phenotypic heterogeneity [40].

The locus of the gene was first identified due to its proximity to the gene for chronic granulomatous disease, a disorder characterized by immune compromise and vulnerability to infections. Some boys with this disorder have large deletions involving both genes; as improved control of infections results in increased survival into adulthood, they are liable to develop MLS.

Although the majority of MLS subjects are male, occasionally female mutation carriers may develop mild symptoms, probably due to X chromosome inactivation [9,41].

Pathology

Neurodegeneration in both core NA syndromes affects predominantly the caudate nuclei, putamen and globus pallidus [9,36,42–46]. Neuropathological findings consist of gliosis of these regions, but no inclusion bodies of any nature have been detected despite examination with antibodies against a number of protein markers of neurodegeneration. In ChAc the thalamus [42,43] and substantia nigra [9] are additionally involved. The nigral involvement most likely accounts for the clinical findings of parkinsonism.

In both conditions neuropathological findings in the cortex are minimal. In MLS very mild gliosis is reported [46]. In ChAc no significant abnormalities are reported on pathological examination [36]; however, mesial temporal atrophy has been found on neuroimaging of patients with temporal lobe seizures [21].

Management

So far no curative treatment is known for these disorders and management is purely symptomatic. In both MLS and ChAc, seizures and psychiatric manifestations should be managed according to established principles. As in Huntington disease, treatment of neuropsychiatric issues, particularly depression, can have a major impact upon quality of life, and these symptoms may be more amenable to pharmacotherapy than others.

Medical management

In some patients, peripheral neuromuscular abnormalities can be more debilitating than trunk or limb chorea. If necessary, chorea can be reduced by decreasing dopaminergic function using atypical antipsychotic agents (such as tiapride, clozapine, quetiapine) or dopamine-depleting agents such as tetrabenazine. Tics may respond to levetiracetam. Parkinsonism is not reported to respond to levodopa, although it is probably worth a therapeutic trial.

Dystonic tongue protrusion during eating in ChAc may be treated with local botulinum toxin injections into the genioglossus muscle [47].

Seizures usually respond to standard anticonvulsants, including phenytoin, clobazam, and valproate, although lamotrigine and carbamazepine may worsen the involuntary movements [15]. Anticonvulsants may have the benefit of multiple parallel effects upon involuntary movements, psychiatric symptoms, peripheral neuropathic paraesthesias and seizures.

In MLS, transfusion with Kell+ blood may result in the generation of anti-Kell antibodies by the patient, and subsequent Kell+ transfusions will be hemolysed (as with the rhesus reaction in rhesus-negative neonates). Blood transfusion problems should be anticipated and banking of the patient's own blood for autologous transfusion is recommended.

Cardiac complications should be considered in MLS and heart function should be monitored regularly. Annual monitoring by echocardiography and appropriate therapy may reduce mortality due to cardiac factors.

Paramedical management

As with many of the choreas and other basal ganglia disorders, weight loss is often a significant problem. Patients with ChAc in particular should undergo periodic evaluation of speech and swallowing by a speech therapist in order to minimize problems due to dysphagia and weight loss. Bite guards can be helpful in reducing the jaw closure dystonia, and have been reported to reduce obsessive-compulsive symptoms, suggesting a common pathophysiology [48]. Dysarthria can become severe and may require the use of assistive communication devices.

Physical and occupational therapists can assist with difficulties with gait, balance and activities of daily living. Ideally, a multidisciplinary team approach should be employed to identify realistic goals of therapy and to optimize patient function despite progression of neurodegeneration [47].

Neurosurgical interventions

Results of deep brain stimulation have been variable, and the optimal site and stimulation parameters remain to be determined. Lesioning may be beneficial if long-term hardware management is likely to be problematic. In general neurosurgical options should be considered experimental and tailored to individual cases. Results of surgical therapy in ChAc [49,50] and

MLS [51] have been mixed, and the optimal target is not yet clear. Benefits have been observed with stimulation of both the posterior ventral oral (Vop) thalamus [49,51] and globus pallidus interna (GPi) [51]. Thalamic stimulation in one ChAc patient resulted in a dramatic and sustained reduction in truncal spasms, but no clear effect upon dysarthria or on hypotonia [51]. High-frequency stimulation (130 Hz) of the GPi worsened speech and chorea but improved dystonia, belching, dyskinetic breathing and tongue-biting [51]. Low-frequency stimulation (40 Hz) improved chorea but not dystonia.

Conclusions

Identification of the causative genes for the NA syndromes has resulted in recognition of the molecular heterogeneity of this group of neurodegenerative disorders, and has facilitated genetic counseling for affected families.

Much remains to be learned regarding the molecular mechanisms that cause neurodegeneration in these conditions. The similarities in central and peripheral nervous system pathology and nonneurological manifestations between MLS and ChAc are striking and suggest a final common pathological pathway. The relationship between the acanthocytosis and neurodegeneration is obscure. We hypothesize that impaired membrane synthesis and maintenance may be a common cause, and may ultimately be related to the etiology of the neurodegeneration. We anticipate that elucidation of molecular pathophysiology will ultimately lead to prevention and reversal of disease at the cellular level.

Acknowledgment

The Advocacy for Neuroacanthocytosis Patients (www.naadvocacy.org) supported much of the work summarized here and development and performance of the chorein Western blot test.

References

1. Rampoldi L, Dobson-Stone C, Rubio JP et al. A conserved sorting-associated protein is mutant in chorea-acanthocytosis. Nat Genet 2001; 28: 119–20.

2. Ueno S, Maruki Y, Nakamura M et al. The gene encoding a newly discovered protein, chorein, is mutated in chorea-acanthocytosis. Nat Genet 2001; 28: 121–2.

3. Dobson-Stone C, Danek A, Rampoldi L et al. Mutational spectrum of the CHAC gene in patients with chorea-acanthocytosis. Eur J Hum Genet 2002; 10: 773–81.

4. Ho M, Chelly J, Carter N *et al.* Isolation of the gene for McLeod syndrome that encodes a novel membrane transport protein. *Cell* 1994; **77**: 869–80.

5. Levine IM. An hereditary neurologic disease with acanthocytosis. *Neurology* 1964; **14**: 272.

6. Critchley EM, Clark DB, Wikler A. Acanthocytosis and neurological disorder without betalipoproteinemia. *Arch Neurol* 1968; **18**: 134–40.

7. Critchley EM, Nicholson JT, Betts JJ *et al.* Acanthocytosis, normolipoproteinaemia and multiple tics. *Postgrad Med J* 1970; **46**: 698–701.

8. Velayos-Baeza A, Holinski-Feder E, Nietzel B. Chorea-acanthocytosis genotype in Critchley's original Kentucky neuroacanthocytosis kindred. *Arch Neurol* in press.

9. Hardie RJ, Pullon HW, Harding AE *et al.* Neuroacanthocytosis. A clinical, haematological and pathological study of 19 cases. *Brain* 1991; **114**: 13–49.

10. Gandhi S, Hardie RJ, Lees AJ. An update on the Hardie neuroacanthocytosis series. In: Walker RH, Saiki S, Danek A, eds. *Neuroacanthocytosis Syndromes II.* Berlin, Heidelberg: Springer-Verlag; 2008: 43–51.

11. Hayflick SJ, Westaway SK, Levinson B *et al.* Genetic, clinical, and radiographic delineation of Hallervorden–Spatz syndrome. *N Engl J Med* 2003; **348**: 33–40.

12. Walker RH, Rasmussen A, Rudnicki D *et al.* Huntington's disease-like 2 can present as chorea-acanthocytosis. *Neurology* 2003; **61**: 1002–4.

13. Tschopp L, Raina G, Salazar Z *et al.* Neuroacanthocytosis and carbamazepine responsive paroxysmal dyskinesias. *Parkinsonism Relat Disord* 2008; **14**: 440–2.

14. Mukoyama M, Kazui H, Sunohara N *et al.* Mitochondrial myopathy, encephalopathy, lactic acidosis, and stroke-like episodes with acanthocytosis: a clinicopathological study of a unique case. *J Neurol* 1986; **233**: 228–32.

15. Al-Asmi A, Jansen AC, Badhwar A *et al.* Familial temporal lobe epilepsy as a presenting feature of choreoacanthocytosis. *Epilepsia* 2005; **46**: 1256–63.

16. Dobson-Stone C, Velayos-Baeza A, Jansen A *et al.* Identification of a *VPS13A* founder mutation in French Canadian families with chorea-acanthocytosis. *Neurogenetics* 2005; **6**: 151–8.

17. Rampoldi L, Danek A, Monaco AP. Clinical features and molecular bases of neuroacanthocytosis. *J Mol Med* 2002; **80**: 475–91.

18. Lossos A, Dobson-Stone C, Monaco AP *et al.* Early clinical heterogeneity in choreoacanthocytosis. *Arch Neurol* 2005; **62**: 611–14.

19. Walker RH, Jung HH, Dobson-Stone C *et al.* Neurologic phenotypes associated with acanthocytosis. *Neurology* 2007; **68**: 92–8.

20. Walterfang M, Yucel M, Walker R *et al.* Adolescent obsessive compulsive disorder heralding chorea-acanthocytosis. *Mov Disord* 2008; **23**: 422–5.

21. Scheid R, Bader B, Ott DV *et al.* Development of mesial temporal lobe epilepsy in chorea-acanthocytosis. *Neurology* 2009; **73**: 1419–22.

22. Saiki S, Hirose G, Sakai K *et al.* Chorea-acanthocytosis associated with Tourettism. *Mov Disord* 2004; **19**: 833–6.

23. Bader B, Walker RH, Vogel M *et al.* Tongue protrusion and feeding dystonia: a hallmark of chorea-acanthocytosis. *Mov Disord* 2010; **25**(1): 127–9.

24. Walker RH, Liu Q, Ichiba M *et al.* Self-mutilation in chorea-acanthocytosis: manifestation of movement disorder or psychopathology? *Mov Disord* 2006; **21**: 2268–9.

25. Hewer E, Danek A, Schoser BG *et al.* McLeod myopathy revisited: more neurogenic and less benign. *Brain* 2007; **130**: 3285–96.

26. Jung HH, Brandner S. Malignant McLeod myopathy. *Muscle Nerve* 2002; **26**: 424–7.

27. Danek A, Rubio JP, Rampoldi L *et al.* McLeod neuroacanthocytosis: genotype and phenotype. *Ann Neurol* 2001; **50**: 755–64.

28. Oechslin E, Kaup D, Jenni R *et al.* Cardiac abnormalities in McLeod syndrome. *Int J Cardiol* 2009; **132**: 130–2.

29. Storch A, Kornhass M, Schwarz J. Testing for acanthocytosis: a prospective reader-blinded study in movement disorder patients. *J Neurol* 2005; **252**: 84–90.

30. Sorrentino G, De Renzo A, Miniello S *et al.* Late appearance of acanthocytes during the course of chorea-acanthocytosis. *J Neurol Sci* 1999; **163**: 175–8.

31. Dobson-Stone C, Velayos-Baeza A, Filippone LA *et al.* Chorein detection for the diagnosis of chorea-acanthocytosis. *Ann Neurol* 2004; **56**: 299–302.

32. Allen FH, Krabbe SM, Corcoran PA. A new phenotype (McLeod) in the Kell blood-group system. *Vox Sang* 1961; **6**: 555–60.

33. Redman CM, Russo D, Lee S. Kell, Kx and the McLeod syndrome. *Baillières Best Pract Res Clin Haematol* 1999; **12**: 621–35.

34. Henkel K, Danek A, Grafman J *et al.* Head of the caudate nucleus is most vulnerable in chorea-acanthocytosis: a voxel-based morphometry study. *Mov Disord* 2006; **21**: 1728–31.

35. Saiki S, Sakai K, Kitagawa Y *et al.* Mutation in the *CHAC* gene in a family of autosomal dominant chorea-acanthocytosis. *Neurology* 2003; **61**: 1614–16.

36. Bader B, Arzberger T, Heinsen H *et al.* Neuropathology of chorea-acanthocytosis. In: Walker RH, Saiki S, Danek A, eds. *Neuroacanthocytosis Syndromes II.* Berlin, Heidelberg: Springer-Verlag; 2008: 187–95.

37. Lee S, Sha Q, Wu X *et al.* Expression Profiles of Mouse Kell, XK, and XPLAC mRNA. *J Histochem Cytochem* 2007; **55**: 365–74.

38. Claperon A, Hattab C, Armand V *et al.* The Kell and XK proteins of the Kell blood group are not co-expressed in the central nervous system. *Brain Res* 2007; **1147**: 12–24.

39. Walker RH, Danek A, Uttner I *et al.* McLeod phenotype without the McLeod syndrome. *Transfusion* 2006; **47**: 299–305.

40. Walker RH, Jung HH, Tison F *et al.* Phenotypic variation among brothers with the McLeod neuroacanthocytosis syndrome. *Mov Disord* 2007; **22**: 244–8.

41. Jung HH, Hergersberg M, Kneifel S *et al.* McLeod syndrome: a novel mutation, predominant psychiatric manifestations, and distinct striatal imaging findings. *Ann Neurol* 2001; **49**: 384–92.

42. Alonso ME, Teixeira F, Jimenez G *et al.* Chorea-acanthocytosis: report of a family and neuropathological study of two cases. *Can J Neurol Sci* 1989; **16**: 426–31.

43. Vital A, Bouillot S, Burbaud P *et al.* Chorea-acanthocytosis: neuropathology of brain and peripheral nerve. *Clin Neuropathol* 2002; **21**: 77–81.

44. Brin MF, Hays A, Symmans WA *et al.* Neuropathology of McLeod phenotype is like chorea-acanthocytosis (CA). *Can J Neurol Sci* 1993; **20**(Suppl 4): 234.

45. Rinne JO, Daniel SE, Scaravilli F *et al.* Nigral degeneration in neuroacanthocytosis. *Neurology* 1994; **44**: 1629–32.

46. Geser F, Tolnay M, Jung HH. The Neuropathology of McLeod Syndrome. In: Walker RH, Saiki S, Danek A, eds. *Neuroacanthocytosis Syndromes II.* Berlin, Heidelberg: Springer-Verlag; 2008: 197–203.

47. McIntosh J. Multidisciplinary neurorehabilitation in chorea-acanthocytosis; A case study. In: Walker RH, Saiki S, Danek A, editors. Neuroacanthocytosis Syndromes II. Berlin Heidelberg, Germany, Springer-Verlag. 2008; 271–284.

48. Fontenelle LF, Leite MA. Treatment-resistant self-mutilation, tics, and obsessive-compulsive disorder in neuroacanthocytosis: a mouth guard as a therapeutic approach. *J Clin Psychiatry* 2008; **69**: 1186–7.

49. Burbaud P, Rougier A, Ferrer X *et al.* Improvement of severe trunk spasms by bilateral high-frequency stimulation of the motor thalamus in a patient with chorea-acanthocytosis. *Mov Disord* 2002; **17**: 204–7.

50. Wihl G, Volkmann J, Allert N *et al.* Deep brain stimulation of the internal pallidum did not improve chorea in a patient with neuro-acanthocytosis. *Mov Disord* 2001; **16**: 572–5.

51. Burbaud P. Deep brain stimulation in neuroacanthocytosis. *Mov Disord* 2005; **20**: 1681–2.

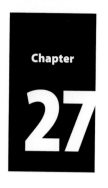

Chapter

27

The boundaries between epilepsy and movement disorders

Eissa Ibrahim Al Eissa and Selim R. Benbadis

Introduction

In this chapter we will cover conditions that are at the border zone between movement disorders and epilepsy. Many of these are at times difficult to diagnose as epileptic or movement disorders, and include myoclonus, epilepsia partialis continua, paroxysmal nonepileptic movement disorders, and sleep-related movement disorders or epilepsies. We will also cover psychogenic disorders, facial movements and abnormal movements in the ICU setting.

Myoclonus

Myoclonus comprises sudden, brief shocklike involuntary movements caused by contractions or inhibition of muscles that are irregular in rhythm and amplitude. It is a descriptive term, not a diagnosis on its own. These jerks typically last 10–50 ms, and rarely longer than 100 ms. They typically consist of a contraction and produce positive myoclonus, but they can also be inhibitory and produce negative myoclonus [1].

The main classification of myoclonus is between epileptic or nonepileptic. Epileptic myoclonus is by definition cortical. Nonepileptic myoclonus can be seen in metabolic abnormalities and diseases of the brainstem or spinal cord. Since myoclonus is often associated with abnormalities in inhibitory transmission, antiepileptic drugs as are often used for both epileptic and nonepileptic myoclonus [2].

Myoclonus can also be subdivided into myoclonus simplex or myoclonus multiplex. *Myoclonus simplex* (also called segmental myoclonus) describes muscular contractions that occur singly or repeatedly in a restricted group of muscles in the leg or arm. *Myoclonus multiplex* (also called term polymyoclonus) describes widespread, lightning-like arrhythmic contractions.

Nonepileptic myoclonus

Hypnogogic myoclonic jerks (sleep starts) are considered normal (physiologic) sleep-related phenomena, and consist of brief contractions of groups of muscles in one limb or the whole body. They occur at sleep transition. Visual hallucinations, dreams, or a sensation of falling are common. Fatigue, anxiety, sleep deprivation and high intake of caffeine are precipitating factors [3]. These common hypnic jerks have a prevalence of 70%, affecting both sexes equally with adults being more affected [4].

Fragmentary hypnic myoclonus comprises repetitive brief twitches occurring asynchronously and asymmetrically affecting any part of the body. They are minor movements of the fingers and toes or twitching of the corners of the mouth. They persist in all stages of sleep. Males are mostly affected and the condition is usually associated with other sleep disorders such as periodic leg movements, narcolepsy and intermittent hypersomnia [3,5].

Epileptic myoclonus

Epileptic myoclonic jerks (myoclonic seizures) are associated transient (less than 100 ms) abnormal excessive or synchronous neuronal activity in the brain resulting in involuntary single or multiple muscular jerks. By definition, EEG shows a spike or polyspike discharge associated with the jerk.

Idiopathic generalized epilepsies, including and especially juvenile myoclonic epilepsy (JME), include myoclonic seizures together with generalized tonic-clonic seizures and typical absence seizures. These epilepsies are genetically determined and typically patients are completely normal other than the seizures. Ictal EEG (during a jerk) typically shows a generalized polyspike. Eyelid myoclonias consists of jerks of the

---

Uncommon Causes of Movement Disorders, ed. Néstor Gálvez-Jiménez and Paul J. Tuite. Published by Cambridge University Press. © Cambridge University Press 2011.

muscles around the eye, and are particularly common with some absence seizures ("eyelid fluttering"). They are also a prominent part of *Jeavons syndrome*, which is characterized by eyelid myoclonia with and without absences, and sensitivity to light and eye closure.

Progressive myoclonus epilepsies are a group of symptomatic generalized epilepsies in which myoclonic seizures are prominent and associated with other neurologic symptoms and signs (dementia, ataxia, etc.). Causes include myoclonic epilepsy with ragged red fibers (MERFF), Lafora body disease, Unverricht–Lundborg disease and ceroid lipofuscinosis, as well as cherry-red spot myoclonus syndrome.

Unclear as to epileptic or not

It should be noted that the epileptic or nonepileptic nature of myoclonus can be difficult to ascertain due to some limitations of surface EEG. Thus, many common conditions inconsistently show a cortical EEG discharge associated with the myoclonic jerks. For this reason, the nature (myoclonic) is best ascertained with good video recordings simultaneously with EEG.

Many myoclonic jerks (cortical or not) occur in systemic encephalopathies. Anoxic encephalopathy is probably the most common cause of symptomatic cortical myoclonus [6]. Other metabolic causes include hepatic encephalopathy and uremic encephalopathy. Creutzfeldt–Jakob disease is characterized by myoclonic jerks early on, but many other degenerative disease can include myoclonus late in the course (Wilson disease, Alzheimer disease, Lewy body dementia, and corticobasal ganglionic degeneration). Other possible causes include viral encephalitis, AIDS dementia, Whipple disease and tetanus. Drug toxicity can also cause myoclonus, including haloperidol, lithium and cyclosporin overdose.

Epilepsia partialis continua

Epilepsia partialis continua (EPC) refers to partial motor status epilepticus, i.e., continuous focal jerking of a body part, usually localized to a distal limb or face due to their large homunculus representation, occurring over hours, days or even longer [7]. EPC is usually symptomatic and causes include cortical dysplasia, tumor, focal infectious, vascular lesions and Rasmussen syndrome [8]. EEG abnormalities can show focal discrete spikes, sharp waves or just slow activity, or periodic lateralized epileptiform discharges (PLEDs). In the same study [8], it was found that interictal EEG was abnormal in 80% of the patients. Ictal EEG was recorded in 11 patients and was abnormal in 9 (82%) of them [8]. While two-thirds of patients have EEG abnormalities that correlate with the jerks [3], ictal EEG is quite frequently normal, as is the case in all "simple partial" seizures. Therefore, again, the diagnosis should not be rejected on the basis of normal ictal EEG, and video recordings are most useful. When the EEG is normal, diagnostic dilemmas include psychogenic attacks and organic movement disorders. For example, hemifacial spasm (HFS) can be difficult to distinguish from EPC as both involve unilateral, irregular twitching of facial muscles. However, HFS tends to affect the upper face (blepharospasm), whereas focal seizures affect the perioral area (homunculus). EPC can be very refractory to treatment, and since it is relatively focal and limited, should not be treated too aggressively.

Facial movements

Abnormal movements of the face can be difficult to diagnose. Possible diagnoses include "simple partial" motor seizures, psychogenic movements, and organic movement disorders such as hemifacial spasms, tics or myokemia.

In *simple partial motor seizures*, consciousness is retained. In general, focal motor seizures can be clonic, tonic, or versive. The majority of the focal motor seizures are those affecting the face and fingers, because these parts of the body have larger cortical representation. Clonic motor seizures of the face consist of rhythmic abrupt "unnatural" jerks, comparable to the type elicited with electrical cortical stimulation. This is difficult to describe in words but is easy to recognize on video recordings. Since EEG is frequently normal in such "simple partial" seizures, the entire diagnosis often relies on the clinical (live or video) observation.

Hemifacial spasm, usually lasting longer than clonic seizures, eventually causes sustained prolonged muscular tonic contraction.

Tics are sporadic, repetitive movements of skeletal muscles (motor tics), respiratory, nasopharyngeal, or laryngeal muscles as in phonatory tics. They are stereotyped but voluntary, following an irresistible urge to move, and are suppressible for some time. Tics are particularly common between ages 5 and 10 years [9]. The ability of the patient to temporally control their tics is a useful diagnostic feature. They do not evolve (unlike seizures) and disappear in sleep.

Paroxysmal (nonepileptic) movements disorders

Paroxysmal spasmodic torticollis occurs in attacks that last for hours or days (much longer than seizures), caused by sustained tonic contraction of the neck muscles. Consciousness is preserved.

Stereotypies, complex tics, mannerisms and self stimulatory behavior can be seen especially in developmentally delayed individuals. They last seconds at a time and are repetitive. Examples are hand clapping, truncal rocking, hand twirling, complex hand-to-mouth routines such as feeding, blowing and touching. While the complex motor tic is performed in response to an inner urge, stereotypy is most commonly seen in Rett syndrome, autism, or Asperger syndrome. Self-stimulating behaviors begin early in childhood and affect girls more than boys. Attacks involve behavior such as the patient crossing her legs and forcing her groin against the furniture.

The movements of *paroxysmal dyskinesia* were in the past considered movement-induced seizures because these are involuntary movements and showed good response to antiepileptic drugs. These attacks are tonic, often twisting contraction, chorea, athetosis or ballistic without loss of conscious. Some patients describe bizarre sensations such as numbness, burning, feeling of stiffness, crawling sensation, or vibratory sensation before appearance of the attacks. These attacks are usually aborted by sleep or by lying flat. One side of the body is usually involved, but sometimes the movements can be bilateral. In all these types of dyskinesias, alteration of the level of consciousness never occurs. Demirkiran and Jankovic label these movements as *paroxysmal kinesiogenic dyskinesia*.

These dyskinetic movements can be triggered by sudden movement, so-called *paroxysmal kinesiogenic dyskinesia* (PKD). *Paroxysmal nonkinesiogenic dyskinesia* (PNKD) is not triggered by movement, but alcohol, coffee, tea and psychological stress are known precipitating factors. Attacks that are triggered by prolonged exercise are termed *paroxysmal exertional dyskinesia*.

Attacks of PKD differ from PNKD in triggering factors and duration; in PKD the attacks are usually brief and last for seconds up to 5 minutes. In PNKD the duration range from 5 minutes to 4 hours, and sometimes attacks can last longer than a day. In paroxysmal exertional dyskinesia the duration of attacks is typically from 5 to 30 minutes.

These dyskinetic movements can occur during sleep, when they are labeled *hypnogenic paroxysmal dyskinesia*. The condition is familial, and attacks can occur in the day time, triggered by sudden movement. Attacks start in early childhood and with time will disappear, occurring during sleep and leaving the child with kinesigenic dyskinesia that shows good response to antiepileptic drugs. The explanation for the good response to antiepileptic drugs is that these movement disorders are mostly channelopathies [10].

Hyperekplexia is a disorder of exaggerated startle reaction to sudden visual, auditory, or propriocptive stimuli. This exaggerated reflex results in sustained tonic contractions. It can be either an inherited disorder caused by a mutation in α1 subunit of the inhibitory glycine receptor or secondary to cortical lesion. EEG shows no epileptiform changes and during the attacks is obscured by muscular artifacts.

Abnormal postures: In focal tonic seizures, different postures can be assumed resulting from sustained contraction of the limb. The *M2e posture* described by Ajmone-Marsan is seen in seizures arising from the supplementary motor area (SMA). It consists of abduction, elevation and external rotation of the contralateral limb with flexed elbow. In versive seizures tonic contraction of the head and eye muscles results in sustained forceful deviation to one side.

Hereditary geniospasm is an unusual movement disorder that causes episodes of involuntary tremor of the chin and the lower lip. Episodes start in early life and genetic factor is noted. Stress is found to be the most precipitating factor.

Nocturnal episodes: seizures vs. parasomnias vs. paroxysmal movements disorders

Non-REM arousal disorders

Non-REM arousal disorders are disorders of partial arousal, i.e., sleepwalking, sleep terrors and confusional arousal. The non-REM parasomnias are most common between ages 4 and 12 years, and night terrors are particularly common. They are often familial, and are worsened by stress, sleep deprivation and intercurrent illnesses [9].

REM sleep behavior disorder

First described by Schenck and colleagues over 20 years ago [11], this disorder typically affects older men. The episodes arise out of REM sleep and consist of violent motor behaviors (acting out the dreams), such as punching, kicking or hitting. Thus, the episodes can resemble frontal lobe seizures. The diagnosis is usually not difficult, but will occasionally require EEG-video monitoring.

Sleep-related movement disorders

Rhythmic movement disorder (RMD) is described in children below 5 years of age. The affected children rhythmically bang their head against the pillow or rock from one side to another every second for a few minutes. It is easy to differentiate it from epilepsy that these movements are voluntary and can usually be stopped on request (similarly to tics).

Sleep bruxism is a sleep related nonepileptic behavioral disorder that occurs at any stage of sleep but mostly in stage II. Featuring teeth grinding and clenching, it may occur in the day time. Other features such as abnormal wear of the teeth, temporomandibular joint discomfort and masseter muscle hypertrophy are found. Bruxism is of unknown etiology and anxiety is considered a precipitating factor. It is common in children, especially those with learning disabilities and psychiatric disorders [4].

Nocturnal epileptic seizures

Nocturnal epileptic seizures are most typically frontal lobe seizures. The following features can help distinguish them from sleep disorders [12]: duration is brief, often less than 1 minute; they occur in repetitive clusters and are stereotyped; and they typically arise from stage II sleep. Motor activity in nonepileptic events is complex and sustained.

Nocturnal paroxysmal dystonia

Initially nocturnal paroxysmal dystonia (NPD) was considered a movement disorder, but recently it has been suggested that it is epileptic in nature, even though EEG changes are often not detectable on surface EEG [13]. Some authors consider NPD as a type of parasomnia, and official classifications of sleep disorder consider NPD within parasomnias [14].

Zucconi classified these motor behaviors as minimal, minor, or major. Minimal activity includes scratching or rubbing the nose and the head, limb flexion, facial grimacing, chewing, moaning with duration of 5–10 seconds. Minor activity has involvement of more body segments in pelvic thrusting and swinging.

Major attacks include sudden raising the head and body from the bed accompanied by dystonic or clonic movements, fear expression and panic attacks with complex behavior, with duration 5–30 seconds [15]. Eighty percent of patients showed some epileptiform abnormalities during sleep [15]. Currently, most authors consider NPD as a form of partial epilepsy [16]. This is supported by the following observations: most patients have a history of nocturnal generalized convulsive disorder; EEG abnormalities are found in most patients; and symptoms are controlled by antiepileptic drugs. Thus nocturnal paroxysmal dystonia is a form of frontal lobe epilepsy. These seizures often arise from the SMA. The role of genetics is well accepted in some forms of frontal lobe epilepsies. An inherited form of nocturnal paroxysmal dystonia is described as autosomal dominant nocturnal frontal lobe epilepsy (ADNFLE), which is caused by a single gene inheritance pattern that was first described in six families by Scheffer [17].

Psychogenic disorders

Psychogenic nonepileptic seizures are very common at referral epilepsy centers, but psychogenic movement disorders are the second most manifestation of psychopathology seen in neurology. The psychopathology is the same and, depending on the manifestations, patients may present to the epileptologist or the movement disorder specialist. Predictors of psychogenic symptoms include response to suggestion, coexisting unexplained "chronic pain" (including "fibromyalgia") [18].

Nonepileptic movements in the ICU setting

Abnormal movements in the ICU setting have been poorly studied but are frequent in practice. Seizures are often considered but, with the increased use of video-EEG recording, it is clear that most often these abnormal behaviors are not epileptic [19].

References

1. Marsden CD, Hallett M, Fahn S. The nosology and pathophysiology of myoclonus. In: Marsden CD, Fahn S, eds. *Movement Disorders*. London: Butterworths; 1982: 196.

2. Krauss G, Mathews G. Similarities in mechanisms and treatments for epileptic and nonepileptic myoclonus. *Epilepsy Curr* 2003; 3(1): 19–21.

3. Panayiotopoulos CP. *A Clinical Guide to Epileptic Syndromes and Their Treatment*. 2nd ed. London: Springer-Verlag; 2007.

4. Walters AS. Clinical identification of the simple sleep-related movement disorders. *Chest* 2007; **131**: 1260–6.

5. Vetrugno R, Plazzi G, Provini F *et al*. Excessive fragmentary hypnic myoclonus: clinical and neurophysiological findings. *Sleep Med* 2002; **3**: 73–6.

6. Jumao-as A, Brenner RP. Myoclonic status epilepticus. *Neurology* 1990; **40**: 1199.

7. Cockerell OC, Rothwell J, Thompson PD, Marsden CD, Shorvon SD. Clinical and physiological features of epilepsia partialis continua. Cases ascertained in the UK. *Brain* 1996; **119**(Pt 2): 393–407.

8. Pandian J D. *et al*. Epilepsia partialis continua: a clinical and electroencephalography study. *Seizure* 2002; **11**: 437–41.

9. Wyllie E, Benbadis SR, Kotagal P. Psychogenic seizures and other nonepileptic paroxysmal events in children. *Epilepsy Behav* 2002, 3: 46–50.

10. Engel J, Pedley TA. In: *Epilepsy: A Comprehensive Textbook*. 2nd ed. Alphen aan den Rijn: Wolters Kluwer; 2008: Chapters 44, 49.

11. Schenck CH, Bundle SR, Ettinger MG, Mahowald MW. Chronic behavioural disorders of human REM sleep: a new category of parasomnias. *Sleep* 1996; **9**: 293–308.

12. Derry CP, Duncan JS, Berkovic SF. Paroxysmal motor disorders of sleep: the clinical spectrum and differentiation from epilepsy. *Epilepsia* 2006; **47**: 1775.

13. Lugaresi E, Cirignotta F. Hypnogenic paroxysmal dystonia; epileptic seizure or a new syndrome. *Sleep* 1981; 4: 129–38.

14. Thorpy MJ. Classification and nomenclature of sleep disorders. In: Thorpy MJ, ed. *Handbook of Sleep Disorders*. New York: Marcel Dekker; 1990: 155–76.

15. Zucconi M, Oldani A, Ferini L, Bizzozero D, Smirne S. Nocturnal paroxysmal arousals with motor behaviours during sleep: frontal lobe epilepsy or parasomnia? *J Clin Neurophysiol* 1997; **14**(6): 513–22.

16. Hirsch E, Sellal F, Maton B *et al*. Nocturnal paroxysmal dystonia: a clinical form of focal epilepsy. *Neurophysiol Clin* 1994; **24**(3): 207–17.

17. Scheffer IE, Bhatia KP, Lopes-Cendes I, *et al*. Autosomal dominant frontal epilepsy misdiagnosed as sleep disorder. *Lancet* 1994, **343**(8896): 515–171.

18. Benbadis SR. Psychogenic nonepileptic seizures. In: Wyllie E, ed. *The Treatment of Epilepsy: Principles and Practice*, 5th ed. Philadelphia: Lippincott, Williams & Wilkins; 2010: 486–94.

19. Benbadis IE, Bhatia KP, Lopes-Cendes I, *et al*. Autosomal dominant frontal epilepsy misdiagnosed as sleep disorder. *Lancet* 1994, **343**(8896): 515–171.

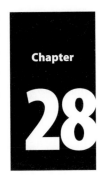

Cerebrovascular diseases and movement disorders

Sarkis Morales-Vidal, Ninith Kartha, Rima M. Dafer,
Michael J. Schneck and Jose Biller

History and terminology

Poststroke movement disorders (PSMDs) may occur at onset of stroke or subsequently. Several types of movement disorders have been associated with cerebrovascular disorders including parkinsonism, chorea, ballismus, tremor, myoclonus, athetosis, dystonia, hemifacial spasm, "limb shaking TIAs," and other miscellaneous movement disorders. Reported frequency of PSMDs ranges from 1% to 3.7% [1]. Hemichorea and hemidystonia are the most commonly observed PSMDs [1]. PSMD affects both sexes equally; advanced age plays a direct risk for the development of these disorders. Most patients have motor deficits at presentation that often improve before appearance of the PSMD [2,3]. Although several cerebrovascular risk factors have been shown to be less frequent among patients with Parkinson disease (PD), patients with PD have neither a protective effect against stroke nor a greater risk of death following stroke [4].

Hyperkinetic movement disorders, particularly chorea, occur early after stroke compared with parkinsonism [5]. Poststroke dystonia may develop at stroke presentation or after a delay of many years following stroke [5].

Applied vascular anatomy

The basal ganglia (BG) include the corpus striatum, the substantia nigra, the subthalamic nucleus of Luys and the ventral tegmental area. The corpus striatum comprises the neostriatum (putamen, caudate nucleus and nucleus accumbens) and the paleostriatum (globus pallidus). The globus pallidus comprises a medial or internal (GPi) segment, and a lateral or external (GPe) segment. Other anatomical structures relevant to our discussion include the thalamus and the triangle of Guillain–Mollaret (Trelles pathway) connecting the dentate nucleus of one side with the red nucleus and

the inferior olive on the opposite side, via the superior cerebellar peduncle [6].

The main arterial blood supply of the striatum derives from branches of the lateral lenticulostriate arteries (LSA) arising from the M1 and M2 segments of the middle cerebral artery (MCA), and from the recurrent artery of Heubner (RAH) arising from the proximal (A2) segment of the anterior cerebral artery (ACA) [7]. Other arterial contributors include branches from the ACA and from the anterior communicating artery (AComA), and direct perforators from the MCA [6]. The anterior-ventral surface of the striatum is supplied by the RAH. The medial LSA supplies the medial portion of the caudate nucleus, putamen, internal capsule and lateral border of the globus pallidus externa (Gpe). The main thalamic blood supply originates from the posterior communicating arteries (PComA) and the perimesencephalic segment of the posterior cerebral arteries (PCA). The subthalamic nucleus is supplied by the anterior choroidal artery (AChoA) and the posterior choroidal artery (PChoA). The main blood supply of the dentate nucleus is by the superior cerebellar artery (SCA); the red nucleus by perforators of the basilar artery (BA) and short circumferentials of the PCA; the central tegmental tract by short circumferentials of the BA as well as branches from the anterior inferior cerebellar artery (AICA) and the SCA; and the inferior olivary complex is supplied by branches from the vertebral artery (VA) and the posterior inferior cerebellar artery (PICA). Figure 28.1 illustrates the main arterial blood supply of the basal ganglia and thalamus.

Clinical findings

A variety of either hyperkinetic or hypokinetic movement disorders may be secondary to a spectrum of cerebrovascular disorders (Table 28.1). Discrete lesions of the anterolateral segment of the caudate nucleus cause

Uncommon Causes of Movement Disorders, ed. Néstor Gálvez-Jiménez and Paul J. Tuite. Published by Cambridge University Press. © Cambridge University Press 2011.

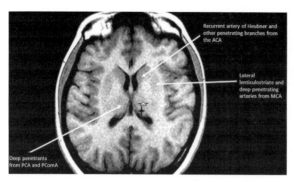

Figure 28.1. Main arterial blood supply of the caudate nucleus, lenticular nucleus and thalamus. White and black stars represent areas supplied by the thalamogeniculate artery and posterior choroidal artery.

contralateral choreoathetosis. Unilateral lesions of the globus pallidus may cause contralateral hemidystonia, hemiparkinsonism, or tremors. Bilateral globus pallidus lesions may cause dystonia or parkinsonism. Lesions of the substantia nigra may cause parkinsonism. Lesions of the subthalamic nucleus produce contralateral hemiballismus.

Deep lesions involving the BG, thalamus and brain stem causing PSMDs are more likely to be ischemic [5]. However, dyskinesias following thalamic vascular insults are more commonly hemorrhagic [1]. Most thalamic strokes causing hemiballismus are ischemic [1]. Poststroke tremors often result from involvement of the posterior thalamus or dentato-rubro-thalamic pathways [1]. In the thalamic syndrome of Dejerine–Roussy, patients exhibit transient contralateral choreoathetoid or ballistic movements. Unilateral or bilateral BG strokes are the most common causes of poststroke parkinsonism. Segmental myoclonus may follow strokes involving the thalamus, midbrain, or pons [8,9]. Palatal myoclonus (palatal tremor) results from involvement of the Guillain–Mollaret triangle (Trelles pathway), particularly following pontine or medullary strokes [5].

Hyperkinetic disorders

Chorea and ballismus are a continuum of hyperkinetic disorders. Chorea (hemichorea) and ballismus (hemiballismus) due to vascular causes (vascular chorea) are among the most common causes of new-onset hemibody hyperkinesias among elderly patients. Vascular hemichorea is often due to striatal (caudate and putamen) lesions. Hemichorea may result from a

contralateral putaminal hemorrhage [10]. Transient hemichorea may rarely be the manifestation of a transient ischemic attack (TIA) [11]. Post-cardiac surgery chorea (post-pump chorea) is one of the most common causes of chorea in children [12]. Subcortical white matter ischemia may also cause chorea [13]. Bilateral manifestations do not exclude brain ischemia as a cause of generalized chorea or ballismus, as exemplified by instances of bilateral lacunar infarcts of the striatum and frontal white matter [14]. Among elderly subjects, generalized chorea could be the presentation of bilateral chronic subdural hematomas or cerebral amyloid angiopathy (CAA) [15]. Rarely chorea may be attributed to migraine. Hemicrania choreatica refers to a form of migraine associated with chorea [16]. Hemichorea-hemiballismus associated with ipsilateral pain may be due to an anterior parietal artery territory stroke [17]. Cerebrovascular causes of corticosteroid-responsive chorea and ballismus include moyamoya disease, post-cardiac surgery, and a wide range of cerebral vasculitides. Chorea is also the most common movement disorder observed in patients with the anti-phospholipid antibody syndrome (APAS). Cerebral aneurysms and central nervous system (CNS) vascular malformations can present with chorea [18]. Watershed infarctions have also been reported to cause hemichorea [19]. Athetosis from vascular lesions has been reported in association with damage of the striatum with sparing of the motor cortex. Athetosis can also be the initial presentation of perinatal anoxia.

At least 20 lacunar syndromes have been defined, including hemiballismus [20]. Hemiballismus is most commonly due to lesions of the contralateral subthalamic nucleus of Luys. Rarely, hemiballismus results from a disconnection between the parietal cortex and BG due to stroke. Cerebrovascular lesions of the posterior subthalamus may manifest as hemiballismus of the contralateral lower extremity [20]. The vascular lesions responsible for hemiballismus are complex. It is uncertain whether the occluded vessels arise from the posterior thalamoperforators, PChoA or AChoA [21].

Dystonia associated with cerebrovascular disease may be focal or segmental or present as hemidystonia. Dystonia may be accompanied by tremors (dystonic tremor), myoclonic jerks (dystonic myoclonus), or athetoid movements [5]. Dystonia may result from strokes involving the lentiform nucleus, caudate, subthalamus, cerebellum, pontomesencephalic region, or spinal cord [22]. Bilateral putaminal hemorrhages

Table 28.1. Clinico-vascular correlation of different movement disorders.

Movement abnormality	Localization	Arterial supply	Common causes	Uncommon causes
Parkinsonism	Substantia nigra	VB circulation	IS	CM
	Putamen	RAH, lateral-LstA	IS, ICH	SAH, SDH, AVM, DAVF, CM, Moyamoya, HHT, vasculitis
	Globus pallidus	Lateral-LstA, AChoA	IS, ICH	SAH, SDH, AVM, DAVF, CM, Moyamoya, HHT, vasculitis
	Diffuse white matter	ICA/VB circulation	Small-vessel disease (lacunar state)	CADASIL
Chorea	Caudate	RAH, lateral-LstA	IS, ICH	SAH, unruptured giant aneurysm, AVM, CCAD, Moyamoya, migraine, RCVS, cardiac (e.g., RF, post-cardiac transplantation, post-cardiopulmonary bypass, papillary fibroelastoma, post-cardiac arrest, PANDAS, Morvan "fibrillary chorea"), hypercoagulable states (e.g., APAS, SLE, pregnancy, OCPs), bleeding diathesis (e.g., Henoch–Schönlein purpura), vasculitis (SLE, Churg–Strauss syndrome, Sydenham chorea, Behçet disease, PACNS, HSP, juvenile idiopathic arthritis, Takayasu arteritis, juvenile ankylosing spondylitis, familial Mediterranean fever, scleroderma, sarcoidosis, Wegener granulomatosis, Kawasaki disease, drug-induced vasculitis (e.g., antirheumatic drugs, chemotherapeutic agents))
	Putamen	RAH, lateral-LstA	IS, ICH	As above
	Globus pallidus (externa and interna)	Lateral-LstA, AChoA	IS, ICH	As above
	Thalamus	AChoA, PChoA	IS, ICH	—
	Subthalamic nucleus	AChoA, PChoA	IS, ICH	—
	Midbrain and pons	BA, PCA, SCA, AICA	IS	—
	Diffuse white matter disease (involving white matter connections of basal ganglia)	ICA/VB	—	CADASIL

Table 28.1. (cont.)

Movement abnormality	Localization	Arterial supply	Common causes	Uncommon causes
Ballismus	Subthalamic nucleus	AChoA, PChoA	IS, ICH	—
	Caudate	RAH, lateral LstA	IS, ICH	SAH, AVM, CCAD, Moyamoya, migraine, RCVS, cardiac (e.g., RF, post-cardiac transplantation, post-cardiopulmonary bypass, papillary fibroelastoma, post-cardiac arrest, PANDAS, Morvan "fibrillary chorea"), hypercoagulable states (e.g., APAS, SLE, pregnancy, OCPs), bleeding diathesis (e.g., Henoch–Schönlein purpura), unruptured giant aneurysm
	Putamen	RAH, lateral-LstA	IS, ICH	As above
	Globus pallidus (externa and interna)	lateral-LstA, AChoA	IS, ICH	As above
	Thalamus	Thalamoperforators	IS, ICH	—
Athetosis	Putamen	RAH, lateral-LstA	IS, ICH	SAH, AVM, CCAD, Moyamoya, migraine, RCVS, cardiac (e.g., RF, post-cardiac transplantation, post-cardiopulmonary bypass, papillary fibroelastoma, post-cardiac arrest, PANDAS, Morvan "fibrillary chorea"), hypercoagulable states (e.g., APAS, SLE, pregnancy, OCPs), bleeding diathesis (e.g., Henoch–Schönlein purpura), unruptured giant aneurysm
	Globus pallidus	Lateral-LstA, AChoA	IS, ICH	As above
	Thalamus	Thalamoperforators	IS, ICH	—
Dystonia	Putamen	RAH, lateral-LstA	IS	SAH, unruptured aneurysm, AVM, CM, postanoxic syndrome, hemiplegic migraine, methylphenidate poisoning, post-cardiac arrest, hypercoagulable states (e.g., APAS, pregnancy), vasculitis
	Globus pallidus	Lateral-LstA, AChoA	IS	As above
	Thalamus	Thalamoperforators	IS, ICH	IPH after DBS; after gamma knife surgery, CM
	Midbrain and pons	BA, PCA, SCA, AICA	IS, ICH	CM, persistent primitive trigeminal artery

		Anterior and posterior cerebrovascular circulation	IS	
Tremor	Diffuse white matter disease (involving white matter connections of extrapyramidal structures)		IS	CADASIL, CM in centrum semiovale
	Putamen	RAH, lateral-LstA	IS, ICH	Familial meningocerebrovascular amyloidosis, cardiac (thyrotoxic cardiomyopathy, after cardiac catheterization, post heart transplant), hypercoagulable states (e.g., APAS, pregnancy, OCPs), vasculitis
	Globus pallidus (externa and interna)	Lateral-LstA, AChoA	IS, ICH	As above
	Thalamus	Thalamoperforators	IS, ICH	—
	Subthalamic nucleus	AChoA, PChoA	IS, ICH	—
	Midbrain	BA, PCA, SCA, AICA	IS, ICH	CM, after CM removal, CCF, midbrain infarction due to cryptococcal meningitis
	Cerebellum	PICA, AICA, SCA	IS, ICH	
	Diffuse white matter disease	ICA/VB	IS (small-vessel disease)	Moyamoya
Myoclonus	Cortical	ICA/PCA	IS, ICH	AVM, CVT, MELAS, pseudoxanthoma elasticum, hypercoagulable states, vasculitis
		ICA/VB	IS, ICH	AVM, giant aneurysm of the BA, CVT, CADASIL, MELAS, pseudoxanthoma elasticum, hypercoagulable states, vasculitis
	Spinal	ASA/PSA	ASA infarction	Spinal AVM, spinal AVF
Hemifacial spasm	Cerebellopontine angle	VB circulation	Tortuosity of AICA or PICA	AVM, dolichoectatic BA, aneurysms
	Intrapontine	VB circulation	Lacunar infarction	—
	Intrapetrosal	VB circulation	—	Hemangioma of the geniculate ganglion
Tics	BG	ICA/VB circulation	—	IS, AVM

AChoA, anterior choroidal artery; AICA, anterior inferior cerebellar artery; APAP, automatic positive airway pressure; ASA, anterior spinal artery; AVF, arteriovenous fistula; AVM, arteriovenous malformation; BA, basilar artery; BG, basal artery; CADASIL, cerebral autosomal dominant arteriopathy with subcortical infarcts and leukoencephalopathy; CCAD, cervicocephalic arterial dissection; CM, cavernous malformations; CPA, cerebellopontine angle; CVT, cerebral venous thrombosis; DAVF, dural arteriovenous fistula; HHT, hereditary hemorrhagic telangiectasia; HSP, Henoch–Schönlein purpura; ICA, internal carotid artery; ICH, intracranial hemorrhage; IPH, idiopathic pulmonary hypertension; IS, ischemic stroke; LstA, lenticulostriate artery; MELAS, mitochondrial encephalopathy, lactic acidosis, and stroke-like episodes; OCPs, oral contraceptives; PACNS, primary angiitis of the central nervous system; PANDAS, pediatric autoimmune neuropsychiatric disorders associated with streptococcal infections; PChoA, posterior choroidal artery; PICA, posterior inferior cerebellar artery; PSA, posterior spinal artery; RAH, recurrent artery of Heubner; RCVS, reversible cerebral vasoconstriction syndrome; RF, rheumatic fever; SAH, subarachnoid hemorrhage; SCA, superior cerebellar artery; SLE, systemic lupus erythematosus; VB, vertebrobasilar.

may cause retrocollis [23]. Stroke and perinatal complications are also among the most common causes of the hemidystonia-hemiatrophy syndrome [24]. Acute orofacial dyskinesias may be the initial manifestation of bilateral thalamocapsular infarctions or strokes involving striatronigral pathways [25]. Facial dystonia may be the initial manifestation of CADASIL (cerebral autosomal dominant arteriopathy with subcortical ischemic strokes and leukoencephalopathy) [26]. Dystonic-like movements ("painful spasms") may occur with putaminal infarction [27]. Unexplained chorea-acanthocytosis may be due to Fabry disease [28]. The 3697G>A/ND1 mutation, known to cause MELAS, has also been described in a family with spastic dystonias associated with Leber hereditary optic atrophy [29].

Poststroke tremors may be multifocal or segmental in distribution. Tremors may be due to strokes or an underlying CNS vascular malformation [30]. Acute onset of head tremor may follow a paramedian pontomesencephalic infarct [31]. Resting tremor in patients with Parkinson disease may improve following infarction in the territory of the inferolateral and tuberothalamic arteries [32]. Acute onset of a "parkinsonian tremor" can be the initial manifestation of a stroke involving the medial aspect of the substantia nigra [33]. Benedikt syndrome may cause contralateral involuntary movements, including intention tremor, hemichorea, or hemiathetosis, due to destruction of the red nucleus [6]. Claude syndrome is other well recognized brain stem syndrome that may be associated with contralateral tremors [6]. An unusual example of orthostatic tremor was described in a 49-year-old man with a pontine cavernous malformation [34].

Poststroke myoclonus is mostly segmental (palatal and spinal myoclonus) or focal, and may result from a wide array of vascular lesions affecting the cerebral cortex, thalamus, brain stem, or spinal cord [1]. Focal action myoclonus of the jaw and tongue may follow an ischemic stroke [2]. Spinal myoclonus can occur as a consequence of ischemic myelopathy [6]. Approximately 40% of cases of palatal myoclonus are due to brain stem strokes involving the Guillain–Mollaret triangle (Trelles pathway). Because of its rhythmicity, palatal tremor is a better term than palatal myoclonus. Most vascular causes of palatal tremor are secondary to interruption of the central tegmental tract. Palatal tremor has also been reported in a case of the "eight-and-a-half-syndrome" and in a patient with an intracranial arteriovenous malformation

associated with pseudoxanthoma elasticum [35]. Isolated lesions of the inferior cerebellar peduncle do not cause tremor, as the inferior olivary nucleus does not have direct connections with the dentate nucleus; rather its fibers project first to the cerebellar cortex (olivocerebellar tract) and then to the dentate nucleus [36,37]. Cerebrovascular insults involving the Guillain–Mollaret triangle can be ischemic or hemorrhagic. Hemorrhagic lesions could result from hypertension or diffuse axonal injury. Olivary hypertrophy may be evident on MRI studies, as observed in a young hypertensive patient with a dentatorubral tremor due to a pontine hemorrhage [38].

Tics are rarely caused by strokes. However, craniocervical motor tics in association with hemidystonia have been described in children with subcortical strokes [39]. Tics could also be the initial presentation of a CNS vascular malformation [39,40].

Hemifacial spasm results from compression of the facial nerve at the brain stem junction. In most instances, the facial nerve is compressed by blood vessels adjacent to the nerve exit zone [41]. Of 1688 cases of hemifacial spasms reviewed by Digre and colleagues, 539 had an identified cause. Of those, 94% were due to vascular compression of the facial nerve [42]. In most instances, an arterial vascular loop compressed the facial nerve, but other vascular anomalies (e.g., the dolichoectatic basilar artery) were described. Three characteristic patterns of vessel configuration may lead to hemifacial spasm [43]. In type I, the ipsilateral VA is dominant and sigmoidal in course. In type II, the contralateral VA is dominant with the BA curving toward the affected side; and in type III, the BA remains near the midline or curves toward the unaffected side. Endoscopic data demonstrate that the most common offending vessels are the PICA, followed by the VA and the AICA respectively [44].

"Limb shaking TIAs" are characterized by repetitive, involuntary, "shaking" or trembling movements of seconds to few minutes in duration, often precipitated by sitting or standing. Limb shaking TIAs are often associated with severe unilateral or bilateral carotid artery stenosis [45]. Stenosis of the intracranial internal carotid artery and proximal MCA was the main cause of limb shaking TIAs in a Chinese cohort [46]. Limb shaking TIAs have been induced by hyperventilation in patients with Moyamoya disease [47]. New onset of restless legs syndrome (RLS) after a cerebrovascular insult result from strokes involving the basal ganglia, internal capsule, or thalamus [48].

Hypokinetic manifestations

Hypokinetic movement disorders are rare following acute stroke. The best-known hypokinetic syndrome associated with cerebrovascular diseases is vascular parkinsonism. McDonald Critchley first described arteriosclerotic parkinsonism in 1929 [49]. Vascular parkinsonism (VP) is also known as lower-body parkinsonism, arteriosclerotic pseudoparkinsonism, or arteriosclerotic parkinsonism. Diagnostic criteria for VP remain controversial. Zijlmans and colleagues proposed three main variables: (1) parkinsonism, (2) cerebrovascular disease (by brain imaging or presence of focal signs or symptoms consistent with stroke), and (3) relationship between onset of parkinsonism and cerebrovascular disease [50]. Winikates and Jankovic proposed clinical, neuroimaging and pathological criteria for diagnosis of VP; parkinsonism plus a vascular score ≥2 or more is considered diagnostic of VP [51].

Clinical syndromes associated with VP include lower-body parkinsonism, parkinsonism associated with a multi-infarct state, parkinsonism indistinguishable from PD, unilateral parkinsonism ("pure parkinsonism"), PSP-like syndrome, and an "overlap syndrome"(combination of PD and VP). The classic type is lower-body parkinsonism often presenting with prominent gait disorder, rare occurrence of resting tremor, and variable response to levodopa. Patients with VP have predominant involvement of the lower body, frequent falls, postural instability, upper motor neuron findings, dementia, urinary incontinence and pseudobulbar palsy. Parkinsonism associated with a multi-infarct state may present with additional features, including gait disorder, pseudobulbar features, urinary incontinence, dementia, and cortical and subcortical infarcts. Unilateral parkinsonism has also been reported with infarcts involving the subcortical gray matter, while a PSP-like syndrome has been associated with multi-infarct states. Clinical and pathological differences between VP and PD are summarized in Table 28.2 [52]. Patients with VP are more likely to be hypertensive [53]. Rarely hemiparkinsonism is a presentation of PSMD [7]. Parkinsonism due to subcortical arteriosclerotic encephalopathy (Binswanger disease), may also respond to levodopa therapy [54].

Acute onset of freezing of gait may be due to an acute bilateral pedunculopontine nuclei infarction [55]. Parkinsonism with a PSP phenotype and VP has been reported with CADASIL [56,57]. Parkinsonism may also be the initial presentation of Fabry disease [58].

Table 28.2. Differences between vascular parkinsonism and Parkinson disease.

	Vascular parkinsonism	Parkinson disease
Resting tremor	4%	73%
Action tremor	12.5%	—
Upper motor neuron signs	62.5%	0%
Hemiparesis	37.5%	0%
Pseudobulbar palsy	50%	—
Dysphagia or dysarthria	50%	27%
Dementia	71%	43%
Levodopa response	12.50%	>90%
Gait abnormality	100%	77%
Asymmetry of limb rigidity	29%	73%
Pathological evidence of cerebrovascular disease	100%	37%

Adapted from reference 52.

Ancillary investigations

Targeted investigations are directed to the suspected cerebrovascular etiology. Magnetic resonance imaging (MRI) may be limited by motion artifacts in patients with hyperkinesias. Motion artifacts may obscure the normal anatomy and be mistaken for underlying pathology. Motion artifacts on MRI are seen only in the *phase*-encoding direction, giving an "up and down" or truncation appearance. The right-to-left motion artifact is seen in the *frequency*-encoding direction, since the *frequency*-encoding step takes much less time (milliseconds) than a *phase*-encoding step (of the order of seconds); this type of motion artifact is not common. The role of dopamine transporter imaging in the diagnosis of VP remains a controversial topic. Most patients with VP have a reduced presynaptic dopaminergic function. The asymmetry index has been proposed as a criterion for the diagnosis of VP [59]. For further details, the reader is referred to standard neurology textbooks.

PSMD and selective management issues

Adverse cerebrovascular effects of drugs and other therapeutic interventions commonly used in the

Table 28.3. Commonly used drugs in the management of movement disorders and potential cardiovascular (CV) adverse effects.

Drugs commonly used in the treatment of movement disorders	Common (or well known) CV adverse effects	Uncommon CV adverse effects
Dopamine agonists – ergots: bromocriptine, cabergoline, pergolide	Syncope and other cerebrovascular effects of arterial hypotension	Ischemic stroke. Arrhythmia, myocardial infarction, fibrotic heart-valve reactions
Dopamine agonists – non ergots: pramipexole, ropinirole, rotigotine	Syncope and other cerebrovascular effects of hypotension	Although not an ergot, there have been postmarketing reports of possible fibrotic complications with pramipexole. Ropinirole: hypertension in 5%, atrial fibrillation in 2%
Dopamine agonists – other: apomorphine	Syncope and other cerebrovascular effects of hypotension	
MAO-B inhibitors: selegiline, rasagiline	Syncope and other cerebrovascular effects of hypotension	Arrhythmias
Catechol-O-methyltransferase inhibitors: entacapone, tolcapone	Syncope and other cerebrovascular effects of hypotension	Cerebral ischemia (<1%)
NMDA-glutamate antagonists: amantadine	Syncope and other cerebrovascular effects of hypotension	
Mineralocorticoids: fludrocortisones, midodrine	Supine hypertension	Hypertension. Myocardial rupture in patient with history of myocardial infarction

MAO-B inhibitors, monoamine oxidase B inhibitors.

Table 28.4. Other therapeutic interventions use in movement disorders and associated cerebrovascular complications.

Intervention	Common (or well-known) cerebrovascular adverse effects	Uncommon cerebrovascular adverse effects
DBS (thalamic or pallidal)	ICH (3.1%)	CVT (0.1%)
DBS (subthalamic)	ICH (3.9%)	Hypoxic brain injury from increase risk of suicide
ECT for refractory psychosis		Ischemic stroke ICH

DBS, deep brain stimulation. ICH, intracranial hemorrhage. CVT, cerebral venous thrombosis. ECT, electroconvulsive therapy.

treatment of movement disorders are summarized in Table 28.3 and Table 28.4, respectively. Deep brain stimulation (DBS) with targets in the contralateral ventromedial (Vm) nucleus of the thalamus is commonly used for the treatment of Parkinson disease-associated tremor and essential tremor. Successful treatment of a debilitating intention tremor associated with Benedikt syndrome via DBS of the lenticular fasciculus was reported in a 55-year-old man with a protracted tremor [60]. However, DBS has been rarely associated with hemorrhagic and ischemic cerebrovascular complications [61].

Certain medications used in patients with cerebrovascular disease may have deleterious extrapyramidal side-effects. Calcium-channel blockers can cause hyperkinetic and hypokinetic movement disorders [62]. Hydrochlorothiazide decreases amantadine clearance; this may result in amantadine toxicity [63]. Corticosteroid therapy has been reported to be effective in cases of post-cardiac transplantation chorea as well as chorea associated with moyamoya [64,65]. Aspirin has been reported to improve chorea in some patients [66].

Conclusions

Movement disorders may be the initial presentation of a wide array of cerebrovascular diseases. Poststroke hyperkinesias occur earlier in contrast to hypokinetic PSMDs. Most hyperkinetic PSMDs are self-limiting.

References

1. Alarcón F, Zijlmans JC, Dueñas G, Cevallos N. Poststroke movement disorders: report of 56 patients. *J Neurol Neurosurg Psychiatry* 2004; **75**(11): 1568–74.

2. Ghika-Schmid F, Ghika J, Regli F, Bogousslavsky J. Hyperkinetic movement disorders during and after acute stroke: The Lausanne Stroke Registry. *J Neurol Sci* 1997; **146**(2): 109–16.

3. Kim JS. Delay onset mixed involuntary movements after thalamic stroke. Clinical, radiological and pathophysiological findings. *Brain* 2001; **124**: 299–309.

4. Jellinger KA. Prevalence of cerebrovascular lesions in Parkinson's disease: a postmortem study. *Acta Neuropathol* 2003; **105**: 415–19.

5. Handley A, Medcalf P, Hellier K, Dutta D. Movement disorders after stroke. *Age Ageing* 2009; **38**: 260–6.

6. Brazis PW. Masdeu JC. Biller J. *Localization in Clinical Neurology*. 5th ed. Philadelphia: Lippincott Williams & Wilkins; 2008.

7. Feekes JA, Cassell MD. The vascular supply of the functional compartments of the human striatum. *Brain* 2006; **129**(8): 2189–201. doi: 10.1093/brain/awl158.

8. Kim JS. Involuntary movements after anterior cerebral artery territory infarction. *Stroke* 2001; **32**: 258.

9. Ghika J. Bogousslavsky J. *Abnormal Movements. Stroke Syndromes.* 2nd ed. Cambridge: Cambridge University Press; 2001; 162–81.

10. Jones HR Jr, Baker RA, Kott HS. Hypertensive putaminal hemorrhage presenting with hemichorea. *Stroke* 985; **16**(1): 130.

11. Margolin DI, Marsden CD. Episodic dyskinesias and transient cerebral ischemia. *Neurology* 1982; **32**(12): 1379–80.

12. Curless RG, Katz DA, Perryman RA, Ferrer PL, Gelblum J, Weiner WJ. Choreoathetosis after surgery for congenital heart disease. *J Pediatr* 1994; **124**(5 Pt 1): 737–9.

13. Fukui T, Hasegawa Y, Seriyama S, Takeuchi T, Sugita K, Tsukagoshi H. Hemiballism-hemichorea induced by subcortical ischemia. *Can J Neurol Sci* 1993; **20**(4): 324–8.

14. Tabaton M, Mancardi G, Loeb C. Generalized chorea due to bilateral small, deep cerebral infarcts. *Neurology* 1985; **35**(4): 588–9.

15. Bae SH, Vates TS Jr, Kenton EJ. Generalized chorea associated with chronic subdural hematomas. *Ann Neurol* 1980; **8**(4): 449–50.

16. Bruyn GW, Ferrari MD. Chorea and migraine: "Hemicrania choreatica"? *Cephalalgia* 1984; **4**(2): 119–24.

17. Rossetti AO, Ghika JA, Vingerhoets F, Novy J, Bogousslavsky J. Neurogenic pain and abnormal movements contralateral to an anterior parietal artery stroke. *Arch Neurol* 2003; **60**(7): 1004–6.

18. Barreiro De Madariaga LM, Sian J, Casas Parrera I, Micheli F. Arm chorea secondary to an unruptured giant aneurysm. *Mov Disord* 2003; **18**(11): 1397–9.

19. Lee MS, Lyoo CH, Lee HJ, Kim YD. Hemichoreoathetosis following posterior parietal watershed infarction: was striatal hypoperfusion really to blame? *Mov Disord* 2000; **15**(1): 178–9.

20. Ohinshi J. A case of monoballism in unilateral lower extremity – somatotopic relation in subthalamic nucleus. *Rinsho Shinkeigaku* 1992; **32**: 506–10.

21. Biller B, Graff-Radoford NR, Smoker WRK, Adams Jr. HP, Johnston P. MR imaging in "lacunar" hemiballismus. *J Comput Assist Tomogr* **10**(5): 793–7.

22. Loher TJ, Krauss JK. Dystonia associated with pontomesencephalic lesions *Mov Disord* 2009; **24**(2): 157–67.

23. Shimpo T. Retrocollis and oculogyric crisis in association with bilateral putaminal hemorrhages. *Rinsho Shinkeigaku* 1993; **33**(1): 40–4.

24. Wijemanne S, Jankovic J. Hemidystonia-hemiatrophy syndrome. *Mov Disord* 2009; **15**; **24**(4): 583–9.

25. Combarros O, Gutiérrez A, Pascual J, Berciano J. Oral dyskinesias associated with bilateral thalamocapsular infarction. *J Neurol Neurosurg Psychiatry* 1990; **53**: 168–9.

26. Miranda M, Dichgans M, Slachevsky A *et al.* CADASIL presenting with a movement disorder: a clinical study of a Chilean kindred. *Mov Disord* 2006; **21**(7): 1008–12.

27. Merchut M, Brumlik J. Painful tonic spasms caused by putaminal infarction. *Stroke* 1986; **17**: 1319–21.

28. Ichiba M, Nakamura M, Kusumoto A *et al.* Clinical and molecular genetic assessment of a chorea acanthocytosis pedigree. *J Neurol Sci* 2007; **263**: 124–32.

29. Spruijt L, Smeets HJ, Hendrickx A *et al.* A MELAS-associated ND1 mutation causing Leber hereditary optic neuropathy and spastic dystonia. *Arch Neurol* 2007; **64**(6): 890–3.

30. Diederich NJ, Verhagen Metman L, Bakay RA, Alesch F. Ventral intermediate thalamic stimulation in complex

tremor syndromes. *Stereotact Funct Neurosurg* 2008; **86**: 167–72.

31. Jong S. Kim. Head tremor and stroke. *Cerebrovasc Dis* 1997; **7**: 175–9.

32. Choi SM, Lee SH, Park MS, Kim BC, Kim MK, Cho KH. Disappearance of resting tremor after thalamic stroke involving the territory of the tuberothalamic artery. *Parkinsonism Relat Disord* 2008; **14**(4): 373–5.

33. Gonzalez-Alegre P. Monomelic parkinsonian tremor caused by contralateral substantia nigra stroke. *Parkinsonism Relat Disord* 2007; **13**(3): 182–4.

34. Benito-León J. Symptomatic orthostatic tremor in pontine lesions. *Neurology* 1997; **49**: 1439–41.

35. Chalk JB, Patterson MC, Pender MP. An intracranial arteriovenous malformation and palatal myoclonus related to pseudoxanthoma elasticum. *Aust N Z J Med* 1989; **19**(2): 141–3.

36. Lapresle J. La voie dento-olivaire: sa mise en evidence, son trajet, sa signification. *Bull Acad Natl Med* 1984; **168**: 336–41.

37. Trelles JO. Les myoclonies velo-palatines: sonsideration anatomiques et physiologiques. *Rev Neurol* 1968; **119**: 165–71.

38. Salamon-Murayama N. Case 17: Hypertrophic olivary degeneration secondary to pontine hemorrhage. *Radiology* 1999; **213**: 814–17.

39. Kwak CH, Jankovic J. Tourettism and dystonia after subcortical stroke. *Mov Disord* 2002; **17**(4): 821–5.

40. Yochelson MR, David RG. New-onset tic disorder following acute hemorrhage of an arteriovenous malformation. *J Child Neurol* 2000; **15**(11): 769–71.

41. Wilkins RH. Hemifacial spasm: a review. *Surg Neurol* 1991; **36**: 251–77.

42. Digre K, Corbett JJ. Hemifacial spasm: differential diagnosis, mechanism, and treatment. *Adv Neurol* 1988; **49**: 151–76.

43. Nagatani T, Inao S, Suzuki Y, Yoshida J. Perforating branches from offending arteries in hemifacial spasm: anatomical correlation with vertebrobasilar configuration. *J Neurol Neurosurg Psychiatry* 1999; **67**: 73–7. doi: 10.1136/jnnp.67.1.

44. Magnan J, Caces F, Locatelli P, Chays A. Hemifacial spasm: endoscopic vascular decompression. *Otolaryngol Head Neck Surg* 1997; **117**(4): 308–14.

45. Baquis GD, Pessin MS, Scott RM. Limb shaking – a carotid TIA. *Stroke* 1985; **16**: 444–8.

46. Ni J, Gao S, Cui LY *et al.* Characteristics of cerebral artery lesions in patients with limb-shaking transient ischemic attacks and its treatment. *Zhongguo Yi Xue Ke Xue Yuan Xue Bao* 2009; **31**(3): 344–8.

47. Kim HY, Chung CS, Lee J, Han DH, Lee KH. Hyperventilation-induced limb shaking TIA in Moyamoya disease. *Neurology* 2003; **60**(1): 137–9.

48. Lee SJ, Kim JS, Song IU, An JY, Kim YI, Lee KS. Poststroke restless legs syndrome and lesion location: anatomical considerations. *Mov Disord* 24(1): 77–84.

49. Critchley M. Arteriosclerotic parkinsonism. *Brain* 1929; **52**(23): 833–83.

50. Zijlmans JC, Daniel SE, Hughes AJ, Revesz T, Lees AJ. Clinicopathological investigation of vascular parkinsonism, including clinical criteria for diagnosis. *Mov Disord* 2004; **19**: 630–40.

51. Winikates J, Jankovic J. Clinical correlates of vascular parkinsonism. *Arch Neurol* 1999; **56**: 98–102.

52. Yamanouchi H, Nagura H. Neurological signs and frontal white matter lesions in vascular parkinsonism: a clinicopathologic study. *Stroke* 1997; **28**: 965–9.

53. Zijlmans J, Evans A, Fontes F *et al.* [123I]FP-CIT SPECT study in vascular parkinsonism and Parkinson's disease. *Mov Disord* 2007; **22**: 1278–85.

54. Mark MH, Sage JI, Walters AS, Duvoisin RC, Miller DC. Binswanger's disease presenting as levodopa-responsive parkinsonism: clinicopathologic study of three cases. *Mov Disord* 10(4): 450–4.

55. Kuo SH, Kenney C, Jankovic J. Bilateral pedunculopontine nuclei strokes presenting as freezing of gait. *Mov Dis* 2008; **23**(4): 616–19.

56. Wegner F, Strecker K, Schwarz J *et al.* Vascular parkinsonism in a CADASIL case with an intact nigrostriatal dopaminergic system. *J Neurol* 2007; **254**(12): 1743–5

57. Van Gerpen JA, Ahlskog JE, Petty GW. Progressive supranuclear palsy phenotype secondary to CADASIL. *Parkinsonism Relat Disord* 2003; **9**(6): 367–9.

58. Buechner S, Teresa M, De Cristofaro R, Ramat S, Borsini W. Parkinsonism and Anderson Fabry's disease: a case report. *Mov Disord* 2006; **21**(1): 103–7.

59. Scherfler C, Schwarz J, Antonini A *et al.* Role of DAT-SPECT in the diagnostic work up of parkinsonism. *Mov Disord* 2007; **22**(9): 1229–38.

60. Bandt SK, Anderson D, Biller J. Deep brain stimulation as an effective treatment option for post-midbrain infarction-related tremor as it presents with Benedikt syndrome. *J Neurosurg* 2008; **109**(4): 635–9.

61. Pahwa R, Factor SA, Lyons KE *et al.* Practice Parameter: Treatment of Parkinson disease with motor fluctuations and dyskinesia (an evidence-based review). Report of the Quality Standards Subcommittee of the American Academy of Neurology. *Neurology* 2006; **66**(7): 983–95.

62. Garcia-Ruiz P. Calcium channel blocker-induced parkinsonism: clinical features and comparison with Parkinson's disease. *Parkinsonism Relat Disord* 1998; **4**(4): 211–14.

63. Wilson TW, Rajput AH. Amantadine-dyazide interaction. *Can Med Assoc J* 1983; **129**(9): 974–5.

64. Tariq M, Khan HA, Moutaery KA, Deeb SA. Dipyridamole potentiates 1-methyl-4-phenyl-1,2,3,6-tetrahydropyridine (MPTP)-induced experimental Parkinsonism in mice. *Parkinsonism Relat Disord* 1998; **4**(1): 43–50.

65. Blunt SB, Brooks DJ, Kennard C. Steroid-responsive chorea in childhood following cardiac transplantation. *Mov Disord* 1994; **9**(1): 112–14.

66. Oates JA, Lovett JK, Gutowski NJ. An aspirin responsive non-progressive chronic chorea. *J Neurol Neurosurg Psychiatry* 2006; **77**(2): 277–8.

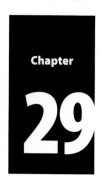

Chapter

29

Neuro-ophthalmologic alterations in patients with movement disorders

Jan Kassubek and Elmar H. Pinkhardt

Introduction

Neuro-ophthalmologic disorders may arise from all areas of the neuro-ophthalmologic tracts. They may be expressed simply as loss of vision or double vision or as complex syndromes or systemic illnesses, depending on the location and type of lesion. Although neuro-ophthalmologic manifestations in movement disorders are manifold, the particular deficits that can be observed in the different entities of movement disorders are closely related to the major neuropathological changes of the single diseases with alterations of brain stem areas, basal ganglia and cerebellar structures. A substantial influence of cortical areas on oculomotor function has to be assumed. Hence the main focus in neuro-ophthalmologic changes in association with movement disorders is oculomotor dysfunction rather than alterations of vision [1]. In order to gain a better understanding of these disturbances, it is important to visualize the basic neurophysiologic characteristics of oculomotor function so that a short survey of the neurophysiologic background of eye movement generation will be given, before movement disorders with prominent neuro-ophthalmologic manifestations will be described in detail.

Neurophysiology of eye movement control

In general the brain areas and related functional brain pathways that are predominantly perturbed in movement disorders – at least with respect to major elements of the clinical presentation – are the basal ganglia, their connections to higher cortical regions and cerebellar areas that have to be considered as most important for alterations of saccadic eye movements and smooth pursuit [2]. Smooth pursuit eye movements (SPEM) and saccadic eye movements are generally seen as two distinct systems; nevertheless they may be assumed as different outcomes from a shared cascade of sensori-motor functions [2–5]. According to saccade generation, brain stem neurons in the pontine paramedian reticular formation (PPRF) and in the rostral interstitial nucleus of the medial longitudinal fasciculus (riMLF) play a substantial role [2]. Saccade generation is triggered by signals from cerebellar areas (predominantly the dorsal vermis and caudal fastigial nucleus) as well as the bilateral superior colliculus (SC). In addition, cortical areas influence saccade generation, namely, the saccade subregion of the frontal eye field, the supplementary eye field, the dorsolateral prefrontal cortex (DLPFC), the parietal eye field and area 7a in the parietal cortex; furthermore, cerebellar structures are involved in the regulation and correction of saccades [6–10]. Brain structures that are necessary for SPEM are the striate cortex with projections to extrastriate areas including area V5, the frontal eye fields, and their subcortical projections such as the posterior limb of the internal capsule, the midbrain and the basal pontine nuclei as well as the ventral paraflocculus and caudal vermis of the cerebellum [11,12].

Parkinson disease

As we know today, the neurobiological changes in Parkinson disease (PD) go far beyond a mere loss of dopaminergic neurons in the substantia nigra [13], since in fact the neuropathological process is distributed throughout the entire nervous system. Braak and co-workers have established a staging scheme with PD-related pathology and progression in a topographically predictable sequence. In stages 1–2, inclusion body pathology includes the medulla oblongata and pontine tegmentum as well as the olfactory system/olfactory bulb. The typical motor impairment in PD does not appear before stages 3–4 when the substantia

Uncommon Causes of Movement Disorders, ed. Néstor Gálvez-Jiménez and Paul J. Tuite. Published by Cambridge University Press. © Cambridge University Press 2011.

nigra and other nuclear grays of the midbrain and fore-brain become the focus of disease progression. In the stages 5–6, the process enters the mature neocortex, and the disease manifests itself in all of its clinical dimensions [14–17]. Although not fully understood yet, the pathology of PD involves, among others, noradrenergic and serotonergic projections to the striatum as well as to cortical areas. The neuropathology beyond the dopaminergic system may be seen as the basis for several non-motor clinical features of PD [18], including a substantial impact on oculomotor dysfunction in PD.

The major eye movement pathology in PD can be found in the saccadic system. A distinction between visually triggered reflexive (exogenous) and voluntary (endogenous) saccades is made. Visually triggered (exogenous) saccades are mediated by the superior colliculus, with important inputs from the visual and posterior parietal cortices [19–21]. Voluntary saccades rely upon pathways including frontal cortical areas and the basal ganglia [22–25]. On the one hand, reflexive saccades are described as nearly normal in PD; on the other, a PD-associated disinhibition of reflexive saccades generation is postulated. Voluntary saccades show increased latency, sometimes hypometria, and impaired voluntary suppression of unwanted saccades [8,26–29]. Regarding predominant neuropathology of PD, it seems to be proven that the substantia nigra pars reticulata (SNr) and related brain stem areas play a crucial role in eye movement pathology via an altered dopamine-mediated function of the SC due to impaired SNr input [17, 27,28,30]. The SNr contains saccade-related neurons in monkeys and in cats [26,27] and shows a strong interaction with the SC. Nevertheless, changes in the basal ganglia network and its connections to the SC cannot fully explain the manifold manifestations of eye movement pathology in PD. Amador and co-workers [26,29] suggest a "tonic inhibition model of orienting" that proposes a voluntary system including prefrontal cortex and basal ganglia that exerts tonic inhibition on a reflexive system including the SC and brain stem while the voluntary system modulates reflexive saccades and attention. Within this model, a deficit in the voluntary system predicts both impaired performance in voluntary saccades and decreased inhibition of reflexive saccades. Additionally, Van Stockum et al. [31] describe a pattern of correlation between eye movement measurements and neuropsychological data that suggests more than one source of saccadic disinhibition in PD. They speculate that some aspects of saccadic impairment may be associated with an attention deficit in terms of altered cognitive function. Chan et al. [30] propose cognitive alterations, namely, deficits in the DLFPC, to be crucial in saccadic dysfunction in that they point out that the DLPFC receives significant input from SNr via the thalamus. Thus, PD-associated loss of input to the striatum leads to the disruption of this prefrontal cortex–basal ganglia circuitry, resulting in impairment in both automatic response suppression and working memory processes involved in the generation of voluntary saccades. However, the question remains open whether the frontal brain deficits in PD patients performing oculomotor tasks are the result of the striatal pathophysiology alone or whether this includes additional direct pathology of frontal cortical areas.

SPEM may also be altered in PD. It may be assumed that SPEM deficits and saccadic deficits in PD arise from the same pathological changes [32]. Notably, there does not seem to be a fundamental inability in PD patients to generate normal SPEM. Pinkhardt et al. [33] showed that most PD patients were indeed able to perform normal smooth pursuit – yet with repeatedly interspersed anticipatory saccades that moved the eyes ahead of the target toward its future anticipated position. Hence, in contrast to disorders with the pathology of the olivo-ponto-cerebellar circuits like multiple system atrophy (MSA) (see below), the saccades within SPEM in PD were not necessitated by a low SPEM gain but were the cause of it. These results support the view that anticipatory saccades during tracking of targets arise from the inability of PD patients to inhibit inherent response tendencies, which is again considered one of the core functions of the DLPFC [32,34]. Thus, disinhibition of frontostriatal circuits may add substantially to SPEM pathology as well as saccadic dysfunction in PD. Although more frequently associated with atypical Parkinsonian syndromes such as progressive supranuclear palsy (PSP) and MSA, square-wave jerks (SWJ) are also observed in PD [4]. Square-wave jerks seem to occur more frequently in PD patients with more severe freezing, postural instability and falls, hence SWJ presumably are correlated with non-motor symptoms outside the dopaminergic pathways in PD.

In summary, the neuropathology of neuro-ophthalmologic changes in PD appears to be complex. On the one hand, there is no doubt that PD-associated dopaminergic depletion with loss of dopaminergic input to the striatum will lead to the disruption of a prefrontal-basal ganglial circuitry that is crucial to various aspects of oculomotor function. On the other hand, an impaired nondopaminergic top-down mechanism of oculomotor control from higher cerebral cortical areas, predominantly frontal and parietal areas, to basal ganglia structures such as the striatum has to be assumed [30] that might be closely linked to cognitive dysfunction in PD.

With respect to the amount of nondopaminergically driven influences on oculomotor function in PD, it is important to consider possible alterations of pharmacological (in particular dopaminergic) therapy or surgical therapy (deep brain stimulation) on eye movement pathology. The literature about the effects of levodopa treatment on eye movement deficits in PD is heterogeneous. Moreover, there are a number of methodological concerns that limit the interpretation and comparability of these studies. Among other things, the use of different testing procedures, failure to counterbalance "on" and "off" medication order of testing, as well as the use of different medications and withdrawal regimes are challenging. Both vast positive effects on latency, gain or amplitude of saccades [35,36] and no effect of dopaminergic drugs [37,38] have been reported in recent literature. Hood et al. [39] reported a significantly increased response time for reflexive pro-saccades and a reduced error rate for voluntary anti-saccades with dopaminergic treatment. They conclude that – in accordance with the tonic inhibition model – levodopa improves function of the voluntary frontostriatal system. Michell et al. [40], who used a testing paradigm that was neither merely reflexive nor voluntary, described a prolongation of saccadic latency distribution due to levodopa treatment, but with a high intersubject variability. They hypothesize that the longer latency of saccades is based on a complex interaction of cortical and subcortical regions of the brain with a predominant effect of dopamine in the frontal or parietal eye fields. In summary, the effects of dopamine on eye movement deficits in PD remain incompletely understood.

Few studies have yet been performed to investigate the influence of deep brain stimulation (DBS) on oculomotor function in PD. Rivaud-Pechoux et al. [41] report a positive effect of stimulation of the subthalamic nucleus (STN) on memorized saccade deficits. They attribute this effect to a modulation of neuronal activity in the DLPFC by STN stimulation. Sauleau et al. [42] elicited beneficial effects on eye and head movements with improvement in gain and latency of voluntary orienting saccades as well as in visually triggered saccades. The authors concluded

that deep brain stimulation of the STN improves the abnormal STN activity in late stages of PD that affects the functioning of the nigrostriatal pathways (i.e., SNr influences on the SC). The most relevant connections might be considered the glutaminergic STN projections to the SNr, which contain neurons that decrease their activity in association with saccades (43,44) and in turn generate SC disinhibition that again is part of the descending pathway from the cortex to the striatum. Alternatively, a positive influence on the parietal cortex–SC pathway might be assumed. Temel et al. [45] examined saccadic latency and found a markedly improved saccadic latency after DBS of the STN, whereas dopaminergic medication increased the latency. Recently, Temel et al. [46] examined the therapeutic effect of DBS by means of saccadic latency distribution changes. They found, both at the group level and for each individual patient, that median latency was shorter with STN stimulation. They concluded that electrical stimulation of the STN enhances both the descending facilitation that passes from the cortex to the colliculus via the basal ganglia and also the tonic background inhibition that suppresses unwanted early responses. However, the high interindividual variability of oculomotor symptoms in PD, its only loose correlation with the severity of major dopaminergic deficits (i.e., motor symptoms), the varying reports about the effect of dopaminergic medication on oculomotor function, and growing evidence for a possibly nondopaminergic influence of frontal lobe pathology remain incompletely understood and need further investigation.

Multiple system atrophy

In multiple system atrophy (MSA), a cerebellar subtype (MSA-C) with predominant olivopontocerebellar atrophy (OPCA) and a parkinsonian subtype (MSA-P) with mainly striatonigral degeneration (SND) are distinguished [47]. With respect to oculomotor disturbances, it is important to know that signs of cerebellar dysfunction in a predominantly akinetic rigid patient are common since simultaneous SND and OPCD may be observed in 49% of all MSA patients. Eye movement alterations in MSA are in close correspondence with the underlying focus of pathoanatomical distribution of the disease; hence clinical evidence of prominent oculomotor deficits point to a predominant OPCD. The cerebellar vermis, the vestibulocerebellum and the corresponding pontine nuclei are vital elements of the oculomotor pathway, i.e., dysfunctions of these structures as evident in MSA reduce SPEM gain and necessitate catch-up saccades [4,33,48].

According to Anderson *et al.* [49], pathologies described as unique to MSA (in comparison with the other major parkinsonian syndromes like PD, PSP or corticobasal syndrome [CBS]) are positioning downbeat nystagmus and gaze-evoked nystagmus. SPEM impairment that occurs in all parkinsonian syndromes though with different neuropathological background can be observed in the great majority of MSA patients. Other common findings are excessive square-wave jerks, mild to moderate saccadic hypometria, and impaired vestibulo-ocular reflex suppression (VORS). Positioning downbeat nystagmus (DBN) was present in 40% of patients, including some patients who had no other signs of cerebellar involvement. In particular, the presence of cerebellar-type eye movement disorders, including gaze-evoked nystagmus, abnormal VORS and positioning DBN, points to MSA in a differential diagnostic approach to other parkinsonian syndromes. With respect to the often challenging differential diagnosis of early MSA versus PD, a close inspection of the saccadic component of pursuit tracking may help. A recent study by Pinkhardt *et al.* [33] revealed that saccades within SPEM in MSA typically correct for positioning errors that accumulate during SPEM (catch-up saccades), whereas saccades in PD are often directed toward an anticipated target position (anticipatory saccades). These differences are described as large enough to warrant their use as diagnostic criteria between these disorders.

Tauopathies with parkinsonism

Tauopathies are a group of neurodegenerative diseases with prominent tau pathology in the central nervous system. The diseases can be subdivided into groups with predominant parkinsonism, dementia with signs of frontal lobe dysfunction, or motor neuron pathology. There is ongoing discussion whether these diseases share fundamental overlapping pathogenetic aspects or whether the term tauopathy is justified simply for practical reasons because the clinical phenotypes are related. The clinical spectrum of tauopathies comprises among others progressive supranuclear palsy, corticobasal degeneration, frontotemporal dementia (with parkinsonism), Pick disease and Niemann–Pick disease type C [50]. Ocular motor abnormalities play an important role in the differential diagnoses of these diseases.

Progressive supranuclear palsy

The eponymous vertical gaze palsy is a core clinical feature in the diagnosis of progressive supranuclear palsy (PSP) [51,52]. Nevertheless, the clinical feature described as "vertical gaze palsy" proves to be a reduction of vertical and also – to a lower degree – of horizontal saccadic maximum velocity and gain if examined carefully, e.g., via video-oculography [53]. Regarding the pathophysiology of slow vertical saccades in PSP, two hypotheses have been proposed. First, consistent with the distribution of neuropathological findings in the midbrain in PSP [54], it is proposed that the burst neurons in the rostral interstitial nucleus of the medial longitudinal fasciculus (riMLF) cannot generate an adequate saccadic command. Second, it is suggested that omnipause neurons cause slow vertical saccades, presumably by disrupting the normal activation sequence of burst neurons [55]. The findings of a more pronounced slowing of vertical saccades in comparison with horizontal saccades in PSP are consistent with the proposed dysfunction of burst neurons in the riMLF, since it is known that riMLF pathology causes loss of vertical saccades whereas horizontal saccades are less affected [56].

Recent literature suggests a further differentiation of the clinical PSP syndrome into Richardson syndrome (RS), which corresponds well to "classical" PSP, and a clinically milder syndrome formerly characterized as atypical PSP with asymmetric onset, tremor and initial response to levodopa, which is now described as PSP-parkinsonism (PSP-P) [52,57,58]. Neuropathological studies underline this distinction by showing that PSP-P differs from RS by its restricted, mild tau pathology. Noticeably, a clinically assessable vertical gaze palsy is not described as a leading symptom in PSP-P [57]. Nevertheless, similar oculomotor deficits have been shown in both RS and PSP-P, with a prominent decreased saccadic velocity (vertical > horizontal) as well as decreased gain of saccades and SPEM, already in the early course of the disease when motor symptoms of PSP-P still are very similar to PD [53].

Corticobasal syndrome

Corticobasal syndrome (CBS), or corticobasal degeneration, has been reported to be associated with increased saccadic latency. Slow vertical saccades may occur as the disease advances, but usually this is less pronounced than is seen with PSP. Similarly to patients with PSP, patients with atypical CBS features (corticobasal syndrome) exhibit clinically evident abnormalities of vertical saccades and early slowing of horizontal saccade velocity but no increase in saccade latency or early SWJ. An early decreased saccade velocity, early presence of SWJ, preservation of saccade latency, and paresis of vertical saccades strongly favor the diagnosis of PSP [41].

Frontotemporal lobe degeneration

Frontotemporal lobe degeneration (FTLD) manifests as one of three clinical syndromes. The frontal lobe variant is known as frontotemporal dementia (FTD), the temporal lobe variant with semantic memory loss, is known as semantic dementia (SD) and a third variant exhibits progressive nonfluent aphasia (PA). Patients with FTD and PA have deficits in performing anti-saccades and smooth pursuit eye movements. In these patients neuropathology lies predominantly in dorsal frontal lobe structures. A direct correlation is suggested between correct responses in an anti-saccade task and frontal lobe gray matter volume – most likely alterations in the DLPFC. However, patients with brain alterations limited to the anterior temporal lobe as in SD show an oculomotor performance that is similar to that of age-matched control subjects [59,60].

Frontotemporal dementia with parkinsonism

In FTD with parkinsonism linked to chromosome 17 (FTDP-17), an increasing number of mutations cause a wide spectrum of clinical presentations [50]. To the present, knowledge of oculomotor alterations in this disease remains limited; nevertheless, Moon *et al.* [61] report that a kind of vertical saccadic impairment was observed in 9 of 11 patients on bedside examination and could be verified as distinctive slowing of vertical saccades in comparison with controls by use of videooculography. Similarly to PSP, involvement of the burst neurons in the dorsal midbrain in patients with FTD-P is suggested. Future studies are needed to investigate the involvement of the dorsal midbrain in patients with FTD-P.

Niemann-Pick disease type C

Apart from cerebellar ataxia, different types of movement disorders and behavioral and cognitive deficits, vertical supranuclear ophthalmoplegia is one of the core clinical features of Niemann–Pick disease type C (NPC). Vertical eye movements are lost much earlier in the course of the illness than horizontal ones due to greater cell loss in the riMLF compared with the paramedian pontine reticular formation (PPRF) where horizontal saccades are generated [62–64]. Additional impairment of saccade control is described in NPC. Reduced reflexive saccade gain is described, most probably due to damage to the dorsal vermis of the cerebellum that is known to occur in NPC [65], but, surprisingly, saccade latency may be abnormally short in some patients with NPC, associated with anti-saccade errors. The neuropathological background for both of these alterations of oculomotor function might arise from frontal eye field pathology or pathological changes in pathways from the posterior parietal cortex to the superior colliculus [64]. In conclusion, both brain stem and frontal control of eye movements are impaired in adult NPC. The severity of these changes seems to reflect other illness variables in NPC.

Huntington disease

Huntington disease (HD) is caused by a CAG trinucleotide expansion of the IT15 gene, and the age of disease onset is determined by the number of CAG repeats. Oculomotor deficits in HD are more prominent in patients with early clinical onset, hence in patients with a higher number of CAG repeats [66]. Even presymptomatic gene carriers may demonstrate abnormalities in eye movement control [67,68]. The oculomotor deficits that are described in HD comprise alterations of fixation and saccades as well as smooth pursuit [69]. Impaired initiation of volitional saccades is considered to be a cardinal symptom of HD [70], and also a slowing of saccade velocity can be observed in many HD patients. Both parameters are progressive in the course of the disease. Saccade initiation may become affected to such an extent that patients have to utilize head movements in order to shift gaze, and even moderately impaired patients show an altered pattern of eye–head coordination in comparison with healthy subjects. Interestingly, the eye–head coordination itself is not at all affected in HD patients [69]. A variable pattern of brain structures is suggested to be involved in oculomotor pathology in HD. In accordance with HD-associated neurodegeneration in general, which is most prominent in the caudate nucleus, the caudate nucleus in turn is part of (fronto-)corticostriatal oculomotor pathways. Likewise, pontine degeneration could be at least partially responsible for the saccade slowing in early-affected HD patients; nevertheless, little is known about HD-neuropathology of pontine substructures that are part of oculomotor pathways like the paramedian pontine reticular formation, the raphe interpositus nucleus, or the medial longitudinal fasciculus. In presymptomatic carriers of the HD mutation, oculomotor abnormalities can be found that may point to a selective vulnerability of white matter tracts between the frontal cortex and the caudate nucleus in the presymptomatic phase, since the severity of the impairment of the voluntary-guided saccades seems to be correlated with altered connectivity between the frontal cortex and caudate body [71].

Choreoacanthocytosis

Oculomotor abnormalities have not been reviewed systematically in choreocanthocytosis (ChAc). Gradstein *et al.* [72] studied three patients and, although the study was limited due to the small cohort, the oculomotor findings suggest a brain stem involvement as an additional site of neurodegeneration outside the basal ganglia in ChAc. The patients exhibited hypometric horizontal and vertical saccades, decreased saccadic peak velocity as well as SWJ.

Pantothenate kinase-associated neurodegeneration

The main clinical characteristics of pantothenate kinase-associated neurodegeneration (PKAN) (formerly known as Hallervorden–Spatz syndrome) are dystonia, parkinsonism, iron accumulation in the brain, and sometimes retinopathy or optic neuropathy. In neuropathological investigations, the cardinal disease feature is the basal ganglial iron accumulation and loss of melanin, predominantly in the globus pallidus and SNr. Recently, Egan *et al.* reported Adie-like pupils, abnormal vertical saccades and saccadic pursuits to be very common in PKAN. These findings suggest that midbrain degeneration occurs in PKAN more frequently than previously thought. It may be that allelic differences contribute to the variable clinical expressions of ocular and oculomotor deficits in PKAN [73,74].

Wilson disease

Already in the first description by Wilson and then later Lennox *et al.* [75] there was reported some kind of "gaze distractibility" in patients with Wilson disease

(WD). Nevertheless, a wide range of eye movement alterations with diplopia, accommodation deficits, squint, upward gaze palsy, abnormal SPEM and external ophthalmoplegia have been reported in single cases of WD. More recently Lesniak *et al.* [76] as well as Ingster-Moati *et al.* [77] have investigated eye movement control in neurologically symptomatic and asymptomatic WD patients. They found that WD is associated with an impairment of voluntary control of saccades and with disturbed smooth pursuit eye movements while reflexive saccades seem to be preserved. They suggest an abnormal top-down inhibition of eye movements with concurrent intact reflexive saccades. The pattern of oculomotor disturbance in WD recalls the predominant findings of eye movement deficits in PD. Neurological, cognitive and psychopathological symptoms in WD are usually related to changes in the basal ganglia and other brain structures such as thalamus, midbrain, cerebellum, brain stem and prefrontal cortex [78]. Additionally, WD appears to be associated with a pre- and postsynaptic dopaminergic deficit with alterations of basal ganglia function [79,80]. Taking these observations into account, it may well be that the neuropathological mechanism underlying oculomotor disturbances in WD comprises alterations of frontal cortical pathology as well as damage to the basal ganglia [76].

Spinocerebellar ataxias

The heterogeneous group of spinocerebellar ataxias (SCAs) is frequently linked with oculomotor disturbances [81]. Especially in SCA2, a severe saccadic slowing occurs early in the course of the disease [82] and remains more prominent in comparison with other SCA subtypes. Altogether, oculomotor abnormalities are best described for SCA subtypes 1, 2, 3 and 6. In SCA1, a saccade slowing is also described. SCA6 exhibits downbeat nystagmus with impaired smooth pursuit but normal saccade velocities. Besides the deficits described above, SCA3 and SCA6 are more frequently linked with diplopia. SCA7 is commonly associated with progressive macular dystrophy, resulting in blindness as well as ophthalmoplegia. It is assumed that also for the oculomotor abnormalities in SCA subtypes that exhibit a CAG repeat pathology (SCA1, 2, 3, 6 and 7) in most instances, the size of the CAG repeat correlates with the severity of oculomotor symptoms (81,83,84). In SCA17, which is a rare type of autosomal dominant spinocerebellar ataxia caused by a CAG/CAA expansion, patients are reported to show a distinct pattern of oculomotor abnormalities, characterized by impairment of smooth pursuit, defects in the accuracy of saccades, normal saccade velocity, hyperreflexia of vestibulo-ocular reflexes, and absence of nystagmus [85].

In a pathophysiologic approach, Buttner *et al.* [81] conclude that the oculomotor findings in several common SCA subtypes are useful for clinical diagnosis and for investigating the mechanism of system specificity within the SCA syndromes, as specific neuropathological mechanisms can be linked to those diseases with pure cerebellar involvement in SCA6, pontine involvement in SCA1 and SCA2, and vestibular nerve or nuclei involvement in SCA3.

Tourette syndrome

Although the etiology of Tourette syndrome (TS) is still unknown, it has long been suspected that basal ganglia circuits are involved in its pathophysiology. Thus, alterations in cortico-striato-thalamo-cortical circuits and dopaminergic neurotransmission might play a major role in the pathophysiology of TS [86]. As basal ganglia circuits are important in saccade generation as well, it has been postulated that TS patients may exhibit an abnormal control of saccadic eye movements. Saccadic reaction times for pro- and anti-saccades are found to be elevated among TS patients. Additionally, eye movements made prior to a "go" signal in a delayed saccade task are seen to be increased in TS, indicating that the ability to inhibit or delay planned motor programs is significantly impaired in TS [87–90]. These findings are consistent with TS patients' difficulties in preventing unwanted movements [91].

Summary

In summary, oculomotor changes occur ubiquitously in the heterogeneous group of common and uncommon movement disorders. The oculomotor deficits are closely related to the specific neuropathological pattern of each disease. Nevertheless, as oculomotor function and movement generation in general share essential complex cerebral pathways with involvement of basal ganglial, cerebellar, brain stem and cortical areas, a large number of oculomotor deficits with pathology of saccade generation/control as well as SPEM deficits are phenotypically similar in several entities. Hence the differential diagnostic value of oculomotor function in these diseases seems to be limited with respect to bedside examination. Nevertheless, via thorough oculomotor investigation, i.e., by use of more subtle

techniques of acquisition of oculomotor function such as video-oculography (VOG), it is possible to elicit subtle differences that may substantially guide early differential diagnosis. In a comparison of the currently available methods of testing, VOG offers the best compromise between ease of use and accuracy of testing. As one example, the different type of saccadic pathology with anticipatory saccades in PD and catch-up saccades in MSA elicited via VOG reveal the different neuropathological backgrounds of these phenotypically similar alterations of SPEM, with predominant cerebellar pathology in MSA and fronto-striato-nigral pathology in PD, even in the early course of the disease. Thus, VOG-guided investigations of oculomotor alterations are a valuable differential diagnostic tool in movement disorders on the one hand, and on the other might help to deepen our pathoanatomical understanding of functional networks deficits in the course of the particular diseases.

References

1. Hamilton SR. Neuro-ophthalmology of movement disorders. *Curr Opin Ophthalmol* 2000; **11**(6): 403–7.

2. Wong A. *Eye Movement Disorders*. 14th ed. Oxford: Oxford University Press; 2008.

3. Bronstein AM, Mossman S, Luxon LM. The neck-eye reflex in patients with reduced vestibular and optokinetic function. *Brain* 1991; **114**(Pt 1A): 1–11.

4. Leigh RJ, Zee DS. *The Neurology of Eye Movements*. 4th ed. Oxford: Oxford University Press; 2006.

5. Waterston JA, Barnes GR, Grealy MA, Collins S. Abnormalities of smooth eye and head movement control in Parkinson's disease. *Ann Neurol* 1996; **39**(6): 749–60.

6. Izawa Y, Suzuki H, Shinoda Y. Response properties of fixation neurons and their location in the frontal eye field in the monkey. *J Neurophysiol* 2009; **102**(4): 2410–22.

7. McDowell JE, Dyckman KA, Austin BP, Clementz BA. Neurophysiology and neuroanatomy of reflexive and volitional saccades: evidence from studies of humans. *Brain Cogn* 2008; **68**(3): 255–70.

8. Mikami A, Ito S, Kubota K. Visual response properties of dorsolateral prefrontal neurons during visual fixation task. *J Neurophysiol* 1982; **47**(4): 593–605.

9. Muri RM, Nyffeler T. Neurophysiology and neuroanatomy of reflexive and volitional saccades as revealed by lesion studies with neurological patients and transcranial magnetic stimulation (TMS). *Brain Cogn* 2008; **68**(3): 284–92.

10. Vidailhet M, Rivaud S, Gouider-Khouja N *et al.* Eye movements in parkinsonian syndromes. *Ann Neurol* 1994; **35**(4): 420–6.

11. Cazzoli D, Muri RM, Hess CW, Nyffeler T. Horizontal and vertical dimensions of visual extinction: a theta burst stimulation study. *Neuroscience* 2009; **164**(4): 1609–14.

12. Dieterich M, Muller-Schunk S, Stephan T, Bense S, Seelos K, Yousry TA. Functional magnetic resonance imaging activations of cortical eye fields during saccades, smooth pursuit, and optokinetic nystagmus. *Ann N Y Acad Sci* 2009; **1164**: 282–92.

13. Poewe W. The natural history of Parkinson's disease. *J Neurol* 2006; **253**(Suppl 7): VII2–6.

14. Braak H, Bohl JR, Muller CM, Rub U, de Vos RA, Del Tredici K. Stanley Fahn Lecture 2005: The staging procedure for the inclusion body pathology associated with sporadic Parkinson's disease reconsidered. *Mov Disord* 2006; **21**(12): 2042–51.

15. Braak H, Del Tredici K. Invited Article: Nervous system pathology in sporadic Parkinson disease. *Neurology* 2008; **70**(20): 1916–25.

16. Braak H, Muller CM, Rub U *et al.* Pathology associated with sporadic Parkinson's disease – where does it end? *J Neural Transm Suppl* 2006; (70): 89–97.

17. Lang AE, Obeso JA. Challenges in Parkinson's disease: restoration of the nigrostriatal dopamine system is not enough. *Lancet Neurol* 2004; **3**(5): 309–16.

18. Salman MS, Sharpe JA, Lillakas L, Steinbach MJ. Square wave jerks in children and adolescents. *Pediatr Neurol* 2008; **38**(1): 16–19.

19. Serra A, Dell'Osso LF, Jacobs JB, Burnstine RA. Combined gaze-angle and vergence variation in infantile nystagmus: two therapies that improve the high-visual-acuity field and methods to measure it. *Invest Ophthalmol Vis Sci* 2006; **47**(6): 2451–60.

20. Sprenger A, Neppert B, Koster S *et al.* Long-term eye movement recordings with a scleral search coil-eyelid protection device allows new applications. *J Neurosci Methods* 2008; **170**(2): 305–9.

21. van der Geest JN, Frens MA. Recording eye movements with video-oculography and scleral search coils: a direct comparison of two methods. *J Neurosci Methods* 2002; **114**(2): 185–95.

22. Eggert T. Eye movement recordings: methods. *Dev Ophthalmol* 2007; **40**: 15–34.

23. Houben MM, Goumans J, van der Steen J. Recording three-dimensional eye movements: scleral search coils versus video oculography. *Invest Ophthalmol Vis Sci* 2006; **47**(1): 179–87.

24. Kimmig H, Greenlee MW, Gondan M, Schira M, Kassubek J, Mergner T. Relationship between saccadic eye movements and cortical activity as measured by fMRI: quantitative and qualitative aspects. *Exp Brain Res* 2001; **141**(2): 184–94.

25. Kimmig H, Ohlendorf S, Speck O *et al.* fMRI evidence for sensorimotor transformations in human cortex during smooth pursuit eye movements. *Neuropsychologia* 2008; **46**(8): 2203–13.

26. Amador SC, Hood AJ, Schiess MC, Izor R, Sereno AB. Dissociating cognitive deficits involved in voluntary eye movement dysfunctions in Parkinson's disease patients. *Neuropsychologia* 2006; **44**(8): 1475–82.

27. Armstrong IT, Chan F, Riopelle RJ, Munoz DP. Control of saccades in Parkinson's disease. *Brain Cogn* 2002; **49**(2): 198–201.

28. Briand KA, Strallow D, Hening W, Poizner H, Sereno AB. Control of voluntary and reflexive saccades in Parkinson's disease. *Exp Brain Res* 1999; **129**(1): 38–48.

29. Rieger JW, Kim A, Argyelan M *et al.* Cortical functional anatomy of voluntary saccades in Parkinson disease. *Clin EEG Neurosci* 2008; **39**(4): 169–74.

30. Chan F, Armstrong IT, Pari G, Riopelle RJ, Munoz DP. Deficits in saccadic eye-movement control in Parkinson's disease. *Neuropsychologia* 2005; **43**(5): 784–96.

31. van Stockum S, MacAskill M, Anderson T, Dalrymple-Alford J. Don't look now or look away: two sources of saccadic disinhibition in Parkinson's disease? *Neuropsychologia* 2008; **46**(13): 3108–15.

32. Pierrot-Deseilligny C, Muri RM, Nyffeler T, Milea D. The role of the human dorsolateral prefrontal cortex in ocular motor behavior. *Ann N Y Acad Sci* 2005; **1039**: 239–51.

33. Pinkhardt EH, Kassubek J, Sussmuth S, Ludolph AC, Becker W, Jurgens R. Comparison of smooth pursuit eye movement deficits in multiple system atrophy and Parkinson's disease. *J Neurol* 2009; **256**(9): 1438–46.

34. Pierrot-Deseilligny C, Muri RM, Ploner CJ, Gaymard B, Demeret S, Rivaud-Pechoux S. Decisional role of the dorsolateral prefrontal cortex in ocular motor behaviour. *Brain* 2003; **126**(Pt 6): 1460–73.

35. Rascol O, Clanet M, Montastruc JL *et al.* Abnormal ocular movements in Parkinson's disease: evidence for involvement of dopaminergic systems. *Brain* 1989; **112**(Pt 5): 1193–214.

36. Vermersch AI, Rivaud S, Vidailhet M *et al.* Sequences of memory-guided saccades in Parkinson's disease. *Ann Neurol* 1994; **35**(4): 487–90.

37. Crevits L, Versijpt J, Hanse M, De Ridder K. Antisaccadic effects of a dopamine agonist as add-on therapy in advanced Parkinson's patients. *Neuropsychobiology* 2000; **42**(4): 202–6.

38. Gibson JM, Kennard C. Quantitative study of "on-off" fluctuations in the ocular motor system in Parkinson's disease. *Adv Neurol* 1987; **45**: 329–33.

39. Hood AJ, Amador SC, Cain AE *et al.* Levodopa slows prosaccades and improves antisaccades: an eye movement study in Parkinson's disease. *J Neurol Neurosurg Psychiatry* 2007; **78**(6): 565–70.

40. Michell AW, Xu Z, Fritz D *et al*. Saccadic latency distributions in Parkinson's disease and the effects of L-dopa. *Exp Brain Res* 2006; **174**(1): 7–18.

41. Rivaud-Pechoux S, Vidailhet M, Gallouedec G, Litvan I, Gaymard B, Pierrot-Deseilligny C. Longitudinal ocular motor study in corticobasal degeneration and progressive supranuclear palsy. *Neurology* 2000; **54**(5): 1029–32.

42. Sauleau P, Pollak P, Krack P *et al*. Subthalamic stimulation improves orienting gaze movements in Parkinson's disease. *Clin Neurophysiol* 2008; **119**(8): 1857–63.

43. Hikosaka O. Role of basal ganglia in saccades. *Rev Neurol (Paris)* 1989; **145**(8–9): 580–6.

44. Hikosaka O, Takikawa Y, Kawagoe R. Role of the basal ganglia in the control of purposive saccadic eye movements. *Physiol Rev* 2000; **80**(3): 953–78.

45. Temel Y, Visser-Vandewalle V, Carpenter RH. Saccadic latency during electrical stimulation of the human subthalamic nucleus. *Curr Biol* 2008; **18**(10): R412–4.

46. Temel Y, Visser-Vandewalle V, Carpenter RH. Saccadometry: a novel clinical tool for quantification of the motor effects of subthalamic nucleus stimulation in Parkinson's disease. *Exp Neurol* 2009; **216**(2): 481–9.

47. Yoshida M, Sone M. Mechanism of neuronal degeneration of multiple system atrophy. *Brain Nerve* 2009; **61**(9): 1051–60.

48. Pierrot-Deseilligny C, Muri RM, Ploner CJ, Gaymard B, Rivaud-Pechoux S. Cortical control of ocular saccades in humans: a model for motricity. *Prog Brain Res* 2003; **142**: 3–17.

49. Anderson T, Luxon L, Quinn N, Daniel S, Marsden CD, Bronstein A. Oculomotor function in multiple system atrophy: clinical and laboratory features in 30 patients. *Mov Disord* 2008; **23**(7): 977–84.

50. Ludolph AC, Kassubek J, Landwehrmeyer BG *et al*. Tauopathies with parkinsonism: clinical spectrum, neuropathologic basis, biological markers, and treatment options. *Eur J Neurol* 2009; **16**(3): 297–309.

51. Steele JC, Richardson JC, Olszewski J. Progressive supranuclear palsy: a heterogeneous degeneration involving the brain stem, basal ganglia and cerebellum with vertical gaze and pseudobulbar palsy, nuchal dystonia and dementia. *Arch Neurol* 1964; **10**: 333–59.

52. Williams DR, Lees AJ, Wherrett JR, Steele JC. J. Clifford Richardson and 50 years of progressive supranuclear palsy. *Neurology* 2008; **70**(7): 566–73.

53. Pinkhardt EH, Jurgens R, Becker W, Valdarno F, Ludolph AC, Kassubek J. Differential diagnostic value of eye movement recording in PSP-parkinsonism, Richardson's syndrome, and idiopathic Parkinson's disease. *J Neurol* 2008; **255**(12): 1916–25.

54. Morris HR, Wood NW, Lees AJ. Progressive supranuclear palsy (Steele–Richardson–Olszewski disease). *Postgrad Med J* 1999; **75**(888): 579–84.

55. Revesz T, Sangha H, Daniel SE. The nucleus raphe interpositus in the Steele-Richardson–Olszewski syndrome (progressive supranuclear palsy). *Brain* 1996; **119**(Pt 4): 1137–43.

56. Suzuki Y, Buttner-Ennever JA, Straumann D, Hepp K, Hess BJ, Henn V. Deficits in torsional and vertical rapid eye movements and shift of Listing's plane after uni- and bilateral lesions of the rostral interstitial nucleus of the medial longitudinal fasciculus. *Exp Brain Res* 1995; **106**(2): 215–32.

57. Williams DR, de Silva R, Paviour DC *et al*. Characteristics of two distinct clinical phenotypes in pathologically proven progressive supranuclear palsy: Richardson's syndrome and PSP-parkinsonism. *Brain* 2005; **128**(Pt 6): 1247–58.

58. Williams DR, Holton JL, Strand C *et al*. Pathological tau burden and distribution distinguishes progressive supranuclear palsy-parkinsonism from Richardson's syndrome. *Brain* 2007; **130**(Pt 6): 1566–76.

59. Boxer AL, Garbutt S, Rankin KP *et al*. Medial versus lateral frontal lobe contributions to voluntary saccade control as revealed by the study of patients with frontal lobe degeneration. *J Neurosci* 2006; **26**(23): 6354–63.

60. Garbutt S, Matlin A, Hellmuth J *et al*. Oculomotor function in frontotemporal lobar degeneration, related disorders and Alzheimer's disease. *Brain* 2008; **131**(Pt 5): 1268–81.

61. Moon SY, Lee BH, Seo SW, Kang SJ, Na DL. Slow vertical saccades in the frontotemporal dementia with motor neuron disease. *J Neurol* 2008; **255**(9): 1337–43.

62. Abel LA, Walterfang M, Fietz M, Bowman EA, Velakoulis D. Saccades in adult Niemann–Pick disease type C reflect frontal, brainstem, and biochemical deficits. *Neurology* 2009; **72**(12): 1083–6.

63. Rottach KG, von Maydell RD, Das VE *et al*. Evidence for independent feedback control of horizontal and vertical saccades from Niemann–Pick type C disease. *Vision Res* 1997; **37**(24): 3627–38.

64. Solomon D, Winkelman AC, Zee DS, Gray L, Buttner-Ennever J. Niemann–Pick type C disease in two affected sisters: ocular motor recordings and brain-stem neuropathology. *Ann N Y Acad Sci* 2005; **1039**: 436–45.

65. Walterfang M, Fietz M, Abel L, Bowman E, Mocellin R, Velakoulis D. Gender dimorphism in siblings with schizophrenia-like psychosis due to Niemann–Pick disease type C. *J Inherit Metab Dis* 2009 Jul 17. doi:10.1007/s10545-009-1173-1.

66. Bithell A, Johnson R, Buckley NJ. Transcriptional dysregulation of coding and non-coding genes in cellular models of Huntington's disease. *Biochem Soc Trans* 2009; **37**(Pt 6): 1270–5.

67. Tabrizi SJ, Langbehn DR, Leavitt BR *et al*. Biological and clinical manifestations of Huntington's disease in the longitudinal TRACK-HD study: cross-sectional

analysis of baseline data. *Lancet Neurol* 2009; **8**(9): 791–801.

68. Kirkwood SC, Siemers E, Stout JC *et al.* Longitudinal cognitive and motor changes among presymptomatic Huntington disease gene carriers. *Arch Neurol* 1999; **56**(5): 563–8.

69. Becker W, Jurgens R, Kassubek J, Ecker D, Kramer B, Landwehrmeyer B. Eye–head coordination in moderately affected Huntington's disease patients: do head movements facilitate gaze shifts? *Exp Brain Res* 2009; **192**(1): 97–112.

70. Leigh RJ, Newman SA, Folstein SE, Lasker AG, Jensen BA. Abnormal ocular motor control in Huntington's disease. *Neurology* 1983; **33**(10): 1268–75.

71. Kloppel S, Draganski B, Golding CV *et al.* White matter connections reflect changes in voluntary-guided saccades in pre-symptomatic Huntington's disease. *Brain* 2008; **131**(Pt 1): 196–204.

72. Gradstein L, Danek A, Grafman J, Fitzgibbon EJ. Eye movements in chorea-acanthocytosis. *Invest Ophthalmol Vis Sci* 2005; **46**(6): 1979–87.

73. Egan RA, Weleber RG, Hogarth P *et al.* Neuro-ophthalmologic and electroretinographic findings in pantothenate kinase-associated neurodegeneration (formerly Hallervorden–Spatz syndrome). *Am J Ophthalmol* 2005; **140**(2): 267–74.

74. Hayflick SJ. Unraveling the Hallervorden–Spatz syndrome: pantothenate kinase-associated neurodegeneration is the name. *Curr Opin Pediatr* 2003; **15**(6): 572–7.

75. Lennox G, Jones R. Gaze distractibility in Wilson's disease. *Ann Neurol* 1989; **25**(4): 415–7.

76. Lesniak M, Czlonkowska A, Seniow J. Abnormal antisaccades and smooth pursuit eye movements in patients with Wilson's disease. *Mov Disord* 2008; **23**(14): 2067–73.

77. Ingster-Moati I, Bui Quoc E, Pless M *et al.* Ocular motility and Wilson's disease: a study on 34 patients. *J Neurol Neurosurg Psychiatry* 2007; **78**(11): 1199–201.

78. Oder W, Prayer L, Grimm G *et al.* Wilson's disease: evidence of subgroups derived from clinical findings and brain lesions. *Neurology* 1993; **43**(1): 120–4.

79. Barthel H, Hermann W, Kluge R *et al.* Concordant pre- and postsynaptic deficits of dopaminergic neurotransmission in neurologic Wilson disease. *AJNR Am J Neuroradiol* 2003; **24**(2): 234–8.

80. Kitzberger R, Madl C, Ferenci P. Wilson disease. *Metab Brain Dis* 2005; **20**(4): 295–302.

81. Buttner N, Geschwind D, Jen JC, Perlman S, Pulst SM, Baloh RW. Oculomotor phenotypes in autosomal dominant ataxias. *Arch Neurol* 1998; **55**(10): 1353–7.

82. Wadia N, Pang J, Desai J, Mankodi A, Desai M, Chamberlain S. A clinicogenetic analysis of six Indian spinocerebellar ataxia (SCA2) pedigrees. The significance of slow saccades in diagnosis. *Brain* 1998; **121**(Pt 12): 2341–55.

83. Ohyagi Y, Yamada T, Okayama A *et al.* Vergence disorders in patients with spinocerebellar ataxia 3/Machado–Joseph disease: a synoptophore study. *J Neurol Sci* 2000; **173**(2): 120–3.

84. Schols L, Amoiridis G, Buttner T, Przuntek H, Epplen JT, Riess O. Autosomal dominant cerebellar ataxia: phenotypic differences in genetically defined subtypes? *Ann Neurol* 1997; **42**(6): 924–32.

85. Mariotti C, Alpini D, Fancellu R *et al.* Spinocerebellar ataxia type 17 (SCA17): oculomotor phenotype and clinical characterization of 15 Italian patients. *J Neurol* 2007; **254**(11): 1538–46.

86. Gilbert DL, Christian BT, Gelfand MJ, Shi B, Mantil J, Sallee FR. Altered mesolimbocortical and thalamic dopamine in Tourette syndrome. *Neurology* 2006; **67**(9): 1695–7.

87. LeVasseur AL, Flanagan JR, Riopelle RJ, Munoz DP. Control of volitional and reflexive saccades in Tourette's syndrome. *Brain* 2001; **124**(Pt 10): 2045–58.

88. Munoz DP, Le Vasseur AL, Flanagan JR. Control of volitional and reflexive saccades in Tourette's syndrome. *Prog Brain Res* 2002; **140**: 467–81.

89. Nomura Y, Fukuda H, Terao Y, Hikosaka O, Segawa M. Abnormalities of voluntary saccades in Gilles de la Tourette's syndrome: pathophysiological consideration. *Brain Dev* 2003; **25**(Suppl 1): S48–54.

90. Thomalla G, Siebner HR, Jonas M *et al.* Structural changes in the somatosensory system correlate with tic severity in Gilles de la Tourette syndrome. *Brain* 2009; **132**(Pt 3): 765–77.

91. Mueller SC, Jackson GM, Dhalla R, Datsopoulos S, Hollis CP. Enhanced cognitive control in young people with Tourette's syndrome. *Curr Biol* 2006; **16**(6): 570–3.

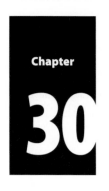

Demyelinating diseases and movement disorders

Daniel Kantor

Introduction

Demyelinating diseases of the central nervous system (CNS) are a common cause of neurological disability. While multiple sclerosis (MS) is the most common form of CNS demyelinating disease, other examples include other autoimmune processes, as well as infectious, toxic/metabolic and vascular processes. Demyelinating diseases, as opposed to dysmyelinating diseases (which usually present in childhood due to a biochemical abnormality of myelin formation), most commonly affect young adults.

While most people with an autoimmune demyelinating disease are genetically predisposed to develop a disruption of their CNS myelin, other causes of demyelination may occur sporadically. Besides MS, other autoimmune causes of CNS demyelination include variants of MS, neuromyelitis optica (Device disease or NMO), clinically isolated syndrome (CIS), acute disseminated encephalomyelitis (ADEM) and acute hemorrhagic leukoencephalopathy. Infectious causes of demyelination are usually synonymous with progressive multifocal leukoencephalopathy (PML) from the JC virus. Toxic and metabolic causes of demyelination include carbon monoxide, mercury intoxication (Minamata disease), vitamin B_{12} deficiency, hypoxia, Marchiafava–Bignami syndrome, alcohol/tobacco amblyopia and central pontine myelinolysis (CPM). Binswanger disease is synonymous with vascular demyelination.

A growing body of evidence (from animal studies, human biopsy and autopsy tissue and paraclinical testing, such as optical coherence tomography or OCT [1]) suggests that central demyelinating diseases involve not only damage to the oligodendrocytes but also primary and secondary damage to the axons themselves [2].

Conversely, there is an increasing realization that many classically neurodegenerative diseases have prominent inflammatory and demyelinating components. This chapter concentrates on primary CNS demyelinating diseases rather than neurodegenerative or other causes of axonal loss followed by secondary demyelination.

History

Jean-Martin Charcot lectured the Société des Biologie in 1868 on the characteristics of *sclerosé en plaque* (disseminated sclerosis, later to be termed multiple sclerosis) on the distinct neurologic and pathological features distinguishing Parkinson tremor from that of MS and other neurologic diseases[3,4], He later described the triad of intention tremor, nystagmus and scanning speech. This need to differentiate Parkinson disease from MS is exemplified in the description by Marshall Hall in his 1836 "Lectures on the Nervous System and its Diseases" of presumed paralysis agitans (Parkinson disease) in a 28-year-old man with weakness of his right arm and leg and a tremor of his arm that was worse with movement [5].

Movement disorders in MS had been reported years earlier in the description of Mrs. Margaret Gatty, a popular Victorian author of children's books, who developed a facial "tic." This, along with the other varied symptoms of MS, highlight the potential for different movement disorders in MS, ranging from tremors to tics to dystonia to cerebellar ataxias (mimicking the spinocerebellar ataxias).

Although it has become well recognized as a common MS symptom, paroxysmal limb dystonia was described most fully by Matthews [6]. While the most common presumed cause of these tonic spasms is spinal in origin (suggesting a form of spasticity as opposed to an actual movement disorder), Maimon *et al.* described a case of tonic spasms caused by a new MRI T2 hyperintensity in the contralateral internal capsule,

Uncommon Causes of Movement Disorders, ed. Néstor Gálvez-Jiménez and Paul J. Tuite. Published by Cambridge University Press. © Cambridge University Press 2011.

which resolved with the resolution of the demyelinating plaque [7].

Clinical findings

Multiple sclerosis is a chronic autoimmune disease of the CNS causing both demyelination and axonal loss. There are 2.5 million MS patients worldwide and 450 000 Americans with MS; 85% of whom start out as relapsing-remitting (RRMS), while 50% of those with RRMS progress to secondary-progressive MS (SPMS). Primary-progressive MS (PPMS) makes up the other 15% of patients, in which patients start out with progressive disease but do not have identifiable relapses.

Multiple sclerosis is characterized by a variable clinical course and presentation. The initial demyelinating event (often only diagnosed in retrospect) is termed a clinically isolated syndrome (CIS). Otherwise normal baseline MRI is predictive in assessing the risk for future demyelinating events (which would then be termed multiple sclerosis). Some patients have a long latency between their initial demyelinating event and future exacerbations (relapses or attacks).

The most common initial demyelinating events involve the spinal cord, optic nerve and brain stem/cerebellum (Figure 30.1). RRMS patients often develop discrete neurological deficits, such as gait difficulties, partial transverse myelitis, optic neuritis, or vertigo and ataxia. Although their symptoms usually improve, RRMS patients may accrue disability with each exacerbation. SPMS patients become progressively disabled, even between relapses (if any). PPMS patients become progressively disabled from the onset, without identifiable relapses or remissions.

The variable nature of MS translates into a wide range of neurological signs and symptoms, some of which may explain abnormal movement disorders.

Just as primary movement disorders encompass a range of abnormalities from absence of movement to abnormal involuntary movements, movement disorders secondary to demyelinating disease may manifest themselves in a myriad of ways. As opposed to conditions such as Parkinson disease, movement disorders secondary to demyelinating diseases do not usually involve the basal ganglia.

Tremor is the most common movement disorder caused by MS and is most commonly thought to result from demyelination in the cerebellum and its pathways [8]. Tremor is often the most disabling symptom of MS, in the form of resting (rubral tremor secondary to midbrain lesions) and postural/intention tremor (lesions of

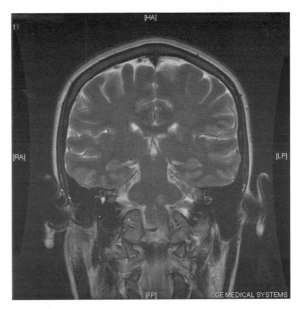

Figure 30.1. T2-weighted coronal brain MRI revealing a brainstem lesion in an MS patient.

the cerebellum and its connections) [9]. Head tremor (titubation) may be seen as a cerebellar sign of MS.

Exaggerated physiologic tremor may be precipitated by stress, fatigue, anxiety, emotion, thyrotoxicosis, Cushing disease and multiple medications. MS patients are especially prone to these aggravating factors. Two-thirds of MS patient suffer from fatigue that is often debilitating. Chronic illness, in general, carries with it the accompanied health-related, family-related and financial stresses. Anxiety may be worsened by the unpredictability of a relapsing-remitting disease, along with the possibility of progression of disability. Many MS patients also have thyroid problems, most commonly hypothyroidism, requiring chronic oral thyroid replacement and the disease-modifying agents for MS may also precipitate thyroid abnormalities. Overcorrection of thyroid hormone (which often occurs because MS patients focus on their neurological diagnosis and sometimes neglect other aspects of their general medical care) may lead to thyrotoxicosis. Long-term exposure to steroids may cause Cushing disease; the use of medications such as adrencorticosteroids (for MS relapses), dopamine agonists (for RLS), amphetamines and caffeine (for MS-related fatigue), valproic acid and lithium (for headaches and mood stabilization) and tricyclic antidepressants (for sleep and neuropathic pain) may lead to exaggerated physiologic tremor.

Chorea is a rare symptom of MS, neurosarcoidosis and neuro-Behçet disease. As opposed to the insidious onset of primary chorea, chorea that has an abrupt or subacute onset or with a relapsing-remitting pattern may suggest the possibility of a secondary cause, such as an exacerbation of a demyelinating disorder. Chorea that waxes and wanes as brief episodes (minutes to hours) throughout the day may suggest the presence of a paroxysmal dyskinesia. Often believed to be a variant of chorea, hemiballismus may be caused by a focal demyelinating lesion in the contralateral subthalamic nucleus or striatum [10].

Paroxysmal tonic spasms (dystonia) usually affect the upper extremities for a few seconds and are reported in 10–14% of MS patients. While these painful spasms are usually spontaneous, they may also be triggered by movement, touch or hyperventilation [11].

Negative movement symptoms are a rarer and underappreciated symptom of MS. At the time of Twomey and Espir's description of paroxysmal akinesia as "sudden loss of power of a limb or limbs described by the patients as 'knees locking,' 'legs collapsing,' 'legs don't go,' or 'unexpected falls' followed by rapid recovery," only 18 such cases had been described in the medical literature [12].

Approximately 30% of MS patients suffer from speech or voice impairments and spasmodic dysphonia is a symptom of MS thought to be caused by abnormal tone in the muscles of phonation. Voice tremors are present in MS patients with associated postural tremor. Very rarely, eructation has been reported as a symptom of MS.

Greater than 30% of MS patients meet diagnostic criteria for restless legs syndrome (RLS) and RLS is associated with a greater overall MS impairment and MRI involvement of the cervical spinal cord. Manconi et al. found that RLS correlated with abnormalities in MRI diffusion tensor and fractional anisotropy independent of T2 lesions, suggesting that RLS arises from "a loss of alignment of axons" rather than direct cord demyelination [13]. Clinically, it is important to differentiate the urge to move in RLS from MS-related central neuropathic pain and spasticity (which may also be confused with periodic limb movements of sleep). Practitioners often discount an urge to move and discomfort as central neuropathic pain, and leg movements during sleep as secondary to hypertonicity and clonus. This can have unfortunate consequences for treatment (pain medications and muscle relaxants as opposed to dopamine agonists and correction of iron

deficiency) and may lead to further daytime fatigue [14].

Other miscellaneous rhythmic disorders caused by MS include rhythmic movements of dystonia, rhythmic myoclonus (spinal myoclonus), clonus and nystagmus. Hemifacial spasm and other paroxysmal symptoms may be explained by ephaptic transmission of nerve impulses. Hemifacial spasm has been reported secondary to demyelinating lesions in the area of the facial nucleus [15].

Depending on the location and size of the demyelinating lesions, other causes of autoimmune demyelination lead to similar movement disorders as seen in MS. Neuromyelitis optica is a disabling demyelinating disease with predominately selective damage to the optic nerves and the spinal cord. This extensive and longitudinal demyelination may lead to a higher incidence of spinal myoclonus.

Natural history

Movement disorders in patients with demyelinating diseases may result from a new demyelinating lesion or may be a paroxysmal symptom, with no identifiable lesion. The natural history of the abnormal movements is tied to the recovery from the causative demyelinating event.

Cerebellar abnormalities are a common presenting sign of MS, appearing as an initial symptom in 11% of patients and in 82% throughout the course of their disease. While cerebellar symptoms may present acutely during an MS exacerbation, these symptoms often remain as residua of these discrete relapses. There is an increasing realization that even MS patients with a relapsing-remitting form of the disease do not return to neurologic baseline and 42% may accrue disability with each relapse [16]. Initial cerebellar symptoms are a poor prognostic indicator for the future course of MS.

The variable clinical course of MS and the lack of a biomarker to predict the clinical outcome make it difficult to predict the prognosis for any individual patient. Factors such as older age at onset, male sex, initial motor and cerebellar signs and large MRI T2 lesion load predict a worse outcome. As opposed to earlier thinking, approximately 25% of patients with no other MRI changes at the time of an initial single demyelinating event (CIS), will be diagnosed with MS over a 15-year period. The natural history of MS and CIS has been changed by the introduction of disease-modifying agents. They are FDA approved for the reduction of relapses and there is data to suggest the reduction in disability as well. Unfortunately, there have been multiple unsuccessful negative trials in the treatment of PPMS.

Neuromyelitis optica carries a worse prognosis, with many of the patients developing sustained disability secondary to the longitudinal nature of the cervical and thoracic cord demyelination. Tumefactive MS (Marburg variant) presents with a large MRI T2 hyperintensity, explained mostly by edema. This edema is usually rapidly responsive to corticosteroids, and therefore many patients with Marburg variant have an ultimately milder clinical course (aside from the transient damage cause by the large lesion).

Laboratory investigations

In a patient with a central demyelinating disease, the presence of a movement disorder needs to be investigated to ensure that there is not another source for these abnormalities. Patients with demyelinating diseases are often on multiple medications for their symptoms, some of which may cause or exacerbate abnormal movements. The temporal relationship between the initiation (and change in dosage) of the likely medication culprit needs to be assessed against the onset of the movement disorder. Acutely, the laboratory and other diagnostic investigations are focused on ensuring that a new exacerbation is not occurring. Exacerbations are investigated through history taking, physical (especially signs of infection) and neurological examination (new abnormalities) and, sometimes, MRI. A new or expanding T2 hyperintensity or gadolinium-enhancing lesion on MRI suggests that a new exacerbation of the underlying disorder is the proximal cause of the new movement disorder.

While evaluating for causes of new signs and symptoms, there is a need to perform laboratory investigations focused on infectious causes (complete blood count with differential and urinalysis with urine Gram stain and culture) and metabolic (chemistry and liver function tests) causes of pseudo-exacerbations. Other focused investigations, such as chest radiographs in patients with new respiratory symptoms, may help to rule out infections. Uhthoff's phenomenon is a clinical description of the suboptimal, heat-sensitive conduction in demyelinated central fibers. A rise in temperature of as little as 0.5°C above normal will cause conduction failure in some fibers [17]. For this reason, any process that increases the core body temperature of MS (or other CNS disease) patients, may cause an uncovering of prior symptoms.

Table 30.1. MRI criteria for dissemination in space (S).

At least three of the following:
1 Gd-enhancing lesion or 9 T2-hyperintense lesions if there is no Gd-enhancing lesion
At least 1 infratentorial lesion
At least 1 juxtacortical lesion
At least 3 periventricular lesions

Note: A spinal cord lesion can be considered equivalent to a brain infratentorial lesion. An enhancing spinal cord lesion is considered equivalent to an enhancing brain lesion. Individual spinal cord lesions can contribute together with brain lesions to reach the required number of T2 lesions.

Table 30.2. MRI criteria for dissemination in time (T).

Gd-enhancement ≥3 months after onset of initial clinical event if not at site corresponding to initial event.
New T2 lesion seen as compared with reference scan with imaging done at least 30 days after onset of initial clinical event.

Clinical presentation	Paraclinical tests needed	
	Space &	Time
2 attacks; 2 locations	No	No
2 attacks; 1 location	MRI (S) *or* 2 MRI lesions +CSF	No
1 attack; 2 locations	No	MRI (T) *or* 2nd attack
1 attack; 1 location	MRI (S) *or* 2 MRI lesions +CSF	MRI (T) *or* 2nd attack
Insidious progression (1 year) suggestive of MS	2 of the following: + brain MRI (9 T2 lesions) *or* 4 T2 lesions & + VEP + spine MRI (2 focal T2 lesions) + CSF (oligoclonal bands or elevated IgG index)	

Figure 30.2. Modified McDonald Criteria (2005) [19].

The cornerstone of the diagnosis is different, not otherwise explained, neurological events consistent with a central demyelinating event and separated in time and space (Tables 30.1 and 30.2). Diagnostic criteria have advanced from the Schumacher criteria through the most recent modified McDonald criteria (Figure 30.2) [18,19].

Multiple sclerosis is a diagnosis of exclusion. Aside from an in-depth history and physical examination, laboratory studies, MRI and paraclinical studies are used to establish a diagnosis of MS. The differential diagnosis of MS is vast and therefore laboratory testing includes both serum and cerebrospinal fluid (CSF) evaluation. The differential diagnosis includes infection (Lyme disease, syphilis, PML, HIV, HTLV-1),

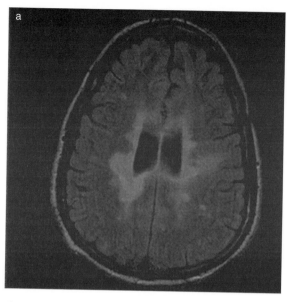
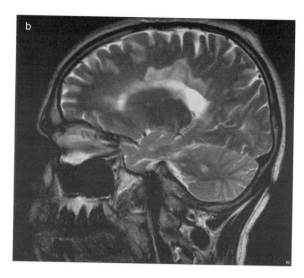

Figure 30.3. (a) Fluid attenuated inversion recovery (FLAIR) axial brain MRI revealing demyelinating lesions consistent with MS. (b) FLAIR sagittal brain MRI revealing demyelinating lesions consistent with MS.

inflammatory causes (systemic lupus erythematosus, Sjögren syndrome, vasculitis, sarcoidosis, Behçhet disease), metabolic causes (vitamin B_{12} deficiency, lysosomal disorders, adrenoleukodystrophy, mitochondrial disorders, other genetic disorders), neoplasm (CNS lymphoma), and spinal disease (vascular malformation, degenerative spinal disease).

Screening serum tests are directed by the history and regional differences, but they usually include complete blood count, liver function tests, thyroid studies, vitamin B_{12} levels, anti-nuclear antibodies (ANA), syphilis serology and Lyme titers. CSF is investigated for cell count, protein, glucose, syphilis, angiotensin-converting enzyme, Lyme antibodies or polymerase chain reaction, myelin basic protein, IgG index/synthetic rate, and oligoclonal banding.

Cranial and spinal cord (cervical and thoracic) MRI is performed to look for classic void T2-weighted hyperintense lesions, with predisposition to certain locations (such as the periventricular, corpus callosal, juxtacortical and infrantentorial areas) (Figure 30.3).

Paraclinical tests include evoked potentials (visual, brain stem and somatosensory). Evoked potentials are the CNS electrical events generated by peripheral stimulation of a sensory organ. The utility of evoked potentials (responses) is that they may detect subclinical damage in the conduction of electrical impulses in the nervous system. A delayed response suggests that there is underlying demyelination of portions of the

nervous system. When this delay occurs in the central portions of the testing, it may suggest CNS demyelination, possibly from MS or another similar demyelinating disease.

Genetics

There is no known specific genetic predisposition for a patient with central demyelinating disease to develop a movement disorder.

Multiple sclerosis is thought of as an autoimmune central demyelinating disease in a genetically predisposed individual with a so far unknown environmental exposure. Twin and sibling studies suggest that there is a genetic susceptibility to the disease, but the concordance in monozygotic twins is only approximately 30% [20]. Siblings of MS patients have a 2.6% risk, parents a risk of 1.8%, and children a risk of 1.5%. Recent studies have suggested the role of HLA and IL2RA susceptibility genes, however there is no consensus regarding the role of DQB1*0602 in the pathogenesis of MS [21–23].

Pathology

In early MS lesions there is a marked hypercellularity with macrophage infiltration and astrocytosis accompanied by perivenous inflammation with lymphocytes and plasma cells. There is debate whether myelin breakdown leads to cellular changes or vice versa. This is followed by demyelination with oligodendrocyte loss and extensive gliosis. Remyelination may be incomplete, contributing to suboptimal nerve fiber function.

The pathophysiology of MS-related tremor appears to be different from that of Parkinson tremor [24]. MS-related tremors may involve more than the cerebello-thalamo-cortical loop, and may involve affect both the cerebellar receiving area (VIM) and the pallidal receiving area (VOA/VOP). VOP is also considered by some investigators as a cerebellar receiving area, with tremor-related cells [25]. The correlations between tremor amplitude and MRI T2 lesion load in the contralateral pons and between the severity of tremor in the bilateral arms and greater lesion load in the pons (but not cerebellum) bilaterally suggest that MS-related intention tremor is related to dysfunction of cerebellar inflow and/or outflow pathways [26].

Only a few cases of MS-related paroxysmal kinesigenic dyskinesia have been reported in the medical literature, and even fewer have been reported as the presenting sign of MS. There is no one site in the brain responsible for all of these cases (subcortical parietal, thalamic, high cervical [27,28]), suggesting the possibility that the proximity of the motor fibers could be an important underlying anatomical factor [29]. This would allow a single lesion to have an effect on a large population of axons, and would also favor radial spreading of ephaptic activation.

Movement disorders in central demyelinating diseases may be related to a focal site of demyelination (which is increasingly being recognized in the gray matter) or may be related to underlying neurodegeneration and axonal loss. A case of parkinsonism/dystonia syndrome secondary to multiple sclerosis with anti-basal ganglia antibodies (ABGA) in a PPMS patient demonstrates the role of neurodegeneration in movement disorders associated with MS. Serial brain MRIs failed to reveal a basal ganglia or midbrain lesion; instead there were progressive diffuse atrophy and periventricular white matter abnormalities [30].

Although MS is the most common demyelinating disease, other forms of demyelination may also cause movement disorders. Other causes of demyelination include central pontine and extrapontine myelinolysis. First described in 1959 by Adams, Victor and Mancall, central pontine myelinolysis (CPM) is characterized primarily by symmetric destruction of the myelin sheath in the basis pontis, usually after rapid correction of serum sodium levels [31]. Seiser et al. reported a woman with CPM and extrapontine myelinolysis who developed parkinsonism. The parkinsonism resolved over 4 months, but 4 months later she developed persistent retrocollis, spasmodic dysphonia and focal hand dystonia [32]. It has been postulated that the reason for late-stage movement disorders is that, although myelin destruction occurs at the onset of myelinolysis (due to osmotic demyelination), there is an ineffective reorganization of neuronal structures. This may cause progressive treatment-refractory movement disorders [33].

Unlike MS, in which associated movement disorders may not be related to a specific demyelinating lesion, abnormal movements in CPM and extrapontine myelinolysis generally stem from the site of myelinolysis. Late-onset dystonia, chorea and parkinsonism have been reported as a sequela to extrapontine myelinolysis affecting the bilateral striate and thalami [34]. In a patient with CPM, dystonia was not associated with striatal lesions on MRI, but cerebellar ataxia was explained by cerebellar atrophy and extension of myelinolysis to the middle cerebellar peduncle [35]. Another patient developed progressive asymmetric parkinsonism with ideomotor apraxia and cortical sensory deficits [36].

Management

The treatment of demyelinating diseases is focused on disease-modifying agents, symptomatic treatment and rescue therapy to shorten the length of an exacerbation (resolve the new demyelinating lesion).

Since 1993, four injectable disease-modifying agents (three beta interferons and glatiramer acetate) and one intravenous monoclonal antibody (natalizumab) have been approved by the FDA for relapsing-remitting MS. Mitoxantrone is a chemotherapeutic agent approved for secondary progressive and worsening relapsing-remitting MS. The use of these immunomodulators and immunosuppressants has reduced the number and severity of relapses, and thus reduced the chances of a new demyelinating lesion developing to cause movement disorders.

Corticosteroids are the gold-standard of treatment to hasten the recovery from a demyelinating event. Prior to the introduction of intravenous methylprednisolone (usually 1000 mg daily for 3–5 days with or without an oral prednisone taper), adrenocorticotropic hormone (ACTH) was administered intramuscularly. Other treatments, with less evidence to support their use, include intravenous immunoglobulin (IVIg) and plasmapheresis. Approaches to hasten the recovery from an MS exacerbation may control the new MS-related movement disorder.

Symptomatic treatment of movement disorders stemming from demyelinating disease is similar to the medications used to treat the symptoms of primary movement disorders.

MS-related RLS, just as other forms of RLS, responds to dopamine agonists. Spasmodic dysphonia may be responsive to botulinum toxin injections and a case of eructation was responsive to 4-aminopyridine [37]. The mechanism, presumably, was prolongation of action potentials and resultant improved neuronal conduction in demyelinated axons.

MS-related tremor is less responsive to medications used in the treatment of other causes of tremor. Muscle relaxants, antiepileptic drugs and beta blockers have historically been the mainstay of treatment. Medications used (often with only limited or no success) for the treatment of MS-related tremor include: baclofen, propranolol, clonazepam, carbamazepine, primidone, levetiracetam, topiramate, isoniazid (combined with pyridoxine), glutethimide, cannabis and ondansetron [38–40].

Other strategies include cooling to reduce core body temperature as well as physical and occupational therapy with the addition of small weights to mask the symptoms [41]. Surgical approaches include thalamotomy, and a growing interest in the use of deep brain stimulation in the suppression of MS-related Holmes tremor [42–44]. An ongoing NIH-funded study of dual ipsilateral thalamic deep brain stimulation (DBS) represents the first prospective blinded study of the efficacy and safety of surgical treatments for MS-related tremor [45]. Previously, the same investigators had success in the placement of two ipsilateral thalamic DBS electrodes (one at the ventralis intermedius nucleus/ventralis oralis posterior nucleus border [VIM] and one at the ventralis oralis anterior nucleus/ventralis oralis posterior nucleus border [VOA/VOP]). Electromagnetic fields were used to treat a parkinsonian syndrome associated with MS. The mechanism of action was presumed to be related to augmentation of dopaminergic and serotonergic neurotransmission in the basal ganglia [46].

Conclusion

Demyelinating diseases of the CNS are an uncommon cause of movement disorders; however, because of the high prevalence of such disease, they should be included in the differential diagnosis for almost any movement disorder.

Multiple sclerosis is, by far, the most common central demyelinating disease and, as such, abnormalities associated with MS open a window into the spectrum of movement disorders caused by demyelinating disorders. No area of the CNS is spared from demyelinating diseases, thus explaining the wide variety of movement disorders associated with them. The presence of a movement disorder in a patient with a demyelinating disease should not automatically be attributed to the demyelinating disease. Patients with demyelinating diseases may have coexistent primary movement disorders or may have another coexistent secondary cause for the movement disorder (such as stroke or medications).

Central pontine and extrapontine myelinolysis differ from MS in that they are acquired acutely (without a known genetic predisposition) and there is a two-phase movement disorder. The initial movement disorder is usually related to the site of osmotic demyelination, as opposed to movement disorders in MS, which may not be correlated to a focal demyelinating lesion. There are several explanations for the lack of correlation in MS between MRI demyelinating lesions and known structural sources of movement disorders: (1) MRI is not entirely sensitive for the detection of demyelinating lesions; (2) normal-appearing white matter in an MS patient is not entirely normal due to inflammatory cell infiltration, demyelination and axonal loss; (3) demyelination causes abnormalities in neuronal networks; (4) demyelination occurs not only in the white matter but in the gray matter as well; (5) current MRI techniques fail to image most cortical and gray matter MS lesions; (6) gray matter atrophy, which is currently thought of as the best correlate with disability, and axonal loss (both primary and secondary) may explain many of the associated movement disorders.

The initial work-up for a newly presenting movement disorders, especially in a young person, should include a through history and examination looking for potential symptoms and signs of MS, with further investigation by MRI if clinically warranted.

References

1. Frohman EM, Fujimoto JG, Frohman TC, Calabresi PA, Cutter G, Balcer LJ. Optical coherence tomography: a window into the mechanisms of multiple sclerosis. *Nat Clin Pract Neurol* 2008; **4**(12): 664–75.

2. Trapp BD, Peterson J, Ransohoff TM *et al.* Axonal transections in the lesions of multiple sclerosis. *N Engl J Med* 1998; **338**: 278–85.

3. Charcot JM. Histologie de le sclérose en plaques. *Gaz Hôp Paris* 1868; **141**: 554–5, 557–8, 566.

4. Charcot JM. Histologie de le sclérose en plaques. *Gaz Hôp Civils Milit (Paris)* 1868; **41**: 554–5, 557–8, 556.

5. Hall M. *On Diseases and Derangements of the Nervous System in Their Primary Forms and in Their Modifications by Age, Sex, Constitution, Hereditary Predisposition, Excesses, General Disorder and Organic Disease.* London: Balliére; 1841.

6. Matthews WB. Tonic seizures in disseminated sclerosis. Brain 1958; **81**: 193–206.

7. Maimon D, Reder AT, Finocchiaro F, Recupero E. Internal capsule plaque and tonic spasms in multiple sclerosis. *Arch Neurol* 1991; **48**: 427–9.

8. Pittock SJ, McClelland R, Mayr WT *et al.* Prevalence of tremor in multiple sclerosis and associated disability in the Olmsted County population. *Mov Disord* 2004; **19**: 1482–5.

9. Zeldowicz L. Paroxysmal motor episodes as early manifestations of multiple sclerosis. *Can Med Assoc J* 1961; **84**: 937–41.

10. Lee MS, Marsden CD. Movement disorders following lesions of the thalamus or subthalamic region. *Mov Disord* 1994; **9**: 493–507.

11. Zenzola A, De Mari M, De Blasi R *et al.* Paroxysmal dystonia with thalamic lesion in multiple sclerosis. *Arch Neurol Sci* 2001; **22**: 391–4.

12. Twomey JA, Espir MLE. Paroxysmal symptoms as the first manifestation of multiple sclerosis. *J Neurol Neurosurg Psychiatry* 1980; **43**: 296–304.

13. Rae-Grant AD, Eckert N, Bartz S *et al.* Sensory symptoms in multiple sclerosis: a hidden reservoir of morbidity. *Mult Scler* 1999; **5**: 179–83.

14. Deriu M, Cossu G, Molari A *et al.* Restless legs syndrome in multiple sclerosis: a case–control study. *Mov Disord* 2009; **24**: 697–701.

15. Telischi FF, Grobman LR, Sheramata WA *et al.* Hemifacial spasm. Occurrence in multiple sclerosis. *Arch Otolaryngol Head Neck Surg* 1991; **117**: 554–6.

16. Lipton FD *et al.* Effect of relapses on development of residual deficit in multiple sclerosis. *Neurology* 2003; **61**: 1528–32.

17. Rasminsky M. The effects of temperature on conduction in demyelinated single nerve fibres. *Arch Neurol* 1972; **28**: 287–92.

18. Schumaker GA, Beebe G, Kibler RF *et al.* Problems of experimental trials of therapy in multiple sclerosis. Report by the panel on the evaluation of experimental trials of therapy in multiple sclerosis. *Ann NY Acad Sci* 1965; **122**: 552–68.

19. Polman CH, Reingold SC, Edan G *et al.* Diagnostic criteria for multiple sclerosis: 2005 revisions to the "McDonald Criteria." *Ann Neurol* 2005; **58**: 840–6.

20. Compston A, Confavreux C, Lassmann H *et al.* The genetics of multiple sclerosis. In: Compston A, McDonald IR, Noseworthy J *et al.*, eds. *McAlpine's Multiple Sclerosis.* 4th ed. Philadelphia: Churchill Livingstone/Elsevier, 2005: 113–81.

21. International Multiple Sclerosis Genetics Consortium, Hafler D, Compston A *et al.* Risk alleles for multiple sclerosis identified by a genomewide study. *N Engl J Med* 2007; **357**: 851–62.

22. Allen M, Sandelberg-Wolheim M, Sjogren K *et al.* Association of susceptibility to multiple sclerosis in Sweden with HLA class II DRB1 and DQB1 alleles. *Hum Immunol* 1994; **39**: 41–8.

23. Boon M, Nolte IM, Bruinenberg M *et al.* Mapping of a susceptibility gene for multiple sclerosis to the 51 kb interval between G%11525 and D651666 using a new method of haplotype sharing analysis. *Neurogenetics* 2001; **3**: 221–30.

24. Deuschl G, Wilms H, Krack P, Wurker M, Heiss WD: Function of the cerebellum in Parkinsonian rest tremor and Holmes' tremor. *Ann Neurol* 1999; **46**: 126–8.

25. Fernandez Gonzalez F, Seijo F, Salvador C *et al.* Applied neurophysiology in the deep brain stimulation treatment of multiple sclerosis tremor. *Rev Neurol* 2001; **32**: 559–67.

26. Feys P, Maes F, Nuttin B *et al.* Relationship between multiple sclerosis intention tremor severity and lesion load in the brainstem. *Neuroreport* 2005; **16**: 1379–82.

27. Riley DE. Paroxysmal kinesigenic dystonia associated with a medullary lesion. *Mov Disord* 1996; **11**: 738–40.

28. Fragoso YD, Araujo MG, Branco NL. Kinesigenic paroxysmal hemidyskinesia as the initial presentation of multiple sclerosis. *MedGenMed* 2006; **8**: 3.

29. Spissu A, Cannas A, Ferrigno P *et al.* Anatomic correlates of painful tonic spasms in multiple sclerosis. *Mov Disord* 2001; **14**: 331–5.

30. Delgado S, Baez S, Singer C *et al.* Parkinsonism/dystonia syndrome secondary to multiple sclerosis with antibasal ganglia antibodies. *Mov Disord* 2009; **24**: 309–11.

31. Adams RD, Victor M, Mancall EL. Central pontine myelinolysis: a hitherto undescribed disease occurring in alcoholic and malnourished patients. *Arch Neurol Psychiatry* 1959; **81**: 154–72.

32. Seiser A, Schwarz S, Aichinger-Steiner MM *et al.* Parkinsonism and dystonia in central pontine and extrapontine myelinolysis. *J Neurol Neurosurg Psychiatry* 1998; **65**: 119–21.

33. Seah AB, Chan LL, Wong MC, Tan EK. Evolving spectrum of movement disorders in extrapontine and central pontine myelinolysis. *Parkinsonism Relat Disord* 2002; **9**: 117–19.

34. Ezpeleta D, de Andrés C, Giménez-Roldán S. Abnormal movements in a case of extrapontine myelinolysis. Review of the literature. *Rev Neurol* 1998; **26**: 215–20.

35. Gille M, Jacquemin C, Kiame G *et al*. Central pontine myelinolysis with cerebellar ataxia and dystonia. *Rev Neurol (Paris)* 1993; **149**: 344–6.

36. Shamim A, Siddiqui BK, Josephs KA. The corticobasal syndrome triggered by central pontine myelinolysis. *Eur J Neurol* 2006; **13**: 82–4.

37. Kantor D. 4-Aminopyridine as a treatment for intractable eructation: The First Case Report – American Academy of Neurology 61st Annual Meeting. Seattle, April 2009 (Poster P07.146).

38. Striano P, Coppola A, Vacca G *et al*. Levetiracetam for cerebellar tremor in multiple sclerosis: an open-label pilot tolerability and efficacy study. *J Neurol* 2006; **253**: 762–6.

39. Hallet M, Lindsey J, Adelstein B, Riley P. Controlled trial of isoniazid therapy for severe postural cerebellar tremor in multiple sclerosis. *Neurology* 1985; **35**: 1374–7.

40. Rice G, Dickey C, Lesaux J *et al*. Ondansteron for disabling cerebellar tremor. *Ann Neurol* 1995; **38**: 973.

41. Feys P, Helsen W, Liu X *et al*. Effects of peripheral cooling on intention tremor in multiple sclerosis. *J Neurol Neurosurg Psychiatry* 2005; **76**: 373–9.

42. Hooper J and Whittle IR. Long term outcome after thalamotomy for movement disorders in multiple sclerosis. *Lancet* 1998; **352**: 1984.

43. Hooper J, Taylor R, Pentland B, Whittle IR. A prospective study of thalamic deep brain stimulation for the treatment of movement disorders in multiple sclerosis. *Br J Neurosurg* 2002; **16**: 102–9.

44. Berk C, Carr J, Sinden M, Martzke J, Honey CR. Thalamic deep brain stimulation for the treatment of tremor due to multiple sclerosis: a prospective study of tremor and quality of life. *J Neurosurg* 2002; **97**: 815–20.

45. Foote KD *et al*. Use of two DBS electrodes to treat post-traumatic tremor. NIH K23 NS052557–01. datalab-1.ics.uci.edu/nih/crisp/2007/getdoc.php?did=55670 (accessed December 23, 2010).

46. Sandyk R. Reversal of an acute parkinsonian syndrome associated with multiple sclerosis by application of weak electromagnetic fields. *Int J Neurosci* 1996; **86**: 33–45.

Index